P SEDMAN
OCTOBER 1992

Nutrient Modulation of the Immune Response

Nutrient Modulation of the Immune Response

edited by

Susanna Cunningham-Rundles
The New York Hospital
Cornell University Medical Center
New York, New York

Marcel Dekker, Inc.   New York • Basel • Hong Kong

Library of Congress Cataloging-in-Publication Data

Nutrient modulation of the immune response / edited by Susanna
 Cunningham-Rundles.
    p. cm.
  Includes bibliographical references and index.
  ISBN 0-8247-8448-0 (alk. paper)
  1. Immunity--Nutritional aspects. 2. Immune response--Regulation.
 I. Cunningham-Rundles, Susanna.
  [DNLM: 1. Immunity, Cellular--physiology. 2. Nutrition-
 -physiology.   QW 568 N976]
 QR185.2.N86 1992
 616.07'9--dc20
 DNLM/DLC
 for Library of Congress   92-49727
                                                               CIP

This book is printed on acid-free paper.

Copyright © 1993 by Marcel Dekker, Inc. All Rights Reserved.

Neither this book nor any part may be reproduced or transmitted in any form or by any means, electronic or mechanical, including photocopying, microfilming, and recording, or by any information storage and retrieval system, without permission in writing from the publisher.

Marcel Dekker, Inc.
270 Madison Avenue, New York, New York 10016

Current printing (last digit):
10 9 8 7 6 5 4 3 2 1

PRINTED IN THE UNITED STATES OF AMERICA

Preface

The significance of nutrition as a key factor in host defense against pathogens has been widely recognized for centuries. However, the specificity of this interaction at the level of the immune system has been unclear. While emerging knowledge on the importance of an intact immune system in disease resistance has stimulated study of nutrition and immunity, the means whereby particular nutrients affect the balance of immune response, apart from indirect support at the substrate level, has been a critical issue.

Protein calorie malnutrition, or severe acquired nutrient deficiency, is clearly associated with susceptibility to infections and increased morbidity. However, in human settings, dietary deficiencies of this magnitude do not occur in isolation. Increased levels of environmental pathogens, contaminated water, and a wide range of factors associated with chronic deprivation and poverty are also present and act to undermine health, including the integrity of the immune system. Furthermore, since immune reactions require a rapid increase in cellular activation and proliferation, it is expected that malnutrition could prevent substrate availability and, therefore, indirectly impair or even entirely block immune response. While key investigations during the late 1960s and 1970s on protein calorie malnutrition and associated infections showed strong correlations with impaired immune response, the question of specific, direct interaction was difficult to address. Now, with the aid of new technological advances using monoclonal antibodies to define cellular differences related to lineage, function, and activation state and with the development of molecular techniques during the 1980s, it is possible to approach these critical questions concerning the specificity of nutrient interaction in human immune response and the effect of more subtle differences in nutrient density.

Work described in this book strongly supports a direct role for nutrients as important cofactors and regulators of immune response. While some effects observed are related to experimental depletion or use of high-dose "pharmacological" concentrations of nutrients, others occur at usual dietary levels reflecting plausible physiological mechanisms. Studies in the development of certain pathological states, specifically autoimmune disease and cancer, suggest that excess of certain nutrients may promote or enhance development of disease. The investigations presented in this book reflect the efforts of many individuals working in different settings and taken as a whole provide compelling evidence that nutrient modulation of immune response can provide a fundamental approach to preventive medicine in the future.

Susanna Cunningham-Rundles

Contents

Preface   *iii*
Contributors   *ix*

PART I.   EXPRESSION OF NUTRIENT INTERACTION IN IMMUNE FUNCTION

1. Immunoregulatory and Prodifferentiating Effects of 1,25-Dihydroxyvitamin D_3 in Human Mononuclear Cells   3
   Stanley C. Jordan, H. Phillip Koeffler, Jaques Lemire, R. Sakai, and J. S. Adams

2. Nutritional Deficiencies and Immunoregulatory Cytokines   31
   Janis Randall Simpson and Laurie Hoffman-Goetz

3. The Role of Arginine as an Immune Modulator   47
   Adrian Barbul

4. Retinoids, Carotenoids, and Macrophage Activation   63
   Ronald R. Watson, Rao H. Prabhala, and David L. Earnest

5. Vitamin C and Phagocytes   75
   Reto Muggli

6. Interaction of Vitamin C in Lymphocyte Activation: Current Status and Possible Mechanisms of Action   91
   Ward F. Cunningham-Rundles, Yitshal Berner, and Susanna Cunningham-Rundles

	7. The Immunoregulatory Properties of Iron *Christopher F. Bryan and Marvin J. Stone*	105
	8. The Role of Metals in the Production of Toxic Oxygen Metabolites by Mononuclear Phagocytes *Joan M. Cook-Mills and Pamela J. Fraker*	127
	9. Zinc Deficiency, Chromatin Structure, and Gene Expression *C. Elizabeth Castro and J. Sanders Sevall*	141

PART II. EFFECT OF NUTRITIONAL CONDITIONING ON IMMUNE RESPONSE

10.	The Influence of Nutrition on Experimental Autoimmune Disease *W. John W. Morrow, Jacques Homsy, Christian Swanson, and Jay A. Levy*	153
11.	Cholesterol, Apolipoprotein E, and Immune Cell Function *Linda K. Curtiss*	169
12.	Oxygenated Derivatives of Cholesterol: Their Possible Role in Lymphocyte Activation and Differentiation *Hans-Jörg Heiniger and Harry W. Chen*	183
13.	Prostaglandins, Fatty Acids, and Arthritis *Robert B. Zurier*	201
14.	Vitamin E and the Immune Response *Simin Nikbin Meydani and Jeffrey B. Blumberg*	223
15.	Copper and Immunity *Tim R. Kramer and W. Thomas Johnson*	239
16.	Modulation of Differentiation Antigen Expression and Function of Immune Cells Following Short and Prolonged Alcohol Intake During Murine Retroviral Infection *Ronald R. Watson, Maria C. Lopez, Olalekan E. Odeleye, and Hamid Darban*	255
17.	The Effect of Experimental Zinc Deficiency on Development of the Immune System *Kimberly G. Vruwink, Carl L. Keen, M. Eric Gershwin, Jean Pierre Mareschi, and Lucille S. Hurley*	263

PART III. NUTRIENT MODULATION OF IMMUNE RESPONSE IN HUMAN DEVELOPMENT AND DISEASE

18.	Malnutrition and the Thymus Gland *Gerald T. Keusch*	283

Contents

19. Maturation of the Immune System in Breast-Fed and Bottle-Fed Infants — 301
    Susan Stephens

20. Gliadin, Intestinal Hypersensitivity, and Food Protein-Sensitive Enteropathy — 319
    Riccardo Troncone, Karl Ziegler, Stephan Strobel, and Anne Ferguson

21. Macromolecular Antigen Absorption from the Gastrointestinal Tract in Humoral Immunodeficiency — 339
    Charlotte Cunningham-Rundles

22. Natural Killer Activity in Protein-Calorie Malnutrition — 359
    Lekan Samusa Salimonu

23. Modification of Lymphocyte Function by Fatty Acids—Biological and Clinical Implications — 369
    Pierre J. Guillou, Peter C. Sedman, John R. Monson, and Thomas G. Brennan

24. Acquired Zinc Deficiency and Immune Dysfunction in Sickle Cell Anemia — 393
    Ananda S. Prasad

25. Effect of Therapeutic Chelation on Immune Response in Transfusion Dependent Thalassemia — 411
    Susanna Cunningham-Rundles, John Thomas Pinto, Patricia J. Giardina, and Margaret W. Hilgartner

26. Stimulation of Breast Cancer-Specific Cellular Immunity by High-Dose Vitamin E and Vitamin A: Adjuvant Therapeutic Implications — 423
    Maurice M. Black and Reinhard E. Zachrau

27. Malnutrition and Lymphocyte Subpopulation Responses in Humans — 441
    Sudhir Gupta

28. Influence of Nutrition on Immunocompetence in the Elderly — 455
    Ranjit K. Chandra

PART IV. ISSUES AND IMPLICATIONS IN NUTRIENT IMMUNE INTERACTIONS

29. Issues in Retinoid and Carotenoid Research — 469
    Adrianne Bendich

30. Impact of Infectious Disease on the Interaction Between Nutrition and Immunity — 475
    William R. Beisel

31.	Nutritional Indications for Cancer Prevention—Calorie Restriction *Ellen Lorenz and Robert A. Good*	481
32.	Circulation and Distribution of Iron: A Key to Immune Interaction *Maria de Sousa*	491
33.	Rationale for the Mechanism of Zinc Interaction in the Immune System *Mireille Dardenne and Jean-François Bach*	501
34.	Interactions Between Cytokine Production and Inflammation: Implications for Therapies Aimed at Modulating the Host Defense to Infection *Lyle L. Moldawer and Stephen F. Lowry*	511
35.	Human Milk Antibodies and Their Importance for the Infant *Lars Å. Hanson, Ingegerd Adlerberth, Barbro U. M. Carlsson, Mirjana Hahn-Zoric, F. Jalil, Lotta Mellander, D. M. Roberton, and S. Zaman*	525
36.	Dietary Antigens and Regulation of the Mucosal Immune Response *Warren Strober*	533

Index   *541*

Contributors

J. S. Adams   Cedars-Sinai Medical Center, UCLA School of Medicine, Los Angeles, California

Ingegerd Adlerberth   Department of Clinical Immunology, University of Göteborg, Göteborg, Sweden

Jean-François Bach, M.D., D.Sc.   INSERM U25, Hôpital Necker, Paris, France

Adrian Barbul, M.D., FACS   Department of Surgery, Sinai Hospital of Baltimore, Baltimore, Maryland

William R. Beisel, M.D., FACP   Department of Immunology and Infectious Diseases, The Johns Hopkins School of Hygiene and Public Health, Baltimore, Maryland

Adrianne Bendich, Ph.D.   Human Nutrition Research, Hoffmann-La Roche, Inc., Nutley, New Jersey

Yitshal Berner   Memorial Sloan-Kettering Cancer Center, New York, New York, and Department of Nutrition and Biochemistry, Hebrew University, Rehovoth, Israel

Maurice M. Black, M.D.   Department of Pathology and Institute of Breast Diseases, New York Medical College, Valhalla, New York

Jeffrey B. Blumberg, Ph.D.   Antioxidant Research Laboratory, USDA Human Nutrition Research Center on Aging, Tufts University, Boston, Massachusetts

Thomas G. Brennan   St. James University Hospital, Leeds, West Yorkshire, England

Christopher F. Bryan, Ph.D.   Histocompatibility and Flow Cytometry Laboratory, Midwest Organ Bank, Inc., Westwood, Kansas

Contributors

Barbro U. M. Carlsson, B.Sc., Ph.D. Department of Clinical Immunology, University of Göteborg, Göteborg, Sweden

C. Elizabeth Castro, Ph.D. Department of Food Science and Human Nutrition, University of Hawaii at Manoa, Honolulu, Hawaii

Ranjit K. Chandra Department of Pediatric Research, Medicine, and Biochemistry, and WHO Center for Nutritional Immunology, Health Sciences Center, Memorial University of Newfoundland, St. John's, Newfoundland, Canada

Harry W. Chen Department of Cardiovascular Science, Du Pont Merck Pharmaceutical Company, Wilmington, Delaware

Joan M. Cook-Mills Department of Biochemistry, Michigan State University, East Lansing, Michigan

Charlotte Cunningham-Rundles, M.D., Ph.D. Departments of Medicine and Pediatrics, The Mount Sinai School of Medicine, New York, New York

Susanna Cunningham-Rundles, Ph.D. Division of Hematology/Oncology, Department of Pediatrics, The New York Hospital, Cornell University Medical Center, New York, New York

Ward F. Cunningham-Rundles Department of Clinical Immunology, The Mount Sinai School of Medicine, and Department of Internal Medicine, Beth Israel Hospital, New York, New York

Linda K. Curtiss, Ph.D. Department of Immunology, The Scripps Research Institute, La Jolla, California

Hamid Darban, Ph.D. Department of Family and Community Medicine, Arizona Health Sciences Center, University of Arizona College of Medicine, Tucson, Arizona

Mireille Dardenne, M.D. Department of Research, CNRS URA 1461, Hôpital Necker, Paris, France

Maria de Sousa, M.D., Ph.D., FRCPath Department of Molecular Pathology and Immunology, Abel Salazar Institute for Biomedical Sciences, Oporto, Portugal

David L. Earnest Department of Internal Medicine, Arizona Health Sciences Center, University of Arizona College of Medicine, Tucson, Arizona

Anne Ferguson, Ph.D., FRCP, FRCPath Department of Medicine, University of Edinburgh, and Western General Hospital, Edinburgh, Scotland

Pamela J. Fraker, Ph.D. Department of Biochemistry, Michigan State University, East Lansing, Michigan

M. Eric Gershwin, M.D. Department of Internal Medicine, University of California, Davis, California

Patricia J. Giardina, M.D. Division of Hematology/Oncology, Department of Pediatrics, The New York Hospital, Cornell University Medical Center, New York, New York

Robert A. Good, Ph.D., M.D., D.Sc. Department of Pediatrics, All Children's Hospital and University of South Florida, St. Petersburg, Florida

Contributors

Pierre J. Guillou, B.Sc., M.D., FRCS Academic Surgical Unit, St. Mary's Hospital, Imperial College of Science, Technology, and Medicine, London, England

Sudhir Gupta, M.D., Ph.D. Department of Medicine, Division of Basic and Clinical Immunology, University of California, Irvine, California

Mirjana Hahn-Zoric, Ph.D. Department of Clinical Immunology, University of Göteborg, Göteborg, Sweden

Lars Å. Hanson, M.D., Ph.D. Department of Clinical Immunology, University of Göteborg, Göteborg, Sweden

Hans-Jörg Heiniger, DVM, Ph.D. Central Laboratory, Blood Transfusion Services, Swiss Red Cross, Bern, Switzerland

Margaret W. Hilgartner, M.D. Division of Hematology/Oncology, Department of Pediatrics, The New York Hospital, Cornell University Medical Center, New York, New York

Laurie Hoffman-Goetz, Ph.D. Department of Health Studies, University of Waterloo, Waterloo, Ontario, Canada

Jacques Homsy Cancer Research Institute, University of California School of Medicine, San Francisco, California

Lucille S. Hurley Department of Nutrition, University of California, Davis, California, and BSN Groupe, Paris, France

F. Jalil Department of Social and Preventive Pediatrics, King Edward Medical College, Lahore, Pakistan

W. Thomas Johnson, Ph.D. Grand Forks Human Nutrition Research Center, U.S. Department of Agriculture, Grand Forks, North Dakota

Stanley C. Jordan, M.D. Department of Pediatrics, Cedars-Sinai Medical Center, UCLA School of Medicine, Los Angeles, California

Carl L. Keen Department of Nutrition, University of California, Davis, California

Gerald T. Keusch, M.D. Division of Geographic Medicine and Infectious Disease, Department of Medicine, New England Medical Center, Boston, Massachusetts

H. Phillip Koeffler, M.D. Division of Hematology/Oncology, and Department of Medicine, Cedars-Sinai Medical Center, UCLA School of Medicine, Los Angeles, California

Tim R. Kramer, Ph.D. Vitamin and Mineral Nutrition Laboratory, Beltsville Human Nutrition Research Center, U.S. Department of Agriculture, Beltsville, Maryland

Jaques Lemire Division of Pediatric Nephrology, Department of Pediatrics, University of California—San Diego, San Diego, California

Jay A. Levy, M.D. Cancer Research Institute, Department of Medicine, University of California School of Medicine, San Francisco, California

Maria C. Lopez, Ph.D. Department of Family and Community Medicine, Arizona Health Sciences Center, University of Arizona College of Medicine, Tucson, Arizona

Ellen Lorenz, B.A. Division of Allergy and Immunology, Department of Pediatrics, All Children's Hospital, St. Petersburg, Florida

Stephen F. Lowry, M.D. Laboratory of Surgical Metabolism, New York Hospital, Cornell University Medical Center, New York, New York

Jean Pierre Mareschi International Scientific Affairs, Department of Science, BSN Groupe, Paris, France

Lotta Mellander, M.D., Ph.D. Department of Pediatrics, East Hospital, Göteborg, Sweden

Simin Nikbin Meydani Nutritional Immunology Laboratory, USDA Human Nutrition Research Center on Aging, Tufts University, Boston, Massachusetts

Lyle L. Moldawer, Ph.D. Department of Surgery, The New York Hospital, Cornell University Medical Center, New York, New York

John R. Monson Academic Surgical Unit, St. Mary's Hospital, Imperial College of Science, Technology, and Medicine, London, England

W. John W. Morrow, Ph.D. Cancer Research Institute and Department of Laboratory Medicine, University of California School of Medicine, San Francisco, California

Reto Muggli, Ph.D. Human Nutrition Research, Vitamins and Fine Chemicals Division, F. Hoffmann-LaRoche, Ltd., Basel, Switzerland

Olalekan E. Odeleye, Ph.D. Department of Family and Community Medicine, Arizona Health Sciences Center, University of Arizona College of Medicine, Tucson, Arizona

John Thomas Pinto, Ph.D. Department of Molecular Pharmacology and Therapeutics, Memorial Sloan-Kettering Cancer Center, New York, New York

Rao H. Prabhala, Ph.D. Department of Microbiology, Chicago College of Osteopathic Medicine, Downer's Grove, Illinois

Ananda S. Prasad, M.D., Ph.D. Department of Internal Medicine, Wayne State University School of Medicine, Detroit, Michigan

D. M. Roberton Department of Pediatrics, Children's Hospital, Adelaide, Australia

R. Sakai Pediatric Renal Immunology Laboratory, Division of Pediatric Nephrology, Department of Pediatrics, Cedars-Sinai Medical Center, UCLA School of Medicine, Los Angeles, California

Lekan Samusa Salimonu, Ph.D. Subdepartment of Immunology, Department of Chemical Pathology, University College Hospital, Ibadan, Nigeria

Peter C. Sedman, MB, ChB, FRCS(Ed) Department of Surgery, St. James University Hospital, Leeds, West Yorkshire, England

J. Sanders Sevall, Ph.D. Department of Research and Development, Specialty Laboratories, Inc., Santa Monica, California

Janis Randall Simpson, Ph.D. Department of Health Studies, University of Waterloo, Waterloo, Ontario, Canada

Contributors

Susan Stephens Immunomodulation Research, Celltech, Ltd., Slough, Berkshire, England

Marvin J. Stone, S.M., M.D. Departments of Oncology and Immunology, Charles A. Sammons Cancer Center, Baylor University Medical Center, Dallas, Texas

Stephan Strobel, M.D., Ph.D., MRCP Division of Cell and Molecular Biology, and Hose Defence Unit, Institute of Child Health and Hospital for Sick Children, London, England

Warren Strober, M.D. Mucosal Immunity Section, Laboratory of Clinical Immunology, National Institute of Allergy and Infectious Diseases, National Institutes of Health, Bethesda, Maryland

Christian Swanson, M.A., M.D. Department of Surgery, University of California School of Medicine, Davis, California

Riccardo Troncone, M.D. Department of Pediatrics, University of Naples, Naples, Italy

Kimberly G. Vruwink Department of Nutrition, University of California, Davis, California

Ronald R. Watson, Ph.D. Specialized Alcohol Research Center, Department of Family and Community Medicine, Arizona Health Sciences Center, University of Arizona College of Medicine, Tucson, Arizona

Reinhard E. Zachrau, M.D. Department of Pathology and Institute of Breast Diseases, New York Medical College, Valhalla, New York

S. Zaman Department of Social and Preventive Pediatrics, King Edward Medical College, Lahore, Pakistan

Karl Ziegler, M.D. Abteilung Gastroenterologie, Innere Medizin, Freie Universität Berlin, Berlin, Germany

Robert B. Zurier, M.D. Division of Rheumatology, Department of Medicine, University of Massachusetts Medical Center, Worcester, Massachusetts

Nutrient Modulation of the Immune Response

Part I
Expression of Nutrient Interaction in Immune Function

Part 1

1
Immunoregulatory and Prodifferentiating Effects of 1,25-Dihydroxyvitamin D_3 in Human Mononuclear Cells

Stanley C. Jordan, R. Sakai, H. Phillip Koeffler, and J. S. Adams
Cedars-Sinai Medical Center, UCLA School of Medicine, Los Angeles, California

Jaques Lemire
University of California–San Diego, San Diego, California

INTRODUCTION

Vitamin D is classically recognized as a hormone which regulates mineral ion homeostasis in mammalian and avian species. The nutritional importance of vitamin D in the maintenance of normal, human bone metabolism was unfortunately demonstrated with epidemic frequency in the urban centers of industrialized Europe and America in the nineteenth and early twentieth centuries. In these smoke-laden, sunlight-deprived environments, rickets, vitamin D-deficient bone disease in growing children, was a major source of childhood morbidity and mortality. The utility of simple sunlight exposure in curing rachitic bone disease was first demonstrated by Huldschinsky in 1919 (1), who suggested that environmental sunlight exposure resulted in the endogenous production of a potent "antirachitic substance." We now know that this substance is vitamin D_3, a secosterol which is produced in sun-exposed skin (2). As shown in Figure 1, 7-dehydrocholesterol (provitamin D_3) in the lower epidermis and upper dermis absorbs a photon of solar ultraviolet B radiation, resulting in the photochemical conversion of 7-dehydrocholesterol to previtamin D_3. Previtamin D_3 undergoes thermal isomerization to vitamin D_3, which then enters the general circulation bound to vitamin D-binding protein. Once in the plasma, vitamin D_3 is subject to a sequence of metabolic modifications which alters the biological potency of the

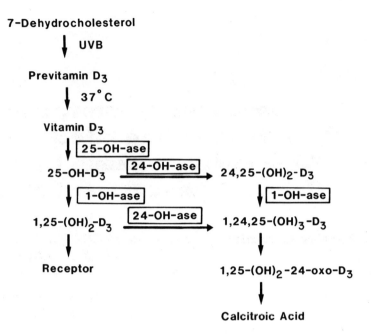

Figure 1 The biochemical pathway for conversion of 7-dehydrocholesterol to 1,25-(OH)$_2$-D$_3$ and metabolite is shown. (See text for details.)

hormone. The first important metabolic step occurs in the liver where vitamin D$_3$ is hydroxylated to 25-hydroxyvitamin D$_3$ (25-OH-D$_3$), the most plentiful circulating vitamin D$_3$ metabolite. A second, stringently regulated hydroxylation reaction takes place primarily in the kidney where 25-OH-D$_3$ is converted to 1,25-dihydroxyvitamin D$_3$ (1,25-[OH]$_2$-D$_3$). 1,25-Dihydroxyvitamin D$_3$ is generally agreed to be the active form of the hormone; its biological effects are mediated through the interaction with a nuclear binding protein (receptor) which binds 1,25-(OH)$_2$-D$_3$ specifically and with high affinity (3,4). In the two classic receptor-possessing target tissues for 1,25-(OH)$_2$-D$_3$, the proximal small intestine and bone, binding of hormone to receptor promotes intestinal calcium absorption (5) and facilitates the normal mineralization of bone (6,7), respectively.

Current dogma holds that regulation of calcium and phosphorus homeostasis by 1,25-(OH)$_2$-D$_3$ is determined by the circulating concentration of hormone to which target tissues are exposed (8). In turn, the plasma concentration of 1,25-(OH)$_2$-D$_3$ is thought to be controlled primarily by the activity of the renal 25-OH-D$_3$-1α-hydroxylase and by the availability of substrate 25-OH-D$_3$ to the enzyme (9). The renal 1α-hydroxylase is a ferrodoxin-requiring, cytochrome p-450 nicotinamide dinucleotide phosphate reductase mainly confined to the mitochondria of proximal renal tubule epithelial cells (10). In vivo, the human renal 25-OH-D$_3$-1α-hydroxylase is most reliably stimulated by an increase in the plasma parathyroid hormone concentration and by a drop in the serum phosphorus concentration. Downregulation of the 1α-hydroxylase is encountered during periods of hyperphosphatemia in human subjects (11) and after administration of supraphysiological concentrations of 1,25-(OH)$_2$-D$_3$

to animals (12). The latter effect may, in part, be due to 1,25-$(OH)_2$-D_3 24-hydroxylase stimulation of 25-OH-D_3 activity (13) (see Fig. 1). The 24-hydroxylase enzyme, which is found in kidney (14) as well as in a variety of extrarenal cell types (15), can metabolize 25-OH-D_3 to 24,25-dihydroxyvitamin D_3 (24,25-$[OH]_2$-D_3), a compound with no substantiated specific biological effects (9). As depicted in Figure 1, 1,25-$(OH)_2$-D_3 is also an acceptable substrate for the 24-hydroxylase producing 1,24,25-trihydroxyvitamin D_3 (1,24,25-$[OH]_3$) (15). This metabolite is a precursor to the 24-oxo metabolite which, in turn, is susceptible to side-chain cleavage into water-soluble, excretable compounds (16).

IS 1,25-DIHYDROXYVITAMIN D_3 AN IMMUNOREGULATORY HORMONE?

The possibility that 1,25-$(OH)_2$-D_3 may modulate the mammalian immune response was raised by three somewhat divergent lines of evidence. First was the observation that a number of mouse and human cultured cell lines of immune cell origin as well as activated human lymphocytes possess the high-affinity receptor for 1,25-$(OH)_2$-D_3 (17). Second was the observation that mouse and human receptor-containing myeloid leukemia cells could be induced to differentiate when exposed to 1,25-$(OH)_2$-D_3 (18). And, third was the finding that pulmonary alveolar macrophages isolated from hypercalcemic patients with sarcoidosis were capable of synthesizing 1,25-$(OH)_2$-D_3 (19,20). Collectively, these data (all acquired in vitro) suggested that immunologically active cells were capable of synthesizing the active metabolite of vitamin D, whereas other cells of immune origin were responsive to the hormone. In addition, a number of solid tumor primary cultures and cell lines, e.g., colon and breast have 1,25-OH_2-D_3 receptors (21,22). As will be expanded upon in subsequent sections of this chapter, the control of the immunological actions of 1,25-$(OH)_2$-D_3 and control of the calcium-phosphorus regulatory actions of the sterol are dissimilar. In the latter case, regulation is apparently achieved by altering circulating concentrations of 1,25-$(OH)_2$-D_3 through stimulation or inhibition of the renal 25-OH-D_3-1α-hydroxylase. The immunological actions of the hormone (monokine), on the other hand, are likely to be regulated by changes in the local production of 1,25-$(OH)_2$-D_3 as well as by expression of receptor in "activated," neighboring target cells. A number of RNA polymerase II-transcribed genes are regulated by 1,25-$(OH)_2$-D_3 and classification of these genes on fucntional grounds has led to the formulation of a gene circuitry hypothesis which links these interactions to a postulated DNA replication-differentiation switch (23).

1,25-DIHYDROXYVITAMIN D_3 REGULATION OF NORMAL AND LEUKEMIC MYELOID CELL DIFFERENTIATION IN VITRO

A diagram of the human hematopoietic system with its stem cells is shown in Figure 2. In vitro clonogenic studies in the murine and human systems have shown that several lymphokines, known as colony-stimulating factors (CSF), induce proliferation and differentiation of hematopoietic stem cells. The myeloid stem cell, known as the granulocyte-monocyte colony-forming cell (GM-CFC), can differentiate to either macrophage colonies when grown in the presence of macrophage or granulocyte-macrophage colony stimulating factors (CSF) or to granulocyte colonies in the presence

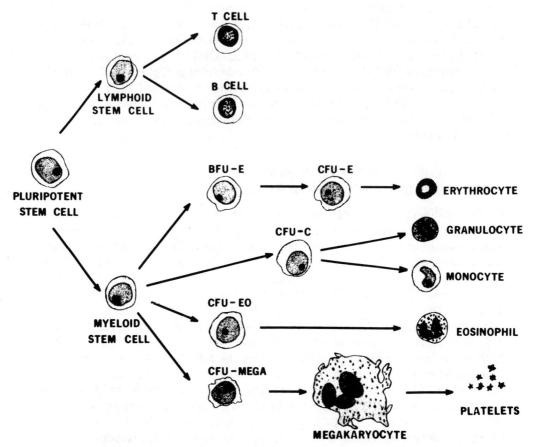

Figure 2 Hematopoietic system. Abbreviations: BFU-E, erythrocyte burst-forming unit; CFU-E, erythrocyte colony-forming unit; CFU-C, colony-forming unit in culture (synonymous with GM-CFC, granulocyte-monocyte colony-forming cell); CFU-EO, eosinophil colony-forming unit; CFU-MEGA, megakaryocyte colony-forming unit).

of granulocyte or granulocyte-macrophage CSF. Few studies have examined the ability of other physiological substances to influence differentiation of myeloid stem cells. Recently, 1,25-$(OH)_2$-D_3 was found to induce cells from both a murine myeloid leukemia line known as M1 (18) and a human promyelocytic leukemia line (HL-60) (24–27) to differentiate to monocyte-macrophage–like cells (Fig. 3) (Table 1). When the cells are cultured in 1,25-$(OH)_2$-D_3 (10^{-7} to 10^{-10} M), they become adherent to charged surfaces, develop long filamented pseudopodia, stain positively for nonspecific acid esterase (NAE), reduce nitro-blue tetrazolium (NBT), and acquire the ability to phagocytose yeast. The HL-60 cells cultured with 1,25-$(OH)_2$-D_3 also acquire the capacity to bind and degrade bone matrix in vitro (25). The effective dose (ED_{50}) that induces approximately 50% of the cells to differentiate is about 6×10^{-9} M.

The mechanism by which HL-60 cells are induced to differentiate by 1,25-$(OH)_2$-D_3 is not clear. These cells contain cellular receptors for 1,25-$(OH)_2$-D_3 as shown by sucrose density gradient analysis, by DNA cellulose chromatography, and by a specific

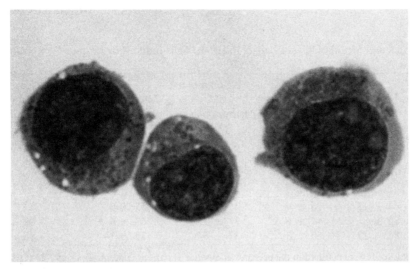

(a)

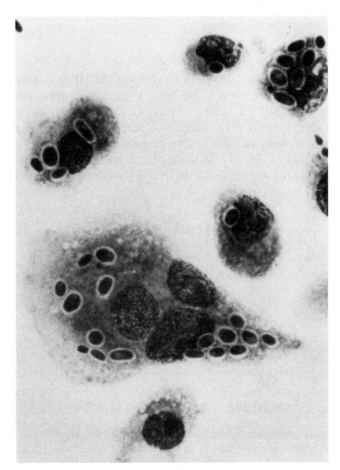

(b)

Figure 3 (a) HL-60 promyelocytes. (b) HL-60 cells induced to macrophage-like cells after exposure to 10^{-7} mol/L 1,25-dihydroxyvitamin D_3 for 7 days. Cells are adherent and have phagocytosed *Candida albicans*.

Table 1 Functional and Morphological Changes in HL-60 Cells Induced by Various Concentrations of 1,25-$(OH)_2$-D_3[a]

Added concentration of 1,25-$(OH)_2$-D_3[b] (M)	NBT reduction (%)	Phagocytic cells (%)	Myeloblasts and promyeloblasts (%)	Intermediate[c] to mature cells (%)	Nonspecific acid esterase–positive (%)
0	2 ± 3	2 ± 2	99 ± 2	1 ± 2	2
10^{-11}	10 ± 2	2 ± 3	95 ± 3	5 ± 4	3
10^{-10}	18 ± 11	13 ± 7	82 ± 5	18 ± 7	10
10^{-9}	37 ± 19	20 ± 7	66 ± 9	23 ± 6	25
10^{-8}	64 ± 13	26 ± 4	45 ± 12	55 ± 9	54
10^{-7}	82 ± 8	44 ± 9	32 ± 5	67 ± 6	82
10^{-6}	86 ± 12	60 ± 3	27 ± 6	78 ± 14	98

[a]HL-60 and HL-60 blast cells were cultured in the presence or absence of various concentrations of 1,25-$(OH)_2$-D_3; after 7 days, cells were assessed for the various differentiation parameters. All data are expressed as the percentage of total cells assayed and the data represent the mean ± standard deviation of triplicate assays.
[b]Basal 1,25-$(OH)_2$-D_3 in 10% fetal bovine serum is 1.6×10^{-11} M.
[c]Intermediate to mature cells include monocytes and macrophages.

monoclonal antibody which recognizes the 1,25-$(OH)_2$-D_3 receptor (24,27). Scatchard analysis shows that the HL-60 has about 4000 1,25-$(OH)_2$-D_3 cellular receptors per cell with a dissociation constant (K_d) of 5.4×10^{-9} M (Fig. 4). Further indirect evidence that the vitamin D_3 analogs mediate their induction of differentiation through 1,25-$(OH)_2$-D_3 cellular receptors is shown in Figure 5. We have found that 1,25-$(OH)_2$-D_3 can inhibit clonal proliferation of HL-60 cells when plated in soft agar. We examined the effect of six vitamin D_3 compounds on the clonal growth of HL-60 and

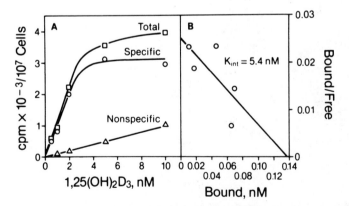

Figure 4 Determination of the equilibrium dissociation constant of 1,25-$(OH)_2$-D_3 internalization in intact HL-60 cells. Saturation analysis (A) was determined by incubating intact cells under normal growth conditions for 4 hr with 10% serum along with various concentrations of titrated 1,25-$(OH)_2$-D_3 in the presence (△) or absence (□) of 100-fold excess nonradioactive 1,25-$(OH)_2$-D_3. Specific binding (○) was transformed by Scatchard analysis and then the data line-fitted by linear regression. (B) to yield a K_{int} = 5.4 nM (abscissa intercept = 4000 molecules/cell, r = 0.71).

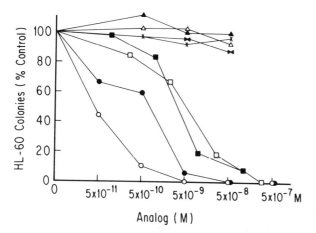

Figure 5 Effect of various concentrations of different analogs of vitamin D on clonal growth of HL-60 promyelocytes. The analogs are: ●, $1\alpha,25\text{-(OH)}_2\text{-D}_3$; ■, $1\alpha\text{-24S},25\text{-(OH)}_3\text{-D}_3$; ▲, $24S,25\text{-(OH)}_2\text{-D}_3$; △, $1\alpha\text{-(OH)-D}_3$; ○, $24,24\text{-F}_2\text{-}1\alpha,25\text{-(OH)}_2\text{-D}_3$; □, $1\alpha,24,25\text{(OH)}_3\text{-D}_3$; x, $24R,25\text{-(OH)}_2\text{-D}_3$; ►◄, 25-(OH)-D_3. Cells were plated in soft agar with various vitamin D analogs and the number of colonies enumerated after 10 days of culture. Results are expressed as a percent of control cells not exposed to the vitamin D analog. Each point represents the mean of three experiments with triplicate dishes per point.

found that the inhibition of growth by these analogs paralleled their known ability to bind to the cellular $1,25\text{-(OH)}_2\text{-D}_3$ receptor. The rank order of potency for the compounds was: $24,24\text{-F}_2\text{-}1\alpha\text{-}25\text{-(OH)}_2\text{-D}_3 > 1,25\text{-(OH)}_2\text{-D}_3 > ,24R,25\text{-(OH)}_3\text{-D}_3 = 1,24S,25\text{-(OH)}_3\text{-D}_3$ (28). In contrast, 1-OH-D_3, 25-OH-D_3, and $24S,25\text{-(OH)}_2\text{-D}_3$ had no effect on clonal growth.

$1,25\text{-(OH)}_2\text{-D}_3$ can also preferentially induce differentiation of normal human myeloid stem cells toward macrophages. An initial study found that an increased percentage of monocytes and macrophages were present when $1,25\text{-(OH)}_2\text{-D}_3$ was added to bone marrow cells in liquid culture for 5 days when compared to control flasks containing no $1,25\text{-(OH)}_2\text{-D}_3$ (25). To further investigate this observation, $1,25\text{-(OH)}_2\text{-D}_3$ was added to soft agar cultures containing normal human bone marrow in the presence of GM-CSF (Table 2) (29). The GM-CFC stem cells proliferated and differentiated in soft agar and formed colonies. These colonies were plucked, cytochemically stained, examined by light microscopy, and the absolute number of monocyte, granulocyte, and combined monocyte and granulocyte colonies was determined. $1,25\text{-(OH)}_2\text{-D}_3$-induced human myeloid GM-CFC to differentiate to colonies containing macrophages. Nearly 95% of the colonies were composed of only macrophages in culture plates containing 10^{-8} M $1,25\text{-(OH)}_2\text{-D}_3$, and 55% of the colonies were composed of only macrophages in the plates containing 10^{-9} M $1,25\text{-(OH)}_2\text{-D}_3$. Control dishes of normal human bone marrow GM-CFC not exposed to $1,25\text{-(OH)}_2\text{-D}_3$ differentiated to approximately 55% neutrophil, 10% mixed neutrophil-macrophage, and 25% macrophage colonies. $1,25\text{-(OH)}_2\text{-D}_3$ increased the absolute number of macrophage colonies rather than merely increasing the relative proportion of macrophage colonies by selectively inhibiting granulocytic differentiation of GM-CFC (Table 2). Plates containing either 10^{-8} or 10^{-9} M $1,25\text{-(OH)}_2\text{-D}_3$

Table 2 Effects of 1,25-$(OH)_2$-D_3 on Differentiation and Proliferation of Human Myeloid Colony-Forming Cells

Cell source[a]	(1,25[OH]$_2$-D_3) (M)	No. of colonies (% of control)[a]	Colony morphology[b] (%)			
			N	NM	M	B
Normal	0	100	56 ± 8	10 ± 1	34 ± 4	0
volunteers	10^{-10}	102 ± 6	58 ± 5	6 ± 1	36 ± 3	0
(7)	10^{-9}	120 ± 5	29 ± 4	5 ± 1	56 ± 4	0
	10^{-8}	101 ± 5	2 ± 1	2 ± 1	96 ± 2	0
	10^{-7}	78 ± 6	0	0	100	0

[a]Marrow cells were obtained from seven normal volunteers and the light density, nonadherent, mononuclear cells were cultured in the presence of colony stimulating factor and various concentrations of the vitamin D metabolite 1,25-$(OH)_2$-D_3. Colonies were counted on day 10 of culture. Normal control cultures contained a mean of 94 ± 8 (± SE) myeloid colonies.
[b]Colony morphology was evaluated on day 10 of culture by dual esterase and luxol fast blue staining. N, neutrophilic colonies; NM, neutrophil-macrophage mixed colonies; M, monocyte-macrophage colonies, B, blast cells colonies.

developed 90 and 65 macrophage colonies, respectively, per 1×10^5 cultured marrow cells. In contrast, only 35 macrophage colonies per 1×10^5 cultured marrow cells developed in control plates containing no 1,25-$(OH)_2$-D_3.

The paucity of GM-CFC in the bone marrow (approximately $1/2 \times 10^3$ marrow cells) prevents purification of these cells in attempts to determine if they contain 1,25-$(OH)_2$-D_3 receptors. Nevertheless, extrapolation of data obtained from the HL-60 promyelocytes suggests that 1,25-$(OH)_2$-D_3 induces macrophage differentiation of hematopoietic progenitor cells by binding of the active vitamin D metabolite to the 1,25-$(OH)_2$-D_3 receptors, which presumably binds to DNA and alters transcriptional control. Differentiation may be regulated by 1,25-$(OH)_2$-D_3 itself, by local shifts in calcium transport mediated by 1,25-$(OH)_2$-D_3, or by induction of differentiation-inducing protein(s) by accessory cells in the culture plates.

The hypothesis that 1,25-$(OH)_2$-D_3 may be a possible differentiation inducer of GM-CFC to macrophages is appealing because of the known ability of 1,25-$(OH)_2$-D_3 to modulate bone resorption. Osteoclasts resorb bone. Evidence suggests that osteoclasts may develop from monocyte-macrophage cells (30), and one study suggested that 1,25-$(OH)_2$-D_3 may modulate the number of osteoclasts (31). Therefore, 1,25-$(OH)_2$-D_3 might modulate bone resorption by inducing GM-CFC to differentiate to monocytes and macrophages and eventually to osteoclasts. In addition, the monocytes and macrophages can resorb bone directly in vitro (32).

The plasma concentration of 1,25-$(OH)_2$-D_3 in humans is approximately 7.7×10^{-11} M (33). Concentrations of $\geq 10^{-9}$ M 1,25-$(OH)_2$-D_3 induce macrophage differentiation of myeloid progenitor cells in vitro. Therefore, 1,25-$(OH)_2$-D_3 may not have a physiological role in the induction of differentiation of human myeloid stem cells to macrophages. Likewise, patients who received superphysiological doses of 1,25-$(OH)_2$-D_3 hve not been reported to have an increased concentration of blood monocytes (34). Also, patients with vitamin D–resistant rickets have not been reported to have low monocyte or macrophage levels (35). The true hematopoietic role of vitamin D metabolites in vivo is unknown. A search for analogs that could promote myelocytic leukemic cells to benign monocytes has shown that some analogs may be even more effective than vitamin D_3, whereas being less active in mobilizing calcium from bone (36).

The effect of 1,25-$(OH)_2$-D_3 on both clonal proliferation and differentiation of cells from eight myeloid leukemic lines is shown on Figure 6 and Tables 3 and 4 (28). The 50% inhibition of colony formation of the responsive lines occurred in the concentration range of 3×10^{-8} to 4×10^{-10} M 1,25-$(OH)_2$-D_3. These concentrations are comparable to the concentrations required for induction of differentiation in liquid culture (20,27,37,38). Cell lines which were induced to differentiate by 1,25-$(OH)_2$-D_3 were always inhibited in their clonal growth by 1,25-$(OH)_2$-D_3. Differentiation was measured by their ability to reduce nitroblue tetrazolium (NBT), which is a measure of maturation. The responsive cells were relatively more mature (HL-60, U-937 THPI, HEL, MI) than the unresponsive cells (KGIA, KG-1, HL-60 blast, K562). Our experiments are supportive of the concept that myeloid blast cells have limited capabilities for replication when induced to differentiate. The vitamin D-responsive progenitor cells differentiated in vitro and lost their potential for clonal growth. The vitamin D-unresponsive leukemic cells did not differentiate and remained in the proliferative pool, giving rise to colonies of similar cells. Thus, the single noted enhancement of osteogenic sarcoma cell growth in the nude mouse (39), appears to us and others (22) to be a rare event perhaps associated with certain cell types or in particular settings.

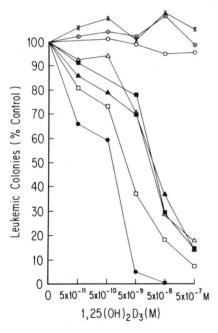

Figure 6 Effect of various concentrations of 1,25-$(OH)_2$-D_3 on clonal growth of myeloid cell lines (●, HL-60; □, U937; △, M1; ▲, THP; □HEL, ●HL-60 blast; x, Kg-1A; ʘ, K562). Cells were plated in soft agar containing different concentrations of 1,25-$(OH)_2$-D_3 and the number of colonies were enumerated on day 12 of culture. Results are expressed as a percent of control cells not exposed to 1,25-$(OH)_2$-D_3. Each point represents the mean of three experiments with triplicate dishes per point.

Table 3 Effects of 1α-25-(OH)$_2$-D$_3$ on Clonal Growth of Cells Freshly Isolated from Myeloid Leukemia Lines

Cell line	Description	50% Inhibitory concentration M 1α,25-(OH)$_2$-D$_3$
HL-60	Human promyelocytes	8×10^{-10}
U937	Human monoblasts/histiocytes	4×10^{-9}
HEL	Bipotent[a]	2×10^{-8}
THP-1	Human monoblasts	3×10^{-8}
M1	Mouse myeloid leukemia	1×10^{-8}
HL-60 blast	Human early myeloblasts	No inhibition
KG-1A	Human early myeloblasts	No inhibition
KG-1	Human myeloblasts	No inhibition[b]
K562	Bipotent[a]	No inhibition

[a]Monoblast and erythroblast characteristics.
[b]Stimulation at suboptimal concentrations of CSF.

We also examined the effect of 1,25-(OH)$_2$-D$_3$ on the clonal growth of leukemic blast cells harvested from the peripheral blood or bone marrow of 14 individuals with myeloid leukemia (Table 5). Ten of the 14 leukemic patients had neoplastic cells that were at least 50% inhibited in their colony formation in the presence of 5×10^{-7} M 1,25-(OH)$_2$-D$_3$, and 5 of the 14 leukemic patients had a 50% inhibition of leukemic colony formation at 5×10^{-9} M 1,25-(OH)$_2$-D$_3$ (Table 5). Clonal growth of acute myelogenous leukemia (AML) and chronic myelogenous leukemia cells was inhibited approximately equally by 1,25-(OH)$_2$-D$_3$. However, 1,25-(OH)$_2$-D$_3$ stimulated the clonal proliferation of blast cells from a single AML patient by greater than 400%. This 33-year-old patient had very immature acute myeloblastic leukemia cells. On the other hand, 1,25-(OH)$_2$-D$_3$ had little effect on clonal growth of normal myeloid stem cells (GM-CFC) harvested from 12 myeloid leukemia patients who were in remission. The GM-CFC from leukemic patients in remission were not inhibited more than 30% at any concentration of the 1,25-(OH)$_2$-D$_3$ (5×10^{-7}–5×10^{-11} M) employed.

Table 4 Effect of 1α,25-(OH)-D$_3$ on the Ability of Cells from Leukemic Lines to Reduce NBT

Cell line	Percentage NBT-positive cells							
	HL-60	HL-60 blast	KG-1	KG-1a	U937	HEL	THPI	M1
Control	2 ± 2	0 ± 1	0 ± 0	0 ± 0	1 ± 1	3 ± 2	35 ± 5	2 ± 1
1,25-(OH)$_2$-D$_3$	60 ± 7	1 ± 1	0 ± 0	0 ± 0	49 ± 8	27 ± 9	48 ± 5	16 ± 3

Results represent the mean of four separate experiments ($\pm$SD). Cells cultured in liquid media containing 5×10^{-7} M 1α,25-(OH)$_2$-D$_3$ for 5 days, washed, and tested for their ability to reduce nitroblue tetrazolium (NBT).

Table 5 Effect of 1α,25-(OH)-D$_3$ on Clonal Growth of Myeloid Leukemia Cells Freshly Obtained from Patients

Patient	Diagnosis[a]	Age yr	Cell source	L-CFC[b]	1,25-(OH)$_2$-D$_3$ ED$_{50}$[c]
M.F.	AML	64	B	22 ± 5	2×10^{-9} M
W.P.	AML	44	B	72 ± 34	No effect
W.M.	AML	33	M	12 ± 4	Stimulation[d]
P.O.	AML	50	M	810 ± 91	5×10^{-11} M
C.L.	AML	42	M	23 ± 4	5×10^{-7} M
B.T.	AML	40	M	131 ± 34	5×10^{-11} M
K.R.	AML	44	M	16 ± 2	No effect
M.L.	AML	31	M	22 ± 3	4×10^{-9} M
W.D.	AML	37	M	112 ± 20	2×10^{-8} M
B.A.	CML	11	B	295 ± 89	No effect
H.J.	CML	12	B	36 ± 12	4×10^{-9} M
M.D.	CML	27	M	60 ± 11	8×10^{-9} M
C.A.	CML	34	B	129 ± 3	6×10^{-9} M
G.S.	CML-BC	25	B	337 ± 45	1×10^{-7} M

[a]CML-BC, chronic myelogenous leukemia, blast crisis; B, peripheral blood; M, bone marrow.
[b]L-CFC, leukemic colony-forming cells per 2×10^5 cells plated in soft agar with maximally stimulated concentrations of CSF.
[c]ED$_{50}$, effective dose that inhibited 50% clonal growth of leukemic cells.
[d]Stimulation: 62 colonies formed in the presence of 1α,25-(OH)$_2$-D$_3$ (5×10^{-8} M).

Why 1,25-(OH)$_2$-D$_3$ preferentially inhibits the in vitro proliferation of leukemic cells but not normal human myeloid stem cells is not clear. Differences in receptor number or affinity or the activation of different genes and metabolic pathways may account for this effect. Since 1,25-(OH)$_2$-D$_3$ has been found to induce fibronectin in human cancer and transformed cell lines, this has also been postulated as a mechanism of action (40).

Further studies suggest that 1,25-(OH)$_2$-D$_3$ can act as a hematopoietic cofactor that promotes clonal growth of certain myeloid stem cells (28). In the presence of submaximal concentrations of CSF, 1,25-(OH)$_2$-D$_3$ stimulated the clonal growth of normal human bone marrow GM-CFC. A similar result was obtained with the human AML cell line known as KG-1 which is dependent on CSF for its clonal growth. 1,25-(OH)$_2$-D$_3$ did not stimulate the marrow or KG-1 cells to produce detectable CSF. The increased clonal growth in the presence of 1,25-(OH)$_2$-D$_3$ and submaximal concentrations of CSF may reflect an increased responsiveness to CSF due to effects on the number and/or affinity of CSF receptors on the target cells.

In contrast to these results, occasionally it seems that certain lymphomas may produce 1,25-(OH)$_2$-D$_3$ and in some cases this may be linked to retroviral transformation (41). However, the circumstances triggering this production are unknown.

A CLINICAL STUDY OF 1,25-DIHYDROXYVITAMIN D$_3$ ADMINISTRATION TO PATIENTS WITH MYELODYSPLASTIC SYNDROMES

Because of the ability of the vitamin D metabolite to induce differentiation and to inhibit the clonal proliferation of some human acute myelogenous leukemia cells, we initiated a trial of administering 1,25-(OH)$_2$-D$_3$ to patients with myelodysplastic syndromes. Previous studies have shown that administration of 1,25-(OH)$_2$-D$_3$ significantly prolongs the life of mice injected with the M1 transplantable murine leukemia cells (42). We chose to study myelodysplastic patients because the tempo of their disease allows scrutiny of therapeutic maneuvers. These patients, most of whom have their leukemic clone established in vitro, demonstrate ineffective hematopoiesis in vivo with anemia, thrombocytopenia, leukopenia, and often an increased number of marrow blast cells. We administered at least 2 mcg of 1,25-(OH)$_2$-D$_3$ daily to the patients (normal calcitropic dose is 0.25 mcg daily). Figure 7 summarizes the alteration of their granulocyte, red cell, platelet, blast cell, and calcium concentrations during the study. All patients received weekly escalating doses of 1,25-(OH)$_2$-D$_3$ until a daily dose of 2 mcg was reached. The median duration of therapy with 1,25-(OH)$_2$-D$_3$ was 12 weeks (range 4 to >20). The concentration of granulocytes, monocytes, and plate-

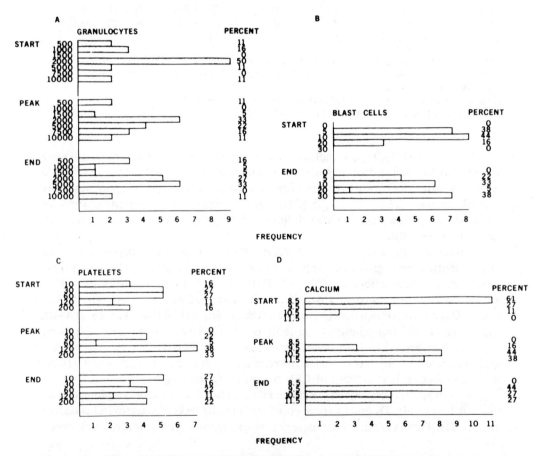

Figure 7 Effect of administration of 1,25-dihydroxyvitamin D$_3$ on hematopoiesis in meylodysplastic (preleukemia) patients. Panel A. Effect of 1,25-(OH)$_2$-D$_3$ on peripheral blood granulocyte concentrations (per microliter of blood). Panel B. Effect of 1,25-(OH)$_2$-D$_3$ on percent of bone marrow myeloblasts. Panel C. Effect of 1,25-(OH)$_2$-D$_3$ on peripheral blood platelet concentrations (per microliter of blood). Panel D. Effect of 1,25-(OH)$_2$-D$_3$ on serum calcium concentrations (mg/dl); normal range of serum calcium is 8.2–10.5 mg/dl.

lets in the blood did not differ significantly between the beginning and the end of the study. The percent of myeloblasts in the marrow rose from a beginning median value of 10% (range 3–20%) to a significantly ($p < 0.0136$) elevated ending median value of 15% (range 4–70%). Seven patients had an improvement of either their absolute granulocyte, monocyte, or platelet blood concentrations for >4 sequential weeks of treatment. Wilcoxian statistics compared values for the patients at the end of the treatment period with the baseline values, and showed no significant improvement in any of the parameters. Of 19 patients in the study, 6 progressed to acute myelogenous leukemia by the end of the study.

The preleukemic patients received at least 2 mcg/day of 1,25-$(OH)_2$-D_3. This dose results in serum 1,25-$(OH)_2$-D_3 concentrations of about 2.0×10^{-10} M in normal individuals (43). A concentration of 2×10^{-10} M 1,25-$(OH)_2$-D_3 induces maturation of <20% of HL-60 promyelocytes in vitro (26,27,44,45). Theoretically, the obtainment of higher serum concentrations of 1,25-$(OH)_2$-D_3 in our preleukemic patients would have been desirable. During the study, however, 9 of 18 patients became hypercalcemic. Somewhat higher concentrations of 1,25-$(OH)_2$-D_3 could have been given if the patients had been placed on a low-calcium diet. In the future, vitamin D analogs (22,36) that induce hematopoietic cell differentiation without inducing hypercalcemia might be medically useful compounds for selected patients with preleukemia and leukemia. In addition, intravenous 1,25-$(OH)_2$-D_3 could be used to achieve higher serum levels without inducing severe hypercalcemia.

1,25-DIHYDROXYVITAMIN D_3 AS AN IMMUNOREGULATOR IN VITRO

The identification of 1,25-$(OH)_2$-D_3 receptors in activated T and B lymphocytes from normal individuals (46) suggests that immunoregulatory processes could be altered by the interaction of the sterol with its specific, high-affinity receptor in these cells. We and others have devoted an extensive effort to defining the immunoregulatory potential of 1,25-$(OH)_2$-D_3 on human peripheral blood mononuclear cell (PBM) functions. It is now clear that these immunoregulatory consequences are the result of the interaction of 1,25-$(OH)_2$-D_3 with its receptor in activated T and B cells. This discovery has triggered new investigations into the mechanism(s) of immunoregulation exerted by the sterol. Data obtained from our laboratory and others (18,47,48) show that 1,25-$(OH)_2$-D_3 induces a number of immunoinhibitory functions in lymphocytes, which include: (a) the inhibition of interleukin 2 (IL-2) production by mitogen and antigen-activated PBM, (b) the inhibition of cytotoxic T-cell generation in the mixed lymphocyte culture, and (c) the inhibition of PBM proliferation and immunoglobulin (Ig) production by mitogen and antigen-activated PBM. These inhibitory effects are significantly reduced by the addition of vitamin D-binding protein or its analogs (49). The specific cellular target(s) and mechanism of action of 1,25-$(OH)_2$-D_3 in regulating lymphocyte responses to mitogen and antigen are the subject of considerable debate and extensive investigation. That which follows are the experimental results that form the current state of our understanding of the effects of 1,25-$(OH)_2$-D_3 on human T- and B-lymphocyte functions in vitro.

After the identification of 1,25-$(OH)_2$-D_3 receptors in activated T and B lymphocytes (46), we designed a study to determine if the expression of these receptors in activated cells had any functional significance. Our initial studies using PBM showed that the addition of $1,25\text{-}(OH)_2\text{-}D_3$ to mitogen or antigen-activated PBM resulted in a dose-dependent inhibition of DNA synthesis and total DNA content at concentrations ranging from 10^{-10} to 10^{-9} M. The half-maximal inhibition of [^{3}H]thymidine incorporation occurred at 10^{-11} to 10^{-10} M in cells activated with the mitogen phytohemagglutinin (PHA) and pokeweed mitogen (PWM), and 10^{-10} to 10^{-9} M $1,25\text{-}(OH)_2\text{-}D_3$ in cultures activated with dermatophyton-0 (47) (Fig. 8). These initial studies indicated that $1,25\text{-}(OH)_2\text{-}D_3$ had an inhibitory effect on DNA synthesis by activated PBMs. This effect was dose dependent with an effect seen at concentrations as low as 10^{-10} M $1,25\text{-}(OH)_2\text{-}D_3$. Experiments conducted incubating activated PBMs with $25\text{-}OH\text{-}D_3$ and $24,25\text{-}(OH)_2\text{-}D_3$ showed that the suppressive effect was specific for $1,25\text{-}(OH)_2\text{-}D_3$, since the half-maximal effect of $1,25\text{-}(OH)_2\text{-}D_3$ was present at concentrations of the hormone 100 to 1000 times less than concentrations of $24,25\text{-}(OH)_2\text{-}D_3$ and $25\text{-}OH\text{-}D_3$, respectively. These results are consistent with a $1,25\text{-}(OH)_2\text{-}D_3$ receptor-mediated effect on PBM DNA synthesis, with the suppressive effects of

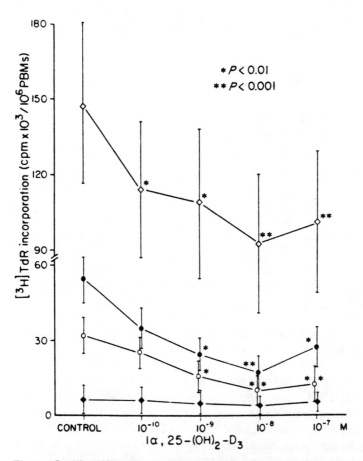

Figure 8 The effect of $1,25\text{-}(OH)_2\text{-}D_3$ on in vitro DNA synthesis by normal human PBMs unstimulated (◆) and stimulated with either PHA (◇), PWM (●) or dermatophyton-0 (○). Each point represents the mean value of four normal human subjects assayed in triplicate. (Reproduced with permission.)

the various metabolites reflecting their affinity for the 1,25-(OH)$_2$-D$_3$ receptor (47). Since 10^{-9} M 1,25-(OH)$_2$-D$_3$ is a receptor-saturating concentration of the hormone in a serum-free environment, it is not surprising that maximal inhibition was seen at 10^{-8} to 10^{-7} M 1,25-(OH)$_2$-D$_3$. Since 1,25-(OH)$_2$-D$_3$ exerted a specific receptor-mediated antiproliferative effect on PBM DNA synthesis, we undertook experiments to determine the specific cellular target(s) in the PBM population that were affected by incubation with 1,25-(OH)$_2$-D$_3$. In these experiments, normal human PBMs were fractionated into T-lymphocyte–enriched and B-lymphocyte–enriched populations by nylon wool column separation techniques (50). The nonadherent cell population (T-lymphocyte enriched) was subsequently submitted for immunofluorescence staining and cell separation into T-helper/inducer (Leu3a+, T_H, CD4) or T-suppressor/cytotoxic (Leu2a+, T_S, CD8) populations. Our initial experiments showed that the inhibitory effect of 10^{-8} M 1,25-(OH)$_2$-D$_3$ on DNA synthesis by human T and B lymphocytes was limited to the T_H cell population (Fig. 9). Synthesis of DNA by activated T_H cells was suppressed by 56.2 ± 7.1% when cultured with 10^{-8} M 1,25-(OH)$_2$-D$_3$. Preincubation of T_S- and B-enriched lymphocytes with 10^{-8} M 1,25-(OH)$_2$-D$_3$ showed minimal or no inhibition of DNA synthesis in these cell populations. The establishment of an antiproliferative effect of 1,25-(OH)$_2$-D$_3$ on human PBM which was specific for the T_H cell subset led to the investigation of 1,25-(OH)$_2$-D$_3$ in mediating other T_H cell functions such as IL-2 production and T_H cell–directed B-cell immunoglobulin synthesis.

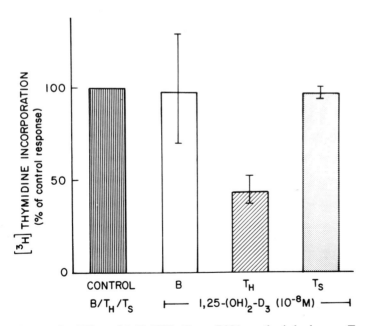

Figure 9 Effect of 1,25-(OH)$_2$-D$_3$ on DNA synthesis by human T and B lymphocytes. The results are expressed as the percentage of the response of 1,25-(OH)$_2$-D$_3$-treated lymphocyte subsets to that of identical cultures not exposed to the hormone. Each value represents the mean (± SEM) of cells from four normal human subjects assayed in triplicate. (Reproduced with permission.)

To evaluate the effect of 1,25-$(OH)_2$-D_3 on IL-2 production, supernatants from mitogen-activated PBMs cultured with or without 10^{-8} M 1,25-$(OH)_2$-D_3 were assayed for their ability to stimulate proliferation of the IL-2–dependent CTLL-2 cells in a standard IL-2 assay. The supernatants from 1,25-$(OH)_2$-D_3–treated PBMs showed an 85.1 ± 4.2% reduction in IL-2 production when compared to mitogen-activated controls. 24,25-$(OH)_2$-D_2 and 25-OH-D_3 incubated at similar concentrations showed no inhibitory effect on IL-2 production (50) (Fig. 10). 1,25-$(OH)_2$-D_3 was shown to have no inhibitory effect on the IL-2 detector cell CTLL-2 at all concentrations tested. Tsoukas et al. (17) and Iho et al. (51) have demonstrated a similar inhibitory effect of 1,25-$(OH)_2$-D_3 on IL-2 synthesis.

We also evaluated the effect of 1,25-$(OH)_2$-D_3 on IL-2 receptor expression (Tac) by PBM using the monoclonal antibody anti-Tac (kindly provided by Dr. T. Waldmann of the National Institutes of Health, Bethesda, Maryland). Interestingly, 1,25-$(OH)_2$-D_3 showed no inhibitory effect on Tac expression by mitogen-activated PBM. Further experiments were performed using fluorescein-activated cell-sorted (FACS) Leu3a+ and Leu2a+ cells which were activated with mitogen in the presence or

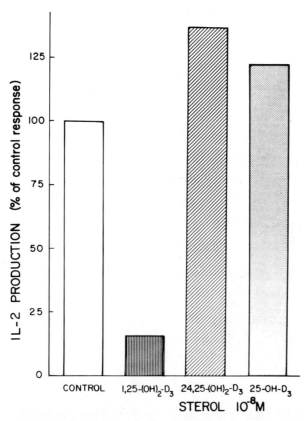

Figure 10 Interleukin 2 (IL-2) production by human PBMs from four normal donors activated with the mitogen PHA with or without a receptor saturating concentration (10^{-8} M) of vitamin D metabolites [1,25-$[OH]_2$-D_3, 24,25-$[OH]_2$-D_3, or 25-OH-D_3). Data is represented as percent mitogen-activated control response.

absence of 1,25-(OH)$_2$-D$_3$. These experiments showed that Tac receptor expression was not inhibited on Leu3a+ or Leu2a+ cells by 1,25-(OH)$_2$-D$_3$. These data indicate that 1,25-(OH)$_2$-D$_3$ exerts a specific receptor-mediated inhibitory effect on IL-2 synthesis by activated T$_H$ cells without interfering with other immune activation signals such as Tac expression. These data have been confirmed by Provvedini and Mandagas (52), who interestingly found that receptor distribution was equivalent on both sets of cells.

To determine if 1,25-(OH)$_2$-D$_3$ exerted an effect on Ig production by PBM, we investigated both mitogen- (PWM) and antigen- (tetanus toxoid) induced IgG and IgM production by PBM incubated with or without 1,25-(OH)$_2$-D$_3$. Initial data (Fig. 11) were similar to the dose-related antiproliferative effect of 1,25-(OH)$_2$-D$_3$ (47). Suppression of mitogen- and antigen-induced Ig production was similar with maximal inhibition evident at 10^{-8} to 10^{-7} M 1,25-(OH)$_2$-D$_3$. Inhibition of Ig production

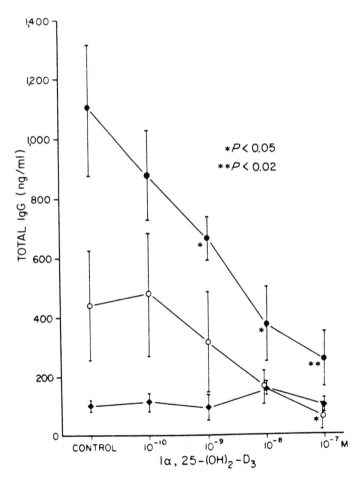

Figure 11 The effect of 1,25-(OH)$_2$-D$_3$ on IgG production in vitro by normal human PBMs unstimulated (◆) and stimulated with either PWM (●) or dermatophyton-0 (○). Each data point represents the mean value of four normal human subjects. The results are expressed in nanograms per milliliters. (Reproduced with permission.)

occurred only at high doses of 24,25-$(OH)_2$-D_3 (10^{-7} M) and no identifiable inhibitory effect was seen when cells were incubated with 25-OH-D_3. Iho et al. (53) have confirmed our earlier findings. Since our previous data indicated that the T_H cell was the specific cellular target for 1,25-$(OH)_2$-D_3, we undertook experiments to determine the mechanisms by which Ig synthesis was inhibited when activated PBMs were incubated with 1,25-$(OH)_2$-D_3. Enriched T_H-, T_S- and B-lymphocyte populations obtained by FACS were cultured separately, (24 hr), mitogen activated, and incubated with or without 10^{-8} M 1,25-$(OH)_2$-D_3. After the 24-hr incubation, the B-cell–enriched population was incubated with analogus T_H, T_S, or T_H + T_S and activated with PWM. Immunoglobulin production was determined at 12 days, and is illustrated in (Fig. 12). Briefly, 1,25-$(OH)_2$-D_3 treatment of B-enriched cells did not affect Ig production. However, a significant inhibition of Ig production was noted when mitogen-activated, 1,25-$(OH)_2$-D_3–treated T_H cells were incubated with untreated B-enriched cells. In sum, the only significant inhibitory effect seen on Ig synthesis was in cultures of T_H cells that were mitogen activated to express 1,25-$(OH)_2$-D_3 receptors and incubated with 10^{-8} M 1,25-$(OH)_2$-D_3 prior to incubation with B-enriched lymphocytes. These data strongly suggest that the immunosuppressive effect of 1,25-$(OH)_2$-D_3

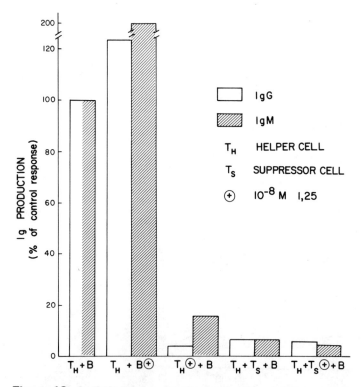

Figure 12 Ig (IgG, IgM) production by B-cell–enriched lymphocytes incubated with FACS T_H, T_S, or T_H + T_S populations which were mitogen activated (to suppress 1,25-$(OH)_2$-D_3 receptors) and incubated with a receptor-saturating concentration (10^{-8} M) 1,25-$(OH)_2$-D_3 for 24 hr. After the 24-hr incubation and vigorous washing, the B-cell–enriched population was incubated with T_H, T_S, or T_H + T_S and activated with PWM. Assays for Ig production were performed at 12 days.

in vitro is mediated primarily by the interaction of the sterol with activated T_H cells. Although both B and T cells are known to express receptors for 1,25-$(OH)_2$-D_3, the hormone interactions with B and T_S cells does not appear to have immunoregulatory significance under the experimental conditions tested here. In addition, we have recently performed experiments activating PBMs with the B-cell mitogen protein A. Protein A induces IgM production only, and when B cells were activated in the presence of 10^{-8} M 1,25-$(OH)_2$-D_3, no inhibition of IgM production was noted. These data also strongly suggest that inhibition of mitogen- and antigen-induced Ig production by 1,25-$(OH)_2$-D_3 is mediated through inhibition of T_H-cell activity.

Iho et al. (51) found a similar effect of 1,25-$(OH)_2$-D_3 on T cell–mediated Ig synthesis; however, they also described a direct inhibitory effect on B-cell Ig synthesis. Provvedini et al. (54) have also described a 1,25-$(OH)_2$-D_3 inhibitory effect on Ig production by Epstein-Barr virus- (EBV) activated human B cells. These authors feel that since EBV is a B-lymphotrophic virus, inhibition of Ig production in this system represents direct inhibition of B-cell function and is independent of T-cell participation. Our data and that of others (72) suggest immunoinhibition by 1,25-$(OH)_2$-D_3 occurs through suppression of T_H-cell activity. This is supported by (a) a specific antiproliferative effect on T_H cells by 1,25-$(OH)_2$-D_3, (b) a significant suppression of Ig synthesis by B cells only when incubated with 1,25-$(OH)_2$-D_3–treated T_H cells, and (c) a dramatic and specific reduction of IL-2 production by activated PBM incubated with 1,25-$(OH)_2$-D_3. The specificity of the 1,25-$(OH)_2$-D_3 effect on T_H cells is further strengthened by the lack of an antiproliferative effect of the hormone on T_S cells and a lack of inhibition of T_S function in vitro.

These results suggest that 1,25-$(OH)_2$-D_3 acts on the activated T_H cell to inhibit production of IL-2, resulting in suppression of T_H cell–mediated B-cell Ig synthesis. Clearly, other investigators have shown that under specific experimental conditions, B-cell Ig synthesis is inhibited by 1,25-$(OH)_2$-D_3 without participation of T cells. Further investigation will be required to clarify these issues.

1,25-DIHYDROXYVITAMIN D_3 SYNTHESIS BY HUMAN MONOCYTE/MACROPHAGE CELLS

The observation that macrophages obtained from the lungs of patients with active pulmonary sarcoidosis are capable of synthesizing 1,25-$(OH)_2$-D_3 (55) is important not only to an understanding of the mechanism of hypercalcemia encountered in patients with this disease, but also in suggesting that the hormone has the potential to function as an immunoinhibitory monokine in the microenvironment of the pulmonary alveolus (56). Patients with sarcoidosis have long been known to be prone to develop hypercalciuria and/or hypercalcemia after prolonged sunlight exposure or oral vitamin D administration (56). More recently, investigators have demonstrated that such hypercalcemic episodes are accompanied by an increase in the circulating concentration of 1,25-$(OH)_2$-D (57). In 1981, Barbour et al. (58) reported 1,25-$(OH)_2$-D-mediated hypercalcemia in an anephric individual with sarcoidosis, clearly demonstrating that the source of hormone overproduction in sarcoidosis resided at an extrarenal site. This prompted investigation in many laboratories to discern the cellular source of 1,25-$(OH)_2$-D_3 synthesis in sarcoidosis. Homogenates of a cutaneous lymph node from a patient with sarcoidosis were shown to convert [^{3}H]25-OH-D_3 to a more polar, [^{3}H]1,25-$(OH)_2$-D_3–like metabolite (59); however, extensive chromatographic characterization of the metabolite was not performed and the cellular source of the metabolite remained undetermined. Subsequent experiments by us (19) demonstrated that primary cultures of pulmonary alveolar macrophages from patients with sarcoidosis and disordered calcium homeostatis (hypercalcemia or hypercalciuria) synthesized in vitro a metabolite of [^{3}H]25-OH-D$_3$ that was chromatographically indistinguishable from authentic, crystalline 1,25-(OH)$_2$-D$_3$ on both normal- and reverse-phase (55) high-performance liquid chromatography (HPLC). In addition, the macrophage metabolite was bound with high affinity by both specific receptor for 1,25-(OH)$_2$-D$_3$ and antibody generated against 1,25-(OH)$_2$-D$_3$ in a manner mimicking authentic [^{3}H]1,25-(OH)$_2$-D$_3$ of comparable specific activity (19). Ultraviolet spectroscopy and mass spectroscopy of the macrophage metabolite of 25-OH-D$_3$ have been reported (20) and confirm the identity of the metabolite as 1,25-(OH)$_2$-D$_3$. Evidence suggests that this activation is the result of gamma interferon stimulation (60).

Although the active vitamin D$_3$ compound synthesized by renal epithelial cells is identical to that made by pulmonary alveolar macrophages, there is considerable evidence mounting to suggest that the physiological control mechanisms governing synthesis of 1,25-(OH)$_2$-D$_3$ by the two cell types is not the same in that hormone production is largely independent of the presence of 1,25-(OH)$_2$-D$_3$ and parathyroid hormone. In normal human subjects, an increase in the serum calcium (and phosphorus) elicited by the administration of 1,25-(OH)$_2$-D$_3$ is accompanied by a decrease in the plasma parathyroid hormone concentration and downregulation of the renal 25-OH-D-1α-hydroxylate (61). The net result is a "reflex" decrease in the serum calcium concentration. In hypercalcemic patients with sarcoidosis, on the other hand, parathyroid hormone levels are appropriately depressed with respect to the serum calcium concentration but 1,25-(OH)$_2$-D levels remain elevated. This clinical observation suggests that the extrarenal production of 1,25-(OH)$_2$-D in patients with sarcoidosis is not responsive to those factors which normally maintain a stringent rein on renal 1,25-(OH)$_2$-D synthesis. A survey of the biochemical characteristics of our sarcoid macrophage 1α-hydroxylation reaction has been performed in our laboratory (62). Kinetic analysis of the 25-OH-D$_3$-1α-hydroxylating activity in cultured alveolar macrophages from five different patients with active pulmonary sarcoidosis (four of whom were either hypercalcemic or hypercalciuric at the time of macrophage harvest) showed that the reaction was saturable with a K_m for 25-OH-D$_3$ of 52–210 nM. This value is in the range previously reported for the mammalian renal 25-OH-D$_3$-1α-hydroxylase (12). Also similar to the renal 1α-hydroxylase, the macrophage 1α-hydroxylation reaction prefers substrate vitamin D$_3$ sterol which is hydroxylated at the carbon-25 position in the molecule's side chain. However, the sarcoid macrophage 1α-hydroxylation reaction diverges from the renal cell 1α-hydroxylase on several counts: (a) the macrophage 1α-hydroxylation reaction is not accompanied by significant 24-hydroxylating activity, even at high substrate levels; (b) it is not susceptible to significant inhibition of 1,25-(OH)$_2$-D$_3$ synthesis by preincubation in vitro with concentration of product 1,25-(OH)$_2$-D$_3$ as high as 75 nM; (c) it is very susceptible to inhibition by glucocorticoids; and (d) the velocity of macrophage metabolite synthesis is accelerated under the influence of gamma interferon (IFN-γ), a lymphokine secreted in high concentrations by pulmonary alveolar lymphocytes in patients with sarcoidosis-mediated high-intensity alveolitis (63). Concerning the latter phenomenon, it is also known that incubation of pulmonary alveolar macrophages from normal human hosts can be induced to produce $[^3H]1,25$-$(OH)_2$-D_3 when incubated with $[^3H]25$-OH-D_3 in the presence of IFN-γ (64) or the calcium ionophore A23187 (Adams et al., unpublished results). The mechanism by which sarcoid macrophages are induced to synthesize 1,25-$(OH)_2$-D_3 is as noted previously (60) linked to T-cell activation and gamma interferon production.

It should be pointed out that the extrarenal production of 1,25-$(OH)_2$-D_3 (presumably by cells of the immune system) probably takes place in other human granulomatous diseases, including tuberculosis (65,66), disseminated candidiasis (67), silicone-induced granulomatous disease (68), and leprosy (R. Rude, personal communication), and in patients with lymphoma (69–71). Interestingly, recognition of elevated plasma concentrations of 1,25-$(OH)_2$-D in hypercalcemic patients with human T-cell lymphotrophic virus I (HTLV-I) (69) and HTLV-III–associated lymphoma (Adams et al., unpublished observations and 41) suggests that these retrovirus-mediated diseases may be associated with extrarenal 1,25-$(OH)_2$-D synthesis. The question of whether 1,25-$(OH)_2$-D production in this apparently diverse set of diseases is by design (23) or by pathological "mistake" is intriguing but has not yet been answered.

CONCLUSIONS

Although there is now conclusive evidence establishing 1,25-$(OH)_2$-D_3 as a potent immunoregulatory hormone in vitro (17,47–54), there are no studies to date indicating that the sterol exerts an immunoinhibitory effect in vivo. Among the potent immunoinhibitory effects in vitro are the inhibition of IL-2 production by T_H cells and Ig production by B cells (17,47,50). The mechanism(s) responsible for these immunoinhibitory effects are not completely agreed upon (50–54), but there is no question they exist. In contrast, IL-1 production may be enhanced (73). These changes have also been found to occur at the mRNA level (74–76). The potential for in vivo immunoinhibition by 1,25-$(OH)_2$-D_3 could offer a new approach to the treatment of autoimmune diseases and allograft rejection (two situations in which B- and T-cell hyperactivity are thought to result in tissue injury). 1,25-$(OH)_2$-D_3 has not been used to induce immunoinhibition in humans or exert an immunoinhibitory effect in animal models of autoimmunity or transplantation. Further animal and human studies are needed to determine if 1,25-$(OH)_2$-D_3 has a place as an immunoregulatory hormone in humans.

The recent identification of IFN-γ–stimulated 1,25-$(OH)_2$-D_3 synthesis by pulmonary-alveolar macrophages suggests that 1,25-$(OH)_2$-D_3 may play a role in the regulation of normal immunoregulatory events. These regulatory circuits are outlined in Figure 13. Briefly, antigen or mitogen stimulation of macrophages results in IL-1 production which stimulates T cells to express IL-2 receptors and/or produce IL-2. With activation, the lymphocytes also express functional receptors for 1,25-$(OH)_2$-D_3. Interleukin 2 induces growth and differentiation of T cells. T-Helper cells produce lymphokines that allow growth and differentiation of B cells to antibody-producing plasma cells. Other T cells produce IFN-γ which interacts with the macrophages to stimulate 1,25-$(OH)_2$-D_3 production. 1,25-$(OH)_2$-D_3 could then bind to the 1,25-$(OH)_2$-D_3 receptors on activated T cells to inhibit IL-2 production and possibly production of other lymphokines. To our knowledge, there are few published reports of the in vivo immunoregulatory effects of 1,25-$(OH)_2$-D_3 in animal models or humans, but these provide some potentially important insights. Fujita et al. (77) showed

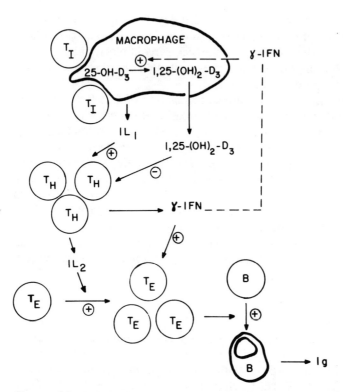

Figure 13 Proposed mechanism(s) for interaction of 1,25-(OH)$_2$-D$_3$ with immunoactive cells. Mitogen-antigen activation of macrophages results in interleukin 1 (IL-1) production which stimulates resting T cells to express IL-2 receptors (Tac) and/or produce IL-2. Gamma interferon (IFN-γ) produced by activated T cells induces 1-hydroxylation of 25-OH-D$_3$ resulting in 1,25-(OH)$_2$-D$_3$ production. The 1,25-(OH)$_2$-D$_3$ subsequently interacts with 1,25-(OH)$_2$-D$_3$ receptors on activated T cells primarily T$_H$) to inhibit IL-2 synthesis and T$_H$-cell–directed Ig production by plasma cells.

that delayed-type hypersensitivity to skin test antigens could be restored in previously anergic elderly osteoporotic patients. Although similar results implying restoration of T-cell immunity have been suggested from studies on the effects of oral administration of 1α-OH-D$_3$ in hemodialyzed patients (78), this is a complex setting from which to draw conclusions. Similar issues arise in the report by Quesada et al. (79) that calcitriol deficiency in the context of renal failure where it becomes difficult to distinguish between primary direct effects and secondary indirect effects (80) if repletion is attempted. In contrast a recent report showing that 1,25-(OH)$_2$-D$_3$ can protect human macrophages from tubercle bacilli (81) suggests that excellent models for these studies can be devised.

As described previously, Koeffler has administered 1,25-(OH)$_2$-D$_3$ orally to patients with myelodysplastic syndromes (44) without significant clinical improvement. The results of that study have been summarized in this chapter. Recently, protocols have been developed to administer 1,25-(OH)$_2$-D$_3$ intravenously. These protocols involve patients with end-stage renal disease and severe renal osteodystrophy. Of interest, is that much larger doses (4–5 μg, three times weekly) can be administered intravenously without inducing significant hypercalcemia. (J. Coburn, personal communication). The therapy is well tolerated and there are no other undesirable side effects. We have studied the plasma of patients receiving intravenous 1,25-$(OH)_2$-D_3 for its ability to inhibit IL-2 and Ig production by autologus PBM and have found that the 3-hr postinfusion plasma inhibits mitogen-stimulated Ig production by >50% when compared to the preinfusion plasma (Jordan et al., unpublished observation). To date, none of the patients have developed hypercalcemia, and the 1,25-$(OH)_2$-D_3 levels achieved in plasma (10^{-9} M, peak) are within the range known to inhibit Ig and IL-2 production in vitro.

In summary, 1,25-$(OH)_2$-D_3 exerts a potent in vitro immunoinhibitory effect on human T- and B-cell functions and prodifferentiating effects on promyelocytic cells. 1,25-$(OH)_2$-D_3 appears to use an important cofactor in hematopoiesis and analogs of vitamin D may be used to produce a differentiation effect on normal versus leukemic growth (82). 1,25-$(OH)_2$-D_3 production by macrophages may regulate in vivo immune reactivity by B and T cells in certain granulomatous and lymphoproliferative disorders and is probably responsible for the hypercalcemia seen in these diseases. The potential use of 1,25-$(OH)_2$-D_3 as an immunoinhibitory or prodifferentiating drug for the treatment of autoimmune disease, promyelocytic leukemia, and allograft rejection are areas of promising investigative efforts for the future.

ACKNOWLEDGMENTS

This work was supported in part by grants from the National Institutes of Health RR0043, AM32568, CA26038, CA32737, CA33936, and CA30512 Bethesda, Maryland, the Dr. Murray Geisler Memorial Leukemia Fund, and the Louis Fagin Leukemia Research Foundation. Dr. Jordan (AM01183) and Dr. Koeffler are recipients of Research Career Development Awards from the National Institutes of Health.

We would also like to recognize Valerie Boyd, Susan Bookstaver, and Barbara Sachs for their excellent secretarial assistance.

REFERENCES

1. Huldschinsky K. Heilung von Rachitis durch kunstliche Hohensonne. Dtsch Med Wochenschr 45:712–713, 1919.
2. Holick MF. The photobiology of vitamin D_3 in man. *In*: Vitamin D: Basic and Clinical Aspects. Edited by R. Kumar. Boston, Martinus Nijhoff, pp 197–216, 1984.
3. Brumbaugh PF, MR Haussler, 1,25-Dihydroxycholecolciferol receptors in intestine. I. Association of 1,25-dihydroxycholecalciferol with intestinal mucossa chromatin. J Biol Chem 249:1251–1257, 1974.
4. Brumbaugh PF, MR Haussler. 1,25-Dihydroxycholecalciferol receptors in intestine. II. Temperature-dependent transfer of hormone to chromatin via a specific cytosol receptor. J Biol Chem 251:2388–2394, 1974.
5. Omdahl J, Holick M, Suda T, Tanaka Y, DeLuca HF. Biological activity of 1,25-dihydroxycholecalciferol. Biochemistry 10:2935–2940, 1971.
6. Tanaka Y, DeLuca HF. Bone mineral mobilization activity of 1,25-dihydroxycholecalciferol, a metabolite of vitamin D. Arch Biochem Biophys 146:574–578, 1971.

7. Tanaka Y, DeLuca HF. Role of 1,25-dihydroxyvitamin D_3 in maintaining serum phosphorus and curing rickets. Proc Natl Acad Sci USA 71:1040–1044, 1974.
8. Aurbach GD, Marx SJ, Spiegel AM. Parathyroid, calcitonin, and the calciferols. *In*: Textbook of Endocrinology. 6th ed, Edited by RH Williams. Philadelphia, Saunders, pp 922–1031, 1981.
9. DeLuca HF, Schnoes HK. Vitamin D: Recent advances. Ann Rev Biochem 52:411–439, 1983.
10. Pedersen JI, Ghazarian JG, Orme-Johnson NR, DeLuca HF. Isolation of chick renal mitochondrial ferrodoxin active in the 25-hydroxyvitamin D_3-1-hydroxylase system. J Biol Chem 251:3933–3941, 1976.
11. Gray RW, Wilz DR, Caldas AE, Lemann J Jr. The importance of phosphate in regulating plasma 1,25-$(OH)_2$-vitamin D levels in humans: Studies in healthy subjects, in calcium-stone formers and in patients with primary hyperparathyroidism. J Clin Endocrinol Metab 45:1008–1016, 1979.
12. Fraser DR. Regulation of the metabolism of vitamin D. Physiol Rev 60:551–613, 1980.
13. Hirst M, Feldman D. Biochem Biophys Res Commun 116:121–127, 1983.
14. Holick MF, Schnoes HK, DeLuca HF, Gray RW, Boyle IT, Suda T. Isolation and identification of 24,25-dihydroxycholecalciferol: A metabolite of vitamin D_3 made in the kidney. Biochemistry 11:4251–4255, 1972.
15. Kleiner-Bossaller A, DeLuca HF. Formation of 1,24,25-trihydroxyvitamin D_3 from 1,25-dihydroxyvitamin D_3. Biochem Biophys Acta 388:489–495, 1974.
16. Kumar R. Metabolism of 1,25-dihydroxyvitamin D_3. Physiol Rev 64:478–504, 1984.
17. Tsoukas CD, Provvedini DM, Manolagas SC. 1,25-Dihydroxyvitamin D_3: A novel immunoregulatory hormone. Science 224:1438–1441, 1984.
18. Abe E, Miyaura C, Sakagamih H, Takeda M, Kouno K, Yamazaki T, Yoshikias S, Suda T. Differentiation of mouse myeloid leukemia cells induced by 1,25-dihydroxyvitamin D_3. Proc Natl Acad Sci USA 78:4990–4999, 1981.
19. Adams JS, Sharma OP, Gacad MA, Singer FR. Metabolism of 25-hydroxyvitamin D_3 by cultured pulmonary alveolar macrophages in sarcoidosis. J Clin Invest 72:1856–1860, 1983.
20. Adams JS, Singer FR, Gacad MA, Sharma OP, Hayes MJ, Vouros P, Holick MF. Isolation and structural identification of 1,25-dihydroxyvitamin D_3 produced by cultured alveolar macrophages in sarcoidosis. J Clin Endocrinol Metab 60:961–966, 1985.
21. Harper KD, Iozzo RU, Haddad JG. Receptors for and bioresponses to 1,25-dihydroxyvitamin D in a human colon carcinoma cell line (HT-29). Metabolism 38(11):1062, 1989.
22. Reichel H, Koeffler HP, Norman AW. The role of the vitamin D endocrine system in health and disease. N Engl J Med 320(15):980, 1989.
23. Minghetti PP, Norman AW. 1,25$(OH)_2$-Vitamin D_3 receptors, gene regulation and genetic circuitry. FASEB J 2(15):3043, 1988.
24. Tanaka H, Abe H, Miyaura C, Kuribayashi T, Konno K, Nishi Y, Suda T. 1,25-Dihydroxyclolecalciferol and a human myeloid leukemia cell line (HL-60). Biochem J 204:713–719, 1982.
25. Bar-Shavit Z, Teitelbaum SL, Reitsma P, Hall A, Pegg LE. Proc Natl Acad Sci USA 80:5907–5911, 1983.
26. McCarthy DM, San Miguel JF, Freake HC, Green PM, Zola H, Catovsky D, Goldman JM. 1,25-Dihydroxyvitamin D_3 inhibits proliferation of human promyelocytic leukemia (HL-60) cells and induces monocyte-macrophage differentiation in HL-60 and normal human bone marrow. Leukemia Res 7:51–55, 1983.
27. Mangelsdorf DJ, Koeffler HP, Donaldson CA, Pike JW, Haussler MR. 1,25-Dihydroxyvitamin D_3-induced differentiation in a human promyelocytic leukemia cell line (HL-60): Receptor-mediated maturation to macrophage-like cells. J Cell Biol 98:391–398, 1984.

28. Munker, Norman RA, Koeffler HP. Vitamin D Compounds: Effects on clonal proliferation and differentiation of human myeloid cells. J Clin Invest 78:1–8, 1986.
29. Koeffler HP, Amatruda T, Ikekawa N, Kobayashi Y, DeLuca HF. 1,25-Dihydroxyvitamin D_3 and its fluorinated analogs induce macrophage differentiation of normal and leukemic myeloid stem cells. Cancer Res 44:5624–5628, 1984.
30. Burger EH, Van der Meer JWM, Van de Gevel JS, Gribnau JC, Thesingh CW, Van Furth R. In vitro formation of osteoclasts from long-term cultures of bone marrow mononuclear phagocytes. J Exp Med 156:1604–1614, 1982.
31. Holtrop ME, Cox KA, Clark MB, Holick MF, Anast CS. 1,25-Dihydroxycholecalcifereol stimulates osteoclasts in rat bones in the absence of parathyroid hormone. Endocrinology 108:2293–2301, 1981.
32. Mundy GR, Altman AJ, Gondek MD, Bandelin JG. Direct resorption of bone by human monocytes. Science 196:1109–1111, 1977.
33. Haussler MR, Baylink MR, Hughes PF, Brumbaugh JE, Wegedal JE, Shen FH, Willsen RL, Counts SJ, Bursac KM, McCain TA. Assays of 1-alpha,25 dihydroxy vitamin D_3: Physiologic and pathologic modulation of circulating hormone levels. Clin Endocrinol 5:157S–165S, 1979.
34. Norman AW. Vitamin D and its clinical relationships. *In*: Vitamin D: The Calcium Homeostasis Steroid Hormone. pp 402–450, 1979.
35. Liberman JA, Eil C, Marx SJ. Resistance to 1,25-dihydroxyvitamin D. J Clin Invest 71:192–200, 1983.
36. Ostrem VK, Tanaka Y, Prahl J, DeLuca HF, Ikekawa N. 24- and 26-Homo-1,25-(dihydroxyvitamin D_3: Preferential activity in inducing differentiation of human leukemia cells HL-60 in vitro. Proc Natl Acad Sci 84:2610, 1987.
37. Rigby WFC, Shen L, Ball ED, Juyre PM, Fanger MW. Differentiation of a human monocytic cell line by 1,25-dihydroxyvitamin D_3 (calcitrol): A morphologic, phenotypic, and functional analysis. Blood 64:1110–1115, 1984.
38. Matsui T, Nakao Y, Kobayashi N. Phenotypic differentiation-linked growth inhibition in human leukemia cells by active vitamin D_3 analogues. Int J Cancer 33:193–202, 1984.
39. Yamaoka K, Marion SL, Gallegos A, Haussler MR. 1,25-Dihydroxyvitamin D_3 enhances the growth of tumors in athymic mice inoculated with receptor rich osteosarcoma cells. Biochem Biophys Res Commun 139:1292, 1986.
40. Franceschi RT, Linson CJ, Peter TC, Romano PR. Regulation of cellular adhesion and fibronectin synthesis by 1α,25-dihydroxyvitamin D_3. J Biol Chem 262:4165.
41. Reichel H, Koeffler HP, Norman NW. 25-Hydroxyvitamin D_3 metabolism by human T-lymphotropic virus-transformed lymphocytes. J Clin Endocrinol Metab 65:519, 1987.
42. Honma Y, Hozumi M, Abe E, Konno K, Fukushima M, Hata S, Nishii Y, DeLuca HF, Suda T. 1,25-dihydroxyvitamin D_3 and 1α-hydroxyvitamin D_3 prolong survival time of mice inoculated with myeloid leukemia cells. Proc Natl Acad Sci USA 80:201–204, 1983.
43. Adams N, Gray R, Lemann J, Cheung H. Effects of calcitriol administration on calcium metabolism in healthy men. Kidney Int 21:90–97, 1982.
44. Koeffler HP. Induction of differentiation of human acute myelogenous leukemia cells: therapeutic implications. Blood 62:709–721, 1983.
45. Miyaura C, Abe E, Kuribauashi T. 1,25-dihydroxyvitamin D_3 induces differentiation of human myeloid leukemia cells. Biochem Biophys Res Commun 102:937–943, 1981.
46. Provvedini D, Tsoukas C, Deftos L, Manolagas SC. 1,25-Dihydroxyvitamin-D_3 receptors in human leukocytes. Science 221:1181–1183, 1983.
47. Lemire J, Adams JS, Sakai R, Jordan SC. 1,25-Dihydroxyvitamin-D_3 suppresses proliferation and immunoglobulin production by normal human peripheral blood mononuclear cells. J Clin Invest 74:657–661, 1984.
48. Rigby W, Stacy T, Fangar W. Inhibition of T-lymphocyte mitogenesis by 1,25-dihydroxyvitamin-D_3 (calcitriol). J Clin Invest 74:1451–1454, 1984.

49. Vanham G, Baelen V, Tan BK, Bouillon R. The effect of vitamin D analogs and of vitamin D-binding-protein on lymphocyte proliferation. J Steroid Biochem 29(4):381, 1988.
50. Lemire J, Adams J, Kermani-Arab V, Bakke A, Sakai R, Jordan SC. 1,25-Dihydroxyvitamin-D_3 suppresses human T helper/inducer lymphocyte activity in vitro. J Immunol 134:3032–3035, 1985.
51. Iho S, Kura F, Sugiyama H, Takahashi T, Hoshino T. The role of monocytes in the suppression of PHA induced proliferation and IL-2 production of mononuclear cells by 1,25-dihydroxyvitamin-D3. Immunol Lett 11:331, 1985.
52. Provvedini DM, Mandagas SC. $1\alpha,25$-Dihydroxyvitamin D_3 receptor distribution and effects in subpopulation of normal human T lymphocytes. J Clin Endocrinol Metab 68(4): 774, 1989.
53. Iho S, Takahashi T, Kura F, Sugiyama H, Hoshino T. The effect of 1,25-dihydroxyvitamin D_3 on in vitro immunoglobulin production in human B cells. J Immunol 136:4427–4431, 1986.
54. Provvedini D, Tsoukas C, Deftos L, Manolagas SC. 1,25-Dihydroxyvitamin D_3-binding macromolecules in human B lymphocytes: Effects on immunoglobulin production. J Immunol 136:2734–2740, 1986.
55. Adams JS, Gacad MA, Singer FR, Sharma OP. Production of 1,25-Dihydroxyvitamin D_3 by pulmonary alveolar macrophages from patients with sarcoidosis. NY Acad Sci 465:587–594, 1986.
56. Singer FR, Adams JS. Abnormal calcium homeostasis in sarcoidosis. N Engl J Med 315: 755–757, 1986.
57. Sandler LM, Winearls CG, Fraher LJ, Clemens TL, Smith R, O'Riordan JLH. Studies of the hypercalcemia of sarcoidosis: Effects of steroids and exogenous vitamin D3 on the circulating concentrations of 1,25-dihydroxyvitamin D3. Q J Med 53:165–180, 1984.
58. Barbour GL, Coburn JW, Slatopolsky E, Norman AW, Horst RL. Hypercalcemia in an anephric patient with sarcoidosis: Evidence for extrarenal generation of 1,25-dihydroxyvitamin D. N Engl J Med 305:440–443, 1981.
59. Mason RS, Frankel T, Chan Y-L, Lissner PD, Posen S. Vitamin D conversion by sarcoid lymph node homogenate. Ann Intern Med 100:59–61, 1984.
60. Reichel H, Koeffler HP, Barbers R, Norman AW. Regulation of 1,25-dihydroxyvitamin D_3 production by cultured alveolar macrophages from normal human donors and from patients with pulmonary sarcoidosis. J Clin Endocrinol Metab 65:1201, 1987.
61. Audran M, Kumar R. The physiology and pathophysiology of vitamin D. Mayo Clin Proc 60:851–866, 1985.
62. Adams JS, Gacad MA. Characterization of 1-hydroxylation of vitamin D_3 sterols by cultured pulmonary alveolar macrophages from patients with sarcoidosis. J Exp Med 161: 755–765, 1985.
63. Nugent K, Monick M, Hunninghake GW. Pulmonary macrophages from patients with active sarcoidosis spontaneously release immune interferon. Clin Res 32:434A, 1984.
64. Koeffler HP, Reichel H, Bishop JE, Norman AW. γ-Interferon stimulates production of 1,25-dihydroxyvitamin D_3 by normal human macrophages. Biochem Biophys Res Commun 127:596–603, 1985.
65. Gkonos PJ, London R, Hendler E. Hypercalcemia and elevated 1,25-Dihydroxyvitamin D levels in a patient with end-stage renal disease and active tuberculosis. N Engl J Med 311:1683–1685, 1985.
66. Bell NH, Shary J, Shaw S, Turner RT. Hypercalcemia associated with increased circulating 1,25-dihydroxyvitamin D in a patient with pulmonary tuberculosis. Calcif Tissue Int 37:588–591, 1985.
67. Kantarjian HM, Saad MF, Estey EH, Sellin RV, Samann NA. Hypercalcemia in disseminated candidiasis. Am J Med 74:721–724, 1983.

68. Kozeny GA, Barbato AL, Bansal VK, Vertuno LL, Hano JL. Hypercalcemia associated with silicone-induced granulomas. N Engl J Med 311:1103–1105.
69. Breslau N, McGuire JL, Zerwekh JE, Frenkel EP, Pak CYC. Hypercalcemia associated with increased serum calcitriol levels in three patients with lymphoma. Ann Int Med 100:1–5, 1984.
70. Davies M, Hayes ME, Mawer EB, Lumb GA. Abnormal vitamin D metabolism in Hodgkin's lymphoma. Lancet 1:1186–1188, 1985.
71. Rosenthal N, Insogna KL, Godsall JW, Smaldone L, Waldron JA, Stewart AF. Elevations in circulating 1,25-dihydroxyvitamin D in three patients with lymphoma-associated hypercalcemia. J Clin Endocrinol Metab 60:29–33, 1985.
72. Matsui T, Nakao Y, Koizumi T, Nakagama T, Fujita T. 1,25-Dihydroxyvitamin D_3 regulates proliferation of activated T-lymphocyte subsets. Life Sci 37:95–101, 1986.
73. Bhalla AK, Amento EP, Krane SM. Differential effects of 1,25-dihydroxyvitamin D_3 on human lymphocytes and monocyte/macrophages: Inhibition of interleukin-2 and augmentation of interleukin-1 production. Cell Immunol 78:311, 1986.
74. Rigby WFC, Denome S, and Fanger MW. Regulation of lymphokine production and human T lymphocyte activation by 1,25-dihydroxyvitamin D_3: Specific inhibition at the level of messenger RNA. J Clin Invest 79:1659, 1987.
75. Rigby WFC, Noelle RJ, Fanger MW. Interleukin 2-independent suppression of T-lymphocyte proliferation and transferrin receptor induction by 1,25-dihydroxyvitamin D_3 (calcitrol). Clin Res 34:505A, 1987.
76. Amento EP. Vitamin D and the immune system. Steroids 49:55, 1987.
77. Fujita T, Matsui T, Nakao Y, Watanabe S. T lymphocyte subsets in osteoporosis: Effect of 1-alpha hydroxyvitamin D_3. Miner Electrolyte Metab 10:375, 1984.
78. Tabata T, Suzuki R, Kikunami K, Matsushita Y, Irsue T, Inoue T, Okamoto T, Miki T, Nishizawa Y, Morii H. The effect of $1\alpha,25$-dihydroxyvitamin D_3 on cell-mediated immunity in hemodialyzed patients. J Clin Endocrinol Metab 63:1218, 1986.
79. Quesada JM, Solana R, Serrano I, Barrio V, Martinez E, Santamaria M, Martin-Malo A. N Engl J Med 321(12):833, 1989.
80. Norman AW, Reichel H, Koeffler HP. Immunologic effects of vitamin D. (Reply to previous.) N Engl J Med 321(12):834, 1989.
81. Crowle AJ, Ross EJ. Comparative abilities of various metabolites of vitamin D to protect cultured human macrophages against tubercle bacilli. J Leukocyte Biol 47(6):545, 1990.
82. Munker R, Norman A, Koeffler H. Vitamin D compounds. Effect on clonal proliferation and differentiation of human myeloid cells. J Clin Invest 78:424, 1986.

2
Nutritional Deficiencies and Immunoregulatory Cytokines

Janis Randall Simpson and Laurie Hoffman-Goetz
University of Waterloo, Waterloo, Ontario, Canada

INTRODUCTION

The immune system, like all systems in the body, is dependent on the availability and utilization of nutrients for optimal maintenance and function of its components (Chandra, 1985). Nutrient deficiencies have been demonstrated to have adverse effects on humoral immunity, phagocytosis, complement systems, and on cell-mediated immunity (Beisel, 1982). Lymphocytes derived from the thymus gland (T cells) are responsible for cell-mediated immunity and also play a role in cooperation with spleen-derived lymphocytes (B cells) in antibody synthesis.

The effects of nutrition on T-cell function have been widely investigated because of their involvement in all aspects of the immune response (Hoffman-Goetz, 1986, 1987). The mechanisms by which altered cell-mediated immunity occurs, however, have not been studied extensively. Some insight into these mechanisms can be gained by studying the effects of malnutrition on regulatory factors such as cytokines. Cytokines are soluble factors released from a variety of cells such as lymphocytes, monocytes, and tissue macrophages. These factors play a key role in initiating and sustaining the immune response. Therefore, an understanding of the effects of nutrient deficiencies on the production and function of these cytokines is essential for an understanding of the role of nutrition in immune function.

The purpose of this chapter is, therefore, to review the literature with respect to the effects of nutritional status on cytokines, with an emphasis on monokines. Implications of research conducted to date along with suggestions for further research are also presented.

CHARACTERISTICS AND FUNCTIONS OF CYTOKINES

Cytokines are soluble, nonimmunoglobulin, hormonelike products of sensitized mononuclear leukocytes (Maizel and Lachman, 1984). Cytokines mediate many aspects of the immune response by regulating motility of target cells (Rocklin et al., 1980) and by providing regulatory signals for target cells (Maizel and Lachman, 1984). Cytokines influence the development of autologous T cells (Strominger, 1989).

Regulation of the immune response by cytokines can be, for example, by enhancement (Dinarello, 1984, 1990; Maizel and Lachman, 1984) or suppression (Beer et al., 1982a, b) of target cell proliferation, or by alteration of the ratios of suppressor to effector cells in lymphoid tissue compartments (Chandra, 1983a). Cytokines also affect immune function by causing a redistribution or recirculation of lymphocytes within the body (Chandra, 1983a) and within developmental organs such as the thymus (Cording et al., 1991).

Many cytokines have been described in the literature and have been assigned names based on function, in part, because purification and detection of these mediators is difficult (Dinarello, 1984; Oppenheim et al., 1986). Some of these functions, originally ascribed to different mediators, are in fact attributed to the same molecular species (Oppenheim et al., 1986). For example, the mediators previously known as endogenous pyrogen (EP), leukocyte-activating factor (LAF), and leukocyte endogenous mediator (LEM) are all now believed to be the same monokine (interleukin 1, IL-1) (Dinarello, 1984; Oppenheim et al., 1986).

Lymphokines

Lymphokines are products of activated lymphocytes, mainly T lymphocytes (Yoshida et al., 1973; Rocklin, 1974), although there is some evidence that B lymphocytes (Yoshida et al., 1973) and macrophages (Sarin and Gallo, 1984) are required as accessory cells for some lymphokine production. Lymphokines can be inhibitory, stimulatory, or inflammatory (Rocklin et al., 1980; Oppenheim and Shevach, 1990).

Macrophage inhibitor factor (MIF), a protein or glycoprotein of 23,000–70,000 molecular weight (Rocklin et al., 1980), was the first lymphokine to be identified (Rocklin, 1974). Macrophage inhibitor factor is produced by T lymphocytes which have been stimulated by antigen; there is some evidence to suggest that some human tumor and some fibroblast cell lines can also produce MIF (Remold et al., 1972, Yoshida et al., 1976).

Macrophage inhibitor factor retards macrophage migration from areas of inflammation, increases macrophage adhesiveness, and increases intracellular tubulin polymerization (Rocklin et al., 1980). The mechanisms by which this takes place have not been clarified, although MIF appears to interact with macrophages at a cell surface receptor. The action of macrophages may be due to an influx or intracellular redistribution of divalent cations such as magnesium (Mg) or calcium (Ca) (Johnson, 1980).

The study of migration inhibition led to the discovery of leukocyte inhibition factor (LIF), which was originally distinguished from MIF in 1974 (Rocklin, 1974). Leukocyte inhibition factor is a protein with a molecular weight of 68,000–158,000 Da and is produced by stimulated lymphocytes. There is evidence that T cells and B cells produce LIF (Chess et al., 1975). Furthermore, some sort of T cell–B cell or

T cell–macrophage cooperation may be involved in LIF production (Weisbart et al., 1978). The primary physiological action of LIF appears to be inhibition of polymorphonuclear (PMN) leukocyte migration by the release of chemotactic inhibitors (Goetzl and Rocklin, 1978).

Interleukin 2 (IL-2) is the name given to a heterogeneous group of factors with molecular weights of 13,000–16,000 Da (Maizel and Lachman, 1984). Activation of a subset of T-helper cells (T_H) by mitogen or antigen causes them to become responsive to IL-1. The activated T cells then produce IL-2, which serves as the mitogenic stimulus for T-cell S-phase entry (Maizel and Lachman, 1984; Saxena et al., 1984a) and production of heat shock or stress proteins (Farrar et al., 1990). Interleukin 2 is capable of sustaining long-term differentiation and proliferation of cultured T cells in vitro and supports generation and proliferation of helper and cytotoxic T lymphocytes in vitro and in vivo (Maizel and Lachman, 1984).

The interferons (IFNs) were first identified by their ability to prevent viral replication and to make new protein and RNA (Trinchieri and Perussia, 1984). The viral interferons, IFN-α and IFN-β are produced primarily by leukocytes and fibroblasts, respectively, whereas immune interferon (IFN-γ) is produced primarily by antigen-specific T cells and possibly by natural killer (NK) cells (Trinchieri and Perussia, 1985). Immune IFN is a protein with a molecular weight of 35,000–70,000 Da.

Except for its role in growth inhibition, IFN-γ appears to be stimulatory with respect to anticellular effects (Trincheri and Perussia, 1985). Immune IFN regulates proliferation, differentiation, and activity of T and B cells and ensures cooperation between T and B cells in the adaptive immune response (Trincheri and Perussia, 1985). Immune interferon modulates the expression of macrophage membrane antigens (Steeg et al., 1985), and also augments LPS induction of IL-1 (Oppenheim, 1986). Immune interferon is believed to be a major endogenous regulator of NK cell activity (Salimonu et al., 1982, 1988). Some of the effects of IFN-γ can also be mediated by the viral interferons (Keller and Calvanico, 1984; Trincheri and Perussia, 1985).

Monokines

Monokines are soluble products of blood monocytes or tissue macrophages which have multiple biological activities. The term *interleukin 1* (IL-1) was originally used to describe the soluble products of mononuclear phagocytes and of a variety of other cells (Oppenheim et al., 1986). Interleukin 1–like activity has been reported for polypeptides with molecular weights of 15,000–17,000 Da (Dinarello, 1984; Oppenheim et al., 1986), although aggregated forms of IL-1 have molecular weights of 75,000 Da (Dinarello, 1984). At least two distinct genes encode products with IL-1 activities, termed IL-α and IL-β. Inducers of IL-1 production include antigens, mitogens, and other lymphokines such as IFN (Oppenheim et al., 1986). Some transformed B and T cells spontaneously produce soluble IL-1–like factors but most normal cells produce IL-1 only in response to stimulants (Oppenheim et al., 1986). The mechanism of IL-1 action is not definitely known, although IL-1 may act as a Ca ionophore stimulating divalent cation flux across cell membranes with resulting changes in intracellular Ca^{2+} levels (Dinarello, 1984; Oppenheim et al., 1986). Many of its activities are mediated through activation of other cytokines.

Some of the biological activities of IL-1 include induction of fever, increases in acute-phase reactant proteins, and shifts in the plasma concentrations of trace minerals (Dinarello, 1984, 1990; Oppenheim et al., 1986). Interleukin 1 also has numerous effects on lymphoid cells such as generation and activation of helper, suppressor, and cytotoxic T cells, induction of lymphokine production and secretion, and induction of prostaglandin E_2 (PGE_2) production by macrophages (Mizel, 1982; Oppenheim et al., 1986; Dinarello, 1990). Some of these effects are mediated by IL-2, which is induced by the production of IL-1. Interleukin 1 also induces maturation of pre-B cells and is a cofactor in clonal expansion of B lymphocytes (Oppenheim et al., 1986), which can also produce IL-1. Interleukin 1 production is suppressed by corticosteroids, cyclosporin, and prostaglandins (Oppenheim et al., 1986).

Tumor necrosis factor (TNF) was originally identified as a factor in the filtrate of growing bacterial cultures which was able to cause spontaneous tumor involution in some cancer patients (Coley, 1891). This factor was subsequently further characterized by Carswell et al. (1975) from mice treated with endotoxin as a tumorolytic agent. Tumor necrosis factor has been found to be a product of the macrophage, structurally related to lymphotoxin, also identified as cachectin, a protein with a molecular weight of 17,000 Da that is one of the major secretory products of the activated macrophage and an important mediator of shock and the inflammatory response (Beutler and Cerami, 1990).

Prostaglandins (PGs) are potent mediators in inflammation, but the role of PGs in the regulation of humoral and cellular immunity has only recently been established (Goodwin and Webb, 1980). Prostaglandins are cyclooxygenase metabolites of arachidonic acid which are released from phospholipids of cell membranes. Prostaglandins are produced by every cell in the body, although PGE_2, an immunoregulatory prostaglandin, is produced primarily by low-density macrophages or monocytes (Bankhurst et al., 1981). Interleukin 1 initiates PGE_2 production by increasing the synthesis of cyclooxygenases as well as by increasing intracellular levels of Ca^{2+} (Bernheim, 1986). In turn, PGE_2 acts as an endogenous mediator of IL-1 production (Kunkel et al., 1985; Bernheim, 1986; Dinarello, 1990).

Prostaglandin E_2 acts on tissues through the activation of membrane-bound adenyl cyclase (cyclic adenosine monophosphate, cAMP) (Goodwin and Webb, 1980) and has a wide variety of effects on lymphocytes and monocytes. Prostaglandin E_2 inhibits cell reactivity by stimulating target cells, which in turn exert suppression (Wasserman et al., 1987). Prostaglandin E_2 suppresses proliferation of lymphocytes in response to mitogen stimulation (Wasserman et al., 1987) and inhibits production of IL-1 (Dinarello, 1983). In addition, PGE_2 suppresses neutrophil activation events (Kunkel et al., 1985), attenuates macrophage Ia region association antigen expression (Kunkel and Chensue, 1984), inhibits IL-2 production (Chouaib and Fradelizi, 1982), and decreases NK cell activity (Wasserman, 1987).

NUTRIENT DEFICIENCIES AND CYTOKINES

Lymphokines

The effects of malnutrition on lymphokines has not been extensively studied even though these products play a key role in the regulation of the immune response. This paucity of data on lymphokine-nutrition interactions may reflect the technical difficulties in obtaining pure preparations of these lymphocyte products and in producing sufficient biologically active samples for analysis. Of the many cytokines released during an immune response, IL-1, tumor necrosis factor (TNF) and interleukin 6 (IL-6) are the major indicators of intermediary metabolism acting together to decrease food intake and to increase resting energy expenditure (Klasing, 1988).

The limited number of reports are equivocal on the effects of nutrient deficiencies on the production and/or action of MIF in animals or in humans. Kramer and Good (1978) reported that MIF activity of lymph node cells from guinea pigs fed protein-deficient diets was normal or augmented. Similarly, Carlomagno and colleagues (1982) reported normal MIF activity of splenic lymphocytes from rats fed protein-deficient diets. In contrast, decreased MIF production by splenic lymphocytes from mice fed protein-deficient diets was documented by Hambor and colleagues (1983). In the latter study, there was no difference in the MIF responsiveness of macrophages from mice fed protein-deficient compared with protein-adequate diets. Interpretation and comparison of these studies is, unfortunately, difficult because different species were used in each study; moreover, in some cases, the results were confounded by omission of a pair-fed control group (Kramer and Good, 1978).

Zinc (Zn) is essential for the normal functioning of the immune system (Carlomagno et al., 1983; Fraker et al., 1986) and may play a role in MIF metabolism. Results of a study by Salvin and coworkers (1987) demonstrated that Zn supplementation (300 ppm Zn sulfate versus 15 ppm Zn sulfate for controls) increased MIF production in vivo in a strain of mice which normally fail to produce MIF. There are a few clinical reports of both decreased MIF function (Ford et al., 1975) and normal or slightly decreased (Chandra, 1980) MIF production and/or function from blood lymphocytes of protein energy–malnourished children. However, the decrease in MIF production reported by Ford and coworkers (1975) is not separable from the effects of recurrent fungal infections.

Similarly, there are conflicting results about the effects of malnutrition in LIF production and/or activity. Chandra (1980) reported normal LIF production in protein energy–malnourished children. Heresi and colleagues (1981) demonstrated no differences in LIF activity between marasmic children and normal children. In contrast, LIF activity was shown to be reduced in patients with kwashiorkor (Lomnitzer et al., 1976). A limitation of these studies was that LIF production and/or activity in response to both B- and T-cell activation was not assessed.

Selenium (Se) deficiency has effects on immune function, possibly because of its role in arachidonic acid metabolism. For example, Se deficiency in goats is associated with impaired PMN random migration and chemotaxis (Aziz et al., 1984). The ability of peripheral blood lymphocytes to produce LIF was decreased in lymphocytes from goats fed diets containing 0.08 mg Se/kg of ration compared with lymphocytes from goats fed Se-adequate diets (0.3 mg Se/kg of ration) (Aziz and Klesius, 1985).

Clinical Se deficiency is believed to exist in Finland where dietary Se intakes (30 μg/day) (Koivistoinen, 1980) are lower than those recommended by the U.S. National Research Council (50–200 μg/day). Selenium supplementation of 40 volunteers with low serum Se concentrations did not affect the production of LIF by peripheral blood lymphocytes (Arvilommi et al., 1983). Selenium deficiency, of the order found in Finland, had little influence on immune functions such as phogocytosis, chemotactic factor generation, and antibody production as measured in this study (Arvilommi et al., 1983).

These is a paucity of data on the effects of nutrient deficiencies on IL-2 production and/or activity. Saxena and colleagues (1984a) reported no effect of protein deficiency on murine splenic lymphocyte production of IL-2. Cytotoxic activity of splenic lymphocytes was, however, lower in cells from mice fed protein-adequate diets compared to those from mice fed protein-deficient diets, suggesting an impairment in a suppressor T-cell population. Recently Petro et al. (1991) reported that protein level is a key regulator of antitumor cytotoxic activity through effects on both tumor growth and development of cytotoxic T lymphocyte activity.

The effects of vitamin and some mineral deficiencies on IL-2 production have been reported by a limited number of investigators. For example, Saxena et al. (1984b) documented decreased splenic IL-2 production and decreased levels of cytotoxic activity in mice fed diets with half the recommended amounts of all vitamins. Aziz and Klesius (1985) reported that Se deficiency in goats did not result in significant differences in peripheral blood IL-2 production. Decreased IL-2 production was demonstrated in vitro in magnesium (Mg) deficiency but not in copper (Cu) or Zn deficiency (Flynn et al., 1984). The interpretation of these results (Flynn et al., 1984) is difficult because in vitro Cu, Mg, and Zn deficiencies all decreased IL-1 production, which induces IL-2 production. Interleukin 2 has been implicated in both positive and negative effects of vitamin supplementation on immune function (Wan et al., 1989; Payette et al., 1990).

There are very few reports on the effects on malnutrition on interferon production. Energy malnutrition (marasmus) in children is associated with a decreased production of total IFN (Schlesinger et al., 1976; Salimonu et al., 1982). Salimonu et al. (1982) also reported impaired NK cell activity in marasmus which was not restored by the addition of supplemental IFN to cell cultures. Unfortunately, only total IFN but not IFN-γ was assessed in this study and, thus, the nature of the immunological lesion remains unclear. Interestingly, vitamin A deficiency, which is associated with increased risk of infectious diseases, has been recently noted to cause decreased natural killer cell activity mediated by decreased IFN production in the rat (Bowman et al., 1991).

Monokines

The effects of nutrient deficiencies on monokine production and activity have been studied more extensively than the effects of malnutrition on lymphokines. Protein deficiency appears to impair the production and/or activity of IL-1 and PGE_2 (Hoffman-Goetz et al., 1981; Hoffman-Goetz, 1982; Bhaskaram and Sivakumar, 1986). In contrast, severe protein-energy malnutrition has been reported to increase IL-1 production (Filteau and Hall, 1991). Protein deficiency has no effect on TNF production (Bradley, 1988), whereas severe protein-energy malnutrition results in increased TNF production (Filteau and Hall, 1991). Protein deficiency also alters the ability of lymphocytes to respond to regulatory signals from IL-1 (Bell and Hoffman-Goetz, 1983; Bell et al., 1986). Indeed, protein deficiency appears to alter the balance between macrophage-produced enhancing factors such as IL-1 and suppressor factors such as PGE_2. The proportion of IL-1–producing and PGE_2-producing macrophages (Shellito and Kaltrieder, 1984; Hoffman-Goetz, 1987) and the ratios of T-cell subsets (Chandra, 1983b; Petro, 1985) may also be changed in protein malnutrition. Impaired production and/or activity of IL-1 in clinical protein deficiency has been documented by a number of investigators (Hoffman-Goetz et al., 1981; Keenan et al., 1982; Kauffman et al., 1986). Experimental protein deficiency and its effects on IL-1 production activity have been studied in rabbits (Hoffman-Goetz, 1982; Hoffman-Goetz et al., 1985), and in guinea pigs (Drabik et al., 1987).

Physiological changes mediated by IL-1 include induction of fever, decreases in plasma concentrations of iron (Fe), and increases in concentrations of a number of acute phase reactant proteins (Dinarello, 1984). Observations of these physiological signs have been used as assays for IL-1 activity in a number of studies in animals and in humans (Dinarello, 1984). For example, Hoffman-Goetz and Kluger (1979) originally documented attenuated fever and no decrease in plasma Fe concentration in rabbits fed 4.5% protein diets following injection with gram-negative bacteria. Interleukin 1 produced from monocytes from normal donor rabbits, however, restored these functions. In contrast, Drabik and colleagues (1987) reported no reversal of the afebrile response in guinea pigs fed 2.5% protein diets following administration of normal IL-1. The protein deficiency was concluded to be more severe in the latter study (Drabik et al., 1987), thus suggesting that severity of protein deficiency is a factor in impaired IL-1 activity. The duration of protein deficiency also appears to affect IL-1 activity. Interleukin 1 produced in vitro from protein-deficient rabbits elicited fever after 4 weeks but not after 6 and 8 weeks of protein restriction (Hoffman-Goetz, 1982).

Impaired production and/or activity of IL-1 in malnourished humans has also been demonstrated. Based on the results of an intact animal assay, Hoffman-Goetz and colleagues (1981) documented decreased activity of IL-1 produced by peripheral blood leukocytes from 12 patients, which was reversed by 7 days of total parenteral nutrition (TPN). Similar findings have been reported by Keenan et al. (1982) and by Kauffman et al. (1986). Other investigators have reported similar results using the more sensitive lymphocyte-activating factor (LAF) assay (Drabik et al., 1985; Bhaskaram and Sivakumar, 1986). For example, Drabik et al. (1985) reported decreased in vitro production of IL-1 by mononuclear cells from protein energy–malnourished patients in response to various stimulants. Likewise, Bhaskaram and Sivakumar (1986) investigated the ability of peripheral blood monocytes from six marasmic children and from five children with kwasiorkor to produce IL-1 or IL-1 activity. Interleukin 1 activity was found to be significantly depressed in children with severe malnutrition compared to controls. However, Bradley et al. (1990) did not find reduced IL-1 or TNF in malnourished nursing home residents despite evidence of decreased resistance to infection.

The mechanisms by which protein deficiency impairs IL-1 activity, however, are not explained by the results of the aforementioned studies. Therefore, a series of experiments was conducted in our laboratory to elucidate the mechanisms involved in the altered IL-1 production and/or activity observed in protein malnutrition (Hoffman-Goetz et al., 1985; Bell et al., 1986; Hoffman-Goetz et al., 1986; Hoffman-Goetz and Keir, 1988).

Male, New Zealand white rabbits were fed one of three diets for 8 weeks: (a) 0% casein diets (PD), (b) 21% casein diets (pair-fed) (PF), or (c) 21% casein diets (ad libitum, AL). Lymphocytes in unfractionated rabbit monocyte-lymphocyte cultures from rabbits fed PD diets had a significantly lower proliferative response to concanavalin A (Con A) compared with lymphocytes from animals fed AL or PF diets (Hoffman-Goetz et al., 1985). Addition of IL-1 prepared from monocytes from control rabbits significantly enhanced the proliferative response to suboptimal concentrations of Con A in lymphocytes cultured from rabbits fed PD diets relative to lymphocyte cultures from animals fed AL or PF diets. The absolute enhancement of the proliferative response in the lymphocyte cultures from rabbits fed protein-restricted diets was, however, significantly less than for the controls. The impaired proliferative response in lymphocytes from protein-malnourished donor rabbits, therefore, was not entirely due to decreased production of IL-1.

Changes in the proportions of T-cell subsets, altered lymphocyte responsiveness, or the presence of inhibitory factors in the lymphocyte cultures were further hypothesized to be responsible for the results observed. An additional series of experiments indicated slight, but not significant, increases in suppressor T-cell (T_S) activity following stimulation with Con A in lymphocytes from donors fed PD diets compared with lymphocytes from control donors (PF) (Hoffman-Goetz et al., 1986); it should be noted that the sample size was small, and therefore replication is necessary both for statistical purposes and for confidence in the data. However, other investigators have also documented increased numbers and activity of T_S in protein malnutrition (Chandra et al., 1983a; Chandra, 1983b; Petro, 1985).

Altered responsiveness of T_S cells to IL-1 was also observed in protein deficiency (Hoffman-Goetz et al., 1986). Enhanced suppression by T_S cells of the fresh, allogenic control lymphocyte response to phylohemagglutinin (PHA) on addition of IL-1 from both control (PF) and protein-malnourished donors was noted. Interleukin 1 was, therefore, produced by monocyte cultures from rabbits fed 0% casein diets. Production of IL-1 from both protein-malnourished and control rabbits was also supported by the presence of a gel-filtered protein band with an isoelectric point similar to that reported for IL-1 by other investigators (Oppenheim et al., 1986; Durum et al., 1990). In contrast, suppression by T_S of fresh allogenic lymphocytes from rabbits fed PD diets was abolished by the addition of IL-1 from both control and protein-malnourished donors to first culture. Lymphocytes from donors fed PD diets were not able to respond to signals from the IL-1 added to the cultures. These results suggest that IL-1 activity is further compromised in protein deficiency by the inability of lymphocytes from protein-malnourished animals to respond appropriately to regulatory signals from monokines, and by the appearance of inhibitory molecules.

In addition to the altered response of T lymphocytes to IL-1 in protein deficiency, Hoffman-Goetz and colleagues (1985) demonstrated that increased PGE_2 production may have a role in the functional T-cell deficits. Monocyte supernatants containing IL-1 and obtained from protein-malnourished rabbits suppressed lymphocyte proliferation to Con A regardless of the source of the monocyte-lymphocyte population (Hoffman-Goetz et al., 1985). Prostaglandin E_2 concentrations were determined to be higher in supernatants from crude monocyte supernatants and from lymphocytes cultured from protein-malnourished rabbits than from control and pair-fed rabbits (Bell et al., 1986). Petro (1985) also observed enhanced production of PGE_2 by macrophages from protein-deficient mice compared with those from control mice, although this study did not include a pair-fed control group.

Altered production of arachidonate metabolites, such as PGE_2, appear to have potent effects on the activity of IL-1. The addition of indomethacin, an inhibitor of arachidonate metabolism, to monocyte cultures from protein-restricted animals increased IL-1 production, which was measured by a thymocyte proliferation assay (Hoffman-Goetz and Keir, 1987). Bhaskaram and Sivakumar (1986) also reported restoration of IL-1 activity by the addition of indomethacin to cultures of blood lymphocytes from malnourished children. Arachidonate metabolites, such as PGE_2, thus appear to be important downregulators of IL-1 activity in malnutrition. The role of other mediators, such as the glucocorticoids, whose concentrations increase in protein energy malnutrition and which interact with IL-1 feedback pathways, have not been investigated.

Kunkel et al. (1985) reported that IL-1 itself induces PGE_2 synthesis in a dose-dependent manner. Macrophages failed to produce significant amounts of PGE_2 at high concentrations of IL-1. Therefore, it is reasonable to hypothesize that depressed production of IL-1 in protein malnutrition may trigger enhanced PGE_2 production which has an inhibitory effect on T-cell responsiveness and on the production of IL-1 (Kunkel and Chensue, 1984) and on IL-2 (Chouaib and Fradelizi, 1982).

Very few studies on the effects of other nutrient deficiencies or excesses on monokine production and/or activity have been conducted. Interleukin 1 activity has been reported to be depressed by in vitro deficiencies of Cu, Mg, and Zn (Flynn et al., 1984). Helyar and Sherman (1987) documented decreased IL-1 production by peritoneal exudate cells from rats fed diets containing 6 or 12 ppm Fe compared with controls fed diets containing 35 ppm Fe. Thus, depressed IL-1 activity in Fe deficiency may be a factor involved in the altered humoral and cell-mediated immunity observed in Fe deficiency.

Some investigators have described the effects of excess nutrients on monokine production and/or activity. For example, Moriguchi and colleagues (1985) documented increased IL-1 production by peritoneal macrophages from mice fed diets containing 650,000 IU vitamin A/kg of diet compared with those from mice fed 3900 IU vitamin A/kg of diet. Koller and colleagues (1986) reported no changes in activity of IL-1 produced by rat peritoneal macrophages following a period of excess Se (0.5, 2.0, or 5.0 ppm sodium selenite added to drinking water). Decreased PGE_2 synthesis was reported in rats which had 5 ppm sodium selenite added to drinking water. The significance of the above finding is unclear, however, as no values were given for the Se content of the drinking water.

CONCLUSIONS

To date, there are only limited and somewhat equivocal data from which to draw definite conclusions regarding the effects of nutrient deficiencies on cytokine production or function in humans. Research that has been conducted, as reviewed above, has focused primarily on the effects of experimental protein deficiency on cytokine production.

Protein deficiency appears to have little biological effect on the production and/or activity of MIF, LIF, or IL-2, although the data are limited and contradictory. Protein deficiency appears to have significant biological effects on the activity of monokines. Decreased IL-1 production, concomitant with increased PGE2 production, has been documented. However, increased IL-1 production in severe protein-energy malnutrition has also been reported, thus emphasizing the need for additional experimental studies in this area. Nevertheless, the balance between IL-1 and other biologically active modulators, such as PGE2, likely plays a major role in the impaired lymphocyte mitogenesis observed in protein (and protein-energy) malnutrition. Increased production of PGE_2 may act as a downregulator of IL-1 production. In addition, an increase in T_S generation and activity may be mediated by enhanced PGE_2 production. Responsiveness of T lymphocytes to monokines is also altered in protein deficiency, although the mechanisms involved in these changes have not yet been elucidated.

It is important to consider that in most of the studies reviewed models of severe protein deficiency were used. A recent study, using a model of moderate protein deficiency, documented increased generation of T_S activity and increased levels of spontaneously generated PGE_2 but unaltered levels of mitogen-stimulated PGE_2 (Petro, 1985). The duration of protein deficiency also appears to be a factor in effecting the changes in concentrations of monokines observed. There is clearly a need for further research on the effects of duration and severity of protein deficiency on cytokine production and/or function.

In the case of arachidonate metabolites such as PGE_2, further research on the effects of nutrients such as dietary fat (Marshall and Johnston, 1985), Zn (Meydani, 1982), and Se (Koller et al., 1986) is warranted given the role that these nutrients play in lipid metabolism. Indeed, the role of eicosanoids and health is a major thrust of nutritional research today, and clearly much more work is needed in defining the interaction with immune system regulatory molecules.

Very little research has been conducted on the effects of energy malnutrition on cytokines. Hoffman-Goetz and colleagues (1981) reported no apparent deficit in IL-1 production and/or function in marasmic patients. Enhanced IL-1 production and heightened proliferative response to Con A by lymphocytes from calorie-restricted rabbits has also been documented (Hoffman-Goetz et al., 1985). Certainly, the effects of energy restriction can confound the interpretation of experimental results, thus emphasizing the need for the inclusion of pair-fed control groups in animal studies (Beisel, 1982).

Redistribution of cells within the body may also affect the production and/or activity of cytokines. For example, the distribution of monokine-producing macrophages within the body may be altered in malnutrition, as has been suggested in sarcoidosis, a disease characterized by depressed in vitro and in vivo delayed-type hypersensitivity (Hudspith et al., 1984). Similarly, the proportions of T-cell subsets among cell compartments may also be altered in malnutrition, thus affecting the response of T cells to immunoregulatory signals (Chandra, 1983a). The effects of nutrient deficiencies and cytokines on such redistributions are unknown at the present time.

Secondary immune deficiency as a result of malnutrition is a global problem. One of the leading causes of immunodeficiency is considered to be protein energy malnutrition (Garre et al., 1987). Clinical malnutrition, however, is a composite of deficiencies of many essential nutrients. In spite of advances made in recent years in elucidating the role of nutrition on immune function, it is evident that relatively little progress has been made in delineating the effects of nutrient deficiencies on cytokines, key modulators of the immune response.

Studies on the role of nutrition on the production and/or activity of lymphokines such as MIF, LIF, IL-2, and IFN are limited and are not definitive, in part because of confounding factors and inadequate experimental control. The role of nutrient deficiencies, especially protein deficiency, on monokines such as IL-1 and PGE_2 have been characterized more fully. Knowledge of the role of single-nutrient deficiencies and their interactions with other nutrients on modulation of cell-mediated immune responses via cytokines is fundamental to understanding the mechanisms involved in dietary-induced immunodeficiency.

REFERENCES

Arvilommi H, Poikonen K, Jokinen I, Muukkonen O, Rasanen L, Foreman J, Huttunen JK (1983). Selenium and immune functions in humans. Infect Immun 41:185-189.

Aziz ES, Kelsius PH, Frandsen JC (1984). Effects of selenium on polymorphonuclear leukocyte function in goats. Am J Vet Res 45:1715-1717.

Aziz ES, Klesius PH (1985). The effect of selenium deficiency in goats on lymphocyte production of leukocyte migration inhibitory factor. Vet Immunol Immunopathol 10:381-390.

Bankhurst AD, Hastain E, Goodwin JS, Peale GT (1981). The nature of the prostaglandin-producing mononuclear cell in human peripheral blood. J Lab Clin Med 97:179-186.

Beer DJ, Dinarello CA, Rosenwasser LJ, Rocklin RE (1982a). Human monocyte-derived soluble product(s) has an accessory function in the generation of histamine- and concanavalin A-induced suppressor T cells. J Clin Invest 70:393-400.

Beer DJ, Rosenwasser DJ, Dinarello CA, Rocklin RE (1982b). Cellular interactions in the generation and expression of histamine-induced suppressor activity. Cell Immunol 69: 101-112.

Beisel WR (1982). Single nutrients and immunity. Am J Clin Nutr 35:417-468.

Bell R, Hoffman-Goetz L (1983). Effect of protein deficiency on endogenous pyrogen-mediated acute phase protein responses. Can J Physiol Pharmacol 61:376-380.

Bell RC, Hoffman-Goetz L, Keir R (1986). Monocyte factors modulate in vitro T-lymphocyte mitogenesis in protein malnutrition. Clin Exp Immunol 63:194-202.

Bernheim HA (1986). Is prostaglandin E_2 involved in the pathogenesis of fever? Effects of interleukin-1 on the release of prostaglandins. Yale J Biol Med 59:151-158.

Beutler B, Cerami A (1990). Cachectin (tumor necrosis factor): an endogenous mediator. *In*: Immunophysiology. JJ Oppenheim and EM Shevach, eds. Oxford University Press, New York, p 226.

Bhaskaram P, Sivakumar B (1986). Interleukin-1 in malnutrition. Arch Dis Child 61:182-185.

Bowman TA, Goonewardene M, Pasatiempo AM, Ross AC, Taylor C (1990). Vitamin A deficiency decreases natural killer cell activity and interferon production in rats. J Nutr 120: 1264-1273.

Bradley SF, Kauffman CA (1988). Protein malnutrition and the febrile response in the Fischer rat. J Leuc Biol 43:36-40.

Bradley SF, Vibhagool A, Fabrick S, Terpenning MS, Kauffman CA (1990). Monokine production by malnourished nursing home patients. Gerontology 36:165-170.

Carding SR, Hayday AC, Bottomly K (1991). Cytokines in T cell development. Immunol Today 12:239-245.

Carlomagno MA, Alito AE, Almiron DI, Gimeno A (1982). T and B lymphocyte function in response to a protein-free diet. Infect Immunol 129:2463-2468.

Carswell EA, Old LJ, Kassel RL, Green S, Firse N, Williamson B (1975). An endotoxin-induced serum factor that causes necrosis of tumors. Proc Natl Acad Sci USA 72:3666-3670.

Chandra RK (1980). Cell-mediated immunity in nutritional imbalance. Fed Proc 39:3088-3092.

Chandra RK (1983a). Numerical and functional deficiency in T helper cells in protein energy malnutrition. Clin Exp Immunol 51:126-132.

Chandra RK (1983b). The nutrition-immunity-infection nexis: The enumeration and functional assessment of lymphocyte subsets in nutritional deficiency. Nutr Res 3:605-615.

Chandra RK (1985). Malnutrition and immune responses. Ann Nestle 43:5-18.

Chess L, Rocklin RE, MacDermott RP, David JR, Schlosman SF (1975). Leukocyte inhibitory factor (LIF): Production by purified human T and B lymphocytes. J Immunol 115:315-317.

Chouaib S, Fradelizi D (1982). The mechanism of inhibition of human Il2 production. J Immunol 129:2463-2468.

Coley WB (1891). Contribution to the knowledge of sarcoma. Ann Sur 15:199-220.

Dinarello CA (1984). Interleukin-1. Rev Infect Dis 6:51-95.

Dinarello CA (1990). Interleukin-1 and its biologically related cytokines. In: Lymphokines and the Immune Response. S Cohen, ed. CRC Press, Boca Raton, Florida, p 181.

Dinarello CA, Marnoy SO, Rosenwasser LJ (1983). Role of arachidonate metabolism in the immunoregulatory function of human leukocytic pyrogen/lymphocyte activating factor/interleukin 1. J Immunol 130:890-895.

Drabik M, Pasulka P, LoPreste G, Moldawer L, Dinarello C, Bistrian, and Blackburn GL (1985). In vitro measurement of lymphocyte activating factor in hospitalized protein-calorie malnourished patients. J Leukocyte Biol 37:698-699.

Drabik MD, Schnure FC, Mok KT, Moldawer LL, Dinarello CA, Blackburn GL, Bistrian BR (1987). Effect of protein depletion and short-term parenteral refeeding on the host response to interleukin 1 administration. J Lab Clin Med 109:509-516.

Durum SK, Oppenheim JJ, Nera R (1990). Immunophysiologic role of interleukin 1. In: Immunophysiology. JJ Oppenheim, EM Shevach, eds. Oxford University Press, New York, p 210.

Farrar WL, Harel-Bellan A, Ferris DK (1990). Lymphoid growth factors: gene regulation and biochemical mechanisms of action. In: Lymphokines and Immune Response. S Cohen, ed. CRC Press, Boca Raton, Florida, p 115.

Filteau SM, Hall NRS (1991). Increased production of tumor necrosis factor and interleukin 1 by peritoneal macrophages from severely malnourished mice. Nutr Res 11:1001-1011.

Flynn A, Loftus MA, Finke JH (1984). Production of interleukin-1 and interleukin-2 in allogeneic mixed lymphocyte cultures under copper, magnesium and zinc deficient conditions. Nutr Res 4:673-679.

Ford GW, Jakeman M, Jose DG, Vorbach EA, Kirke DK (1975). Migration inhibitory factor production by lymphoid cells of Australian aboriginal children with moderate protein-calorie malnutrition. Aust Paediatr J 11:160-164.

Fraker PJ, Gershwin ME, Good RA, Prasad A (1986). Interrelationships between zinc and immune function. Fed Proc 45:1474-1479.

Garre MA, Boles JM, Youinou P (1987). Current concepts in immune derangement due to undernutrition. J Parenter Enteral Nutr 11:309-313.

Goetzl EJ, Rocklin RE (1978). Amplification of the activity of human leukocyte inhibitory (LIF) by the generation of a low molecular weight inhibitor of PMN leukocyte chemotaxis. J Immunol 121:891-896.

Goodwin JS, Webb DR (1980). Regulation of the immune response by prostaglandins. Clin Immunol Immunopathol 15:106–122.

Hambor JE, Fleck L, Stevenson JR (1983). Impairment of macrophage migration inhibitory factor synthesis and macrophage migration in protein-malnourished mice. Cell Immunol 81:303–312.

Helyar L, Sherman AR (1987). Iron deficiency and interleukin 1 production by rat leukocytes. Am J Clin Nutr 46:346–352.

Heresi GP, Saitua MT, Schlesinger L (1981). Leukocyte migration inhibition factor production in marasmic infants. Am J Clin Nutr 34:909–913.

Hoffman-Goetz L (1982). Protein deficiency and endogenous pyrogen fever. Can J Physiol Pharmacol 60:1545–1550.

Hoffman-Goetz L (1986). Malnutrition and immunological function with special reference to cell-mediated immunity. Yearbook Physical Anthropol 29:139–159.

Hoffman-Goetz L (1987). Lymphokines and monokines in protein-energy malnutrition. *In*: Nutrition and Immunology. RK Chandra, ed. New York, Liss, pp 9–23.

Hoffman-Goetz L, Bell RS, Keir R (1985). Effect of protein malnutrition and interleukin 1 on in vitro rabbit lymphocyte mitogenesis. Nutr Res 5:769–780.

Hoffman-Goetz L, Keir R, Young C (1986). Modulation of cellular immunity in malnutrition: Effect of interleukin 1 on suppressor T cell activity. Clin Exp Immunol 65:381–386.

Hoffman-Goetz L, Keir R (1988). Effect of indomethacin on interleukin-1 production in experimental protein malnutrition. Nutr Res 8:89–93.

Hoffman-Goetz L, Kluger MJ (1979). Protein deprivation: Its effects on fever and plasma iron during bacterial infection in rabbits. J Physiol 295:419–430.

Hoffman-Goetz L, Marcon T (1983). Effect of in vitro amino acid supplementation on endogenous pyrogen fever. Nutr Res 3:237–241.

Hoffman-Goetz L, McFarlane D, Bistrian B, Blackburn GL (1981). Febrile and plasma iron responses of rabbits injected with endogenous pyrogen from malnourished patients. Am J Clin Nutr 34:1109–1116.

Hudspith BN, Brostoff J, McNicol MW, Johnson NMcJ (1984). Anergy in sarcoidosis: The role of interleukin-1 and prostaglandins in the depressed in vitro lymphocyte response. Clin Exp Immunol 57:324–330.

Johnson JD, Hand WL, King-Thompson NL (1980). The role of divalent cations in interactions between lymphokines and macrophages. Cell Immunol 53:236–245.

Kauffman CA, Jones PG, Kluger MJ (1986). Fever and malnutrition: Endogenous pyrogen/interleukin-1 in malnourished patients. Am J Clin Nutr 44:449–452.

Keenan RA, Moldawer LL, Yan RD, Kawarmura I, Blackburn GL, Bistrian BR (1982). An altered response by peripheral leukocytes to synthesize or release leykocyte endogenous mediator in critically ill, protein malnourished patients. J Lab Clin Med 100:844–857.

Keller RH, Calvanico NJ (1984). Suppressor macromolecules. CRC Crit Rev Immunol 54:149–199.

Klasing KC (1988). Nutritional aspects of leukocytic cytokines. J Nutr 118(12):1436–1446.

Koivistoinen P (ed) (1980). Mineral element composition of Finnish foods: N, K, Ca, Mg, P, S, Fe, Cu, Mn, Zn, Mo, Co, Ni, Cr, F, Se, Si, Rb, Al, B, Br, Hg, As, Cd, Pb, and ash. Acta Agr Scand (Suppl 22):1–171.

Koller LD, Exon JH, Talcott PA, Osborne CA, Henningsen GM (1986). Immune responses in rats supplemented with selenium. Clin Exp Immunol 63:570–576.

Kramer TM, Good RA (1978). Increased in vitro cell-mediated immunity in protein-malnourished guinea pigs. Clin Immunol Immunopathol 11:212–228.

Kunkel SL, Chensue SW (1984). Prostaglandins and the regulation of immune responses. Adv Inflamm Res 7:93–109.

Kunkel SL, Chensue SWE, Spengler M, Geer J (1985). Effects of arachidonic acid metabolites and their metabolic inhibitors on interleukin-1 production. *In*: The Physiologic, Metabolic, and Immunologic Actions of Interleukin-1. MJ Kluger, JJ Oppenheim, MC Powanda, eds. New York, Liss, pp 297–307.

Lomnitzer R, Rosen EU, Geefhuyssen J, Rabson AR (1976). Defective leukocyte inhibitory factor (LIF) production by lymphocytes in children with kwashiorkor. S Afr Med J 50: 1820–1822.

Maizel AL, Lachman LB (1984). Biology of disease—Control of human lymphocyte proliferation by soluble factors. Lab Invest 50:369–377.

Marshall LA, Johnston PV (1985). The influence of dietary essential fatty acids on rat immunocompetent cell prostaglandin synthesis and mitogen-induced blastogenesis. J Nutr 115:1572–1580.

Meydani SN, Dupont J (1982). Effect of zinc deficiency on prostaglandin synthesis in different organs of the rat. J Nutr 112:1098–1104.

Moriguchi S, Werner L, Watson RR (1985). High dietary vitamin A (retnyl palmitate) and cellular immune functions in mice. Immunology 56:169–177.

Mizel SB (1982). Interleukin 1 and T-cell activation. Immunol Rev 63:51–72.

Oppenheim JJ, Shevach EM (1990). The Role of Cells and Cytokines in Immunity and Inflammation. In: Immunophysiology. JJ Oppenheim, EM Shevach, eds. Oxford University Press, New York, p 226.

Oppenheim JJ, Kovacs EJ, Matsushima K, Durum SK (1986). There is more than one interleukin 1. Immunol Today 7:45–56.

Payette H, Rola-Pleszczynski M, Ghadirian P (1990). Nutrition factors in relation to cellular and regulatory immune variables in a free-living elderly population. Am J Clin Nutr 52(5): 927–932.

Petro TM (1985). Effect of reduced dietary protein intake on regulation of murine in vitro polyclonal T-lymphocyte mitogenesis. Nutr Res 5:263–276.

Petro TM, Schwartz KM, Schmid MJ (1991). Natural and immune anti-tumor interleukin production and lymphocyte cytotoxicity during the course of dietary protein deficiency or excess. Nutr Res 11:679–686.

Remold HG, David RA, David JR (1972). Characterization of migration inhibitory factor (MIF) from guinea pig lymphocytes stimulated with concanavalin A. J Immunol 109: 578–586.

Rocklin RE (1974). Products of activated lymphocytes: Leukocyte inhibitory factor (LIF) distinct from migration inhibitor factor (MIF). J Immunol 112:1461–1466.

Rocklin RE, Bendtzen K, Greineder D (1980). Mediators of immunity: Lymphokines and monokines. Adv Immunol 29:55–136.

Salimonu LS, Ojo-Amaize E, Williams AIO, Johnson AOK, Cooke AR, Adekeunle FA, Alm GV, Wigzell H (1982). Depressed natural killer cell activity in children with protein-calorie malnutrition. Clin Immunol Immunopathol 24:1–7.

Salvin SB, Horecker BL, Pan L-X, Rabin BS (1987). The effect of dietary zinc and prothymosin on cellular immune responses of RF/J mice. Clin Immunol Immunopathol 43: 281–288.

Sarin PS, Gallo RS (1984). Human T-cell growth factor (TCGF). CRC Crit Rev Immunol 4: 279–305.

Saxena QB, Saxena RK, Adler WH (1984a). Effect of protein calorie malnutrition on the levels of natural and inducible cytotoxic activities in mouse spleen cells. Immunology 51:727–733.

Saxena QB, Saxena RK, Adler WH (1984b). Effect of feeding a diet with half of the recommended levels of all vitamins on the natural and inducible levels of cytotoxic activity in mouse spleen cells. Immunology 52:41–48.

Schlesinger L, Ohlbaum A, Grez L, Stekel A (1976). Decreased interferon production by leukocytes in marasmus. Am J Clin Nutr 29:758-761.

Shellito J, Kaltreider HB (1984). Heterogeneity of immunologic function among subfractions of normal rat alveolar macrophages. Am Rev Respir Dis 129:747-753.

Steeg PS, Moore RN, Johnson HM, Oppenheim JJ (1982). Regulation of murine macrophage Ia antigen expression by a lymphokine with immune interferon activity. J Exp Med 156:1780-1793.

Strominger JL (1989). Developmental biology of T cell receptors. Science 244:943-950.

Trinchieri G, Perussia B (1985). Immune interferon: A pleiotropic lymphokine with multiple effects. Immunol Today 6:131-136.

Wan JM, Haw MP, Blackburn GL (1989). Nutrition, immune function, and inflammation: An overview. Proc Nutr Soc 48(3):315-335.

Wasserman J, Hammarstrom S, Petrini B, Blomgren H, von Stedingk L-V, Vedin I (1987). Effects of some prostaglandins and leukotrienes on lymphocytes, monocytes and their activity in vitro. Int Arch Allergy Appl Immunol 83:39-43.

Weisbart R, Yu DTY, Billing R, Fan PT, Clements PJ, Paulus HE (1978). Cellular collaboration in production of human leukocyte migration inhibition factor. Immunology 34:815-820.

Yoshida T, Kuratsuji T, Takada Y, Minowada J, Cohen S (1976). Lymphokine-like factors produced by human lymphoid-cell lines with B or T cell surface markers. J Immunol 117:548-554.

Yoshida T, Sonozaki H, Cohen S (1973). The production of migration inhibition factor by B and T cells of the guinea pig. J Exp Med 138:784-796.

3
The Role of Arginine as an Immune Modulator

Adrian Barbul
Sinai Hospital of Baltimore, Baltimore, Maryland

INTRODUCTION

The use of intravenous postoperative nutritional support is currently under investigation in different clinical settings as a result of the growing recognition that nutrition can play a major role in wound healing and host defense against infection as well as providing essential protein calorie support when normal dietary intake is not feasible (1–6). Metabolic response to injury occurs in the context of rather diverse but often concurrent traumatic events, including major surgical intervention, shock, or infection, and leads to both a clinically significant impact on the neuroendocrine and immune system and in patients who cannot respond to treatment, to acceleration of disease, organ failure, and morbidity. It seems that classic total parenteral nutrient support may be unable to promote a return to normal metabolism when inflammatory processes have produced a kind of autoreactive state as a result of immune suppression (6,7). It now appears that particular nutrients may play a role in specific regulatory processes within the immune system and that certain nutrients, including arginine, glutamine, omega-6 and omega-3 fatty acids, metals such as iron and zinc, and certain vitamins E, C, and A, as discussed in several chapters in this book and elsewhere, may have direct and targeted effects within the immune system and effectively restore normal regulation of the immune system. Alexander (8) has also stressed the need to differentiate between physiological replacement of missing nutrients and pharmacological immune system modulation. The role of nutritional supplementation in the tumor-bearing host, however, has been found to present complex issues, since there may be a danger of supporting tumor growth, either directly through supply of a critical substrate or indirectly through affecting host defense against the tumor negatively through effects on the immune system. Studies have shown that limiting tyrosine and phenylalanine intake in the diet may decrease tumor growth and metastasis, and when given to healthy volunteers caused an increase in natural killer (NK) cell activity and decreased platelet aggregation, which in light of other studies suggests correlation with decreased tumor growth and metastasis (9). Although these data imply that there may be certain amino acids which enhance and others which retard tumor growth, it is essential to recognize that free amino acid pool and amino acid oxidation rates may change in response to intermittent food intake (10) and that those cycles may be further disrupted in the cancer patient.

In cancer patients, immune suppression is often evident prior to any therapeutic interventions which could compromise nutritional status, yet Daly et al. (11) have shown improved delayed-type hypersensitivity with relatively brief nutritional support.

The specificity of nutritional support appears to have particular significance for the cancer patient, since both deficiency or excess may affect the balance of critical immune reactions (12) on subpopulations (13), which may have effects on tumor response. It has been hypothesized that nutritional support will only benefit the cancer patient with an innate, or otherwise determined, strong antitumor response (14).

In the following sections, studies on the role of arginine as a key immunomodulator both in healthy persons and in patients undergoing surgery or with primary immunodeficiency are presented. These studies (15,16) and those of others (17,18) clearly demonstrate the potential significance of this single amino acid in affecting immune response.

BIOCHEMISTRY AND PHYSIOLOGY

Arginine plays a pivotal role in protein synthesis, the biosynthesis of amino acids and derivatives, and the urea cycle. All tissues utilize arginine for cytoplasmic and nuclear protein biosynthesis. Arginine is also an amidine donor for guanidoacetic acid and subsequent creatine synthesis. Arginine is, therefore, indirectly required for the primary storage energy phosphagen, creatine phosphate.

Exogenous arginine is dispensable for the survival of most adult mammals. Limited growth of the young of some species is possible without dietary arginine. An endogenous biosynthetic source must therefore exist to provide for muscle and connective tissue growth. The endogenous synthetic pathway interacts very closely with the urea cycle enzymes of the liver and kidney with the generation of arginine from ornithine via citrulline (19). Normally, some arginine is derived from the diet and some from citrulline as the result of several interorgan reactions; i.e., gut glutamine → circulating citrulline → renal arginine; or hepatic arginine → hepatic ornithine → hepatic citrulline → circulating citrulline → renal arginine → circulating arginine.

The arginase activity in the liver is very high, so that hepatic arginine levels are very low and there is little arginine released (20). Citrulline, a major end product of gut glutamine nitrogen metabolism, is released as such into the circulation. It is estimated that more than 25% of gut glutamine is released as citrulline (21). Approximately 80% of the citrulline released by the gut is taken up by the kidneys, which in turn generate arginine. This arginine is released into the bloodstream for uptake by tissues for protein synthesis (21–23). This is in part due to the lower ratio of renal arginase to arginine synthetase activity when compared to the liver (20). Although the brain also possesses urea cycle enzymes and generates urea from citrulline, it does not contribute appreciably to the body economy of arginine or urea (19). Urea cycle enzymes have also been described in fibroblasts, leukocytes, and rapidly dividing tissues.

Role of Arginine in Nutrition

Rose established that arginine was a semidispensible amino acid (24,25). He noted that arginine was not a necessary dietary component for the maintenance of nitrogen balance in healthy adult rats, but that it was required for optimal nitrogen balance in the young growing rat. Rose interpreted these data as showing that the endogenous synthesis of arginine in the neonate and the young was inadequate to supply the organism with its arginine requirement. Since then these findings have been confirmed in a variety of mammalian species, although it has been somewhat controversial in humans (26,27). It is of interest to note that of the urea cycle–related amino acids, citrulline can replace arginine for growth requirements of growing animals (28); ornithine, which shares many of the biological and pharmacological effects of arginine (see below), cannot replace arginine for growth requirement.

Secretagogic Actions of Arginine

Arginine has multiple and potent secretagogic activities on several endocrine glands. Intravenous administration of arginine to adult humans in doses of 30 g in 30 min (0.5 g/kg in children) causes a marked increase in human pituitary growth hormone secretion (29,30). This also occurs after oral arginine administration (31,32). Ornithine also possesses strong secretagogic activity for human pituitary growth hormone in doses of 12 g/m^2 (33,34). It has been noted that growth hormone release after ornithine infusion is even higher and more sustained than after arginine infusion. Another pituitary effect of arginine in humans is the release of prolactin after an intravenous infusion (35).

Intravenous, oral, or intraduodenal arginine induces a marked insulin release in humans (36,37). Of all amino acids, arginine has the strongest insulinogenic effect and its activity is equivalent to the infusion of all 10 dietary essential amino acids (38). The infusion of arginine in man is followed by a slight hyperglycemia is secondary to a release of glucagon from the β cells of the pancreas (39). More recently, arginine has been found to increase pancreatic somatostatin (40), pancreatic polypeptide (41), and adrenal catecholamine (42) release; all of these may contribute to the insulinogenic response to arginine.

Trauma and Arginine

Based on the concept that nutritional requirements posttrauma approximate those of the growing rather than the adult organism, Seifter et al. (43) have shown that arginine is required for the survival and weight gain of mildly injured rats. The addition of supplemental arginine to either oral or intravenous diets containing adequate amounts of arginine for growth and reproduction lessened the posttraumatic weight loss and accelerated wound-breaking strength gain and the rate of collagen deposition (43,44). The improved weight gain was shown to correlate with better nitrogen retention in normal and injured rats and in humans undergoing mild operative trauma (45–48). Supplemental ornithine also increases nitrogen retention and stimulates wound healing (49). Since ornithine cannot replace arginine for growth requirements, their similar action on posttraumatic catabolism suggests a similar pharmacological mechanism.

IMMUNE EFFECTS OR ARGININE

In Vitro

It has been known for quite some time that arginine is necessary for the growth of cells in tissue culture (50). Of further interest, citrulline can replace arginine for the growth requirement of cells in vitro, whereas ornithine cannot (51). This is analogous to the in vivo situation in animals that have an arginine requirement for optimal growth (28). Mitogenesis of human peripheral blood lymphocytes in response to concanavalin A (Con A) or phytohemagglutinin (PHA) is abrogated if the cultures are carried out in arginine-free medium (52,53); however, no cell death is noted. Normal responses are restored at a concentration of 1.15 mM (52) and 50 μM (53), respectively. Once again, ornithine cannot replace arginine for optimal mitogenic response (J.E. Albina, personal communication). Further evidence for the absolute requirement for arginine in lymphocyte blastogenic responses is provided by using indospicine, a competitive but reversible inhibitor of arginine, which inhibits the PHA response of human peripheral blood lymphocytes in a reversible fashion (54). Since increased arginase activity is noted within 6 hr of incubation with mitogen (55), it has been suggested that arginine is needed to provide the ornithine necessary for polyamine synthesis, which is one of the earliest events noted after mitogenic stimulation (56). The fact that ornithine cannot replace arginine for optimal mitogenic responses suggests that ornithine generation is likely not the reason for the absolute arginine requirement. There is one reported study showing that ornithine can influence B lymphocyte activity in vitro; the addition of 10^{-5} M/L of ornithine to peripheral blood lymphocytes obtained from malnourished subjects increased the production of IgM and IgG in response to pokeweed mitogen stimulation (57).

It has been shown that supranormal supplementation of RPMI 1640 culture medium with arginine (400–1024 mg/L as compared to 200 mg/L in RPMI 1640) increases NK activity and monocyte cytotoxicity accompanied by increased production of monocyte tumor cytotoxic factor (58). Hibbs et al. (59) demonstrated that activated cytotoxic macrophages cause inhibition of DNA synthesis and of mitochondrial respiration in target tumor cells. This was correlated with an arginine-dependent pathway leading to the synthesis of citrulline from arginine via arginine deiminase. Arginine deiminase has not been described previously in mammalian cells. However, arginine deiminase-like activity has been confirmed to be present in secondary mixed leukocyte culture supernatants (60) and in activated rat peritoneal macrophages (61). Hibbs et al. have since shown that this is a unique property of arginine; no other amino acids are required for cytotoxic macrophages to inhibit target tumor cell metabolism (62) and ornithine is not able to substitute for arginine in this situation (J.J. Hibbs Jr., personal communication). This finding is somewhat surprising, since the level of macrophage production of ornithine from arginine has been shown to be directly correlated with immunogenicity (63) and tumor necrosis factor (TNF) can augment the capacity of peritoneal macrophages to convert arginine to ornithine (64).

L-Ornithine has been shown in vitro to inhibit the generation of cytotoxic T lymphocytes in mixed lymphocytes cultures; at the same doses (3–9 mM/L), ornithine did not inhibit proliferation in mixed lymphocyte cultures or generation of interleukin 2 (IL-2) and interferon (INF) in mitogen-stimulated lymphocyte cultures (65, 66). Arginine and putrescine in 10-mM concentrations act similar to ornithine in inhibiting cytotoxic T-cell generation (67). It should be pointed out once more that these are supraphysiological concentrations of the amino acids, and for the present the in vivo relevance of these findings is difficult to appreciate.

IN VIVO EFFECTS OF ARGININE ON IMMUNITY
Animal Studies

In the course of studying the influence of supplemental dietary arginine on wound healing in rats, we noted that arginine increased thymic weight in uninjured rats and mice and minimized the thymic involution that occurs with injury (68). Subsequent studies showed that the gain in thymic weight is due to significant increases in the lymphocyte content on the thymic glands (69,70). Furthermore, the increase in the total number of thymic gland lymphocytes is accompanied by a significant enhancement in the blastogenesis of these lymphocytes in response to mitogens (70,71). Additional experiments have shown that dietary supplements with ornithine also have strong thymotropic activity (72), but citrulline (73), spermine, spermidine, agmatine, or putrescine do not affect thymic size or cellularity (74,75). The experimental data suggest that the thymotropic effects of arginine and ornithine are not mediated directly via polyamine synthesis. Seifter (76) has suggested that the thymic effects may be related to the pituitary secretagogic activity of the two basic amino acids. His view is partly supported by the fact that hypophysectomy abolishes the thymotropic effect or arginine, indicating the need, at the very least, of an intact hypothalamo-pituitary axis (76). The onset of the arginine effect on the thymus is fairly rapid and is dose-limited; i.e., once the effect is achieved, higher supplements do not result in higher immune responses. The thymic effect of 1 week of arginine supplementation in mice lasts for 6 weeks after the cessation of the therapy (77).

Arginine is very effective in abrogating the thymolytic effects of stress, as defined by Hans Selye. This finding has been noted in mice subjected to partial body casting (75), in mice inoculated with the Moloney sarcoma virus (71), in genetically obese, diabetic mice (78), and in rats subjected to dorsal wounding (68) and unilateral or bilateral femoral fractures (70). The effect is also noted when high levels of arginine are used as part of a total parenteral nutrition regimen (79,80).

The trophic action of arginine on the thymus and T lymphocytes results in improved host immunity in a variety of conditions. Arginine enhances allogeneic skin graft rejection in mice (81). In guinea pigs subjected to 30% total body surface third-degree burns, a diet containing 2% arginine of the total nonprotein calories increases survival, improves delayed hypersensitivity responses to dinitrofluorobenzene, and heightens local bacterial containment as assessed by the size of pustules following subdermal staphylococcal injections (82). We have shown that arginine significantly improves the survival of rats subjected to highly lethal peritonitis (83).

Another aspect of host immune modulation by arginine relates to its effects on tumor induction and development. Over the past 50 years, most studies seem to indicate that arginine has a beneficial effect on a variety of tumor models. Arginine lessens tumor incidence following the use of chemical carcinogens such as acetamide (84), 7,12-dimethylbenzanthracene (85–87), and N-methyl-N-nitrosurea (88). It increases the latency period, reduces tumor size, and shortens the time of tumor regression in mice inoculated with the Moloney sarcoma virus (71). In transplantable solid tumor models, arginine has been found to have a positive influence on tumor incidence, latency time, tumor growth and/or metastatic spread, and host survival (89–100). In one study, the positive effect of arginine on tumor growth and metastatic spread was correlated with the enhanced phagocytic activity of alveolar macrophages (100). More recently, the positive effect of arginine supplementation on host-tumor interaction was correlated with increased Con A blastogenesis and IL-2 production by host splenocytes. These responses occurred in both highly immunogenic and in very poorly immunogenic tumor strains (101). Increased host reactivity against tumor antigens as assessed by mixed lymphocyte-tumor cultures were noted in hosts bearing the highly immunogenic tumors. This suggests that the effects of arginine on tumor growth may be mediated by both specific and nonspecific immune enhancement of the tumor-bearing host. The same group of investigators than studied the effects of arginine on tumor growth and antitumor responses in protein-depleted tumor-inoculated mice (102). It was noted that arginine could enhance host nutritional status, retard tumor growth, and augment immune responses in protein-depleted animals bearing immunogenic tumors, but not in animals inoculated with a poorly immunogenic tumor. This suggests that although arginine can positively affect host nonspecific immune responses to nonimmunogenic tumors in well-nourished animals, it can not overcome the immune deficiency of protein malnutrition and the poor immunogenicity of the tumor.

Human Studies

In normal human volunteers, daily oral arginine HCl supplements (30 g) given for 1 week significantly increased peripheral blood lymphocyte (PBL) blastogenesis in response to Con A and PHA (34). The response was evident within 3 days of the start of the supplementation. More recently, the same arginine supplementation was found to significantly decrease the T-suppressor subset and markedly increase the T-helper to T-suppressor ratio (Barbul, A. et al., unpublished data) (Table 1).

Table 1 Effect of Arginine on T-cell Subsets[a]

Subset	Prearginine	Postarginine	p
T lymphocytes (OKT3)	1,594 ± 567	1,621 ± 425	NS
% T lymphocytes	71.3 ± 8.9	70.2 ± 11.6	NS
T helper (OKT4)	1,017 ± 525	1,072 ± 382	NS
% T helper	50.5 ± 11.7	47.9 ± 10.9	NS
T suppressor (OKT8)	562 ± 122	437 ± 118	<0.05
% T suppressor	28.3 ± 10.4	19.9 ± 5.0	<0.05
T_H/T_S	1.86 ± 0.73	2.55 ± 0.88	<0.03

[a]n = 12. Mean ± SD.

In a subsequent study, we have examined the effect of ornithine on the immune responses of healthy human volunteers. Six subjects were given 30 g/day of ornithine HCl in addition to their normal food intake. Peripheral blood lymphocyte responses to Con A, PHA, and allogeneic cells (MLR) were assayed pre-, 3 days, and 7 days postsupplementation. As shown in Figure 1, 7 days of ornithine supplementation significantly enhanced PBL mitogenic responses. Allogeneic responses were higher after 7 days, but not in a statistically significant manner owing to the fairly large standard errors (A. Barbul, unpublished observations).

Both the arginine and ornithine supplements were well tolerated by the volunteers. The most annoying side effect is diarrhea due to the large osmotic load, but this can be controlled by spacing the amino acid intake throughout the day.

We have used arginine clinically in two situations, both involving patients with immune compromise. The first study involved seven patients undergoing major abdominal surgery. The patients, all of whom required intravenous postoperative nutritional support, were divided into two groups. The control group (n = 3) received a standard TPN mixture consisting of 25% dextrose and FreAmine II as the source of amino acids. In addition, they were given 10 g of essential amino acids IV q8h in the form of Nephramine, which does not contain arginine. The control group included a 47-year-old male undergoing an abdominoperineal resection, an 81-year-old male undergoing a right hemicolectomy for perforation with peritonitis, and a 71-year-old male undergoing a cholecystectomy, common bile duct exploration and drainage of a liver abscess.

The experimental group (n = 4) received the same TPN regimen and was given supplementary arginine HCl 10 g/IV every 8 hr. These patients included a 73-year-old female undergoing esophagectomy, a 45-year-old male undergoing an excision of a pancreatic pseudocyst, a 63-year-old male undergoing an esophagogastrectomy, and a 54-year-old diabetic female on steroids who underwent a Hartmann's procedure for perforated diverticulitis with peritonitis.

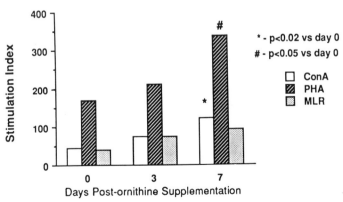

Figure 1 Effect of one week of ornithine supplementation on mitogenic and allogeneic responses of peripheral blood lymphocytes. Data are reported as Mean ± SEM, n = 6 volunteers.

The regimens were not isonitrogenous, given the high nitrogen density of arginine. Some patients received preoperative TPN; however, the amino acid supplements were begun on the day following the operations. Peripheral blood lymphocytes were harvested at 0, 1, 3 and 7 days postoperatively and their mitogenic responses to Con A and PHA were assayed. The results are shown in Figure 2, and demonstrate that arginine supplementation prevented or lessened the postoperative reduction in blastogenesis in response to Con A and PHA. This study was interrupted in 1980 because of the replacement of FreAmine II with FreAmine III. The latter solution contains higher amounts of arginine. These results seem to be very promising and we

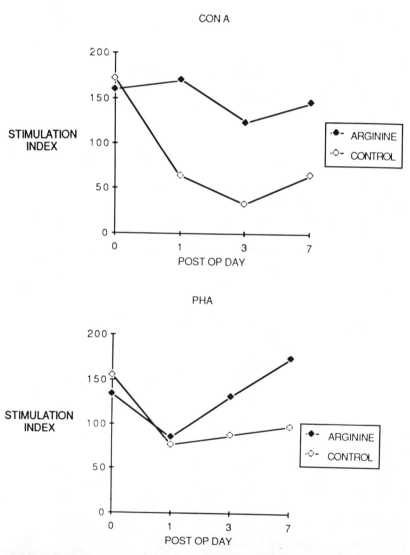

Figure 2 Effect of intravenous arginine (30 grams) on the mitogenic responses of peripheral blood lymphocytes of post-operative patients (n = 4 in the arginine group and n = 3 for controls).

are now in the process of starting a new study on the effect of arginine supplementation in high-risk surgical patients.

We are presently in the process of studying the effect of arginine supplementation in a group of patients who are seropositive for human immunodeficiency virus (HIV) infections. We select patients who have no clinical symptoms referrable to their viral infection, have no previous major infectious complications or lymphadenopathy. As an entrance criterion, all patients have to have a T_H/T_S ratio of less than 0.8, which we chose arbitrarily as a sign of immunesuppression. Patients receive 20 g of arginine free base/day for a 2-week period. All patients have lymphocyte subset studies performed twice before the start of the supplementation (to ensure stable baseline values), at the end of the two weeks of supplementation, and then 2 and 6 weeks later. So far, five patients have been entered in this study. In addition, the last three patients had peripheral blood lymphocyte mitogenic assays performed at the same times as the subset studies.

No changes in T-lymphocyte subsets or ratios are discernible following the arginine supplementation (Table 2). There was, however, a significant enhancement in the mitogenic responses to Con A and PHA observed in all three patients tested (Fig. 3). This enhancement persisted up to 6 weeks postsupplementation in two patients, whereas in the third there was a return to baseline values by that time. Obviously, these are preliminary findings in a small number of patients and no conclusions can be made yet as to the effect of arginine on the immune response of HIV-infected patients. There does not seem to be any effect on the peripheral blood lymphocyte ratios. While the increase in mitogenic responses is marked, how this affects overall

Table 2 Effect of Arginine Supplementation of PBL Subsets in Patients Infected with HIV

	Pre[a]	Post[a]	2 wks Post[a]	6 wks Post[a]
All T (OKT3)	1532 (69.6)	1428 (72.5)	1463 (76.1)	1303 (70.6)
	1694 (77.7)	2368 (79.8)	1644 (79.7)	1533 (80.4)
	926 (66.0)	1328 (73.6)	1145 (80.8)	1696 (82.0)
	321 (63.7)	773 (59.0)	1302 (66.0)	1053 (73.4)
	1356 (63.4)	1667 (65.4)	1554 (64.7)	1771 (60.8)
	1166 (68.1)	1513 (70.1)	1423 (73.5)	1471 (73.4)
T_H (OKT4)	680 (32.0)	657 (33.4)	701 (36.4)	599 (32.5)
	267 (12.2)	385 (13.0)	302 (14.6)	286 (15.0)
	223 (18.3)	285 (15.8)	359 (25.4)	514 (24.8)
	64 (9.6)	86 (5.9)	201 (10.2)	132 (9.2)
	500 (23.3)	658 (25.8)	594 (24.7)	850 (29.2)
	347 (19.1)	623 (18.8)	431 (22.2)	476 (22.1)
T_S (OKT8)	839 (39.6)	751 (38.2)	730 (38)	707 (38.3)
	1166 (53.5)	1718 (57.9)	1202 (58.2)	1137 (59.6)
	870 (39.7)	566 (31.3)	544 (38.4)	923 (44.6)
	218 (43.2)	546 (39.7)	850 (43.1)	822 (57.3)
	634 (29.6)	735 (28.9)	704 (29.3)	846 (29.1)
	745 (41.1)	863 (39.2)	806 (41.4)	887 (45.8)

[a]Numbers/mm³ (%).

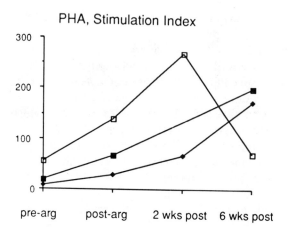

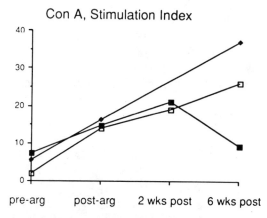

Figure 3 Effect of two weeks of arginine supplementation on the mitogenic responses of three subjects sero-positive for HIV infection.

host antiviral immunity cannot be gauged from these studies. If arginine is to play a role in HIV-infected patients, it is likely to be in adjuvant therapy, perhaps to aid in response to specific antiviral therapies or even conceivably in conjunction with other immunomodulators, or in the context of boosting immunity with a vaccine.

CONCLUSIONS

It is evident that arginine has multiple biological effects that are beneficial in a variety of situations, such as trauma, tumors, infections, and depressed immunity. Perhaps the most striking effect is the one on T cell–mediated immunity, which appears to be of both specific and nonspecific nature. Further work is needed to determine if arginine has biological activity on macrophage, neutrophil, and B-lymphocyte function. Of note is the minimal, if any, side effect of arginine administration, which makes it a very attractive agent for pharmacological use. Lastly, arginine may have a significant role as an adjuvant treatment concomitant with therapies that by themselves impair host immunity or concurrent to other therapeutic modalities.

ACKNOWLEDGMENTS

I wish to express my sincere thanks to Drs. Eli Seifter and Stanley M. Levenson, who first introduced me to the field of arginine research; To Mrs. H.L. Wasserkrug, my long-time collaborator, who patiently helped me in all studies and whose expertise I most gratefully acknowledge; to Drs. D. Sisto, L. Penberthy, R.S. Fishel, S. Shimazu, and H. Madden, all of whom collaborated on some of the reported projects; to Drs. N.N. Yoshimura, R. Tao, and R. Kelly from Kendall McGaw for their analytical support; to Dr. E. Bransom, for referring patients for some the clinical studies; and finally to Dr. G. Efron for his continued nurture and support.

REFERENCES

1. Madden HP, Breslin RJ, Wasserkrug HL, Efron G, Barbul A (1988). Stimulation of T cell immunity by arginine enhances survival in peritonitis. J Surg Res 44(6):658.
2. Yamato S, Ota F, Akiyama M, Takeuchi S, Ikemoto S, Shizuka F, Kishi K, Fukui K, Inoue G (1988). Optimal protein intake estimated by the resistance to streptococcal infection and the nutritional indices in mice. J Nutr Sci Vitaminol 34(4):423.
3. Christou N (1990). Perioperative nutritional support: Immunologic defects. J Parenter Enter Nutr 14(Suppl 5):186S.
4. Bower RH (1990). Nutritional and metabolic support of critically ill patients. J Parenter Enter Nutr 14(Suppl 5):257S.
5. Alexander JW, Gottschlich MM (1990). Nutritional immunomodulation in burn patients. Crit Care Med 18(Suppl 2):S149.
6. Cerra FB (1991). Nutrient modulation of inflammatory and immune function. Am J Surg 161(2):230.
7. Wan JM, Haw MP, Blackburn GL (1989). Nutrition, immune function, and inflammation: An overview. Proceed Nutr Soc 48(3):315.
8. Alexander JW, Peck MD (1990). Future prospects for adjunctive therapy: Pharmacologic and nutritional approaches to immune system modulation. Crit Care Med 18(Suppl 2):S159.
9. Norris JR, Meadows GG, Massey LK, Starkey JR, Sylvester DM, Liu SY (1990). Tyrosine- and phenylalanine-restricted formula diet augments immunocompetence in healthy humans. Am J of Clin Nutr 51(2):188.
10. Arnal M, Obled C, Attaix D, Patureau-Mirand P, Bonin D (1987). Dietary control of protein turnover. Diabet Metabol 13(6):630.
11. Daly JM, Hoffman K, Lieberman M, Leon P, Redmond HP, Shou J, Torosian MH (1990). Nutritional support in the cancer patient. J Parenter Enter Nutr 14(Suppl 5):244S.
12. Petro TM, Schwartz KM, Schmid MJ (1991). Natural and immune anti-tumor interleukin production and lymphocyte cytotoxicity during the course of dietary protein deficiency or excess. Nutr Res 11(6):679.
13. Gogos CA, Kalfarentzos FE, Zoumbos NC (1990). Effect of different types of total parenteral nutrition on T-lymphocyte subpopulation and NK cells. Am J Clin Nutr 51:119.
14. Karpeh MS, Kehne JA, Chois H, Ziegler MM (1987). Tumor immunogenicity, nutritional repletion and cancer. Surgery 102(2):283.
15. Barbul A, Lazaron SA, Efron DT, Wasserkrug HL, Effran G (1990). Arginine enhances wound healing and lymphocyte immune responses in humans. Surgery 108:331.

16. Kirk SJ, Barbul A (1990). Role of arginine in trauma, pepsis and immunity. J Parenter Enter Nutr 14:226S.
17. Daly JM, Reynolds J, Sigal RK, Shou J, Liberman MD (1990). Effect of dietary protein and amino acids on immune function. Crit Care Med 18(Suppl 2):S86.
18. Reynolds JV, Daly JM, Shou J, Sigal R, Ziegler MM, Naji A (1990). Immunologic effects of arginine supplementation in tumor-bearing and non-tumor-bearing hosts. Ann Surg 211(2):202.
19. Ratner S (1973). Enzymes of arginine and urea synthesis. Adv Enzymol 39:1-90.
20. Featherston WR, Rogers QR, Freedland RA (1973). Relative importance of kidney and liver in synthesis of arginine by the rat. Am J Physiol 224:127-129.
21. Windmueller HG, Spaeth AE (1981). Source and fate of circulating citrulline. Am J Physiol 241:473-480.
22. Rogers QR, Freedland RA, Symmons RA (1972). In vivo synthesis and utilization of arginine in the rat. Am J Physiol 223:236-240.
23. Perez GO, Epstein M, Rietberg B, et al. (1978). Metabolism of arginine by the isolated perfused rat kidney. Am J Physiol 4:376-380.
24. Rose WC (1937). The nutritive significance of the amino acids and certain related compounds. Science 86:298-300.
25. Borman A, Wood T, Black H, et al. (1946). The role of arginine in growth with some observations on the effect of arginic acid. J Biol Chem 166:585-594.
26. Nakagawa I, Takahashi T, Suzuki T, et al. (1963). Amino acid requirements of children: Minimal needs of tryptophan, arginine, histidine based on nitrogen balance method. J Nutr 80:305-310.
27. Rose WC (1949). Amino acid requirements of man. Fed Proc 8:546-552.
28. Levenson SM, Rettura G, Barbul A, et al. (1980). Citrulline replaces arginine as dietary essential in rats: Ornithine does not. Fed Proc 39:726, abstr. 2421.
29. Knopf RF, Conn JW, Fajans SS, et al. (1965). Plasma growth hormone response to intravenous administration of amino acids. J Clin Endocrinol 25:1140-1144.
30. Merimee TJ, Rabinowitz D, Riggs L (1967). Plasma growth hormone after arginine infusion: Clinical experiences. N Engl J Med 276:434-439.
31. Elsair J, Poey J, Rochiocioli P, et al. (1980). Effects de l'administration per os, a doses variables, d'aspartate d'arginine et de chlorhydrate d'arginine sur les taux d'hormone de croissance et d'acides gras libres du plasma chez l'enfant normal a jeun. Pathol Biol 28:639-644.
32. Isidori A, LoMonaco A, Cappa M (1981). Study of growth hormone release in man after oral administration of amino acids. Curr Med Res Opin 7:475-481.
33. Evain-Brion D, Donnadieu M, Roger M, et al. (1982). Simultaneous study of somatotrophic and corticotrophic pituitary secretions during ornithine infusion test. Clin Endocrinol 17:119-122.
34. Gourmelen M. Donnadieu M, Schimpff RM, et al. (1972). Effet du chlorohydrate d'ornithine sur le taux plasmatique de l'hormone de croissance (HGH). Ann Endocrinol 33:526-528.
35. Rakoff JS, Siver TM, Sinha YN, et al. (1973). Prolactin and growth hormone release in response to sequential stimulation by arginine and TRF. J Clin Endocrinol 37:641-644.
36. Dupre J, Curtis JD, Waddel RW, et al. (1968). Alimentary factors in the endocrine response to administration of arginine in man. Lancet 1:28-29.
37. Floyd JC Jr, Fajans SS, Conn JW, et al. (1966). Stimulation of insulin secretion by amino acids. J Clin Invest 45:1487-1502.
38. Fajans SS, Floyd JC Jr, Knopf RF, et al. (1967). Effect of amino acids and proteins on insulin secretion in man. Rec Prog Horm Res 23:617-662.
39. Palmer JP, Walter RM, Ensinck JW (1975). Arginine-stimulated acute phase of insulin and glucagon secretion. I. In normal man. Diabetes 24:735-740.

40. Utsumi M, Makimura H, Ishihara K, et al. (1979). Determination of immunoreactive somatostatin in rat plasma and responses to arginine, glucose and glucagon infusion. Diabetologia 17:319–323.
41. Weir CG, Samols E, Loo S, et al. (1979). Somatostatin and pancreatic polypeptide secretion: Effects of glucagon, insulin and arginine. Diabetes 28:35–40.
42. Imms FJ, London DR, Neame RLB (1969). The secretion of catecholamines from the adrenal gland following arginine infusion in the rat. J Physiol (Lond) 200:55–56.
43. Seifter E, Rettura G, Barbul A, et al. (1978). Arginine: An essential amino acid for injured rats. Surgery 84:224–230.
44. Chyun JH, Griminger P (1984). Improvement of nitrogen retention by arginine and glycine supplementation and its relation to collagen synthesis in traumatized mature and aged rats. J Nutr 114:1697–1704.
45. Barbul A, Sisto DA, Wasserkrug HL, et al. (1981). Metabolic and immune effects of arginine in post-injury hyperalimenation. J Trauma 21:970–974.
46. Barbul A, Wasserkrug HL, Penberthy LT, et al. (1984). Optimal levels of arginine in maintenance intravenous hyperalimentation. J PEN 8:281–284.
47. Pui YML, Fisher H (1979). Factorial supplementation with arginine and glycine on nitrogen retention and body weight gain in the traumatized rat. J Nutr 109:240–246.
48. Elsair J, Poey J, Issad H, et al. (1978). Effect of arginine chlorhydrate on nitrogen balance during the three days following routine surgery in man. Biomed Express 29:312–317.
49. Rettura G, Stratford F, Levenson SM, et al. (1983). Improved wound healing, anti-catabolic and thymotropic actions of supplemental ornithine, 17th Mid-Atlantic Reg. Meeting, American Chemical Society, April 6–8.
50. Eagle H (1959). Amino acid metabolism in mammalian cell cultures. Science 130:432–437.
51. Tytell AA, Neuman RE (1960). Growth response of stable and primary cell cultures to l-ornithine, l-citrulline, and l-arginine. Exp Cell Res 20:84–91.
52. Barbul A, Sisto DA, Wasserkrug HL, et al. (1981). Arginine stimulates lymphocyte immune response in healthy humans. Surgery 90:244–251.
53. Chisari FV, Nakamura M, Milich DR, et al. (1985). Production of two distinct and independent hepatic immunoregulatory molecules by the perfused rat liver. Hepatology 5:735–743.
54. Christie GS, de Munk FG, Madsen NP, et al. (1971). The effects of an arginine antagonist on stimulated human lymphocytes in culture. Pathology 3:139–144.
55. Klein D, Morris DR (1978). Increased arginase activity during lymphocyte mitogenesis. Biochem Biophys Res Commun 81:199–204.
56. Bachrach U, Menashe J, Faber J, et al. (1981). Polyamine biosynthesis and metabolism in transformed human lymphocytes. Adv Polyamine Res 3:259–274.
57. Pasquali JJ, Urlacher A, Storck D (1983). La stimulation lymphocytaire in vitro par le pokeweed mitogene chez les sujets normaux et les sujets denutris: Influence des sels d'ornithine. Pathol Biol 31:191–194.
58. Moriguchi S, Mukai K, Hiraoka I, et al. (1987). Functional changes in human lymphocytes and monocytes after in vitro incubation with arginine. Nutr Res 7:719–729.
59. Hibbs JB Jr, Taintor RR, Vavrin Z (1987). Macrophage cytotoxicity: Role for l-arginine deiminase and imino nitrogen oxidation to nitrite. Science 235:473–476.
60. Schneider E, Kamoun PP, Migliore-Samour D, et al. (1987). A new enzymatic pathway of citrullinogenesis in murine hemopoietic cells. Biochem Biophys Res Commun 144:829–835.
61. Albina JE, Mills C, Barbul A, et al. (1988). Arginine metabolism in wounds. Am J Physiol 254:E459.
62. Hibbs JJ Jr, Vavrin Z, Taintor RR (1987). L-Arginine is required for expression of the activated macrophage effector mechanism causing selective metabolic inhibition of target cells. J Immunol 138:550–565.

63. Kriegbaum H, Benninghoff B, Hacker-Shahin B, et al. (1987). Correlation of immunogenicity and production of ornithine by peritoneal macrophages. J Immunol 139:899–904.
64. Droge W, Benninghoff B, Lehmann V (1987). Tumor necrosis factor augments the immunogenicity and the production of l-ornithine by peritoneal macrophages. Lymphokine Res 6:111–117.
65. Janicke R, Droge W (1985). Effect of l-ornithine on proliferative and cytotoxic T-cell responses in allogeneic and syngeneic mixed leukocyte cultures. Cell Immunol 92:359–365.
66. Droge W, Mannel W, Falk V, et al. (1985). Suppression of cytotoxic T lymphocyte activation by l-ornithine. J Immunol 134:3379–3383.
67. Susskind BM, Chandrasekaran J (1987). Inhibition of cytolytic T lymphocyte maturation with ornithine, arginine and putrescine. J Immunol 139:905–912.
68. Barbul A, Rettura G, Levenson SM, et al. (1977). Arginine: Thymotropic and wound healing promoting agent. Surg Forum 28:101–103.
69. Rettura G, Padawer J, Barbul A, et al. (1979). Supplemental arginine increases thymic cellularity in normal and murine sarcoma virus-inoculated mice and increases the resistance of mice to the murine sarcoma virus tumor. JPEN 3:409–416.
70. Barbul A, Wasserkrug HL, Seifter E, et al. (1980). Immunostimulatory effects of arginine in normal and injured rats. J Surg Res 29:228–235.
71. Barbul A, Wasserkrug HL, Sisto DA, et al. (1980). Thymic and immune stimulatory actions of arginine. JPEN 4:446–449.
72. Barbul A, Rettura G, Levenson SM, et al. (1978). Thymotropic actions of arginine, ornithine and growth hormone. Fed Proc 37:264, abstr. 282.
73. Rettura G, Barbul A, Levenson SM, et al. (1979). Citrulline does not share the thymotropic properties of arginine and ornithine. Fed Proc 38:289, abstr. 343.
74. Barbul A, Rettura G, Wasserkrug HL, et al. (1982). Thymotropic actions of arginine and metabolites. J Am Coll Nutr 1:115, abstr. 44.
75. Rettura G, Barbul A, Levenson SM, et al. (1982). Putrescine does not have the thymotropic properties of ornithine and arginine. J Am Coll Nutr 1:423, abstr. 110.
76. Barbul A, Rettura G, Wasserkrug HL, et al. (1983). Wound healing and thymotropic effects of arginine: A pituitary mechanism of action. Am J Clin Nutr 37:786–794.
77. Madden HP, Barbul A, Knud-Hansen JP, et al. (1987). Prolonged thymotropic effect after one week of oral arginine supplementation. Fed Proc 46:588, abstr. 1586.
78. Barbul A, Sisto DA, Wasserkrug HL, et al. (1981). Arginine stimulates thymic immune function and ameliorates the obesity and the hyperglycemia of genetically obese mice. JPEN 5:492–495.
79. Barbul A, Wasserkrug HL, Yoshimura NN, et al. (1984). High arginine levels in intravenous hyperalimentation abrogate posttraumatic immune suppression. J Surg Res 36:620–624.
80. Barbul A, Fishel RS, Shimazu S, et al. (1985). Intravenous hyperalimentation with high arginine levels improves wound healing and immune function. J Surg Res 31:328–334.
81. Rettura G, Levenson SM, Barbul A, et al. (1982). Supplemental arginine and ornithine promote allograft rejection. 183rd Meeting of the American Chemical Society, AGFD, abstr. 11.
82. Saito H, Trocki O, Wang S, et al. (1987). Metabolic and immune effects of dietary arginine supplementation after burn. Arch Surg 122:784–789.
83. Madden HP, Breslin RJ, Wasserkrug HL, et al. (1988). Stimulation of T cell immunity enhances survival in peritonitis. J Surg Res 44:658–663.
84. Weisburger JH, Yamamoto RS, Glass RM, et al. (1969). Prevention by arginine glutamate of the carcinogenicity of acetamide in rats. Toxicol Appl Pharmacol 14:163–175.
85. Takeda Y, Tominaga T, Tei N, et al. (1975). Inhibitory effect of l-arginine on growth of rat mammary tumors induced by 7,12-dimethyl(a)anthracene. Cancer Res 35:2390–2393.

86. Cho-Chung YS, Clair T, Bodwin JS, et al. (1980). Arrest of mammary tumor growth in vivo by l-arginine: Stimulation of NAD-dependent activation of adenylate cyclase. Biochem Biophys Res Commun 95:1306–1313.
87. Burns RA, Milner TA (1981). Effect of arginine, ornithine and lysine on 7,12-dimethylbenzanthracene mammary tumors. Fed Proc 40:948, abstr. 4074.
88. Burns RA, Milner JA (1984). Effect of arginine on the carcinogenicity of 7,12-dimethyl-(a)anthracene and N-methyl-N-nitrosurea. Carcinogenesis 5:1539–1542.
89. Beard HH, Givens E (1944). Further observations upon the effect of subcutaneous injection of amino acids and creatine upon the appearance, growth and regression of the Emge sarcoma in rats. Exp Med Surg 2:125–128.
90. Levy HM, Montanez G, Feaver ER, et al. (1954). Effect of arginine in tumor growth in rats. Cancer Res 14:198–200.
91. Nakanishi K (1969). Studies on tumor growth inhibition of arginine imbalanced diets. Med J Osaka Univ 21:193–204.
92. Nakagawa I, Takahashi T, Suzuki T, et al. (1972). Effects of diets imbalanced by an excess of l-arginine, l-ornithine and l-citrulline on experimental tumor metastases. J Kansai Med Sch 24:21–42.
93. Kojima R, Shimada K, Asano H (1973). Effects of oral administration of arginine on the tumor bearing mice. Exp Anim 22:237–242.
94. Seifter E, Barbul A, Levenson SM, et al. (1980). Supplemental arginine increases survival in mice undergoing local tumor excision. JPEN 5:589, abstr. 38.
95. Pryme IF (1977). The failure of growth of a mouse myeloma tumour during the course of oral administration of l-arginine-hydrochloride. Cancer Lett 1:177–182.
96. Milner JA, Stepanovich LV (1979). Inhibitory effect of dietary arginine on growth of Ehrlich ascites tumor cells in mice. J Nutr 109:489–494.
97. Chany C, Cerutti I (1981). Action inhibitrice du butyrate d'arginine sur le developpement de la tumeur 180/TG de Crocker chez les souris swiss. CR Acad Sci (Paris) 293:367–369.
98. Chany C, Cerutti I, Mace B (1983). Effect of coordinated therapeutic assays using C parvum, interferon and arginine butyrate on spontaneous disease and survival of akr mice. Int J Cancer 32:379–383.
99. Seifter E, Levenson SM, Mendecki J, et al. (1984). Lewis lung tumor: Anti-tumor action of supplemental arginine and vitamin A. 188th National Meeting, American Chemical Society, August 26–31, Philadelphia, Pennsylvania.
100. Tachibana K, Mukai K, Hiraoka I, et al. (1985). Evaluation of the effect of arginine-enriched amino acid solution on tumor growth. JPEN 9:428–434.
101. Reynolds JV, Zhang SM, Thom AK, et al. (1987). Arginine as an immunomodulator. Surg Forum 38:415–418.
102. Reynolds JV, Thom AK, Zeigler M, et al. (1988). Arginine, protein calorie malnutrition and cancer. J Surg Res 45:513–522.

4
Retinoids, Carotenoids, and Macrophage Activation

Ronald R. Watson and David L. Earnest
Arizona Health Sciences Center, University of Arizona College of Medicine, Tucson, Arizona

Rao H. Prabhala
Chicago College of Osteopathic Medicine, Downer's Grove, Illinois

INTRODUCTION

Epidemiological studies have indicated that even relatively mild vitamin A deficiency may be associated with increased infections and morbidity, particularly in infants and children, and that vitamin A deficiency is associated with a decreased immune response. Although mild xerophthalmia in school-age children of developing countries has been associated with clinically significant infections (1), there has been a tendency to place major emphasis on the eye-related problems rather than the implications of the systemic manifestations. The need for studies on the relationship between malnutrition, in particular vitamin A deficiency, and infection in addition to the exclusive implementation of stategies focusing on vaccines, antibiotics, and oral rehydration (2) is of current interest (3). These studies are timely, as methods to study the mechanism of interaction become available. Thus, recent data in an experimental animal model show that normal antibody is impaired even in the early stages of vitamin A deficiency (4). In a related model, vitamin A deficiency was found to decrease natural killer (NK) cell activity and interferon (IFN) production (5). In humans, vitamin A administration has been found to reduce mortality and morbidity from severe measles (6), which is interesting in light of the recent emergence of significant measles infections in the pediatric population in the United States. Excess intake of vitamin A may also depress the immune response to infecting agents; the mechanism is not understood, although it has been suggested that downregulation of nuclear receptors or toxic levels of retinol esters in the blood may be involved (7).

Table 1 Some Factors Altering Anticancer Host Defenses

Enhancement	Suppression
1. Vitamin A (retinoids)	1. Severe nutrient deficiencies
2. Moderate protein or calorie deficiency (animal studies)	2. Emotional stress
3. Drugs (thymosin, etc.)	3. Aging (> 40 years)
4. Selenium and vitamin E	4. Infancy (0–2 years)
5. Exercise	5. Severe burns
	6. Drugs (corticosteroids, cytotytic etc.)
	7. Tumor burden
	8. Vitamin A deficiency

Recently there has been considerable interest in β-carotene, which has immunomodulatory activity as well as being a precursor of vitamin A, which is a cancer-preventing agent. Long-term ingestion of β-carotene has been associated with the decreased incidence of cancer (8,9) and a dose relationship between β-carotene ingestion and plasma level has been established in humans (10). While it seems highly likely that cancer risk assessment needs to be carried out at the micronutrient level in different populations and will involve antioxidant vitamins and β-carotene (11), the relevant parameters of deficiency remain to be unambiguously identified. The studies presented here indicate that detailed analysis of these issues is beginning to come within reach of present laboratory methods.

A variety of dietary components are possible inhibitors of human cancer initiation or promotion. Two related groups include: (a) retinoids, particularly retinol or preformed vitamin A; and (b) carotenoids, provitamin A compounds. The latter group includes β-carotene, which can be convered into retinol in vivo, and others, like canthaxanthin, which cannot. However, all have immunomodulatory effects at physiological levels which may affect cancer growth.

Vitamin A, its precursors, and synthetic derivatives have been reported to affect various aspects of the cellular and humoral immune response. These compounds stimulate or inhibit the immune response depending upon the compound, dosage, and method of administration. Retinoids may act independently or in concert with other immunoaltering conditions to suppress or stimulate host defenses (Table 1). A detailed description of these effects has been reviewed elsewhere by Watson and Rybski (12). In this chapter, we shall briefly summarize the literature, describe recent findings in our laboratory, and suggest areas for special emphasis.

IN VITRO EFFECTS OF RETINOIDS AND CAROTENOIDS ON CELL FUNCTIONS

In vitro studies allow rapid delineation of the direct effects of micronutrients on macrophages or lymphocytes. There has recently developed a wide interest in the immunological and antitumor actions of the natural precursor to retinol, β-carotene. β-Carotene and other carotenoids that can be metabolic precursors of retinol are known as provitamin A. β-Carotene enhances resistance to immunogenic tumors (13–15). This may occur via a stimulatory action on the growth of the thymus gland and resulting enhancement of T-cell functions (12).

We have previously isolated human peripheral blood monocytes and stimulated them in vitro with a number of retinoids and carotenoids and measured the production of tumor cytolytic factor (TCF) (16) and modification of T-cell subsets (17). When β-carotene was introduced into these cultures, incubated for 2 days, and culture supernatants assayed, there was a significant increase in their cytolytic activity. We have tested a number of tumor cell lines with β-carotene–stimulated monocyte culture supernatants from different volunteers, and have shown that in all cases there was a significant amount of TCF found by killing of the tumor cells in vitro (16). However, there was a difference in the cytolytic activity for each person, ranging from 35–85%. The same results were obtained with the murine macrophage cell line J774A.1. This line was maximally stimulated by β-carotene at a very low concentration (10^{-12} M). When we tested the effect of other retinoids on TCF production by either human monocytes or J774A.1, little cytolytic activity was produced. Therefore, we conclude that β-carotene is capable of stimulating the production of a factor which kills up to 80% of tumor cells in vitro (16). Preliminary data suggest that TCF is not tumor necrosis factor type alpha (TNF-α) (16).

To further investigate these in vivo effects of β-carotene, we did in vitro studies much as previously reported (16,17). For example, β-carotene added to tissue culture media containing human lymphoid cells caused release of a cytokine with anti–cancer cell activity (16) or led to expansion of cells with markers of activation (17). We recognize that β-carotene is not soluble in aqueous media, but is in ethanol. Therefore, we approached getting β-carotene to cells in culture as described (16,17), which is similar to the method used by Hazuka et al. (19), who added β-carotene to cancer cells in vitro. We dissolved β-carotene in ethanol, filter sterilized it, and then diluted the ethanol–β-carotene in aqueous tissue culture media (16,17). Control media was ethanol diluted in aqueous media. Although we have not investigated the state of β-carotene in media after ethanol treatment, some appears to be in suspension as

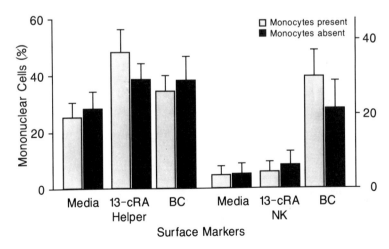

Figure 1 Human peripheral blood lymphoid cells were incubated with BC (β-carotene), 13-cRA (13-*cis* retinoid acid), or media as described elsewhere. Monocytes were removed by adherence prior to incubation in some cultures. They were stained and measured by flow cytometry (17).

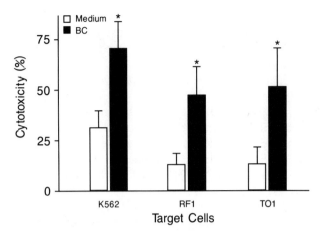

Figure 2 Natural killer cell cytotoxicity for three tumor cell lines was carried out with in vitro exposure of human peripheral blood effector cells to BC or media for 24 hr prior to assay.

small particles of β-carotene, whereas some may be more solubly associated with ethanol droplets (16,17; J. Olson, personal communication). However, β-carotene treated in this fashion does interact with cells in culture (16,17,19). As shown in Figure 1, β-carotene and 13-cRA (13-*cis* retinoic acid) has little effect on the number of cells with markers for T-helper cells. However, β-carotene stimulated the percentage of cells with NK cell markers.

We further studied the action of β-carotene on NK cell numbers by determining that it stimulated NK cell activity in vitro (Fig. 2). There was increased NK activity to three tumor cell lines after lymphocyte exposure to β-carotene, including K562, the accepted target of NK cells. As shown in Figure 3, total T cells, T-helper, and T-suppressor cells did not change significantly. Such increases do not occur with all

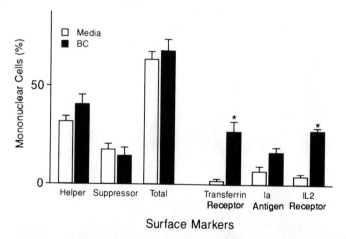

Figure 3 Peripheral blood lymphoid cells were incubated with BC and counted as described elsewhere (17).

lymphoid subsets after short-term exposure in vitro to β-carotene, just as they do not in vivo (18). However, activated cells, those with interleukin 2r (Il-2r) and transferrin receptors on their surface, did significantly increase (Fig. 3).

IN VIVO EFFECTS OF CAROTENOIDS ON LYMPHOCYTES

Carotenoids, especially β-carotene, appear to have a major inhibitory effect on cancer incidence. Epidemiological studies have demonstrated a positive correlation between β-carotene intake and lower cancer risk (14,15).

The postulated anticancer mechanisms for carotenoids include acting as antioxidants by quenching free radicals (20). Modification of host immune defenses may also be an important activity of carotenoids which could play a role in their anticancer effects (12). β-Carotene in vivo can stimulate rat lymphocyte mitogenesis (22). Thus, it may be possible to exploit immunomodulatory effects of carotenoids for the treatment of specific diseases. For instance, β-carotene increases human NK cells (18) and T-helper cell numbers (21). Restoring the number of these cells may be useful in acquired immunodeficiency syndromes such as (AIDS) in which immune cells are in low numbers and defective in mature. Clinical trials with carotenoids to stimulate activation of helper cells, macrophages, and NK cells in AIDS patients would be of great interest owing to their low toxicity. Thus, immunomodulation may be an exciting tool to stimulate the cellular immune system and to understand the role of these dietary agents in cancer prevention.

The percentage of lymphoid cells with surface markers for T-helper and NK cells, and cells with IL-2 and transferrin receptors were significantly and substantially increased in peripheral blood mononuclear cells collected from older human adult volunteers after supplementation of 30 mg/day or more of β-carotene for 2 months. The increase in the percentage of cells with markers of NK cells and in expression of IL-2 receptors was dose dependent (18). The plasma levels of β-carotene were also elevated significantly; however, there was no increase in the amount of retinol present in plasma (Table 2). This indicates that immunomodulation induced by β-carotene may be due to the carotenoid rather than an increased amount, and hance actions, of vitamin A. These results support the role of immunostimulation as a potential mechanism of action of β-carotene with cancer prevention potential. Furthermore, we have found that different carotenoids produce different effects on lymphocyte subpopulations. For example, 13-*cis* retinoic acid caused an increase in T-helper cell surface markers but had no effect on NK cell markers (23).

Table 2 Effects of 2 Months of β-Carotene Supplementation on the Percentage of Various Lymphoid Subsets in Blood of Aged Adults[a]

β-Carotene (mg)	Percentage of lymphoid cell				
	Total T cells (CD3$^+$)	T-helper (CD4$^+$)	T-suppressor (CD8$^+$)	NK cells (CD16$^+$)	Activated lymphocytes (IL-2r$^+$)
0	77.0 ± 10.0	35.0 ± 2.6	19.3 ± 2.1	10.3 ± 3.6	3.8 ± 3.8
45	73.3 ± 9.1	40.5 ± 6.2	16.3 ± 2.9	22.8 ± 5.5	20.5 ± 5.5[a]

[a]Significantly different from unsupplemented controls (p = 0.05).
Source: Modified from Ref. 7, used with permission.

We undertook a pilot study of the clinical and immunological effects of 60 mg/day of β-carotene given for 4 months to 11 HIV-infected (human immunodeficiency virus) patients with follow-up for 2 months after β-carotene was stopped. Patients were in three groups based on T-helper cells, per microliter: 200 (group 1, n = 3, all on azidothymidine, AZT); 200–400 (group 2, n = 4); and 400 (group 3, n = 4). No toxic effects of β-carotene were seen. For patients in groups 2 and 3, after 3 and 4 months of β-carotene therapy there were increases in the lymphocyte marker Leu11b and in IL-2 and transferrin receptors. These increases returned to baseline 2 months after β-carotene was discontinued (42). Mice with a retrovirus infection causing AIDS had increased melanoma growth until treated with canthoxanthin, a carotenoid not converted into vitamin A (43). Canthaxanthin increased NK activity.

DIETARY EFFECTS IN VIVO OF RETINOIDS ON LYMPHOCYTES AND MACROPHAGES

Deficiency in dietary vitamin A reduces macrophage-mediated phagocytosis, mitogen-induced lymphocyte proliferation, delayed-type hypersensitivity reactions, and serum immunoglobulin levels in animals (24). It also leads to a reduction in the size and cellularity of the thymus, spleen, and bursa of Fabricius (25,26). Dietary replenishment for 3 days returned peripheral blood lymphocyte number and the proliferative response to normal (27). In humans, vitamin A deficiency has been reported to reduce the number of peripheral blood lymphocytes without reduction in serum immunoglobulin levels (24).

However, high intakes of vitamin A and their effects should receive more attention and study. Vitamin A in high concentration may directly affect lymphocyte growth or maturation. In addition, it may alter functions of immunoregulatory organs. For example, the thymus size of vitamin A–supplemented mice increased, although production of thymic factors needs to be studied in both animals and humans (12). Dietary supplementation with vitamin A at concentrations greater than necessary for the health of the animal has been reported to increase the rate of mouse skin homograft rejection (28), host-versus-graft reactivity (29), and reverse postburn immunosuppression (30). Repletion also stimulated alveolar macrophage-mediated tumoricidal activity, phagocytosis (31), and delayed-type hypersensitivity (32). These effects may be dose dependent, however, as the increased rate of induction of cytolytic T cells reported by Glaser and Lotan (33) was seen with moderate dosage, whereas high dietary vitamin A suppressed cytolytic T-cell induction. Retinol injected intramuscularly blocked humoral and cellular immunosuppression induced by cyclophosphamide and prednisolone of murine lymphocytes (34). In humans, high dietary vitamin A increased T-cell mitogenesis by lung cancer patients (35) and reversed postoperative immunosuppression (36).

We have found that high dietary intakes (400,000–650,000 IU/kg diet) of vitamin A (retinyl palmitate, RP) modified the functions of peritoneal macrophages (37). Macrophages from mice fed high dietary retinyl palmitate showed higher tumoricidal activities than those from controls. In vitro tumoricidal activity of macrophages increased with increasing content of retinyl palmitate in the diets, reaching 30% lysis by macrophages isolated from mice fed the highest retinyl palmitate diet (650,000 IU/kg). Such increases should have significant effects on any host defense system mediated by macrophage activation.

Interleukin 1 production by peritoneal macrophages can be stimulated by incubation with lipopolysaccharide, and its release assessed by measuring the proliferation of normal mouse thymocytes in vitro. Production of interleukin 1 in vitro showed about a twofold increase using cells from mice fed the highest RP diet compared to controls. Additionally, these macrophages showed an increased ability to phagocytose both nonopsonized and opsonized sheep red blood cells (SRBCs) when compared to controls.

We also found that a high dietary intake of retinyl palmitate (RP) modified both function and morphology of fixed tissue macrophages or Kupffer cells in rat liver. In these studies, both female BN/BiRij and male Sprague-Dawley rats were loaded orally with RP (125,000 IU/kg/dry) for 3 weeks to achieve a hepatic concentration of approximately 7000 μg/g liver. Standard blood tests reflecting liver function were not significantly altered by vitamin A loading, and no significant change in morphology of hepatic parenchymal cells was evident by either light or electron microscopy. In contrast, the hepatic fat- or vitamin A-storing cells were markedly enlarged by the retained retinyl esters (Fig. 4). The Kupffer cells were also significantly different and showed electron microscopic features compatible with cell activation. These included apparent expansion of the cell plasma membrane with prominent micropseudopods and the presence of large phagocytic vacuoles and also wormlike bodies in the cytoplasm (Fig. 5).

The effects of excess hepatic vitamin A on Kupffer cell phagocytic function was evaluated in vivo by measuring blood clearance rates for both colloidal carbon and ^{99m}technetium sulfur colloid. The plasma disappearance rate (k) was significantly more rapid and the $t_{1/2}$ significantly shorter ($p < 0.05$) for these particulate test substances in the vitamin A-loaded animals than in the controls (Table 3). Moreover, a significantly larger amount of the ^{99m}technetium sulfur colloid was retained in the liver in contrast to spleen in the animals treated with retinyl palmitate. This latter observation demonstrates that the enhanced blood clearance of the colloid test substance actually reflects increased phagocytosis by hepatic macrophages.

These morphological and in vivo functional data demonstrate that large amounts of retinyl palmitate activate or stimulate fixed liver macrophages. However, whether such stimulation of liver macrophages is beneficial or potentially harmful is not clear at this time. For example, previous studies in experimental animals show that activation of liver marophages by other immunostimulants such as glucan impart a protective effect against gram-negative bacteremia and also infection with viral hepatitis (38). In other studies, just the opposite was observed; i.e., pretreatment with a variety of reticuloendothelial stimulants, including zymosan, particulate glucan, and BCG, caused increased host susceptibility to certain drugs and to endotoxin (39). We have carried out preliminary studies on the effects of vitamin A loading on liver injury caused by exposure to small amounts of several well-known hepatotoxins. In these studies, we used the same dosage of retinyl palmitate reported above, which caused stimulation of hepatic macrophages but no significant biochemical or microscopic evidence of liver injury. We found that small doses of carbon tetrachloride, allyl alcohol, and endotoxin, which caused only minimal liver abnormality in control animals, produced extensive liver necrosis in animals pretreated with retinyl palmitate (40). Moreover, in these studies vitamin A loading also significantly potentiated liver toxicity of acetaminophen, a commonly used antipyretic analgesic drug.

The exact mechanism responsible for increased liver toxicity of certain xenobiotics in the presence of excess vitamin A is unknown. Conceivably, it may involve

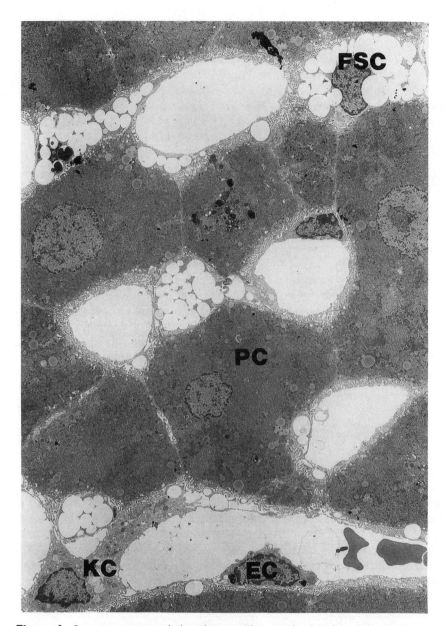

Figure 4 Low-power transmission electron micrograph of rat liver following treatment with a total cumulative dose of 380,000 IU retinyl palmitate administered orally over 3 weeks. Parenchymal cells (PC) and endothelial cells (EC) are essentially normal. Vitamin A– or fat–storing cells (FSC) are markedly enlarged by stored retinyl esters. Hepatic macrophages or Kupffer cells (KC) demonstrated morphological changes compatible with cell activation, which are better seen at higher magnification.

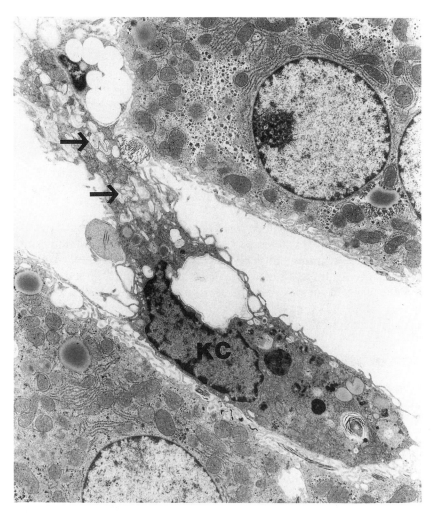

Figure 5 High-power transmission electron micrograph of hepatic Kupffer cells (KC) from the same rat liver as shown in Figure 6. The plasma membrane appears expanded and demonstrates numerous micropseudopods. There are prominent phagocytic vacuoles and also wormlike structures (arrows) in the cytoplasm. (Transmission electron micrographs for Figs. 6 and 7 were obtained by A.M. deLeeuw, Ph.D., at the TNO Institute for Experimental Gerontology, Rijswijk, the Netherlands.)

Table 3 Effect of Treatment with Retinyl Palmitate on Blood Half-Life ($t_{1/2}$) and Phagocytic Index (K) for Colloidal Carbon and Technetium Sulfur Colloid in the Rat

	Control	Retinyl palmitate
Carbon (n = 4)		
$t_{1/2}$ (min)	11.120 ± 0.650	6.500 ± 1.070[a]
K	0.027 ± 0.002	0.046 ± 0.008[a]
Sulfur colloid (n = 10)		
$t_{1/2}$ (min)	1.410 ± 0.010	1.320 ± 0.010[a]
K	0.212 ± 0.001	0.228 ± 0.003[a]

[a]Different from control, $p < 0.05$.

both potentiation of the primary effect of the toxin on liver parenchymal cells as well as some consequence of stimulation of liver macrophages acting either independently or in concert with a more generalized effect of vitamin A on the immune system. Our early data clearly show that excess hepatic vitamin A both stimulates fixed liver macrophages and also potentiates certain types of liver toxicity. Further evaluation of these effects and investigation for a possible causal relationship is certainly needed. Skeletal kinetics are currently under investigation (41).

These combined data suggest that it is critical to monitor the cellular immune system when attempting to achieve immunoenhancement with either retinoid or carotenoid supplementation.

CONCLUSIONS

In summary, altered cellular immune functions could play a major role in the prevention of carcinogenesis with hypovitaminosis A suppressing and hypervitaminosis A sometimes enhancing cellular immunity. Hypervitaminosis A may be able to elevate suppressed immune functions in the cancer patient for optimum functioning of host defenses to pathogens and tumor cells. The use of vitamin A, related retinoids, or carotenoids may inhibit initial malignant cell growth directly or via modulation of cellular immune functions (42).

ACKNOWLEDGMENTS

Research supported in part by grants from the National Institutes of Health, Bethesda, Maryland (CA-27502, AA-08037), Wallace Genetics, Inc., and Phi Beta Psi Sorority.

REFERENCES

1. West KP Jr, Howard GR, Sommer A. Vitamin A and infection: Public Health Implications. Ann Rev Nutr 1989; 9:63–86.
2. Keusch GT, Schrimshaw NS. Selective primary health care: Strategies for control of disease in the developing world XXII. Control of infection to reduce the prevalence of infantile and childhood malnutrition. Rev Infect Dis 1986; 8:272.
3. Vitamin A and malnutrition/infection complex in developing countries (editorial). Lancet 1990; 336(8727):1349.
4. Pasatiempo AMG, Taylor CE, Ross AC. Vitamin A status and the immune response to pneumococcal polysacchoride: Effects of age and early stages of retinol deficiency in rats. J Nutr 1990; 121:556–562.
5. Bowman TA et al. Vitamin A deficiency decreases natural killer cell activity and interferon production in rats. J Nutr 1990; 120:1264.
6. Vitamin A administration reduces mortality and morbidity from severe measles in population nonendemic for hypovitaminosis A. Nutr Rev 1991; 49:89–91.
7. Friedman A et al. Decreased resistance and immune response to Escherichia coli infection in chicks with low or high intakes of vitamin A. J Nutr 1991; 121:395.
8. Menkes MS, Comstock GW, Vuilleumier JP, Helsing KJ, Rider AA, Brookmeyer R. Serum β-carotene, vitamins A and E, selenium, and the risk of lung cancer. N Engl J Med 315: 1250–1254.
9. Fontham ET, Pickle LW, Haenszel W, Correa P, Lin Y, Falk RT. Dietary vitamins A and C and lung cancer risk in Louisiana. Cancer 1988; 62:2267–2273.

10. Ringer TV et al. Beta-carotene's effects on serum lipoproteins and immunologic indices in humans. Am J Clin Nutr 1991; 53:888.
11. Schmidt K. Antioxidant vitamins and β-carotene. Am J Clin Nutr 1991; 53:383S.
12. Watson RR, Rybski J. Immunomodulation by retinoids and carotenoids. In: Nutrition and Immunology. Chandra RK, ed. New York, Liss, 1988; pp 87-99.
13. Mathews-Roth M. Anti-tumor activity of beta-carotene, canthaxanthin and phytoene. Oncology 1982; 39:33.
14. Ritenbaugh C. Carotenoids and cancer. Nutr Today 1987; 1:14-19.
15. Bendich A. The safety of beta-carotene. Nutr Cancer 1988p; 11:207-214.
16. Abril RE, Rybski JA, Scuderi R, Watson RR. Beta-carotene stimulates human monocyte secretion of a novel tumoricidal cytokine. J Leuk Biol 1989; 45:255-261.
17. Prabhala RH, Maxey V, Hicks MJ, Watson RR. Enhancement of the expression of activation markers on human peripheral blood mononuclear cells by in vitro culture with retinoids and carotenoids. J Leuk Biol 1989; 45:249-254.
18. Watson RR, Prabhala RH, Plezia PM, Alberts DS. Effect of beta-carotene on lymphocyte subpopulation in elderly humans: Evidence for a dose response relationship. Am J Clin Nutr 1991; 53:90-94.
19. Hazuka MB, Edwards-Prasad J, Newman F, Kinzie JJ, Prasad KN. Beta-carotene induces morphological differentiation and decreases adenylate cyclase activity in melanoma cells in culture. J Am Coll Nutr 1990; 9:143-149.
20. Bendich A, Olson J. Biological actions of carotenoids. FASEB J 1989; 3:1927-1932.
21. Alexander M, Newmark H, Miller G. Oral beta-carotene can increase the number of OKT4 positive cells in human blood. Immunology 1985; 9:221-224.
22. Bendich A, Shapiro SS. Effect of beta-carotene and canthaxanthin on immune response of the rat. J Nutr 1986; 116:2254-2262.
23. Prabhala RH, Garewal HS, Hicks MJ, Sampliner RE, Watson RR. The effects of 13-cis-retinoic acid and beta-carotene on cellular immunity in humans. Cancer 1991; 67:1556.
24. Vyas D, Chandra R. Vitamin A and immunocompetence. In: Nutrition, Disease Resistance and Immune Function. R. Watson, ed. New York, Marcel Dekker, 1984, pp 325-356.
25. Krishnan S, Bhuyan U, Talwar G, Ramalingaswami V. Effect of vitamin A and protein-calorie undernutrition on immune responses. Immunology 1974; 27:383.
26. Bang B, Foard M, Bang F. The effect of vitamin A deficiency and Newcastle disease on lymphoid cell system in chickens. Proc Soc Exp Biol Med 1973; 143:1140.
27. Nauss K, Mark D, Suskind R. The effect of vitamin A deficiency on the in vitro cellular immune response of rats. J Nutr 1979; 109:1815.
28. Floersheim G, Bollog W. Accelerated rejection of homografts by vitamin A acid. Transplantation 1974; 14:564.
29. Malkovsky M, Edwards A, Hunt R, Palmer L, Medawar P. T-cell-mediated enhancement of host-versus-graft reactivity in mice fed a diet enriched in vitamin A acetate. Nature 1983; 302:338.
30. Fusi S, Kupper T, Green D, Ariyan S. Reversal of postburn immunosuppression by the administration of vitamin A. Surgery 1984; 96:330.
31. Tachibana K, Sone S, Tsubura E, Kishino Y. Stimulatory effect of vitamin A tumoricidal activity of rat alveolar macrophages. Br J Cancer 1984; 49:343.
32. Miller K, Maisey J, Malkovsky M. Enhancement of contact sensitization in mice fed a diet enriched in vitamin A acetate. Int Arch Allergy Appl Immunol 1984; 75:120.
33. Glaser M, Lotan R. Augmentation of specific tumor immunity against a syngeneic SV40-induced sarcoma in mice by retinoic acid. Cell Immunol 1979; 45:175.
34. Nuwayri-Salti N, Murad T. Immunologic and anti-immunosuppressive effects of vitamin A. Pharmacology 1985; 30:181.
35. Micksche M, Cerni C, Kokron O, Titscher R, Wrba H. Stimulation of immune response in lung cancer patients by vitamin A therapy. Oncology 1977; 34:234.

36. Cohen B, Gill G, Cullen P, Morris P. Reversal of postoperative immunosuppression in man by vitamin A. Surg Gynecol Obstetr 1979; 149:658.
37. Moriguchi S, Werner L, Watson RR. High dietary vitamin A and cellular immune functions in mice. Immunology 1985; 56:169–177.
38. DiLuzio N, Browder W, Wilhams D, McNamu R, Jones E. Relationship of Kupffer cell function to final outcome in murine models of lethal E. coli sepsis and viral hepatitis. *In*: Sinuosoidal Liver Cells. Knook DL, Wisse E, eds. Elsevier Biomedical Press, Amsterdam, 1982, pp 393–404.
39. DiLuzio NR, Al-Tuwaijri A, Williams DL, Ketahama A, Browder W. Modulation of host susceptibility to endotoxin by reticuloendothelial system stimulation or depression. *In*: Bacterial Endotoxins and Host Resistance. Agarwa MK, ed. Elsevier Biomedical Press, Amsterdam, 1980, p 71.
40. Sim WW, Earnest DL, Sipes IG, Chvapil M. Hypervitaminosis A potentiates liver toxicity of known hepatotoxins. Hepatology 1983; 3:857.
41. Forsyth KS, Watson RR, Gensler HL. Osteotoxicity after chronic dietary administration of 13-cis-retinoic acid, retinyl palmitate or selenium in mice exposed to tumor initiation and promotion. Life Sci 1989; 45(22):2149.
42. Prabhala RH, Garewal HS, Meyskens FL, Watson RR. Immunomodulation in humans caused by beta-carotene and vitamin A. Nutr Res 1990; 10:1473–1486.
43. Ampel NM, Garewal HS, Watson RR, Prabhala RH, Dols CL. A preliminary trial of beta-carotene in subjects with human immunodeficiency virus. J Nutr 1992; 122:March.
44. Huang D, Watson RR. The effects of canthaxanthin on JB/MS melanoma growth during retroviral pathogenesis induced by LP-BM5 murine leukemia virus. H. Friedman (ed.), Drugs of Abuse, Immunity and Immunodeficiency. Plenum Press, New York, 279–286, 1991.

5
Vitamin C and Phagocytes

Reto Muggli
F. Hoffmann–La Roche, Ltd., Basel, Switzerland

INTRODUCTION

The immune system is a highly sophisticated and flexible defense system, designed by nature to protect the body against pathogenic organisms and any other cell, tissue, organ, or particle which is characterized as nonself. The immune response is a coordinated process consisting of various functional components and varies according to the particular immunogenic challenge. Numerous mechanisms contributing to immunity have been identified, and different cells and tissues are involved in this task. Among them are polymorphonuclear neutrophils (PMNs), eosinophils, and monocytes-macrophages, which have among their functions the phagocytosis and destruction of microorganisms, immune complexes, and foreign particle matter and are, therefore, collectively called professional phagocytes. As these cells maintain high intracellular ascorbate levels against a considerable concentration gradient, it seems reasonable to assume an important role for ascorbate in their proper functioning. Supporting this notion are in vitro and animal studies on particular immune functions, plausible biochemical rationales, and clinical correlates with phagocyte ascorbate levels.

When searching for an involvement of ascorbate in phagocytosis and by that for an involvement of vitamin C in the protection against infections and diseases, the known biochemical functions of the vitamin may serve as guide (1). Vitamin C is an essential nutrient for humans and is required for the optimal functioning of cells, tissues, and organs. Vitamin C functions in one-electron transfer reactions as well as a cofactor in the hydroxylation of aromatic or aliphatic structures, such as occur in the metabolism of lysine, proline, or tyrosine, and facilitates the intestinal absorption of iron. As an important biological redox reagent it is a component of the overall antioxidant defense system which functions to protect against damage from reactive molecules such as free radicals, usually derived from oxygen. The importance of vitamin C as a water-soluble antioxidant has been reviewed by Bendich et al. (2).

Because immunity is an integral response of the organism, any specific effect of vitamin C must be separated from the general effect vitamin C has as an essential nutrient in all cells and tissues. In order to define such a specific role, it may help to review the well-defined metabolic and physiological phenomena which normally accompany the ingestion and degradation of a bacterium by phagocytes, a sequence involving signal recognition, chemotaxis, phagocytosis, secretion of oxygen radicals and hydrolytic enzymes, and finally bacterial killing. Therefore, this chapter will first focus on the known effects of ascorbate on individual phagocyte functions and then try to define more precisely a specific role of the vitamin in phagocytic leukocytes. A full discussion of the role of PMNs and monocytes-macrophages in biology and pathology may be found in certain reviews and textbooks (3–8).

ASCORBATE CONTENT AND UPTAKE BY RESTING AND STIMULATED PHAGOCYTES

Polymorphonuclear neutrophils and monocytes-macrophages are rich in ascorbate (9–12). In order to achieve intracellular concentrations of 1 mmol/L and more (13, 14) at physiological plasma ascorbate levels between 0.03 and 0.06 mmol/L, ascorbate has to be transported against a considerable concentration gradient. For gran-

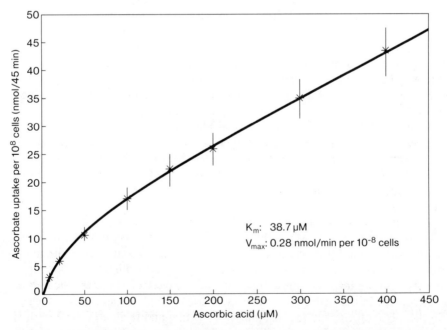

Figure 1 Uptake of ascorbate by PMNs, $\bar{x} \pm$ SEM, n = 8. (From Ref. 12; used with permission.)

ulocytes, a K_m of 38.7 μM, a V_{max} of 0.28 nmol/min per 10^8 cells was determined (Fig. 1); the corresponding values for mononuclear cells were K_m = 100 μM and V_{max} = 0.31 nmol/min per 10^8 cells (12). The uptake occurs primarily by a stereospecific active transport which is temperature- and energy-dependent (15) and is increased by various N-formyl peptides up to threefold (12). Uptake of dehydroascorbate (16–18) most probably serves no physiological role, since the K_m of the process is about 2 mM (19), well above normal circulating plasma levels of dehydroascorbate. Neutrophils store ascorbate in the reduced form (13).

Activation of neutrophils and monocytes with opsonized zymosan or phorbolmyristate acetate in vitro was found to cause no significant change in their total ascorbate (reduced and dehydroascorbate) concentration (13), quite in contrast to macrophages, which loose about half their ascorbate content following functional activation in vitro or after surgical or thermal trauma (14). However, the activation of neutrophils and monocytes can affect the proportion of dehydroascorbate relative to ascorbate; a consistent decrease of the latter, representing oxidation of approximately 30–40% of the ascorbate, was reported (20). The formylated tripeptide fMLP, however, gave no net oxidation, but about 20% of the total ascorbate was lost during the 2-hr incubation. Despite this fact, the authors considered it unlikely that ascorbate is released during stimulation or degranulation.

EFFECT OF VITAMIN C ON PHAGOCYTE FUNCTION

Polymorphonuclear neutrophils and monocytes-macrophages are highly specialized for the performance of their primary function, the phagocytosis and destruction of microorganisms. Phagocytosis refers to the physical act of engulfment, the process by which particles recognized as foreign are taken up by cells and sequestered in an intracellular vacuole (phagosome). The process is initiated by the attraction of the phagocyte to the site of microbial invasion under the influence of chemotactic factors (chemotaxis). Once contact between particle and phagocyte is established and the particle has been recognized as foreign, a cohesive force prevents their separation. This occurs largely through the action of particle-bound opsonins which bind to specific receptors on the surface of the phagocyte. Cellular pseudopods form, and the sequential and circumferential interaction between opsonins and receptors results in the movement of the phagocyte membrane around the particle until engulfment is complete. The vacuole retains its connection to the cell surface by a membraneous stalk for a short period; the opposed membranes fuse and the phagosome is set free in the interior of the cell.

Seconds after specific membrane perturbation by particulate or soluble stimuli and prior to significant particle ingestion, phagocytes exhibit a marked increase in metabolic activity, which has been termed metabolic or respiratory burst. Oxygen consumption is increased manyfold and much, if not all, of the extra oxygen consumed is converted to reactive oxygen metabolites. They are released into the phagosome and used for the killing of phagocytosed microorganisms, but they also are released to the outside of the cell, with the potential for attack on adjacent normal tissue, malignant cells, and invading organisms too large to be ingested, and to the inside of the cell (Fig. 2).

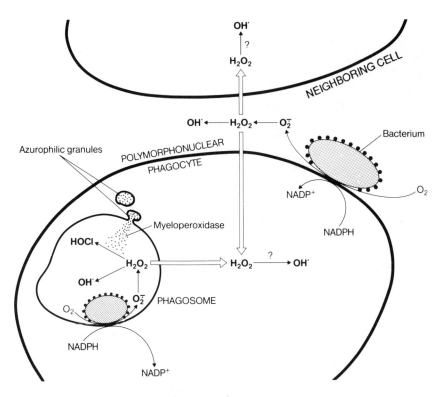

Figure 2 Schematic representation of the generation of reactive oxygen species by polymorphonuclear phagocytes. Membrane perturbation by microorganisms activates an oxidase system in the plasma membrane that converts oxygen into superoxide and hydrogen peroxide. The latter can be converted to the extremely reactive hydroxyl radical and in the presence of myeloperoxidase and chlorine to hypochlorous acid. The low reactivity allows H_2O_2 to pass intact through cell membranes and to be toxic at a distance from the site of its production.

Direct Effects of Vitamin C

Signal Reception and Signal Transduction

Phagocytes respond to stimulation with the activation of a transmembrane NADPH oxidase on the cytoplasmic side of the membrane which reduces oxygen in the extracellular fluid, or in the phagosome when the membrane is invaginated. The earliest evidence of stimulation yet described following the contact of the phagocyte with particulate or soluble stimuli is a change in the transmembrane potential and an increase in free cytoplasmic Ca^{2+}. Although the change in transmembrane potential and the rise in cytosolic free Ca^{2+} may be required, the reactions are not sufficient to induce respiratory burst activity. The metabolic steps of signal transduction then follow the classic pathway, culminating in the activation of protein kinase C, a Ca^{2+}-activated, phospholipid-dependent phosphorylating enzyme. Protein kinase C phosphorylates a variety of proteins, and is considered the immediate precursor enzyme to NADPH oxidase (21). Indeed, suppression of superoxide anion production by PMNs with an inhibitor of protein kinase C implies that protein kinase C may mediate the PMN respiratory burst (22,23).

A second phosphorylating enzyme involved in signal transduction in cells is cyclic AMP–dependent protein kinase. Although cyclic AMP levels of neutrophils increase transiently with stimulation, an effect that precedes superoxide anion production, cyclic AMP seems not to be required for triggering the respiratory burst (8). No change in cyclic GMP levels was observed on neutrophil stimulation (24, 25). Ascorbate caused significant accumulation of cyclic GMP in monocytes but not in PMNs (26).

Chemotaxis

Ascorbate has been found to be important for neutrophil chemotaxis and has been shown by several groups to be immunostimulatory in animals that can synthesize the vitamin as well as in humans, who cannot synthesize vitamin C (27). Incubation of phagocytes with ascorbic acid at neutral pH and at concentrations 10 to 50 times that of normal blood levels augmented both the in vitro random migration and chemotaxis of the cells to leukoattractants one- to threefold, however, without influencing their phagocytic capacity (28). Similar in vitro findings were reported by other researchers (26,27,29–31).

In vivo stimulation of neutrophil motility was observed after the ingestion of 1 g of vitamin C daily (32) or 2-6 g daily (33) by normal adult volunteers and following the intravenous injection of 1 g vitamin C in normal adults (34). Chemotaxis of PMNs could be enhanced by vitamin C supplementation (33) as well as in patients with Chédiak-Higashi syndrome (32) and in patients suffering from chronic granulomatous disease (27). These findings are similar to the reduction in mobility of macrophages from vitamin C–deficient guinea pigs (35).

Phagocytosis

Phagocytes internalize foreign material by invagination of their cell membrane and formation of a phagosome. Secretion of oxygen radicals and enzymes (e.g., the hydrolase lysozyme in PMNs) into the phagosome results in the killing of engulfed microorganisms and degradation of the ingested organic material. There are very few and controversial reports on the effect of ascorbate on phagocytosis. It was demonstrated more than 4 decades ago that deficiency of ascorbate resulted in impaired phagocytosis by leukocytes, a defect which could be reversed by the addition of exogenous ascorbate (36). Greendyke et al. (37) reported that ascorbate stimulated the uptake of sensitized erythrocytes in vitro, whereas others found no effect of physiological concentrations of ascorbate on the erythrophagocytosis by human neutrophils (28,31).

Respiratory Burst and Formation of Oxygen-Derived Reaction Products

Membrane perturbation by particulate and chemical stimuli (e.g., bacteria, aggregated immunoglobulin G, opsonized particles, complement, interleukin 1) of neutrophils, sensitized monocytes, macrophages, and eosinophils triggers the rapid uptake and utilization of oxygen. This respiratory burst of phagocytes is not involved in the generation of metabolic energy for phagocytosis. Rather, the oxygen uptake is due to the activation of a dormant plasma membrane enzyme, NADPH oxidase, which reduces oxygen in the extracellular fluid to superoxide anion (O_2^-). The enzyme is also involved in the production of O_2^- when the membrane is invaginated to form a phagosome (see Fig. 2). In activated neutrophils, after initiation of the respiratory burst, approximately 90% of the consumed oxygen can be linked to the generation of O_2^-. The concomitantly produced $NADP^+$ is regenerated by the hexose monophosphate shunt (HMPS) to NADPH.

The generation of hydrogen peroxide (H_2O_2) is considered crucial for the optimal bactericidal capability of phagocytes and is deduced from data obtained from cells of patients with chronic granulomatous disease of childhood (CGD). The PMNs from CGD patients lack the normal increments in O_2 consumption, H_2O_2 production, and monophosphate shunt activity (5), and show defective killing of ingested bacteria (38,39). In this particular syndrome, the ascorbate content of leukocytes is not significantly different from that of normal cells (10); however, whereas in normal PMNs phagocytosis induces a fall in ascorbate levels, this is not observed when CGD leukocytes are employed (40).

The initial product of the oxygen burst is superoxide anion. Two molecules may interact in a dismutation reaction with the formation of oxygen and H_2O_2:

$$O_2^- + O_2^- + 2H^+ \rightarrow O_2 + H_2O_2 \tag{1}$$

This spontaneous reaction occurs optimally at pH 4.8 (41) and is in all likelihood responsible for the formation of H_2O_2, since most studies of the pH within the phagosome have indicated it to be acidic (42–44), and the release of superoxide dismutase into the phagosome has not been demonstrated.

Although H_2O_2 is not by itself a radical, it is a reactive oxygen metabolite from which secondary oxygen reaction products may be derived (Fig. 3). The low reactivity allows H_2O_2 to pass intact through cell membranes and to be toxic at a distance from the site of its production.

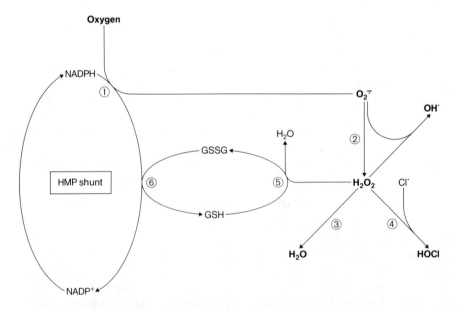

Figure 3 Pathways of oxygen metabolism in the respiratory burst. Enzymes catalyzing individual steps are as follows: 1. NADPH oxidase, 2. spontaneous reaction or superoxide dismutase, 3. glutathione peroxidase, 4. myeloperoxidase, 5. glutathione peroxidase, and 6. glutathione reductase.

The reactions leading to more aggressive microbicidal oxidants are as follows: Hydroxyl radicals (OH$^{\cdot}$) are produced in the iron-catalyzed Haber-Weiss reaction when hydrogen peroxide comes into contact with O_2^- in the presence of traces of iron salts:

$$O_2^- + H_2O_2 \rightarrow OH^{\cdot} + OH^- + O_2 \qquad (2)$$

and hypochlorous acid (HOCl) is formed through the myeloperoxidase-catalyzed oxidation of chlorine by H_2O_2:

$$Cl^- + H_2O_2 \rightarrow HOCl + H_2O \qquad (3)$$

Ascorbate is known to increase in vitro HPMS activity in resting and stimulated phagocytes (28,45–47). The proposed mechanism of the effect is the conversion of ascorbate to dehydroascorbate, which occurs rapidly upon stimulation, followed by, via the glutathione shuttle, the oxidation of NADPH by dehydroascorbate to NADP$^+$, the coenzyme in the rate-limiting initial step of the HMPS (45,48,49). NADP$^+$ is then regenerated in turn by HMPS to NADPH.

Bacterial Killing

Bacterial killing is achieved by reactive oxygen products and hydrolytic enzymes and takes place in the phagocytic vacuole or, in case a particle cannot be completely engulfed, in the cleft between the phagocyte membrane and the particle surface. Depending on the stimulus, O_2^- and the secondary products H_2O_2 and OH$^{\cdot}$ can be detected outside of the phagocyte. As NADPH oxidase is present in the plasma membrane of phagocytes, it becomes part of the wall of the phagosome and can thus discharge O_2^- directly into the vesicle from which hydrogen peroxide can be formed according to reaction 1.

In view of its low reactivity, it is unlikely that O_2^- or H_2O_2 are themselves responsible for bacterial killing, but they can be converted to powerful oxidants by two pathways, one of which utilizes myeloperoxidase. The enzyme is present in neutrophil azurophilic granules and juvenile mononuclear phagocytes. Once the phagocytic vacuole is formed, the azurophilic granules fuse with it and discharge the enzyme myeloperoxidase into the vesicle (see Fig. 2). Present evidence indicates that the function of myeloperoxidase is to catalyze the oxidation of Cl$^-$ by H_2O_2 to generate hypochlorous acid (reaction 3), a very potent agent whose antimicrobicidal activity is 50 times that of H_2O_2. Another lethal agent which utilizes superoxide is the hydroxyl radical, generated by reaction 2. Patients with an inborn error of deficiency of myeloperoxidase in their neutrophils show only minor decreases in resistance to infection, whereas chronic granulomatous disease results from a failure of the respiratory burst, and so the enzyme must be of less importance in bacterial killing than is the respiratory burst. However, neutrophils from these patients do kill bacteria more slowly than normal in vitro and myeloperoxidase may be of special importance in the protection against fungi such as *Candida albicans*.

The role of the ascorbic acid system in the microbicidal activity of intact leukocytes is only incompletely understood. The in vitro exposure of gram-negative organisms to ascorbic acid and H_2O_2 renders them more susceptible to the lytic action of lysozyme (50): on the other hand, ascorbic acid was also reported to have no effect on leukocytic microbicidal activity (51,52). A connection between the antimicrobial activity of phagocytes in vitro and the vitamin C status of healthy individuals could not be established (40,53). However, it was shown to exist in patients with Chédiak-Higashi syndrome, where the microbicidal activity of the PMN against *Staphylococcus aureus* could be restored by giving the patient 50 mg/kg body weight of ascorbic acid daily.

Indirect Effects of Vitamin C

The effect of vitamin C may also be an indirect one by protecting the antioxidant capacity of vitamin E, which is an immunoenhancing nutrient (54). Rats on a diet lacking vitamin E have defective neutrophil chemotaxis that may be corrected by vitamin E supplementation (55). Vitamin E is thought to play a protective role against oxidative damage to cytoplasmic organelles by scavenging oxygen radicals produced by neutrophils (56). The free radical–scavenging action by vitamin E is associated with the production of a vitamin E radical. Vitamin C reacts with the free radical of vitamin E and regenerates the reduced form, while being oxidized. The net result is a decrease in vitamin C and a maintenance of the antioxidant vitamin E level.

CLINICAL CORRELATES WITH PHAGOCYTE ASCORBATE LEVELS

Evidence on the immunostimulatory effect of ascorbate has been successively accumulated during the last couple of years (57,58). It is well established that ascorbate levels are decreased in human granulocytes in various diseases associated with impaired host defense against infection. After surgical and burning events, functions of phagocytes are severely curtailed, and the cells exhibit severely reduced ascorbate levels (14). Such patients often suffer from septic complications, which may in part be due to impaired granulocyte and macrophage functions (59,60). The level of this vitamin rapidly decreases in leukocytes following a viral infection (61–63), and returns to normal after recovery (62).

PUTATIVE ROLE OF VITAMIN C IN PHAGOCYTES

Theoretically, the high ascorbate concentrations in phagocytic leukocytes may serve the function of providing reducing equivalents for the generation of bactericidal products or, alternatively, to protect the cell from the toxic effects of its own bactericidal oxygen derivatives.

Ascorbate in the Generation of Bactericidal Products

There is general agreement that among the oxygen-derived reaction products, the hydroxyl radical $OH^\cdot$ is the most reactive species, which might explain why no enzyme systems involving it as a substrate exist, rather all efforts of the cell are directed at preventing $OH^\cdot$ formation. Hydroxyl radicals are formed in the iron-catalyzed Haber-Weiss reaction. To keep these reactions going, Fe^{3+} must be recycled to Fe^{2+}. This is achieved by the O_2^- radical. Alternatively, it has been proposed that in place of O_2^-, ascorbate performs as the reducing agent (64–68) and gives rise to a O_2^--independent formation of hydroxyl radicals in combination with H_2O_2 and a metal catalyst, and cause efficient killing of bacteria, fungi, and viruses (45,50,69–72).

$$\text{Ascorbate} + H_2O_2 \rightarrow \text{Dehydroascorbate} + OH^\cdot + OH^- \tag{4}$$

Winterbourn (65) presented evidence that ascorbate can be a major contributor to iron-catalyzed $OH^\cdot$ radical production in plasma taken from individuals before and after oral administration of ascorbic acid.

Various observations, however, seem to indicate that this mechanism does not operate in normal circumstances. It has been questioned whether normal body fluids contain suitable metal complexes to act as catalysts for the $OH^\cdot$ radical production. Furthermore, the role of ascorbate as a supplier of reducing equivalents in the generation of bactericidal products is questionable. Stimulation of human neutrophils with fMLP causes superoxide and hydrogen peroxide production without significant ascorbate oxidation, and if reaction 4 were the predominant mechanism for the production of $OH^\cdot$, its formation should be reduced in phagocytes with subnormal ascorbate content, which seems not to be the case. In addition, if ascorbate were to play an active role in the generation of bactericidal products by neutrophils, they would be expected to release ascorbate into the phagolysosome when stimulated; however, no significant loss of ascorbate from neutrophils treated with phorbol myristate or opsonized zymosan was detected (13,14,20). Hence, it is unlikely that a direct reaction between ascorbate and H_2O_2 is involved in the production of $HO^\cdot$ during stimulation and degranulation of phagocytes.

Ascorbate as a Protector of Self-Inflicted Free Radical Damage

NADPH oxidase functions vectorially with production of superoxide on the outside of the cell membrane, which will form the interior of the phagosome. Indeed, most of the superoxide and peroxide is produced on the external surface of the cells (73), suggesting that during the killing of phagocytosed organisms by oxygen-derived radicals, superoxide is produced only in the primary phagosome in close proximity to the ingested microorganism. Yet, activated neutrophils, macrophages, and other cells release O_2^- not only in the phagocyte vacuole, but also into their surrounding tissue fluid (74–77) where it can give rise to hydrogen peroxide and hydroxyl radicals and, as an inadvertent and unfortunate side effect of the process, even into the cytoplasm (78). Whereas tissue damage caused by extracellular reactive oxygen products from activated PMNs or "leakage" from resting PMNs is probably minimized by the efficient radical-trapping antioxidant activity of plasma (79), phagocytic leukocytes need to be protected from heavy intracellular and extracellular oxidative stress during phagocytosis. Neutrophils are susceptible to damage by self-produced oxidants, probably by damage to the plasma membrane (80–82).

Several systems have the potential to protect the cytosol against this danger; e.g., superoxide dismutase, which catalyzes the conversion of superoxide into hydrogen peroxide (83–86), catalase, which facilitates the degradation of hydrogen peroxide into water and oxygen (87–90), and the glutathione peroxidase system, which reduces hydrogen peroxide to water (91–94) (indeed, neutrophils deficient in glutathione reductase activity are much more rapidly inactivated during phagocytosis than normal cells, presumably because hydrogen peroxide can easily diffuse out of the phagocytic vacuole into the cell cytoplasm, and reduced glutathione cannot be regenerated for glutathione peroxidase activity), and the ascorbate redox system.

Reduced ascorbate reacts readily with O_2^- and may therefore function, like superoxide dismutase, in the protection against superoxide toxicity (95–97); even more rapid is the reaction with $OH^{\cdot}$ (98). In both cases, ascorbate is oxidized to dehydroascorbate. Ascorbic acid inhibited the myeloperoxidase from isolated rabbit leukocytes (99) and the myeloperoxidase-mediated iodination in vitro (51,52,100–102) and following ingestion of 2-3g ascorbate (33) or intravenous injection of 1 g ascorbate (34). Therefore, ascorbic acid appears to inhibit the functional activity of the peroxidase in PMNs, thus preventing potential unwanted tissue damage by this enzyme.

Though Winterbourn and Vissers (20) concluded that intracellular ascorbate oxidation is not a necessary accompaniment of superoxide production, it would be expected that the capacity to regenerate oxidized ascorbate by ascorbate reductase may be a determinant of cell capacity to inactivate oxidants and free radicals. In agreement with this notion is the finding of Stankova et al. (103) that PMNs deficient in catalase show an increased uptake and reduction of dehydroascorbate. Apparently, through adaptive regulation, the function served by catalase in intact cells is compensated by ascorbate and dehydroascrobate reductase in acatalasemic neutrophils.

Similarly, granulocytes from a majority of chronic granulocytic leukemic donors have subnormal capacity for ascorbate uptake and reduction, along with decreased resistance to injury by the oxidants and free radicals produced during X irradiation (104). The function of glutathione deficient PMNs is rapidly impaired by oxidants and free radicals generated during phagocytosis (105). More direct evidence is provided by the observation that dehydroascorbate-reducing activity is one of the parameters contributing to the disparity between mature blood neutrophils and lymphocytes in resistance to oxidant and free radical injury following exposure to ionizing radiation (106).

Oberritter et al. (14) reasoned that PMNs needed no protection during or after phagocytosis, since they perish after phagocytosis (107). Therefore, at least in PMNs, ascorbic acid may only play a role in processes preceding phatocytosis, helping the cell to stay viable until it is needed at sites of inflammation and infection. During phagocytosis ascorbic acid is required to maintain important functions, but cell death is not inhibited. Macrophages, however, live much longer and can phagocytose during their whole life span by resynthesis of lysosomal enzymes (107). Macrophages need, therefore, a protecting system not only prior to but also during and after phagocytosis to scavenge damaging radicals originating from phagocytosis. The role of ascorbate in that system is reflected by its high ascorbate content, which is about twice as high as it is in neutrophils and monocytes (13), and by the protection afforded in vitro to rabbit macrophages from phagocytosis-dependent injuries (108). Hence, the high ascorbate concentrations compared to neutrophils and monocytes and the strong consumption during macrophage phagocytosis may be due to a protective action against auto-oxidation. The intracellular pool of ascorbic acid can be replenished by uptake of ascorbate in the wake of phagocytosis (12).

A condition in which insufficient protection of phagocytes may occur is rheumatoid arthritis. Neutrophils and monocytes of patients with rheumatoid arthritis exhibit highly reduced intracellular ascorbate levels as compared to healthy controls. These cells are presumably exposed to chronic challenge, which results in a permanent generation of toxic oxygen radicals, leading to a constant consumption of ascorbic acid in chronic inflammatory events. The diminished chemotaxis of PMNLs in rheumatic patients could be a consequence of the reduced ascorbate levels (109–111).

In view of insufficient radical-scavenging systems, the release of these oxygen species into the extracellular pool (76) damages joints as well as the white blood cells themselves, compromising their viability (66).

It may be legitimate to ask if the antioxidant activity of ascorbate does not interfere with the oxygen-dependent killing capacity of phagocytes. The results presented by Anderson (112,113) demonstrate that ascorbate mediates efficient neutralization of phagocyte-derived, potentially harmful extracellular oxidants, whereas the intracellular and presumably intraphagocytic generation of antimicrobial oxidants remains intact. Thus, ascorbate can decrease the damaging effects of the products of the oxidative burst without decreasing the intracellular concentration of bactericidal molecules; the generation of intracellular reactive oxidants is even potentiated in vitro by extracellular ascorbate.

In summary, the high cellular concentration of ascorbate brought about by a stereospecific active transport and its disease-related fluctuations in phagocytes suggests a role for the vitamin in the immune process. Evidence published to date shows the greatest effect of ascorbate on phagocytic cell mobility and chemotaxis; its effect on bactericidal activity is variable. In addition, the high ascorbate levels in phagocytes protect them against oxidative damage caused by the large amounts of highly reactive oxygen species produced in the respiratory burst when the cells ingest and kill microorganisms. Experimental evidence does not support the theoretical possibility of ascorbate being a major contributor to iron-catalyzed $OH^{\cdot}$ production during the stimulation and degranulation of phagocytes.

REFERENCES

1. Levine M. New concepts in the biology and biochemistry of ascorbic acid. N Engl J Med 1986; 314:892-902.
2. Bendich A, Machlin LJ, Scandurra O, Burton GW, Wayner DDM. The antioxidant role of vitamin C. Adv Free Radical Biol Med 1986; 2:419-444.
3. Roberts R, Gallin JI. The phagocytic cell and its disorders. Ann Allergy 1983; 51:330-343.
4. Gallin JI, Quie PG. Leukocyte chemotaxis: Methods, physiology and clinical implications. New York: Raven Press, 1978.
5. Klebanoff SJ, Clark RA. The neutrophil: Function and clinical disorders. Amsterdam: Elsevier/North Holland, 1978.
6. Davis GM, Gallin JI. The neutrophil. In: Oppenheim JJ, Rosenstreich DL, Potter M, eds. Cellular Functions in Immunity and Inflammation. New York: Elsevier/North-Holland, 1981:77-102.
7. Van Furth R (ed). Mononuclear phagocytes; Parts I + II. The Hague: Martinus Nijhoff, 1980.
8. Klebanoff SJ. Phagocytic cells: Products of oxygen metabolism. In: Gallin JI, Goldstein IM, Snyderman R, eds. Inflammation: Basic Principles and Clinical Correlates. New York: Raven Press, 1988:391-444.
9. Mohanram M, Srikantia SG. Leucocytes and ascorbic acid uptake. Clin Sci 1967; 32:215-222.
10. DeChatelet LR, McCall CE, Cooper MR, Shirley PS. Ascorbic acid levels in phagocytic cells. Proc Soc Exp Biol Med 1974; 145:1170-1173.
11. Evans RM, Currie L, Campbell A. Effect of platelets on apparent leucocyte ascorbic acid content. Ann Clin Biochem 1980; 17:252-255.
12. Moser U. Uptake of ascorbic acid by leukocytes. Ann NY Acad Sci 1987; 498:200-215.

13. Schmidt K, Moser U. Vitamin C—A modulator of host defense mechanism. Int J Vitam Nutr Res 1985; suppl 27:363–379.
14. Oberritter H, Glatthaar B, Moser U, Schmidt KH. Effect of functional stimulation on ascorbate content in phagocytes under physiological and pathological conditions. Int Arch Allergy Appl Immunol 1986; 81:46–50.
15. Moser U, Weber F. Uptake of ascorbic acid by human granulocytes. Int J Vitam Nutr Res 1984; 54:47–53.
16. Bigley RH, Stankova L. Uptake and reduction of oxidized and reduced ascorbate by human leukocytes. J Exp Med 1974; 139:1084–1092.
17. Stankova L, Rigas DA, Bigley RH. Dehydroascorbate uptake and reduction by human blood neutrophils, erythrocytes, and lymphocytes. Ann NY Acad Sci 1975; 258:238–242.
18. Bigley R, Riddle M, Layman D, Stankova L. Human cell dehydroascorbate reductase: Kinetic and functional properties. Biochim Biophys Acta 1981; 659:15–22.
19. Bigley R, Wirth M, Layman D, Riddle M, Stankova L. Interaction between glucose and dehydroascorbate transport in human neutrophils and fibroblasts. Diabetes 1983; 32:545–548.
20. Winterbourn CC, Vissers MCM. Changes in ascorbate levels on stimulation of human neutrophils. Biochim Biophys Acta 1983; 763:175–179.
21. Babior BM. The respiratory burst oxidase. Trends Biochem Sci 1987; 12:241–243.
22. Gennaro R, Florio C, Romeo D. Activation of protein kinase C in neutrophil cytoplasts: Localization of protein substrates and possible relationship with stimulus-response coupling. FEBS Lett 1985; 180:185–190.
23. Pontremoli S, Melloni E, Michetti M, et al. Biochemical responses in activated human neutrophils mediated by protein kinase C and a Ca^{2+}-requiring proteinase. J Biol Chem 1986; 261:8309–8313.
24. Smolen JE, Korchak HM, Weissmann G. Increased levels of cyclic adenosine-3',5'-monophosphate in human polymorphonuclear leukocytes after surface stimulation. J Clin Invest 1980; 65:1077–1085.
25. Simchowitz L, Fischbein LC, Spilberg I, Atkinson JP. Induction of a transient elevation in intracellular levels of adenosine-3',5'-cyclic monophosphate by chemotactic factors: an early event in human neutrophil activation. J Immunol 1980; 124:1482–1491.
26. Sandler JA, Gallin JI, Vaughan M. Effects of serotonin, carbamylcholine, and ascorbic acid on leukocyte cyclic GMP and chemotaxis. J Cell Biol 1975; 67:480–484.
27. Anderson R. Ascorbic acid and immune functions: Mechanism of immunostimulation. In: Counsell JN, Hornig DH, eds. Vitamin C (Ascorbic Acid). London: Applied Science, 1981:249–272.
28. Goetzl EJ, Wasserman SI, Gigli I, Austen KF. Enhancement of random migration and chemotactic response of human leukocytes by ascorbic acid. J Clin Invest 1974; 53:813–818.
29. Anderson R, Theron A. Effects of ascorbate on leucocytes. Part I. Effects of ascorbate on neutrophil motility and intracellular cyclic nucleotide levels in vitro. S Afr Med J 1979; 56:394–400.
30. Dallegri F, Lanzi G, Patrone F. Effects of ascorbic acid on neutrophil locomotion. Int Arch Allergy Appl Immunol 1980; 61:40–45.
31. Anderson R. Effects of ascorbate on leucocytes. Part II. Effects of ascorbic acid and calcium and sodium ascorbate on neutrophil phagocytosis and postphagocytic metabolic activity. S Afr Med J 1979; 56:401–404.
32. Boxer LA, Watanabe AM, Rister M, Besch HR, Allen J, Baehner RL. Correction of leukocyte function in Chediak-Higashi syndrome by ascorbate. N Engl J Med 1976; 295:1041–1045.
33. Anderson R, Oosthuizen R, Maritz R, Theron A, Van Rensburg AJ. The effects of increasing weekly doses of ascorbate on certain cellular and humoral immune functions in normal volunteers. Am J Clin Nutr 1980; 33:71–76.

34. Anderson R. Ascorbate-mediated stimulation of neutrophil motility and lymphocyte transformation by inhibition of the peroxidase/H_2O_2/halide system in vitro and in vivo. Am J Clin Nutr 1981; 34:1906–1911.
35. Ganguly R, Durieux MF, Waldman RH. Macrophage function in vitamin C-deficient guinea pigs. Am J Clin Nutr 1976; 29:762–765.
36. Nungester WJ, Ames AM. The relationship between ascorbic acid and phagocytic activity. J Infect Dis 1948; 83:50–54.
37. Greendyke RM, Brierty RE, Swisher SN, Trabold NC. In vitro studies on erythrophagocytosis. II. Effects of incubating leukocytes with selected cell metabolites. J Lab Clin Med 1964; 63:1016–1026.
38. Holmes B, Quie PG, Windhorst DB, Good RA. Fatal granulomatous disease of childhood. An inborn abnormality of phagocytic function. Lancet 1986; 1:1225–1228.
39. Quie PG, White JG, Holmes B, Good RA. In vitro bactericidal capacity of human polymorphonuclear leukocytes: Diminished activity in chronic granulomatous disease of childhood. J Clin Invest 1967; 46:668–679.
40. Stankova L, Gerhardt NB, Nagel L, Bigley RH. Ascorbate and phagocyte function. Infect Immun 1975; 12:252–256.
41. Behar D, Czapski G, Rabani J, Dorfman LM, Schwarz HA. The acid dissociation constant and decay kinetics of the perhydroxyl radical. J Phys Chem 1970; 74:3209–3213.
42. Roos D, Hamers MN, van Zwieten R, Weening RS. Acidification of the phagocytic vacuole: A possible defect in chronic granulomatous disease? Adv Host Defen Mech 1983; 3:145–193.
43. Jensen MS, Bainton DF. Temporal changes in pH within the phagocytic vacuole of the polymorphonuclear neutrophilic leukocyte. J Cell Biol 1973; 56:379–388.
44. Jacques Y, Bainton DF. Changes in pH within the phagocytic vacuoles of human neutrophils and monocytes. Lab Invest 1978; 39:179–185.
45. DeChatelet LR, Cooper MR, McCall CE. Stimulation of the hexose monophosphate shunt in human neutrophils by ascorbic acid: Mechanism of action. Antimicrob Agents Chemother 1972; 1:12–16.
46. Kraut EH, Metz EN, Sagone AL. In vitro effects of ascorbate on white cell metabolism and the chemiluminescence response. J Reticuloendothel Soc 1980; 27:359–366.
47. Cooper MR, McCall CE, DeChatelet LR. Stimulation of leukocyte hexose monophosphate shunt activity by ascorbic acid. Infect Immun 1971; 3:851–853.
48. Aellig A, Maillard M, Phavorin A, Frei J. The energy metabolism of the leukocyte. Enzyme 1977; 22:196–206.
49. Leibovitz B, Siegel BV. Ascorbic acid, neutrophil function and the immune response. Int J Vitam Res 1978; 48:159–164.
50. Miller TE. Killing and lysis of gram-negative bacteria through the synergistic effect of hydrogen peroxide, ascorbic acid, and lysozyme. J Bacteriol 1969; 98:949–955.
51. McCall CE, DeChatelet LR, Cooper MR, Ashburn P. The effects of ascorbic acid on bactericidal mechanisms of neutrophils. J Infect Dis 1971; 124:194–198.
52. Klebanoff SJ, Hamon CB. Role of myeloperoxidase-mediated antimicrobial systems in intact leukocytes. J Reticuloendothel Soc 1972; 12:170–196.
53. Shilotri PG, Bhat KS. Effect of mega doses of vitamin C on bactericidal activity of leukocytes. Am J Clin Nutr 1977; 30:1077–1081.
54. Bendich A. Antioxidant vitamins and immune response. *In*: Chandra RK, ed. Nutrition and Immunology. New York: Liss, 1988:125–147.
55. Schulman JD, Mudd SH, Schneider JA, et al. Genetic disorders of glutathione and sulfur amino-acid metabolism. Ann Intern Med 1980; 93:330–346.
56. Oski FA. Vitamin E—A radical defense. N Engl J Med 1980; 303:454–455.
57. Thomas WR, Holt PG. Vitamin C and immunity: An assessment of the evidence. Clin Exp Immunol 1978; 32:370–379.

58. Panush RS, Delafuente JC. Vitamins and immunocompetence. World Rev Nutr Diet 1985; 45:97–132.
59. Ward PA. Chemotactic mechanisms in thermal injury. *In*: Ninnemann JL, ed. The immune consequences of thermal injury. Baltimore: Williams & Wilkins, 1981.
60. Miller RL, Elsas LJ II, Priest RE. Ascorbate action on normal and mutant human lysyl hydroxylases from cultured dermal fibroblasts. J Invest Dermatol 1979; 72:241–247.
61. Wilson CWM, Loh HS. Vitamin C and colds. Lancet 1973; 1:1058–1059.
62. Hume R, Weyers E. Changes in leucocyte ascorbic acid during the common cold. Scott Med J 1973; 18:3–7.
63. Greene M, Wilson CWM. Effect of aspirin on ascorbic acid metabolism during colds. Br J Clin Pharmacol 1975; 2:369.
64. Winterbourn CC. Comparison of superoxide with other reducing agents in the biological production of hydroxyl radicals. Biochem J 1979; 182:625–628.
65. Winterbourn CC. Hydroxyl radical production in body fluids. Roles of metal ions, ascorbate and superoxide. Biochem J 1981; 198:125–131.
66. Rowley DA, Halliwell B. Formation of hydroxyl radicals from hydrogen peroxide and iron salts by superoxide- and ascorbate-dependent mechanisms: Relevance to the pathology of rheumatoid disease. Clin Sci 1983; 64:649–653.
67. Rowley DA, Halliwell B. Superoxide-dependent and ascorbate-dependent formation of hydroxyl radicals in the presence of copper salts: A physiologically significant reaction? Arch Biochem Biophys 1983; 225:279–284.
68. Shinar E, Navok T, Chevion M. The analogous mechanisms of enzymatic inactivation induced by ascorbate and superoxide in the presence of copper. J Biol Chem 1983; 258:14778–14783.
69. Ericsson Y, Lundbeck H. Antimicrobial effect in vitro of the ascorbic acid oxidation. I. Effect on bacteria, fungi and viruses in pure cultures. Acta Pathol Microbiol Scand 1955; 37:493–506.
70. Drath DB, Karnovsky ML. Bactericidal activity of metal-mediated peroxide-ascorbate systems. Infect Immun 1974; 10:1077–1083.
71. Karnovsky ML. Biochemical aspects of the functions of polymorphonuclear and mononuclear leukocytes. *In*: Bellanti JA, Dayton DH, eds. The phagocytic cell in host resistance. New York: Raven Press, 1975:25–43.
72. Klebanoff SJ. Antimicrobial systems of the polymorphonuclear leukocyte. *In*: Bellanti JA, Dayton DH, eds. The phagocytic cell in host resistance. New York: Raven Press, 1975:45–59.
73. Roos D. The metabolic response to phagocytosis. *In*: Weissmann G, ed. The cell biology of inflammation. Amsterdam: Elsevier/North-Holland, 1980:337–385. (Glynn LE, Houck JC, Weissmann G, eds. Handbook of inflammation; vol 2).
74. Babior BM. Superoxide production by phagocytes. Biochem Biophys Res Commun 1979; 91:222–226.
75. Homan-Müller JWT, Weening RS, Roos D. Production of hydrogen peroxide by phagocytizing human granulocytes. J Lab Clin Med 1975; 85:198–207.
76. Root RK, Metcalf JA. H_2O_2 release from human granulocytes during phagocytosis. Relationship to superoxide anion formation and cellular catabolism of H_2O_2: Studies with normal and cytochalasin B-treated cells. J Clin Invest 1977; 60:1266–1279.
77. Weening RS, Wever R, Roos D. Quantitative aspects of the production of superoxide radicals by phagocytizing human granulocytes. J Lab Clin Med 1975; 85:245–252.
78. McCord JM, Salin ML. Free radicals and inflammation: Studies on superoxide-mediated NBT reduction by leukocytes. *In*: Brewer GJ, ed. Erythrocyte structure and function. New York: Liss, 1975:731–746. (Brewer GJ, Grover R, Hirschhorn K, Kety SS, Udenfriend S, Uhr JW, eds. Progress in clinical and biological research; vol 1).

79. Wayner DDM, Burton GW, Ingold KU, Barclay LRC, Locke SJ. The relative contributions of vitamin E, urate, ascorbate and proteins to the total peroxyl radical-trapping antioxidant activity of human blood plasma. Biochim Biophys Acta 1987; 924:408–419.
80. Clark RA, Klebanoff SJ. Myeloperoxidase-H_2O_2-halide system: Cytotoxic effect on human blood leukocytes. Blood 1977; 50:65–70.
81. Tsan MF. Phorbol myristate acetate induced neutrophil autotoxicity. J Cell Physiol 1980; 105:327–334.
82. Baehner RL, Boxer LA, Allen JM, Davis J. Autooxidation as a basis for altered function by polymorphonuclear leukocytes. Blood 1977; 50:327–335.
83. Salin ML, McCord JM. Superoxide dismutases in polymorphonuclear leukocytes. J Clin Invest 1974; 54:1005–1009.
84. DeChatelet LR, McCall CE, McPhail LC, Johnston RB Jr. Superoxide dismutase activity in leukocytes. J Clin Invest 1974; 53:1197–1201.
85. Patriarca P, Dri P, Rossi F. Superoxide dismutase in leukocytes. FEBS Lett 1974; 43:247–251.
86. Salin ML, McCord JM. Free radicals and inflammation. Protection of phagocytosing leukocytes by superoxide dismutase. J Clin Invest 1975; 56:1319–1323.
87. Gee JBL, Vassallo CL, Bell P, Kaskin J, Basford RE, Field JB. Catalase-dependent peroxidative metabolism in the alveolar macrophage during phagocytosis. J Clin Invest 1970; 49:1280–1287.
88. Stossel TP, Pollard TD, Mason RJ, Vaughan M. Isolation and properties of phagocytic vesicles from polymorphonuclear leukocytes. J Clin Invest 1971; 50:1745–1757.
89. Roos D, Weening RS, Wyss SR, Aebi HE. Protection of human neutrophils by endogenous catalase. Studies with cells from catalase-deficient individuals. J Clin Invest 1980; 65:1515–1522.
90. Voetman AA, Roos D. Endogenous catalase protects human blood phagocytes against oxidative damage by extracellularly generated hydrogen peroxide. Blood 1980; 56:846–852.
91. Spielberg SP, Boxer LA, Oliver JM, Allen JM, Schulman JD. Oxidative damage to neutrophils in glutathione synthetase deficiency. Br J Haematol 1979; 42:215–223.
92. Reed PW. Glutathione and the hexose monophosphate shunt in phagocytizing and hydrogen peroxide-treated rat leukocytes. J Biol Chem 1969; 244:2459–2464.
93. Vogt MT, Thomas C, Vassallo CL, Basford RE, Gee JBL. Glutathione-dependent peroxidative metabolism in the alveolar macrophage. J Clin Invest 1971; 50:401–410.
94. Noseworthy J Jr, Karnovsky ML. Role of peroxide in the stimulation of the hexose monophosphate shunt during phagocytosis by polymorphonuclear leukocytes. Enzyme 1972; 13:110–131.
95. Nishikimi M. Oxidation of ascorbic acid with superoxide anion generated by the xanthine-xanthine oxidase system. Biochem Biophys Res Commun 1975; 63:463–468.
96. Halliwell B, Foyer CH. Ascorbic acid, metal ions and the superoxide radical. Biochem J 1976; 155:697–700.
97. Allen JF, Hall DO. Superoxide reduction as a mechanism of ascorbate-stimulated oxygen uptake by isolated chloroplasts. Biochem Biophys Res Commun 1973; 52:856–862.
98. Anbar M, Neta P. A compilation of specific bimolecular rate constants for the reactions of hydrated electrons, hydrogen atoms and hydroxyl radicals with inorganic and organic compounds in aqueous solution. Int J Appl Radiat Isot 1967; 18:495–523.
99. Williams RN, Paterson CA, Eakins KE, Bhattacherjee P. Ascorbic acid inhibits the activity of polymorphonuclear leukocytes in inflamed ocular tissue. Eye Res 1984; 39:261–265.
100. Smith WB, Shohet SB, Zagajeski E, Lubin BH. Alteration in human granulocyte function after in vitro incubation with L-ascorbic acid. Ann NY Acad Sci 1975; 258:329–338.

101. Bigley R, Gerhardt NB, Eigner T, Dehlinger A, Niedra J, Stankova L. Effects of ascorbate loading on PMN bacterial iodination and other functions. J Reticuloendothel Soc 1978; 24:1-7.
102. Anderson R. Assessment of oral ascorbate in three children with chronic granulomatous disease and defective neutrophil motility over a 2-year period. Clin Exp Immunol 1981; 43:180-188.
103. Stankova L, Bigley R, Wyss SR, Aebi H. Catalase and dehydroascorbate reductase in human polymorphonuclear leukocytes (PMN): Possible functional relationship. Experientia 1979; 35:852-853.
104. Stankova L, Rigas D, Head C, Gay BT, Bigley R. Determinants of resistance to radiation injury in blood granulocytes from normal donors and from patients with myeloproliferative disorders. Radiat Res 1979; 80:49-60.
105. Roos D, Weening RS, Voetman AA et al. Protection of phagocytic leukocytes by endogenous glutathione: Studies in a family with glutathione reductase deficiency. Blood 1979; 53:851-866.
106. Stankova L, Rigas DA, Keown P, Bigley R. Leukocyte ascorbate and glutathione: Potential capacity for inactivating oxidants and free radicals. J Reticuloendothel Soc 1977; 21:97-102.
107. Bainton DF. The cells of inflammation: A general view. *In*: Weissmann G, ed. The Cell Biology of Inflammation. Amsterdam: Elsevier/North-Holland, 1980:1-52. (Glynn LE, Houck JC, Weissmann G, eds. Handbook of inflammation; vol 2).
108. McGee MP, Myrvik QN. Phagocytosis-induced injury of normal and activated alveolar macrophages. Infect Immun 1979; 26:910-915.
109. Walker JR, Smith MJH. An inhibitor of leucocyte movement in the plasma of patients with rheumatoid arthritis. Ann Rheum Dis 1980; 39:563-565.
110. Hanlon SM, Panayi GS, Laurent R. Defective polymorphonuclear leucocyte chemotaxis in rheumatoid arthritis associated with a serum inhibitor. Ann Rheum Dis 1980; 39:68-74.
111. Mowat AG. Neutrophil chemotaxis in rheumatoid arthritis. Ann Rheum Dis 1978; 37:1-8.
112. Anderson R, Lukey PT, Theron AJ, Dippenaar U. Ascorbate and cysteine-mediated selective neutralisation of extracellular oxidants during N-formyl peptide activation of human phagocytes. Agents Actions 1987; 20:77-86.
113. Anderson R, Lukey PT. A biological role for ascorbate in the selective neutralization of extracellular phagocyte-derived oxidants. Ann NY Acad Sci 1987; 498:229-247.

6
Interaction of Vitamin C in Lymphocyte Activation: Current Status and Possible Mechanisms of Action

Ward F. Cunningham-Rundles
The Mount Sinai School of Medicine and Beth Israel Hospital, New York, New York

Yitshal Berner
Memorial Sloan-Kettering Cancer Center, New York, New York, and Hebrew University, Rehovoth, Israel

Susanna Cunningham-Rundles
The New York Hospital, Cornell University Medical Center, New York, New York

INTRODUCTION

While interest in the role of vitamin C, or ascorbic acid, in the host defense against infections and in the protection against tumor development has been sustained for more than 50 years, there is currently no consensus on the possible specificity of action, and observations have remained largely phenomenological. This gap between the suspected and established role of vitamin C has characterized the history of research on this vitamin. Even the undisputed fact that vitamin C is essential for the prevention of scurvy was not accepted until 40 years after the original observations were reported in 1753 (1).

In part, the controversial nature of vitamin C studies may derive from the fact that ascorbic acid accelerates the hydroxylation reactions of many biosynthetic pathways (2-4). Ascorbic acid is a strong reducing agent which in transferring electrons to enzymes that require prosthetic metal ions in a reduced form provides reducing equivalents in hydroxylation, amidation, and other reactions. However, if ascorbic acid is replaced by other reductants, most of the ascorbic acid–assisted reactions will still go forward, although not maximally.

Ascorbic acid is a 6-carbon molecule closely related biosynthetically to glucose or galactose. Although it is synthesized by amphibians, reptiles, some birds, and most mammals, ascorbic acid is not synthesized by humans, most primates, guinea pigs, and fruit bats, all of which lack one or more of several enzymes, including uronolactonase, glucuronolactone reductase, and gulonolactone oxidase (5,6). Interestingly, one of the missing enzymes, L-gulonolactone oxidase, has been found in the liver of guinea pig embryos (7), suggesting that expression may have been suppressed during embryonic development (8). Furthermore, some guinea pigs appear to be resistant to scurvy and to have some possible residual ability to produce vitamin C. Although there are no comparable data in human studies suggesting that some humans may possibly be able to synthesize a low level of vitamin C, these data suggest that there may be such individuals. Relevant enzyme studies during embryonic development in humans also have not been done.

Ascorbic acid is transported against a concentration gradient to various tissues. The fact that these concentrations may exceed 50 times that of the plasma level in the adrenals, pituitary, central nervous system, spleen, testes, salivary glands, and eye lens has suggested a distinct role for vitamin C in these tissues (9). Ascorbic acid is also highly concentrated in bone marrow and in leukocytes, suggesting a potentially specific need (10).

Several lines of evidence have indicated that vitamin C may interact with vitamin E to reduce the free radicals formed as a result of vitamin E's antioxidant activity (11). Since there is potential for oxidative reactions during the immune response, it has been suggested that vitamin C may affect immune reactions by functioning as an antioxidant (12). As an antioxidant and free radical scavenger, vitamin C has been observed to be an effective detoxifying agent of various poisons and carcinogens (13), as in studies showing that ascorbic acid blocks conversion of nitrates to nitrites and also blocks the formation of nitrosamines from nitrites (14). Reversal of the morphological form of chemically transformed cells to normal-appearing cells in the presence of ascorbic acid has also been noted (15).

Vitamin C levels have been noted to drop during stress in animals who do not make it and to increase in those who can (16,17). The basis of this effect is unknown. Since the acute inflammatory response produces a series of reactions which protect host tissues against endogenous oxidative and hydrolytic agents, vitamin C has been thought to affect oxidative processes involving chemotoxis and phagocytosis during the functional stimulation of leukocytes and macrophages (18). Cameron and Pauling originally proposed that circulating leukocytes might serve as a reservoir for ascorbic acid so that local inflammatory reactions, visualized as excessive "depolymerization" events would be downregulated (19). The effect of vitamin C on phagocytic function is reviewed in Chapter 5.

Since a variety of physiological stress states lead to increased ascorbic acid synthesis in animals that make vitamin C, it has been suggested that this reflects an essential homeostatic response (20). Increased activities which are linked to vitamin C include the enhancement of cAMP, biosynthesis of epinephrine and norepinephrine, effects on drug metabolism, quenching of reactive oxygen and free radicals, production of collagen, and effects on enzymes participating in reactions increasing the viscosity of interstitial substances.

In this chapter, some of the effects of vitamin C on the immune response will be discussed in relationship to recent observations in this laboratory (21) suggesting that vitamin C may act specifically at the level of interleukin 2 (IL-2). However, given the complex nature of the interaction of vitamin C with biological processes at several levels, the relationship of these findings to physiological states will require further investigation.

VITAMIN C DEFICIENCY IN EXPERIMENTAL ANIMAL MODELS

Most of the work on the effect vitamin C on the immune response in animals has been carried out using the guinea pig, since this is the only commonly available animal that does not synthesize vitamin C. A few studies on the need for vitamin C in regenerating lymphoid tissue done in mice as well as guinea pigs (22) following x-irradiation demonstrated a vitamin C requirement that seemed to work through thymic humoral factors, leading to the conclusion that vitamin C was essential either for the production or activity of thymic humoral factors or both. However, there are no recent studies using any of the better-characterized thymic factors. Also, there have been no recent studies in this area using monoclonal antibodies to define lymphocyte subset changes. Although ascorate was reported to be essential for the differentiation of lymphoid organs during the development of cockerals and young rats (23) stressed with steroids, further analysis is needed to establish the mechanism and, therefore, the relationship of these observations to vitamin C requirements during normal development. In fact, pure scurvy seems not to affect either peripheral blood lymphocyte counts or lymphoid structure.

Early studies on the need for vitamin C during immunization showed that guinea pigs were unable to develop tuberculin activity if animals were made ascorbic acid deficient during the immunization period (24). Later studies suggested that this deficient inflammatory response to mycobacterial antigen challenge was related to defective migration of recruited cells to the challenge site. Scorbutic guinea pigs were markedly leukopenic, yet sensitized lymphocytes from these animals were able to transfer delayed-type hypersensitivity to nonscorbutic animals, who could then respond normally to antigen challenge (25). Thus, a defective response to challenge in the scorbutic guinea pig could be assumed to be solely related to defective macrophage migration and alterations in the microarchitecture. However, in other studies, animals presensitized before vitamin C deprivation could still respond after deprivation and animals who were immunized during a period of ascorbate depletion and challenged after repletion could not (24), so it seems likely that there must be significant effects of vitamin C deprivation during the induction phase as well as during the effector phase of delayed-type hypersensitivity (type IV) reactions.

Although early studies on the need for vitamin C during immunization suggested that vitamin C affected antibody responses, later studies did not confirm this, and it now seems that the earlier methods used produced methionine deficiency resulting in low sulphydryl levels in tissues (27,28), and that the conclusions drawn reflected this deficiency rather than that of ascorbic acid.

Initial studies on the effect of vitamin C on complement produced highly contradictory results suggesting no effect, a slight effect, or a highly significant effect, as discussed by Thomas and Holt (29). However, these studies have been more recently repeated using both indirect and direct (30,31) methods for measuring complement in scorbutic guinea pigs compared to pair-fed controls and these newer studies showed a highly significant relationship. Furthermore, Johnston et al. (31) found that the dietary increase of ascorbate that produced tissue-saturating levels produced complement increase (Clq) that was at least 30 times that seen in animals fed either adequate or suboptimal vitamin C. Since Clq is the first component of the classic complement pathway, and these proteins are known to play a key role in host defense against microbial and viral infections, these studies do suggest a specific role for vitamin C in the immune response.

There is also excellent evidence that scorbutic guinea pigs do not develop experimental allergic encephalomyelitis if the diet is started 1 week prior to immunization (32), and that ascorbic acid–deficient guinea pigs show prolonged skin graft survival (33). These findings have been frequently used as evidence that vitamin C has a critical relationship to cell-mediated immunity.

Although delayed-type hypersensitivity reactions are often abnormal in ascorbic acid–deficient guinea pigs, the relationship of this to in vitro T-lymphocyte dysfunction has not been clear. The studies of Fraser et al. (34) suggested that ascorbic acid–deficient animals showed increased B lymphocytes and decreased T lymphocytes, whereas the reverse was seen with very high-dose (250 mg/day) ascorbate supplementation. Probably as a result of these differences, scorbutic animals had a lower response to concanavalin A (Con A) (T-cell response) and a higher response to lipopolysaccharide (B-cell response) compared to ascorbic acid–replete animals. In contrast, results reported by Anthony et al. (28) that T cells were not reduced in the spleen of scorbutic guinea pigs may suggest compartmentalization of lymphocyte subsets during vitamin C deprivation. In part, the changes occurring during vitamin C deficiency may be linked to profound inanition associated with the vitamin C–free diet (Reid-Briggs, Teklad diet). Inanition was found to increase greatly over the 4-week diet period, leading to profound nutritional stress. Approximately 15% of animals would not eat these diets, which may be assumed to skew results obtained by this approach (34). The use of pair-fed controls showed that the addition of vitamin C was strongly protective of the overall health and body weight despite caloric restriction. Other complications in this approach stem from the fact that guinea pigs tend to carry latent *S. hemolyticus* infections and scorbutic guinea pigs are more prone to infections (35). When one considers that the inflammatory process is associated with an increased need for vitamin C, it seems that the interaction between nutritional stress, infection, and potential direct effects of vitamin C on the immune response may be inherently difficult to address in this model.

Vitamin C has been shown to affect phagocyte cell function in several ways, as discussed more extensively in Chapter 5, in animals that do synthesize vitamin C where an increase in the migration and chemotoxis of phagocytes has been observed. Similarly, peritoneal macrophages from ascorbic acid–deficient guinea pigs have been found to show reduced phagocytic motility (37). The effects on phagocytosis, itself, remain controversial. The respiratory burst, however, does appear linked to vitamin C, since regeneration of $NADP^+$ through the hexose monophosphate shunt is increased by ascorbate. Further, as discussed in detail in Chapter 5, ascorbate may participate as a reducing agent in the generation of bacteriocidal products.

Bendich et al. (38) have concentrated on the antioxidant properties of vitamin C in relationship to vitamin E, since vitamin C has been shown to regenerate vitamin E from the tocopherol free radical (39). In several carefully designed experiments (38), these investigators showed that the dietary level of vitamin C did not affect the T- and B-cell mitogen responses of spleen cells from guinea pigs except when vitamin E was also deficient. Since lowering vitamin C without vitamin E supplementation caused a striking reduction in the tissue levels of vitamin E, these authors (38) postulated that previous studies on vitamin C deficiency were also producing a critical vitamin E reduction that might suggest that the principal effect of vitamin C is actually on vitamin E level.

Another indirect effect of vitamin C on the immune response has been proposed by Oh and Nakano (40), who observed that ascorbic acid could detoxify histamine, which normally builds up to an inhibitory level following lymphocyte activation in vitro as a result of histadine decarboxylase activity. Ascorbic acid in a fairly wide concentration range, 10^{-8} to 10^{-4} M, significantly enhanced proliferation in vitro to Con A. Since histamine itself had a positive effect on cell division early in culture and a suppressing effect late in culture, a regulatory role for ascorbate was proposed. These studies may also shed light on some of the controversies in the literature on the effects of vitamin C, since both suppressive and enhancing effects could be related to the nonenzymatic degradation of histamine, which is in itself a biphasic regulator of lymphocyte transformation. Recently, Johnston and Huang (57) have reported that ascorbate lowered histamine levels in guinea pigs, but that both high and low ascorbate were associated with reduced leukocyte chemotaxis compared to the ascorbate-sufficient state.

Although only a few studies have addressed the possibility that vitamin C affects cytokine production, the work of Siegal and Morton (41,42) has shown that dietary vitamin C could enhance interferon production in the mouse after stimulation with the murine leukemia virus, and that this could also be demonstrated in vitro using murine L cells or embryonic fibroblasts (43).

Megadoses of ascorbate have been studied in animal models, but these results are difficult to interpret because of alterations in catabolism. Further, as suggested by the studies of Fraser et al. (34), who found that guinea pigs receiving a megadose of 100 mg/day showed a greater increase in the plasma vitamin C level at 14 days than did animals receiving 250 mg/day. However, at later periods, there appeared to be an accommodation to higher levels of plasma ascorbate, so that the animals supplemented at the higher level eventually achieved a higher level of plasma ascorbate than animals supplemented at the lower level.

In summary, while data in animal models, primarily the guinea pig, suggest that vitamin C is a critical factor in the development of the immune response, some of these relationships appear to operate through the antioxidant activity of ascorbate. In addition, the results appear quite dependent upon experimental conditions. The relationship between the use of vitamin C as an antiscorbutic agent and the use of vitamin C as an enhancer of host defense remain to be defined, and the study of each effect seems likely to require a different experimental approach.

HUMAN VITAMIN C DEFICIENCY

Subclinical ascorbic acid deficiency is relatively common even in affluent societies (44), although scurvy is rare. Although animal model studies have indicated that mild deficiency of vitamin C is associated with altered metabolism, the demonstration of an altered host defense in humans with subtle vitamin C deficiency have been largely epidemiological. Consumption of foods high in vitamin C has been associated with reduced cancer incidence, especially of the stomach and esophagus (8,45,46); the effects, which as discussed previously, have been generally ascribed to nonimmunological mechanisms. The nutritional status of cancer patients is, on the other hand, potentially interrelated with immune mechanisms which do affect host defense against tumor development. For example, in lung cancer patients, in whom immunological defense against tumor extension and metastasis may be a central factor in survival, Anthony and Schorah found strongly reduced levels of vitamin C in their leukocytes, particularly among patients with a relative leukocytosis (47). There are no reported studies on the relationship between the immune response and vitamin C in cancer patients. Hypovitaminosis C has been found to accompany IL-2 therapy and adoptive immunotherapy with lymphokine-activated killer (LAK) cells (48). Interestingly, clinically defined responders showed faster recovery of ascorbate levels than nonresponders. Although this may have had no direct relationship to vitamin C per se, the possible connection warrants further study.

Physiological stress has been recognized to cause a sharp drop in ascorbate levels whether the stress is related to myocardial infraction, surgical trauma, or infection (16,47,49), and may occur partly as a result of leukocyte migration to tissue injury sites. However, now that the role of interleukins in the stress response is becoming clearer, it may be appropriate to look for a more direct relationship between vitamin C and cytokine regulation.

Ascorbic acid deficiency has been achieved experimentally in humans. These studies showed no impairment of the cellular immune response in vitro to T-cell mitogens or in lymphocyte subsets in volunteers who became temporarily scorbutic on the vitamin C–deficient diet (50), and appeared to contradict an earlier single case report of an individual in whom experimental vitamin C deprivation was accompanied by reduced total white cells (51).

VITAMIN C SUPPLEMENTATION IN HUMANS

The question of appropriate vitamin C supplementation in humans has arisen in several settings, including parenteral nutrition, low-birth-weight infants, patients on hemodialysis, and in stress states, including cancer, where low levels of vitamin C have been observed. Yet, in many cases, the complexity of the relationships between infecting agents, other nutrients, and preexisting factors influencing the immune response confuse the interpretation of data. For example, since ascorbic acid enhances iron absorption, relatively low levels of vitamin C can strongly enhance iron uptake from food (52). While increased iron uptake could be beneficial in some cases, there may a risk in the case of iron-replete patients or in patients with iron overload; i.e., thalassemia major, idiopathic hemachromotosis, and sideroblastic anemia. Further iron may influence the immune response in both positive and negative ways (see Chap. 7). In addition, studies have shown that the timing of ascorbate supplementation affects iron uptake only during that period of the day when it is taken and does not affect uptake at later periods (52). Few studies have attempted to control for any of these factors in the effects of supplementation. Plasma losses of ascorbate were found to increase following moderately increased intake (10 × RDA) by Omaye et al. (53), whereas turnover was found to decrease with lowered dietary intake; thus, sudden elevation in vitamin C levels affects a subsequent depletion period via catabolism, absorption, or elimination (16,20). Leukocyte levels have been found to be similarly affected, although not as quickly.

As discussed above, neutrophil motility has been thought to be vitamin C dependent in the guinea pig. Increasing doses of vitamin C in human volunteers were also found to cause increased neutrophil chemotaxis by Anderson et al. (54) when ingestion was greater than 2 g/day. An increased response to phytohemagglutinin (PHA) was also observed in vitro in the Anderson study. In contrast, Goodwin and Garry (55) found no increase in the responses of peripheral blood lymphocytes in vitro to mitogen in elderly persons taking megadoses of vitamins, including vitamin C, in a relatively random- and self-selected fashion, although there was a trend toward increased skin test reactivity. Despite the care with which these data were evaluated, the interpretation that the long-term use of megavitamins may lead to a nonspecific adjuvant effect that disappears with time seems tenuous in this random setting. The relationship between ascorbate needed for the prevention of scurvy and for the other aspects of homeostasis has been discussed by Levine (20), who has suggested that these requirements are intrinsically quite different. Interestingly, a recent study among elderly, institutionalized persons supplemented with vitamins, including vitamin C, and minerals showed that skin test responsiveness was positively affected by supplementation (58).

THE EFFECT OF VITAMIN C IN VITRO ON THE IMMUNE RESPONSE

Data on the effect of vitamin C on the immune response in vitro also have been conflicting. The inhibition of lymphocyte proliferative response to mitogens has been reported at concentrations of ascorbate (55) greater than 15 μg/ml. We have recently examined (21) the effect of vitamin C on peripheral blood mononuclear activation or T-cell mitogens in a standardized microtiter cell assay using a broad range of concentrations of PHA from 70 μg/ml to 3 μg/ml. When the concentration of vitamin C exceeded 15 mg/dl (150 μg/ml), the response to PHA was completely abolished owing to excessive acidity. At 10 mg/dl or lower, no change in pH was observed, but the inhibition of response was seen in all cell donors. When the concentration of vitamin C exceeded 6.0 mg/dl and the concentration of PHA ranged from 40 to 3 μg/dl, this inhibition was statistically significant ($p < 0.01$). Inhibition was also time dependent such that the inhibitory effect of vitamin C on the response to PHA was observed more strongly during the earlier phase of activation before the peak of the proliferative response. Data are shown in Figure 1.

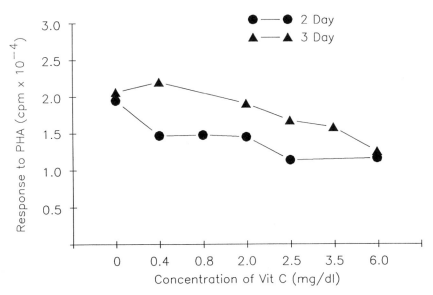

Figure 1 Proliferative response to PHA in the presence of varying concentrations of vitamin C. Concentration of PHA was 12 mg/ml and cultures were pulse labeled for 18 hr with [^{14}C]thymidine after either 48 or 72 hr. Data are shown median counts per minute of each triplicate.

When Con A was used to activate mononuclear cells in vitro, essentially the same inhibitory effect was seen. However, when the T-cell–dependent B lymphocyte activator, pokeweed mitogen (PWM) was used as a lymphocyte stimulant, much less inhibition was seen. Furthermore, at concentrations less than 2.5 mg/dl, a slight enhancement of responsiveness was sometimes observed which, in some experiments, achieved a 20% increment over that of cells cultured in the absence of vitamin C. However, neither inhibition nor enhancement were great enough to achieve statistical significance.

In marked contrast to the effect of vitamin C addition to lymphocytes stimulated with mitogens, when mononuclear cells were activated with influenza A antigen, a strongly augmenting effect was observed. Inhibition was seldom observed even at concentrations of vitamin C greater than 6 mg/dl and never at lower vitamin C concentrations. This augmentation did not affect the mononuclear cell response to the influenza control antigen preparation, which consisted of the matching dilution of supernatant from uninfected cells in which the virus had been grown and which was prepared identically with the viral antigen, as shown in Figure 2. Experiments were then conducted to determine the effect of vitamin C in response to influenza A antigen in vitro in a sequential series of 15 normal controls (21). Of 15 donors tested, 8 responded positively to influenza A antigen in vitro, and 7 donors did not respond. Lymphocyte activation of normal nonresponders to influenza A antigen was not affected by vitamin C at any concentration. In contrast, the levels of response of controls who did show a response to influenza A in vitro was strongly enhanced. The response to influenza A antigen was significantly greater in the presence than in the absence of vitamin C ($p < 0.02$) in the responder group. Interestingly,

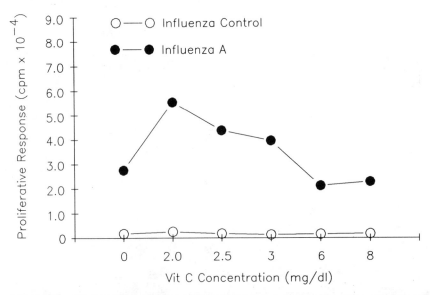

Figure 2 Proliferative response of one cell donor to influenza A antigen and the control virus preparation in the presence and absence of varying concentrations of vitamin C are shown following 6 days of culture with addition of [^{14}C]thymidine during the final 18 hr of culture. Data are given as median triplicate counts per minute.

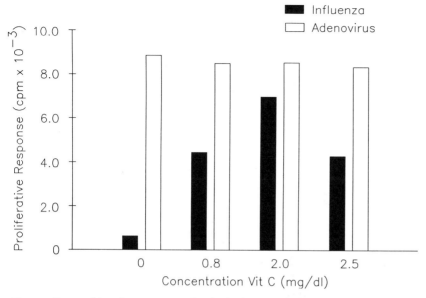

Figure 3 Proliferative response of a single donor to influenza A and adenovirus in parallel in the presence and absence of vitamin C. Culture conditions identical to those described for Figure 2. Data are given as median counts per minute of each triplicate.

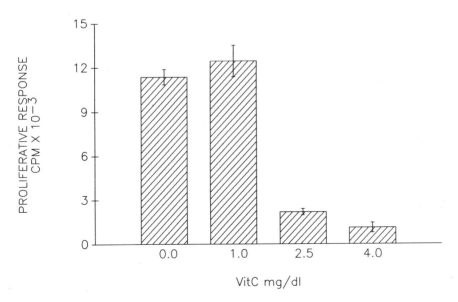

Figure 4 Proliferative response to IL-2 at 21 U/ml in the presence and absence of vitamin C at the noted concentrations. Cultures were incubated for 5 days and then pulse labeled with [^{14}C]thymidine for an additional 18 hr. Data are given as mean counts per minute of triplicate cultures.

Table 1 Effect of Vitamin C[a] on INF-γ[b] Production and Proliferation

Culture	Culture condition	CPM[c]	INF[d]
1	Cells alone	230	0
2	Influenza A	2,300	58
3	Influenza A + Vit C	4,100	59
4	INF-γ	3,800	N.D.
5	INF-γ + Vit C	6,800	N.D.
6	Vit C	200	0

[a]Vitamin C = 0.8 mg/dl.
[b]INF-γ = 100 U/ml.
[c]Counts per min (mean triplicate).
[d]INF-γ in units (per ml in supernatant).

this augmenting effect was not observed as a general phenomenon with all other antigens. For example, as shown in Figure 3, there appeared to be no effect on the response to adenovirus in donors in whom the response to influenza A was strongly affected (representative experiment is shown).

The results obtained appeared to suggest that vitamin C might act through interaction with a regulatory cytokine induced during activation, since vitamin C did not directly cause mitogenesis. We first studied the effect of vitamin C on IL-2 activation of lymphocytes in vitro. As shown in Figure 4, for one representative experiment (n=6), the response to IL-2 was strongly suppressed at 2.5 and 4.0 μg/ml, whereas some enhancement was observed at 1.0 mg/dl vitamin C.

These experiments appeared to indicate a possible basis of the inhibitory effect of vitamin C on the response to T-lymphocyte mitogens. Since IL-2 is known to induce gamma interferon INF-γ, the effect on the production of INF-γ and the response to this cytokine was studied in subsequent studies. Vitamin C did not inhibit the production of INF-γ that accompanied the response to influenza A, but did enhance the proliferative response to INF-γ, as shown in Table 1.

Concentrations of vitamin C inhibitory to the proliferative response to IL-2 did not affect lymphokine activated killer cell induction of tumor cell killing by IL-2. A possible interpretation of this appeared to be that LAK cell induction was critically related to the gamma interferon (INF-γ) response, and further suggested that vitamin C might enhance reactions that develop by means of the INF-γ response or those that are potentially amplified through the proliferative response to this cytokine.

These data and those previously published suggest that while vitamin C may act at more than one level of immune response, at least some of these interactions involve the specific regulation of the cytokine network, and are therefore susceptible to defined experimental approach.

ACKNOWLEDGMENTS

The authors acknowledge the expert technical assistance of Desiree Ehleiter, Theresa Manalo, and Mahasti Hassani. These studies were supported in part by the National Institutes of Health, National Cancer Institute, Bethesda, Maryland, CA52905, and the Children's Blood Foundation, New York, New York.

REFERENCES

1. Lind JA (1953). Treatise On Scurvy. Stewart CP, Cuthrie D, eds. Edinburgh University Press.
2. Peterkofsky B, Udenfriend S (1965). Enzymatic hydroxylation of proline in microsomal polypeptide leading to formation of collagen. Proc Natl Acad Sci USA 53:335.
3. Dunn WA, Retterra G, Seiffer E, Englard S (1984). Carnitine biosynthesis from γbutyrobetaine and from exogenous protein bound G-N-trimethyl-1-Lysine by the perfused guinea pig liver: Effect of ascorbate deficiency on the in situ activity of γbutrobetaine hydroxylase. J Biol Chem 259:10764.
4. Levine M, Morita K, Pollard H (1985). Enhancement of norepinephrine biosynthesis by ascorbic acid in cultured bovine chromaffin cells. J Biol Chem 260:12942.
5. Burns JJ, Peyser P, Moltz A (1956). Missing step in guinea pigs required for the biosynthesis of L-ascorbic acid. Science 124:1148.
6. Chatterjee IB (1973). Evolution and the biosynthesis of ascorbic acid. Science 182:1271.
7. Zloch E, Ginter E (1984). Experimentally proved biosynthesis of vitamin C in a guinea pig. Naturwissen Schaffen 71:533.
8. Block G, Menkes M (1989). Ascorbic acid in cancer prevention. *In*: Nutrition and Cancer Prevention. Noon TE, Micozzi MS, eds. Marcel Dekker, New York, p 341.
9. Hornig D (1975). Distribution of ascorbic acid metabolites and analogues in man and animals. Ann NY Acad Sci 758:103.
10. Moser U, Weber F (1984). Uptake of ascorbic acid by human granulocytes. Int J Vitam Nutr Res 54:47.
11. Niki E, Tsuchiya J, Tanimura R, Kamiya U (1982). Regeneration of vitamin E from alpha-chromo-manoxyl radical by glutathione and vitamin C. Chem Lett 789.
12. Bendich A (1988). Antioxidants, vitamins and immunity. *In*: Nutrition and Immunology. Chandra R, ed., Liss, New York, p 125.
13. Sauberlich HE (1984). Ascorbic acid. *In*: Nutrition Reviews Present Knowledge In Nutrition. The Nutrition Foundation, Washington, D.C.
14. Ranieri R, Weisberger JH (1975). Reduction of carcinogens with ascorbic acid. Ann NY Acad Sci 258:181.
15. Wittes RE (1985). Vitamin C and cancer. N Engl J Med 312:178.
16. Pipkin GE, Schlegel JU, Nishimura R, Schultz GN (1969). Inhibitory effect of L-ascorbate on tumor formation in urinary bladders implanted with 3-hydroxyanthrilic acid. Proc Soc Exp Biol Med 131:522.
17. Kamm JJ, Dashman T, Conney AH, Burns JJ (1973). Protective effect of ascorbic acid on hepatotoxicity caused by sodium nitrite plus aminopyrine. Proc Natl Acad Sci 70:747.
18. Schmidt K, Moser U (1985). Vitamin C—A modulator of host defense mechanism: An overview. Int J Vitam Nutr Res 27(Suppl):363.
19. Cameron E, Pauling L (1973). Ascorbic acid and the glycosaminoglycans. Oncology 27:181.
20. Levine M (1986). New concepts in the biology and biochemistry of ascorbic acid. N Engl J Med 314:892.
21. Cunningham-Rundles S, Berner Y, Cunningham-Rundles WF. Specificity and concentration dependence of vitamin C effect on lymphocyte activation (manuscript submitted).
22. Dietere MP (1971). Further studies on the relationship between vitamin c and thymic humoral factor. Proc Soc Exp Biol Med 136:316.
23. Dieter MP, Breitenbach RP (1971). Vitamin C in lymphoid organs of rats and cockerels treated with corticosterone or testosterone. Proc Soc Exp Biol Med 137:341.
24. Mueller PS, Kies MW (1962). Suppression of tuberculin reaction in the scorbutic guinea pigs. Nature 195:813.

25. Zweiman B, Schoenwetter WF, Hildreth EA (1966). The effect of the scorbutic state on tuberculin hypersensitivity in the guinea pig. I. Passive transfer of tuberculin hypersensitivity. J Immunol 96:296.
26. Stinebring WR, Traketellis AC, Axelrod AE (1963). Studies on systemic reactivity to purified protein derivative (PPD) and endotoxin. J Immunol 91:46.
27. Kumar M, Axelrod AE (1969). Circulating antibody formation in scorbutic guinea pigs. J Nutr 98:41.
28. Anthony LE, Kurahara CC, Taylor KB (1979). Cell medicated cytotoxicity and humoral immune response in ascorbic acid deficient guinea pigs. Am J Clin Nutr 32:1691.
29. Thomas WB, Holt PG (1978). Vitamin C and immunity: An assessment of the evidence. Clin Exp Immunol 32:370.
30. Johnston CS, Carter GD, Haskell BE (1985). The effect of ascorbic acid nutriture on protein bound hydroyproline in guinea pig plasma. J Nutr 115:1089.
31. Johnston CS, Kolb WP, Haskell BE (1987). The effect of vitamin C nutriture on complement component clq concentrations in guinea pig plasma. J Nutr 117:764.
32. Mueller PS, Kies MW, Alvord EC, Shaw CM (1962). Prevention of experimental allergic encephalomyelitis (EAE) by vitamin C deprivation. J Exp Med 115:329.
33. Kalden JR, Guthy EA (1972). Prolonged skin allograft survival in vitamin C deficient guinea pigs. Eur Surg Res 4:114.
34. Fraser RC, Parlovic S, Kurahara CG, Murata A, Peterson NS, Taylor KB, Feigen CA (1978). The effect of variations in vitamin C intake on the cellular immune response of guinea pigs. Am J Clin Nutri 33:839.
35. Reid ME, Briggs GM (1953). Development of a semisynthetic diet for young guinea pigs. J Nutri 51:341.
36. Anderson R, Theron A (1979). Effects of ascorbate on leukocytes III: In vitro and In Vivo Stimulation of abnormal neutrophil motility by ascorbate. S Afr Med J 56:429.
37. Ganguly R, Durieux MF, Waldman RH (1976). Macrophage function in vitamin C deficient guinea pigs. Am J Clin Nutr 29:762.
38. Packer JE, Slater TF, Willson RL (1979). Direct observation of a free radical interaction between vitamin E and vitamin C. Nature 278:737.
39. Bendich A, D'Apolito P, Gabriel E, Machlin CJ (1984). Interaction of dietary vitamin C and vitamin E on guinea pig immune responses to mitogen. J Nutr 114:1588.
40. Oh C, Nakane K (1988). Reversal by ascorbic acid of suppression by endogenous histamine of rat lymphocyte blastogenesis. J Nutr 118:639.
41. Siegel BV, Morton JI (1977). Vitamin C and the immune response. Experentia 33:393.
42. Siegel BV (1974). Enhanced interferon response to murine leukemia virus by ascorbic acid. Infect Immun 10:409.
43. Siegel BV (1975). Enhancement of interferon production by poly (rI) poly (rC) in mouse cell culture by ascorbic acid. Nature 254:531.
44. Ten State Nutrition Survey In The United States 1968-1970—US Center for Disease Control 1972 118. U.S. Department of Health, Education and Welfare Publication No. (HSM)72-8132.
45. Glatthaar BE, Hornig DH, Moser H (1986). The role of ascorbic acid in carcinogenesis. In: Essential Nutrients in Carcinogenesis. Poirer LA, Newberne PM, Pariza MW, eds. Plenum Press, New York, p 357.
46. Burr MC, Samloff IM, Bates CJ, Halliday RM (1987). Atrophic gastritis and vitamin C status in two towns with different stomach cancer death rates. Br J Can 56:163.
47. Anthony HM, Schorah CJ (1982). Severe hypovitaminosis C in lung cancer patients. The utilization of vitamin C in surgical repair and lymphocyte—Related host resistance. Br J Can 46:354.
48. Marcus SC, Dutcher JB, Pietta E, Ciobanu N, Strauman J, Wiernik PH, Hatner SH, Frank O, Baker H (1987). Severe hypovitaminosis C occurring as the result of adoptive

immunotherapy with high dose interleukin 2 and lymphokine activated killer cells. Can Res 47:4028.
49. Hume R, Weyers E, Rowan T, Reid P, Hillis WS (1972). Leukocyte ascorbic acid levels after acute myocardial infarction. Br Heart J 34:238.
50. Kay NE, Holloway DE, Hutton SW, Bone ND, Duane WC (1982). Human T cell function in experimental ascorbic acid deficiency and spontaneous scurvy. Am J Clin Nutr 36: 127.
51. Crandon JH, Land CC, Dill DB (1940). Experimental human scurvy. N Engl J Med 223: 353.
52. Cook JD, Monsen ER (1977). Vitamin C. The common cold, and iron absorption. Am J Clin Nutr 30:235.
53. Omaye ST, Skaala JH, Jacob RA (1986). Plasma ascorbic acid in adult males: Effects of depletion and supplementation. Am J Clin Nutr 44:257.
54. Anderson R, Dosthuizen R, Maritz R, Theron A, Van Resnburg AJ (1980). The effect of increasing weekly doses of ascorbate on certain cellular and humoral immune functions in normal volunteers. Am J Clin Nutri 33:71.
55. Goodwin JS, Garry PJ (1983). Relationship between megadose vitamin supplementation and immunological function in a healthy elderly population. Clin Exp Immunol 51:647.
56. Ramirez I, Riche E, Wang YM, Van Eys J (1980). Effect of ascorbic acid in vitro on lymphocyte reactivity to mitogen. J Nutr 110:2207.
57. Johnston CS, Huang S (1991). Effect of ascorbic acid nurture on blood histamine and neutrophil chemotaxis in guinea pigs. J Nutr 121:126.
58. Subotičarec K, Stavlenič A, Bilič-Pešič L, Gorajščan M, Gorajščan D, Brubachor Buzina R (1989). Nutritional status, grip strength, and immune function in institutionalized elderly. Int J Vitam Nutr Res 59:20.

7
The Immunoregulatory Properties of Iron

Christopher F. Bryan
Midwest Organ Bank, Inc., Westwood, Kansas

Marvin J. Stone
Baylor University Medical Center, Dallas, Texas

CELLULAR IMMUNOREGULATORY PROPERTIES OF IRON

The immunoregulatory properties of iron and its binding proteins have been investigated primarily in vitro. These studies have shown that iron and certain iron-binding proteins influence structural and functional properties of T and B lymphocytes. Furthermore, a variety of immunological abnormalities have been reported in patients with iron deficiency and iron overload. In this chapter, we will critically examine data relating to the hypothesis that iron and iron-containing proteins possess definable immunoregulatory properties. Immune responses may be described conveniently as having afferent, central, and efferent components (1). The afferent limb is concerned with events associated with the transport of antigen to the potentially reacting lymphoid cells; the central limb with the participation of the immunocompetent (antigen-sensitive) cells; and the efferent limb with the expression of the immune response through various effector mechanisms.

Many effector functions are regulated by a group of molecules produced by lymphocytes and monocytes, interleukins, also termed lymphokines, and cytokines. Studying these interactions in the presence of iron has yielded a body of evidence that iron and certain proteins that bind or contain iron have immunoregulatory properties. Studies supporting this conclusion are summarized in Tables 1 and 2, and are described in the following sections.

Lymphocyte Surface Molecules

Antigenic specificity of the T-cell receptor for antigen (TCR) is conferred by a heterodimeric complex of an alpha and a beta molecule which is able to recognize foreign

Table 1 Immunoregulatory Properties of Iron and Iron-Containing Proteins on T-Lymphocyte Surface Molecule Expression

T-lymphocyte surface molecule evaluated	Molecular species of iron	Influence on expression	References
E-Rosette receptor (CD2)	Ferric citrate	Reduction	4,5
EAC-Rosette receptor	Ferric citrate	Reduction	5
EA-Rosette receptor	Ferric citrate	No influence	5
Active E-rosette receptor	Ferric citrate, transferrin, and lactoferrin	Modulation	6
CD3 and CD4	Ferric citrate	Reduction	7
CD8	Ferric citrate	No influence	7
Transferrin receptor (CD71)	Ferric citrate	Enhanced	7
HLA-DR, CD38 and TER	Ferric citrate	No influence	7

Table 2 Immunoregulatory Properties of Iron and Iron-Containing Proteins on Lymphocyte Function

Lymphocyte population evaluated	Functional test evaluated	Molecular species of iron	Influence	References
T	Mixed lymphocyte culture response	Ferric citrate	Suppression	8
		Ferritin	Suppression	9
		Iron salts and hemoglobin	Suppression	10
	Cell-mediated lympholysis			
	sensitization phase	Iron salts and hemoglobin	Suppression	10
	effector phase	Iron salts and hemoglobin	No influence	10
	Lymphocyte proliferation			
	concanavalin A	Ferric citrate and ferritin	Suppression	9, 11
		Hemin	Enhancement	12
	phytohemaglutinin	Ferric citrate, ferritin, and iron salts	Suppression	9–11
		Hemin	Enhancement	12
	pokeweed mitogen	Ferric citrate	Enhancement	11
		Ferritin	No influence	9
B	Antibody production			
	immunoglobulin secretion	Ferric citrate concentration		13
	IgG	high	Enhancement	
		low	Suppression	
	IgM	high	Suppression	
		low	Enhancement	
	IgA	high	Suppression	
		low	Enhancement	
	primary antibody response	Lactoferrin	Suppression	14
NK	Natural killer activity	Ferric citrate	Suppression	15
		Lactoferrin	Enhancement	15
		Transferrin	No influence	15
ADCC	Antibody-dependent cellular cytotoxicity	Lactoferrin	Suppression	15
		Ferric citrate	No influence	15

antigen on antigen-presenting cells in an MHC-restricted manner (2,3). The CD3 complex is the second molecular component of the TCR and comprises five molecules that may influence the transduction of the signal that results in T-cell activation, the CD3/TCR complex.

Initial studies demonstrating the surface molecule-modulating influence of iron were performed by de Sousa et al. These investigators showed that iron in various salts could specifically reduce expression of the T-cell E-rosette receptor (CD2) that binds sheep red blood cells at 4° (4). These and other studies dealing with the effect of iron on T-lymphocyte molecules are summarized in Table 1 (4–7). In subsequent studies (5,6), iron was shown to cause decreased expression of the EAC-rosette receptor, a receptor on T cells that binds the third component of complement. The differential effect and specificity of iron was suggested by its failure to alter the EA-rosette receptor. Definitive evidence that iron modulated lymphocyte surface determinants was provided by showing that active E-rosette receptor expression was downregulated in cultures containing high concentrations of iron (6). When iron-treated lymphocytes were transferred to a culture system with lower iron levels, this receptor was reexpressed. The possibility that the observed effects were due to toxicity was ruled out. Mononuclear cells pretreated with ferric citrate, incubated overnight, washed, and then allowed to respond in the mixed lymphocyte culture (MLC) had functional capabilities no different from untreated cells. However, cells treated with iron and added directly to the MLC had suppressed proliferative capacity (8).

In further experiments (7), the effects were evaluated in lymphocytes induced to mitotic activity by pokeweed mitogen (PWM). Expression of the T-cell surface molecules CD3, CD4, CD8, and the activation-associated markers CD71 (transferrin receptor), CD38, HLA-DR (HLA class II monomorphic determinant), and TER (thermostable erythrocyte rosettes) were evaluated at the time of peak of PWM-induced mitogenesis in the presence and absence of ferric citrate. A differential effect was noted as follows: (a) CD3 and CD4 were decreased in expression by iron, (b) CD71 was increased by iron, and (c) CD8, CD38, HLA-DR, and TER were not influenced. These surface changes were accompanied by the functional observation that the proliferative response of PWM-induced lymphocytes was significantly enhanced by iron, as discussed in detail in the following section.

Lymphocyte Function

Following the observations that iron altered expression of certain T-lymphocyte surface molecules, several series of experiments were designed to determine whether iron altered lymphocyte function. A summary of selected studies bearing on this question is listed in Table 2 (8–15).

The first report of the immunoregulatory influence of iron on a cellular function documented the ability of ferric citrate to differentially suppress the allogeneic response (MLC) (8). From other studies it became known that the MLC response occurs when CD4 helper/inducer T cells recognize class II (DR, DQ, and DP) disparity on stimulator cells (16–19). The inhibitory influence mediated by iron was further shown to be related to the HLA class I phenotype of the cell donor. Essentially, the MLC-responsivity of individuals who carried HLA-A2 was resistant to the inhibitory influence of iron. In contrast, iron inhibition of the MLC response was seen in cell donors who lacked HLA-A2. Other workers have shown that other iron salts, ferritin and hemoglobin, are also capable of suppressing the MLC response (9,10). A genetically restricted inhibition of the MLC was not reported by either of those groups, however.

Cell-mediated lympholysis (CML), a lytic response generally mediated by $CD8^+$ lymphocytes to target cells that express HLA class II antigens used in the priming phase (18,19), also was shown to be suppressed by various iron salts and hemoglobin (10). Furthermore, the inhibitory effect of iron on CML was shown to occur only at the CML-sensitization phase and not at the CML-effector phase.

T-Cell mitogenic (9-12) responses have been shown to be modulated by iron. The mitogen-induced proliferative response to phytohemaglutinin (PHA) and concanavalin A (Con A) was inhibited by iron as ferric citrate, or other iron salts and ferritin. In contrast to these suppressive effects, ferric citrate and hemin were shown to enhance the proliferative response to PWM and Con A, respectively (9,12). Such iron-mediated enhancement was shown to have an effect on T lymphocytes, since it was unaltered by removal of monocytes and did not occur with T-depleted lymphocyte populations. In contrast, the iron chelator, deferoxamine, was found to be a reversible S-phase inhibitor of human T- and B-lymphocyte proliferation (20).

The humoral arm of the immune system has also been examined for a potential immunoregulatory influence of iron. The system used to assess this effect has been immunoglobulin (Ig) secretion in response to PWM (13,21). As shown in Table 2, iron exhibited a differential effect with respect to (a) immunoglobulin class, and (b) concentration. For example, iron at the high concentration was able to enhance IgG secretion and yet suppress IgM secretion. Alternatively, at low concentration the results were reversed in that IgG secretion was suppressed and IgM secretion was increased.

The immunoregulatory effect of iron on specific antibody production to T-dependent and T-independent antigens has been examined by Duncan and McArthur, who demonstrated that lactoferrin, an iron-binding protein produced by neutrophils and found in concentration in secretions, could suppress T-dependent and independent primary antibody responses in the murine system. The evidence that lactoferrin influenced B function was indirect in that lactoferrin needed to be bound to monocyte-specific receptors, to be capable of mediating this suppressive effect. The role of lactoferrin in this study is paralleled by other work showing that myelopoiesis is also regulated by the binding of lactoferrin to monocytes (22).

Natural killer (NK) cell activity (23) and antibody-dependent cellular cytotoxicity (ADCC) are two immune effector functions that have been shown to be influenced by iron (15). Activity was suppressed by ferric citrate, enhanced by lactoferrin, but not influenced by transferrin at the concentration. By contrast, ADCC was suppressed by lactoferrin and not affected by citrate.

IMMUNOLOGICAL ABNORMALITIES ASSOCIATED WITH IRON IN DISEASE

A vast literature has accummulated describing the relation of iron with susceptibility to infectious, and inflammatory and neoplastic diseases (24-28). It seems likely that the ability of microorganisms to compete successfully with the host for iron is a feature of pathogenicity or virulence, and the ability of the host to limit availability of iron to the pathogen is associated with resistance to infection.

The bacteriostatic and fungistatic effects of serum are weakened by the addition of iron (29). Many microorganisms produce iron-binding substances (siderophores) which compete with animal or human hosts for iron. One such compound, deferoxamine, is widely used therapeutically as a chelator of ferric iron in iron overload disorders (20). Payne and Finkelstein (30) classified gram-negative bacteria according to their response the modification in iron levels in a chick embryo model, these results correlate with the nature of the infections they typically produce in humans. There is a good deal of evidence suggesting that increased availability of iron may predispose to infections with a variety of different kinds of organisms. Paradoxically, there are also a number of reports in which increased susceptibility to infection is apparently associated with states of iron deficiency.

One of the responses to infection or inflammation is a prompt drop in the plasma iron concentration (31–33). It has been suggested that fever plays a role in host defense against infection by reducing the ability of pathogenic bacteria to grow well at an elevated temperature in an iron-poor medium (34). Beresford et al. (35) have shown that iron absorption as measured by ^{59}Fe-labeled ferrous ascorbate was profoundly depressed in the presence of fever. This effect was not related to the nutritional state of the host.

A partial explanation for the paradox in susceptibility to infection in the presence of iron excess or deficiency may relate to the availability of iron, which promotes growth and pathogenicity of invading microorganisms on the one hand, and to the effects of iron depletion on lymphocyte function and the immune response on the other (36).

The following sections will deal with the in vivo and clinical correlates of immune function which have been reported in iron-deficiency and iron-overload states. Unfortunately, few well-controlled studies exist. In addition to the possible role of iron in the susceptibility to infection, the availability of iron and its effect on various cell populations of the immune system have been postulated as contributing to the activity of inflammatory diseases such as rheumatoid arthritis (37).

Iron Deficiency

The possibility of enhanced susceptibility to infections in iron-deficient subjects has been subject to debate for more than 50 years. Investigators have attempted to define defects in the immune system of iron-deficient subjects during the past 20 years (36,38).

In 1972, Joynson et al. (39) studied peripheral blood lymphocytes from 12 subjects with iron-deficiency anemia and demonstrated reduced lymphocyte transformation and macrophage inhibition factor (MIF) production after stimulation with *Candida albicans* and purified protein derivative (PPD). Moreover, delayed hypersensitivity skin testing was negative with these antigens in most iron-deficient subjects. Interestingly, treatment with iron reversed the MIF defect but not the lymphocyte transformation defect.

Contrasting evidence on the role of iron deficiency in the susceptibility to infections was reported by Masawe et al. (40), who studied infections in patients with iron deficiency and other anemias in the tropics. African patients with hemoglobin less than 10 g/dl were examined for frequency of infections. Of 67 subjects with iron-deficiency anemia, 5 (7%) had bacterial infections and 16 (24%) had evidence of malaria. Forty-three patients with other types of anemia (mainly secondary to parasitic infection) demonstrated a much higher incidence (65%) of bacterial infections, but only two had malaria. It was noted that malarial attacks in the iron-deficiency group generally developed after iron treatment. Subsequently, Barry and Reeve reported a high incidence of gram-negative sepsis in infants given iron dextran shortly after birth (41). When the injections were stopped, the incidence of sepsis decreased dramatically. These descriptive results suggest that increased iron, particularly sudden increased levels, rather than iron deficiency, may be associated with bacterial infections.

Kulapongs et al. (42) studied cell-mediated immunity and phagocytosis and killing function in a small group of children with severe iron-deficiency anemia. These investigators found no significant defect in lymphocyte response to mitogen and phagocytosis and killing function were abnormal in only one of eight malnourished children.

Chandra and Saraya (43) reported impaired immunocompetence associated with iron deficiency in a larger group of 20 children. Serum immunoglobulins were normal except in those with concurrent infection. Serum C3 levels were normal except in three children with active infection. Serum antibody responses to tetanus and *Salmonella typhimurium* were adequate. Delayed hypersensitivity was decreased, the in vitro response to PHA was impaired, and spontaneous T-cell rosette formation was slightly decreased. Opsonic activity of plasma and phagocytosis by neutrophils were normal. Intracellular killing of bacteria and reduction of nitroblue tetrazolium (NBT) were impaired and correlated with the severity of iron deficiency. Treatment with oral or parenteral iron injection corrected the immunological abnormalities. These authors concluded that iron deficiency was associated with a secondary reduction of immunocompetence, which was reversible.

Murray et al. (44) studied the incidence of malarial attacks in adults in Central Africa with refeeding and attendant hyperferremia. Early hyperferremia, associated with refeeding, led to rapid multiplication of parasites and attacks of malaria.

Srikantia et al. (45) reported a reduction in the cell-mediated immune response and the bacterial activity of leukocytes in Indian children with low hemoglobin but many of the subjects did not have iron deficiency.

Krantman et al. (46) studied 10 iron-deficient children under 3 years of age before and after iron replacement and found mild defects in T-cell immunity, which improved following iron repletion. The authors thus concluded that these subtle defects in cell-mediated immunity in iron-deficient children could be corrected with oral iron replacement.

Warshaw et al. (47) found low levels of serum transferrin, and immunoglobulins in patients with nephrotic syndrome. This led to studies on the effect of hypotransferrinemic serum on lymphocyte proliferation in vitro. Lymphocyte responses were found to be proportional to serum transferrin concentration, suggesting that hypotransferrinemia was associated with poor lymphocyte function and immunity in this syndrome. The percentage of iron saturation was measured in patients with relapsed nephrotic syndrome and was elevated (>50%) in some cases. The relationship of these findings to iron deficiency was not defined, however, as the status of the patients was not presented.

In a brief review of the effects of iron deficiency other than anemia, Dallman et al. (48) cited evidence for a subtle decrease in DNA synthesis by lymphocytes in clinical iron deficiency.

An interesting report on the effects of chronic iron deficiency in patients with polycythemia vera treated exclusively with venesection for periods as long as 15 years showed no increased incidence of bacterial or other infections (49). Lack of problems with infection strongly suggests that any immune system abnormalities present in chronic iron deficiency in adults may be subclinical.

Chandra (50,51) has suggested that conflicting data in the literature might be explained by different methodology and tests conducted, number of subjects, the presence of concommitant recent infection (bacterial or parasitic), cause of the iron deficiency, and criteria for the diagnosis of iron deficiency.

Chandra's own studies have indicated that iron deficiency may result in a slight reduction in circulating T cells, a decrease in delayed hypersensitivity, and a decrease in lymphocyte transformation to mitogens and antigens (50,51). Increased susceptibility to fungal (*Candida*) and viral (herpes simplex) infections was reversed after iron treatment. Similarly, 15 of 16 patients (ages 11–41 years) with recurrent staphylococcal furunculosis and hypoferremia (but not anemia) improved following 1 month of treatment with oral iron supplements (52).

Chandra has suggested that the route of iron administration may influence susceptibility to infection (50) since oral iron does not saturate transferrin but parenteral iron may exceed the iron-binding capacity and, therefore, may increase the virulence of the pathogen.

Children with protein-calorie malnutrition would pose a special problem, since they have reduced levels of transferrin that may correlate with a poor chance for survival. The risk of infection might be reduced if iron administration were delayed for a few days, allowing time for repair of transferrin synthesis (50).

Although unsaturated transferrin is known to inhibit the growth of many microorganisms, and iron loading may have an adverse effect on the survival of experimental animals inoculated with certain bacteria, the clinical importance of these observations remains unclear. It is noteworthy that of six reported cases of congenital atransferrinemia in humans in which transferrin was absent from serum, infections were reported in only one (53). However, Beutler and Fairbanks (54) have suggested that in this disorder other proteins, possibly albumin, may bind and transport the plasma iron. There seems little doubt that iron deficiency in children is associated with subtle defects in cell-mediated immunity and the available data suggest that some, and possibly all, of these defects can be corrected by iron therapy. However, the clinical consequences of iron deficiency with respect to enhanced susceptibility to infection remain obscure, even in children. Moreover, the route, dose, and schedule of iron replacement may pose an even greater hazard for the development of certain infections than iron deficiency. In adults with iron lack, there is little evidence for increase in infections.

There is some circumstantial evidence relating iron deficiency to susceptibility to develop various autoimmune diseases (55). Interestingly, a case of iron deficiency anemia caused by the development of an autoantibody against the transferrin receptor (56,57) was associated with normal immune response and slightly elevated $CD8^+$ T cells.

Primary Iron Overload

Hereditary hemochromatosis (HH) is an HLA-linked, recessively transmitted, disease that involves inappropriately high intestinal iron absorption (58–60). Consequently, accumulation of transferrin-transported iron in the parenchymal cells of organs such as the liver, heart, and pancreas results. The immune system in HH has been evaluated in a few studies (61–66) (Table 3). In our studies (61), a T-lymphocyte receptor abnormality was identified which involved aberrant expression of an epitope of the E-rosette receptor, CD2 (defined by OKT11 and 9.6), as measured by the sheep red blood cell binding assay at 37°C as thermostable erythrocyte rosettes (TER). Previous studies had shown TER receptor expression was associated with activation or early thymocyte differentiation (75), but was not the basis of TER expression in HH. Furthermore, TER expression appeared not to be associated with the iron level (presented in Figure 1). This conclusion was further supported by the observation

Table 3 Immune Evaluation in Iron Overload Disease

Iron overload etiology	Disease evaluated	Lymphoid function/molecule evaluated	Influence	References
Primary	Hereditary hemochromatosis			61–66
	untreated	Lymphocyte proliferation	Suppressed	
		TER lymphocytes	Elevated	
		CD8 lymphocytes	Elevated	
		CD3 and CD4 lymphocytes	Normal	
	treated	Lymphocyte proliferation	Normal	
		TER lymphocytes	Elevated	
		CD8 lymphocytes	Reduced	
		CD3 and CD4 lymphocytes	Normal	
		NK activity	Normal	
		Transferrin receptor expression	Normal	
		PWM-induced Ig secretion	Altered (see text)	
Secondary	Thalassemia intermedia			65–68
		Lymphocyte proliferation	Suppressed	
		Serum IgG and IgM	Elevated	
		B lymphocytes	Reduced	
		T lymphocytes	Normal	
	Thalassemia major			69–71
		CD8 lymphocytes	Elevated	
		CD4 lymphocytes	Reduced	
		Ig-containing B lymphocytes	Elevated	
		NK activity	Suppressed	
		HLA-DR expression	Elevated	
	Sickle cell disease			72, 73
	transfused	CD4:CD8 ratio	Reduced	
		NK activity	Reduced	
	nontransfused	CD4:CD8 ratio	Normal	
		NK activity	Normal	
	Chronic hemodialysis	CD4:CD8 ratio	Reduced	

Abbreviations: TER, thermostable erythrocyte rosette-forming lymphocytes; CD3, pan-T cell population; CD4, helper/inducer T-cell subset; CD8, suppressor/cytotoxic T-cell subset; NK, natural killer cell.

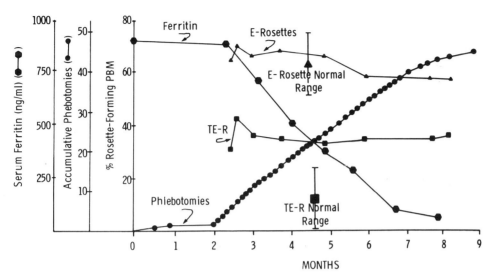

Figure 1 Enumeration of thermostable (37°C) erythrocyte rosette (TER)–forming peripheral blood mononuclear cells (PBM) and conventional E-rosette (4°C) forming PBM in a 67-year-old male, HH patient during treatment. (From Bryan and Leech, unpublished data).

(62) that the absolute number of TER receptor-bearing T cells was elevated to the same level in untreated and treated HH patients. Moreover, it was found that males but not females who were heterozygous for the hemochromatosis gene (siblings, parents, and children of the patient) had significantly elevated TER levels that were intermediate between that of controls and HH patients (Table 4), suggesting that TER expression might be linked to genes involved in HH.

Table 4 Thermostable Erythrocyte Rosettes in Hereditary Hemochromatosis

Group evaluated	TER/mm³	p Value[a]
Controls	202.2 ± 18.0[b]	—
males	205.3 ± 25.4	—
females	207.8 ± 23.8	—
HH untreated	597.2 ± 158.3	1.9×10^{-6}
HH treated	615.0 ± 136.0	1.4×10^{-6}
Heterozygotes	336.9 ± 39.3	1.2×10^{-3}
males	445.7 ± 75.1	9.7×10^{-3}
females	261.9 ± 32.3	NSD[c]

[a] The P value given is for the comparison with the control group except for male heterozygotes where the p value is for the comparison with female heterozygotes.
[b] The mean ± SEM are presented for control individuals, patients with HH who are untreated or treated, and individuals who are heterozygous for the hemochromatosis gene.
[c] Not significantly different.

The biological relevance of the aberrant expression of the TER epitope on HH T cells (HH-CD2/TER epitope) and its clinical significance in HH is unknown. The CD2 molecule has been shown to be involved in regulation of T-cell function (76–82) and in adhesion of cytotoxic T lymphocytes and thymocytes to specific ligands on the target cell and thymic epithelium (78–82).

At least three regulatory properties have been proposed for the CD2 molecule on normal T lymphocytes. The first is in its role in the alternate pathway of antigen-independent T-cell activation distinct from the classic MHC-restricted T-cell antigen receptor, CD3/TCR (76–78). Furthermore, a functional relationship has been reported to exist between the CD2 molecule and the IL-2 receptor (79,80). A second postulated role for the CD2 molecule is in the cytolytic T-lymphocyte effector mechanism (78). A third regulatory function of the CD2 molecule is its ability to behave as a "negative signal receptor" which can depress T-cell proliferation (80,81). The CD2 molecule has also been implicated as the natural receptor for the thymic ligand, LFA 3 (82). Altered expression of the CD2 molecule in HH, in concert with iron, or an iron-modulated cytokine, may be associated with the altered immune function noted in HH patients.

Proliferative response to mitogens (PHA, Con A, and PWM) and in the MLC was found to be significantly reduced in untreated HH patients but was normal in those HH patients who were treated in our studies. Furthermore, the absolute number of CD8 lymphocytes was elevated in untreated HH patients, whereas they were reduced in treated HH patients, as compared to controls. Natural killer cell function was normal in treated HH patients (62), but in recent preliminary experiments we have found low NK activity in one of two untreated HH patients (C.F. Bryan et al., unpublished results). Finally, PWM-induced immunoglobulin secretion was altered in treated HH patients. Increased spontaneous synthesis of total Ig and IgG was noted. Enhanced Ig synthesis in response to suboptimal concentrations of PWM was found, and suppression of Ig synthesis (total Ig and IgG) occurred when optimal and superoptimal PWM concentrations were used. The mechanism(s) are unknown.

Increased expression of the HH-CD2/TER epitope in HH could relate to an HLA-linked gene that is responsible for the activity of liver neuraminidase, which is known to remove sialic acid from an epitope of the T lymphocyte's CD2 molecule and is the basis of the ability of T cells to form TER (77). Such an MHC-linked gene has been identified in one particular mouse strain, SM/J, that is responsible for low activity of liver neuraminidase (83).

Studies have shown that expression of the transferrin receptor is not affected in HH (61,64).

Relationship to the monocyte-macrophage system has also been postulated by Bjorn-Rasmussen (84). Despite the chronic massive iron overload and associated high transferrin saturation and immunological abnormalities described above, infections are rarely found in HH (85). However, Van Asback et al. (85) reported a patient with HH who developed *Listeria* meningitis; monocytes from this patient were shown to have reduced phagocytic capacity which was reversible after a series of therapeutic phlebotomies. These in vitro studies were felt to indicate that iron had a deleterious effect on monocyte and granulocyte phagocytosis. Individuals with HH do have a higher than expected incidence of hepatomas and possibly other extrahepatic neoplasms (86–88). The propensity to develop hepatoma does not appear related to the iron status of the individual, since it remains even after depletion of iron by phlebotomy. Relationship to immune dysfunction is unknown.

Secondary Iron Overload

Most existing data relate to observed immunological abnormalities in patients with thalassemia intermedia or major and are summarized in Table 3 (67-74). Patients with thalassemia intermedia have been studied for mitogenic response to PHA, Con A, and PWM (59), and impaired responses were seen only in patients with serum iron levels higher than 200 μg/dl. No clinically important correlations were found among the patients who displayed poor mitogenic responses and splenectomy had no apparent effect on the response level. In thalassemia major, Grady et al. (69) showed that the percentage of CD8-positive suppressor/cytotoxic cells increased linearly with the number of units of blood transfused irrespective of splenectomy. The percentage of CD4 helper cells varied inversely with increasing transfusion in nonsplenectomized patients, whereas no significant correlation was apparent in those who were splenectomized. Thus, in both groups of patients, the CD4:CD8 ratio declined in a transfusion-related manner. Splenectomized patients displayed a persistent lymphocytosis due to an increase in the number of both T and B cells. The greatest relative increase occurred in the number of B cells and was unrelated to the number of transfusions received. None of the serum parameters usually associated with iron overload or abnormal liver function correlated with observed increases in T-suppressor or surface immunoglobulin–positive cells. These findings corroborated the reports that transfusion of blood products may lead to reduced CD4:CD8 ratios.

The proportion of B cells was increased in terms of cytoplasmic immunoglobulin but not by an increase in immunoglobulin-secreting cells as measured by a reverse hemolytic plaque assay (70). Despite the hyperimmunoglobulinemia (89), in thalassemia there is no correlation with an increased incidence of infection or with serum iron level or transferrin saturation.

Increases in suppressor T cells (CD8-positive) also have been found in multiply transfused sickle-cell patients (72,73), and are not present in nontransfused patients with this disorder. Although such abnormalities lead to a CD4:CD8 ratio like that found in patients with AIDS, the low ratio in multiply transfused patients is primarily due to an elevation in the CD8 population, whereas the low ratio in AIDS patients is due to depletion of CD4 cells. Patients with thalassemia major also have been reported to have a reduction in natural killer cell activity which appeared to be reversible and transfusion-related, possibly as a consequence of iron overload (71-73).

Infections in Patients with Secondary Iron Overload

As noted, iron overload in thalassemia patients does not correlate with a substantial increase in clinically apparent infections. The same circumstance may not apply to other conditions of secondary iron excess. Mossey and Sontheimer (90) retrospectively studied the incidence of infections with *Listeria* in two separate hemodialysis units during a 4-year interval. Four cases of *Listeria* bacteremia were documented; these patients had received between 75 and 200 transfusions of packed red blood cells, which appeared to be suggestive of a causal relationship in light of there being no other etiological factors. Transfusion-related iron overload in dialysis patients also appears to predispose them to *Yersinia* bacteremia (91). Infections with this organism as well as mucormycosis (91) have been associated with deferoxamine therapy (91-93).

Felton et al. (94) reported a relationship between serum iron levels and response to hepatitis B virus. These investigators studied 201 patients on chronic renal dialysis and found that serum iron was higher in those with hepatitis B surface antigen present in their serum than in those without hepatitis B antigen, independent of the transferrin level. These findings also support a possible relationship between high iron levels and the likelihood of hepatitis B infection progressing to primary hepatocellular carcinoma.

IRON ABSORPTION AND THE MAJOR HISTOCOMPATIBILITY COMPLEX

In humans, only two inherited diseases exist that involve inappropriate iron absorption, atransferrinemia and hereditary hemochromatosis (HH). Subsequent discussion in this section will be confined to HH, since only a few cases of atransferrinemia have been reported (53,54). Moreover, HH is linked to the major histocompatibility complex (HLA), a genetic region that has been evaluated extensively regarding its role in the regulation of the immune response and cellular interaction (95).

It is thought that HH is one of the more common inherited diseases. Among caucasians, the frequency of homozygousity (hh) is 0.3–0.5% and the frequency of heterozygousity (Hh) is 10% (95,96). Gene frequency in other populations varies considerably. Hereditary hemochromatosis is an iron overload disorder that results from inappropriate and unregulated intestinal iron absorption (58–60). The absorbed iron is transported through the intestinal cell by the iron-transport molecule, transferrin. A gradual accumulation of iron thus occurs in various organs, especially the liver, heart, and pancreas. Such tissue iron overload generally results in clinically detectable sequelae, which become detectable in men during the fourth or fifth decade of life and still later in women. The diagnosis of HH is made by the demonstration of iron deposition primarily in the parenchymal cells of the liver after other secondary causes have been ruled out. Phlebotomy therapy, which mobilizes the storage iron in the various organs of deposition, is successful in the prolongation of life for patients with HH (97), but the incidence of hepatomas in HH remains elevated in those with cirrhosis. An increased incidence of extrahepatic malignancies (86–88) has also been observed.

Although Sheldon presented familial evidence supporting the genetic nature of HH in 1935, vigorous debate ensued during the following 40 years until in 1976, it was shown that the HLA class I antigens, A3 and B7, were both highly associated with HH. The hemochromatosis gene was found to be recessive and linked to the HLA-A locus. Thus, siblings of an HH patients could be genotyped. For example, siblings of an HH patient who were HLA genotypically identical and possessed both of the HLA-linked h genes should eventually develop the disease. Similarly, siblings who were HLA haploidentical with the HH patient and only possessed one h gene would most likely not develop any clinical evidence of HH. This analysis assumes that an HLA/h gene recombination has not occurred, but one such HLA/h recombination has recently been identified (98). This unusual circumstance enabled the mapping of the h gene to the centromeric side of the HLA-A locus, between the A and B loci.

The basic function of the h gene with respect to iron absorption is, however, unknown. We can, therefore, only pose questions that need to be answered about expression of the h gene. Examples of such questions are as follows: (a) What is the nature of the product(s) of the h gene? (b) How is that gene and/or gene product involved in iron absorption? (c) Why is the h gene located inside the HLA complex within the A and B loci? (d) Is the molecular structure of the h gene related to that of HLA class I genes? Taking this possibility one step further, is there a relationship between the HLA-HT antigen system, which is an HLA-associated antigen system identified on activated T cells, that has been reported to be associated with HLA-A3? (e) What is the tissue distribution of the h gene product? These and other questions undoubtedly will be addressed by investigators in the near future using recombinant DNA technology. One such report has already appeared, in which a 6.2 kilobase Bgl I genomic DNA fragment associated with HH was identified (99). Perhaps that fragment is in linkage disequilibrium with the h gene.

Finally, the possibility that unconventional HLA gene products may be involved in the development of HH is worthy of consideration in view of recent studies in mice. A liver-specific, H-2-linked (H-2 is the mouse major histocompatibility complex) class I gene mRNA with unusual properties has been identified (100). This molecule is structurally different from that of the classic molecules expressed on the surface of a cell in that the transmembrane portion of that mRNA is truncated. Such a structural change makes it likely that its protein molecule is secreted as contrasted with class I molecules, which usually are expressed on the surface membrane. Furthermore, congenic strains of mice of different H-2 types vary with regard to the amount of this unusual mRNA. Twenty-five percent of that mRNA is found in the liver, whereas in other tissues, such as the brain and thymus, that mRNA comprises only background levels of less than 5%. This finding raises the question whether such HLA gene products may be responsible in part for the development of HH.

MECHANISMS INVOLVED IN THE IMMUNOREGULATORY PROPERTIES OF IRON

The molecular mechanism(s) responsible for the previously described immunoregulatory properties of iron and the proteins that bind iron are incompletely understood. The following discussion will review the various mechanisms that may be involved in iron's immunoregulatory effect and emphasize those needing additional information.

Transferrin Receptor Regulation

Bomford and Munro reviewed the role of the transferrin receptor in normal iron transport and iron homeostasis (101). Receptor number increases coincide with the onset of DNA synthesis. Transferrin receptor-specific transcription can be detected within 12 hr of lymphocyte activation. Maximum DNA synthesis peaks much later, however. The mechanism involved in transporting the transferrin-bound iron, via the transferrin receptor, is known to occur by the endocytosis of the transferrin/transferrin receptor complex (102), which is a general mechanism for the transport of various molecules into cells (103,104). In the case of iron, the intracellular endocytic vesicle becomes acidic (pH 5), which causes the iron to be released from transferrin. The apo-transferrin, which is still bound to the transferrin receptor, is returned to the cell surface, and the receptor is ready for additional cycles.

Recent observations regarding the regulation of the transferrin receptor support its important role in immunoregulation. First, expression of the transferrin receptor is closely associated with that of the receptor for interleukin 2 (IL-2) (105,106). Several data from those reports support the interactive role for transferrin and interleukin-2 in immune regulation. The presence of IL-2 receptors is necessary for transferrin receptor induction. Furthermore, DNA synthesis is inhibited by monoclonal antibodies to the IL-2 receptor, only if administered before transferrin receptors have appeared. By contrast, monoclonal antibodies to the transferrin receptor inhibit DNA synthesis but not expression of the IL-2 receptor.

Trowbridge and Lopez (107) and Manger et al. (106) have presented evidence that the transferrin receptor also has a role in the regulation of cell growth and activation. Finally, Lum et al. (108) showed that CD4, helper/inducer, lymphocytes have a second autocrine regulatory loop in addition to that of the IL-2/IL-2 receptor system. The second loop is that of the transferrin/transferrin receptor autocrine system.

Lymphocyte-Monocyte Secretion of Iron-Containing Molecules

Another mechanism that may underlie some of the immunoregulatory properties of iron involves lymphocyte-monocyte secretion of iron-containing molecules. For example, transferrin has been shown to be synthesized by $CD4^+$ and $CD8^+$ lymphocytes. A summary of the studies that have evaluated the synthesis and/or secretion of such lymphokines-monokines is shown in Table 5 (109–114). Furthermore, ferritin has been shown to be synthesized by T cells and monocytes, and may be involved in immunoregulation as is transferrin (113).

Several investigators have examined the monocyte system to evaluate its ability to "handle" iron. Such studies were performed because of the notion that in early

Table 5 Iron-Binding Proteins Produced by Cells of the Immune System

Cell source	Cell population	Protein	Result	References
Hemochromatosis				109,110
untreated	Monocytes	Intracellular ferritin	Elevated	
treated	Monocytes	Intracellular ferritin	Normal	
		Iron uptake	Normal	
		Ferrition synthesis	Normal	
		Ferriton iron incorporation	Normal	
	Lymphocytes	Iron uptake	Normal	
		Ferriton synthesis	Normal	
		Ferriton iron incorporation	Normal	
	PBMC	Ferritin secretion	Reduced	111
Control individuals	PBMC	Ferritin secretion:		112
		HLA-A2 positive	Elevated	
		HLA-A3 positive	Normal	
	T lymphocytes	Ferritin synthesis	—	113
	CD4 lymphocytes	Transferrin synthesis	—	108
	CD8 lymphocytes	Transferrin synthesis	—	114

Abbreviations: PBMC, peripheral blood mononuclear cells.

The Immunoregulatory Properties of Iron

hemochromatosis, the propensity for iron deposition was in the hepatic parenchymal cells as opposed to the reticuloendothelial cells. As shown in Table 5, the majority of studies show that ferritin synthesis and all other evaluated mechanisms of "iron handling" were normal in such patients (109,110). In one study, however, ferritin secretion was examined in a population of unseparated peripheral blood mononuclear cells (111), in contrast to those above that used purified monocytes following activation and treatment with ferric citrate. Normal individuals who possessed the HLA class I antigen A3 had ferritin secretion levels that were less than those who lacked this antigen.

Biochemical Mechanisms Involved in the Immunoregulatory Properties of Iron

The biochemical mechanisms involved at the cell membrane and/or intracellularly which are responsible for the immunoregulatory properties of iron are not known. The observation that PWM-activated lymphocytes display an iron-induced increase in proliferative response and transferrin receptor expression have not been correlated with the biochemical events involved in lymphocyte proliferation (7,11).

Certain biochemical events involved in lymphocyte triggering and subsequent steps that lead to a proliferating cell are known. For instance, once the CD3/TCR receptor complex on T cells is triggered, an increase in cytoplasmic free calcium occurs, which in turn initiates the intracellular events necessary for activation (115). A second example of intracellular biochemical events that occur after antigen-induced lymphocyte triggering involves membrane signal transduction with protein kinase C (116). Furthermore, protein kinase C may be located on a crossover point of many biochemical pathways in hormone activation and cell proliferation that involve calcium, inositol phospholipids, arachidonic acid, prostaglandins, cyclic nucleotides, and tumor promotors.

In view of our knowledge that specific biochemical events occur at either the cell membrane or intracellularly, it would be instructive to know whether any of the immunoregulatory properties of iron discussed in this chapter are the result of an influence by iron at those and/or other points. Of interest with respect to possible intracellular effects that may be mediated by iron is a report by Bomford et al. (117). They showed that once inside an activated lymphocyte, iron is partitioned into three compartments: (a) haem-iron, (b) ferritin-iron, and finally (c) non–haem-iron and non-ferritin-iron. They concluded that iron in those forms may act as a precursor for functional and/or structural compounds. The question of whether such compounds may influence the rate of biochemical events that lead to lymphocyte proliferation is unresolved. An example of how iron may influence an intracellular enzyme is a study by Weintraub et al. (118). These investigators found that prolyl hydroxylase activity, a key enzyme in collagen biosynthesis, was significant elevated in iron-loaded rats as compared to levels in the control group. Information on the influence of iron and its binding proteins on such biochemical events would help to elucidate the mechanism(s) responsible for their immunoregulatory properties.

Iron-Modulated Cytokine(s) or Interleukins

A final mechanism that may influence the immune system in patients with primary or secondary iron overload is that of iron-modulated cytokines, specifically the IL-2 receptor autocrine loop (108). Good et al. (119) have shown that iron is capable of reducing the cloning efficiency of antigen-specific CD4-positive helper cell precursor development, and that iron decreased the rate of proliferative response which resulted in a decrease in final clone size. In interpretation of these data, Good proposed that iron was responsible for a reduction of IL-2 production. These findings appear to relate to the reduced proliferative response exhibited by untreated HH patients compared to treated HH patients with normal or reduced iron stores. Definitive evidence showing that iron is responsible for altering cytokine/interleukin levels remains to be obtained.

CONCLUSIONS

Although a range of immunological abnormalities have been documented in patients with iron deficiency and iron overload, the clinical importance of such abnormalities remains largely undefined. The demonstrated defects noted in patients with iron deficiency appear related to the iron-deficient state, but are subtle and of questionable clinical relevance. Clinical correlation with immunological abnormalities noted in patients with iron overload are likewise vague and difficult to define.

In order to better delineate the immunoregulatory properties of iron in humans, other variables need to be evaluated in a critical manner. These include (a) age of the patient group under study, (b) underlying disease responsible for iron deficiency or excess, (c) associated disorders present (particularly those which may affect the immune system), (d) methodological factors, (e) serial observations during iron repletion and/or removal, and (f) genetic (HLA) factors of the host. Despite the less than clear-cut clinically important immunological consequences of iron deficiency or overload, the immunoregulatory role of iron and its binding proteins clearly has been established and should provide further important insights into the function of the immune system in the future. In addition, improved methods for the study of reticuloendothelial iron kinetics as reported by Bentley et al. (120) and Uchida et al. (121) may better define our understanding of in vivo iron metabolism.

Our own observations, first, that $CD8^+$ T cells are increased in untreated HH patients, and, second, that $CD8^+$ T cells normalize with treatment provide a logical basis for the hypothesis that cellular immunity may be influenced by the high level of iron storage in HH patients (122). In addition, since as we recently reported (123), alterations in cellular immunity can be followed by the development of carcinoma in HH, it seems probable that elevated iron may be an important cofactor in the development of cancer.

ACKNOWLEDGMENTS

We would like to thank Sally Arnold for expert typing and Jennifer Bryan for valuable editorial assistance in the preparation of this chapter. We also thank Dr. Corwin Q. Edwards for his helpful discussion.

REFERENCES

1. Frenkel EP, Stone MJ. The rationale and approach to immunosuppressive therapy. Adv Int Med 17:21, 1971.

2. Meuer SC, Hussey RE, Cantrell DA, Hodgdon JC, Schlossman SF, Smith KA, Reinherz EL. Triggering of the T3-Ti antigen-receptor complex results in clonal T-cell proliferation through an interleukin 2-dependent autocrine pathway. Proc Natl Acad Sci USA 81:1509, 1984.
3. Tsoukas CD, Landgraf B, Bentin J, Valentine M, Lotz M, Vaughan JH, Carson DA. Activation of resting T lymphocytes by anti-CD3 (T3) antibodies in the absence of monocytes. J Immunol 135:1719, 1985.
4. De Sousa M, Nishiya K. Inhibition of E-rosette formation by two iron salts. Cell Immunol 38:203, 1978.
5. Nishiya K, Gupta S, De Sousa M. Differential inhibitory effect of iron on E, EA and EAC rosette formation. Cell Immunol 46:405, 1979.
6. Nishiya K, De Sousa M, Tsoi E, Bognacki JJ, DeHarven E. Regulation of expression of a human lymphoid cell surface marker by iron. Cell Immunol 53:71, 1980.
7. Bryan CF, Leech SH, Bozelka B. The immunoregulatory nature of iron. II. Lymphocyte surface marker expression. J Leuk Biol 40:589, 1986.
8. Bryan CF, Nishiya K, Pollack MS, Dupont B, DeSousa M. Differential inhibition of the MLR by iron: Association with HLA phenotype. Immunogenetics 12:129, 1981.
9. Matzner Y, Hershko C, Polliack A, Konijn AM, Izak G. Suppressive effect of ferritin on in vitro lymphocyte function. Br J Haematol 42:345, 1979.
10. Keown P, Latscha-Descamps B. In vitro suppression of cell-mediated immunity by ferroproteins and ferric salts. Cell Immunol 80:257, 1983.
11. Bryan CF, Leech SM. The immunoregulatory nature of iron. I. Lymphocyte proliferation. Cell Immunol 75:71, 1983.
12. Stenzel KM, Rubin AL, Novogrodsky A. Mitogenic and co-mitogenic properties of hemin. J Immunol 127:2469, 1981.
13. Munn CG, DeSousa M. Iron and B cell differentiation: Effect on secretion of IgG, IgA and IgM by human cells. Fed Proc 41:794, 1982.
14. Duncan RL, McArthur WP. Lactoferrin-mediated modulation of mononuclear cell activities. Cell Immunol 63:308, 1981.
15. Nishiya K, Horwitz DA. Contrasting effects of lactoferrin on human lymphocyte and monocyte natural killer activity and antibody-dependent cell-mediated cytotoxicity. J Immunol 129:2519, 1982.
16. Biddison WE, Rao PE, Talle MA, Goldstein G, Shaw S. Possible involvement of the T4 molecule in T cell recognition of class II HLA antigens: Evidence from studies of proliferative responses to SB antigens. J Immunol 131:152, 1983.
17. Golding H, McCluskey J, Munitz TI, Germain RN, Margulies DH, Singer A. T-cell recognition of a chimaeric class II/class I MHC molecule and the role of L3T4. Nature 317:425, 1985.
18. Spits H, Yssel H, Voordouw A, Vries JE. The role of T8 in the cytotoxic activity of cloned cytotoxic T lymphocyte lines specific for Class II and Class I major histocompatibility complex antigens. J Immunol 134:2294, 1985.
19. Reinherz EL, Meuer SC, Schlossman SF. The human T cell receptor: Analysis with cytotoxic T cell clones. Immunol Rev 74:83, 1983.
20. Lederman HM, Cohen A, Lee JWW, Freedman MH, Gelfand EW. Deferoxamine: A reversible S-phase inhibitor of human lymphocyte proliferation. Blood 64:748, 1984.
21. Ashman RF. Lymphocyte activation. In: Fundamental Immunology. Paul WE, ed. Raven Press, New York, 1984. Chapter 12.
22. Gentile P, Broxmeyer HE. Suppression of mouse myelopoiesis by administration of human lactoferrin in vivo and the comparative action of human transferrin. Blood 61:982, 1983.
23. Roder JC, Pross HF. The biology of the human natural killer cell. J Clin Immunol 2:249, 1982.

24. Weinberg ED. Iron and susceptibility to infectious disease. Science 184:952, 1974.
25. Weinberg ED. Iron withholding: A defense against infection and neoplasia. Physiol Rev 64:65, 1984.
26. Letendre ED. The importance of iron in the pathogenesis of infection and neoplasia. Trends Biochem Sci 9:166, 1985.
27. Ward CG. Influence of iron on infection. Am J Surg 151:291, 1986.
28. Brock JH. Iron and cells of the immune system. *In*: De Sousa M, Brock JH, eds. Iron in immunity, cancer, and inflammation. Chichester: John Wiley, 1989, p 81.
29. Caroline L, Rosner F, Kozinn PJ. Elevated serum iron, low unbound transferrin and Candidiasis in acute leukemia. Blood 34:441, 1969.
30. Payne SM, Finkelstein RA. The critical role of iron in host-bacterial interactions. J Clin Invest 61:1428, 1978.
31. Ballantyne GH. Rapid drop in serum iron concentration as a host defense mechanism. A review of clinical and experimental evidence. Ann Surg 50:405, 1984.
32. Huebers HA, Finch CA. Transferrin: Physiologic behavior and clinical implications. Blood 64:763, 1984.
33. Hunter RL, Bennett B, Towns M, Vogler WR. Transferrin in disease II: Defects in the regulation of transferrin saturation with iron contributes to susceptibility to infection. Am J Clin Pathol 81:748, 1984.
34. Kluger MJ, Rothenberg BA. Fever and reduced iron: Their interaction as a host defense response to bacterial infection. Science 203:374, 1979.
35. Beresford CH, Neale RJ, Brooks OG. Iron absorption and pyrexia. Lancet 1:568, 1971.
36. Cook JD, Lynch SR. The liabilities of iron deficiency. Blood 68:803, 1986.
37. Blake DR, Bacon PA, Dieppe PA, Gutteridge JMC. The importance of iron in rheumatoid disease. Lancet 2:1142, 1981.
38. Bothwell T. The importance of assessing iron status. Hosp Pract 26 (Suppl 3):11, 1991.
39. Joynson DHM, Jacobs A, Walker DM, Dolby AE. Defect of cell-mediated immunity in patients with iron-deficiency anaemia. Lancet 2:1058, 1972.
40. Masawe AEJ, Juindi JM, Swai GBR. Infections in iron-deficiency and other types of anaemia in the tropics. Lancet 2:314, 1974 (see also editorial: Iron and resistance to infection. Lancet 2:325, 1974).
41. Barry DMJ, Reeve AW. Iron and infection in the newborn (letter). Lancet 2:1385, 1974.
42. Kulapongs P, Vithayasai V, Suskind R, Olson RE. Cell-mediated immunity and phagocytosis and killing function in children with severe iron-deficiency anaemia. Lancet 2:689, 1974.
43. Chandra RK, Saraya AK. Impaired immunocompetence associated with iron-deficiency. J Pediatr 86:899, 1975.
44. Murray MJ, Murray AB, Murray NJ, Murray MB. Refeeding-malaria and hyperferraemia. Lancet 1:653, 1975.
45. Srikantia SG, Prasad JS, Bhaskaram C, Krishnamachari KAVR. Anaemia and immune response. Lancet 1:1307, 1976.
46. Krantman HJ, Young SR, Ank BJ, O'Donnell CM, Rachelefsky GS, Stiehm ER. Immune function in pure iron deficiency. Am J Dis Child 136:840, 1982.
47. Warshaw BL, Check IJ, Hymes LC, DiRusso SC. Decreased serum transferrin concentration in children with the nephrotic syndrome: Effect on lymphocyte proliferation and correlation with serum immunoglobulin levels. Clin Immunol Immunopathol 33:210, 1984.
48. Dallman PR, Beutler E, Finch CA. Effects of iron-deficiency exclusive of anaemia (annotation). Br J Haematol 40:179, 1978.
49. Rector WG, Fortuin NJ, Conley CL. Non-hematologic effects of chronic iron deficiency. A study of patients with polycythemia vera treated solely with venesections. Medicine 61:382, 1982.

50. Chandra RK, Vyas D. Functional consequences of iron deficiency. Non erythroid effects. *In*: Critical Reviews in Tropical Medicine. Chandra RK, ed., New York: Plenum Press, Vol. 2, 1984, Chapter 4.
51. Chandra RK. Trace element regulation of immunity and infection. J Am Coll Nutr 4:5, 1985.
52. Weijmer MC, Neering H, Wetten C. Preliminary report: Furunculosis and hypoferraemia. Lancet 336:464, 1990.
53. Heilmeyer L, Keller W, Vivell O, Keiderling W, Betke K, Wohler F, Schultze HE. Congenital transferrin deficiency in a seven year old girl. Ger Med Monthly 6:385, 1961.
54. Beutler E, Fairbanks VF. The effects of iron deficiency. *In*: Iron in Biochemistry and Medicine, II. Jacobs A, Worwood M, eds., London: Academic Press, 1984, Chapter 11.
55. Chisholm M. Tissue changes associated with iron deficiency. Clin Haematol 2:303, 1973.
56. Hyman ES. Acquired iron-deficiency anemia due to impaired iron transport. Lancet 1:91, 1983.
57. Larrick JW, Hyman ES. Acquired iron-deficiency anemia caused by an antibody against the transferrin receptor. N Engl J Med 311:214, 1984.
58. Valberg LS, Ghent CN. Diagnosis and management of hereditary hemochromatosis. Ann Rev Med 36:27, 1985.
59. Fairbanks VF, Baldus WP. Hemochromatosis: The neglected diagnosis. Mayo Clin Proc 61:296, 1986.
60. Bothwell TH, Charlton RW, Motulsky AG. Hemochromatosis. *In*: Scriver CR, Beaudot AL, Sly WS, Valle D, eds. The metabolic basis of inherited disease, ed. 6. New York: McGraw-Hill, 1989, p 1433.
61. Bryan CF, Leech SH, Ducos R, Edwards CQ, Kushner JP, Skolnick MH, Bozelka B, Linn JC, Gaumer R. Thermostable erythrocyte rosette-forming lymphocytes in hereditary hemochromatosis. I. Identification in peripheral blood. J Clin Immunol 4:134, 1984.
62. Bryan CF, Leech SH, Kumar P, Gaumar P, Bozelka B, Morgan J. The immune system in hereditary hemochromatosis: A quantitative and functional assessment of the cellular arm. Am J Med Sci 301(1):55, 1991.
63. Kranwinkel R, Gudino M, Kakaiya R, Harrison L, Lenart S. Intact Immunological Response in Long Term Intensively Phlebotomized Patients with Idiopathic Hemochromatosis. AABB abstract from 1985 Meeting.
64. Ward JH, Kushner JP, Ray FA, Kaplan J. Transferrin receptor function in hereditary hemochromatosis. J Lab Clin Med 103:246, 1984.
65. Good MF, Powell LW, Halliday JW. Iron status and cellular immune competence. Blood Rev 2:43, 1988.
66. De Sousa M. Immune cell functions in iron overload (review). Clin Exp Immunol 75:1, 1989.
67. Kapadia A, De Sousa M, Markenson AL, Miller DR, Good RA, Gupta S. Lymphoid cell sets and serum immunoglobulins in patients with thalassaemia intermedia: Relationship to serum iron and splenectomy. Br J Haematol 45:405, 1980.
68. Munn CG, Markenson AL, Kapadia A, De Sousa M. Impaired T-cell mitogen responses in some patients with thalassemia intermedia. Thymus 3:119, 1981.
69. Grady RW, Akbar AN, Giardina PJ, Hilgartner MW, De Sousa M. Disproportionate lymphoid cell subsets in thalassaemia major: The relative contributions of transfusion and splenectomy. Br J Haematol 59:713, 1985.
70. Akbar AN, Giardina PJ, Hilgartner MW, Grady RW. Immunological abnormalities in thalassaemia major. I. A transfusion-related increase in circulating cytoplasmic immunoglobulin-positive cells. Clin Exp Immunol 62:397, 1985.
71. Akbar AN, Fitzgerald-Bocarsly PA, De Sousa M, Giardina PJ, Hilgartner MW, Grady RW. Decreased natural killer activity in thalassemia major: A possible consequence of iron overload. J Immunol 136:1635, 1986.

72. Gascon P, Zoumbos NC, Young NS. Immunologic abnormalities in patients receiving multiple blood transfusions. Ann Intern Med 100:173, 1984.
73. Kaplan J, Sarnaik S, Gitlin J, Lusher J. Diminished helper/suppressor lymphocyte ratios and natural killer activity in recipients of repeated blood transfusions. Blood 64:308, 1984.
74. Dupont E, Vereerstraeten P, Espinosa O, Tielemans C, Dhaene M, Wybran J. Multiple transfusions and T cell subsets: A role for ferritin? Transplantation 35:508, 1983.
75. Richie E, Patchen M. Correlation between temperature-stable E-rosette formation and lymphocyte commitment to activation. Clin Immunol Immunopathol 11:88, 1978.
76. Meuer SC, Hussey RE, Fabbi M, Fox D, Acuto O, Fitzgerald KA, Hodgdon JC, Protentis JP, Schlossman SF, Reinherz EL. An alternative pathway of T-cell activation: A functional role for the 50 kd T11 sheep erythrocyte receptor protein. Cell 36:897, 1984.
77. Brottier P, Boumsell L, Gelin C, Bernard A. T cell activation via CD2 molecules: Accessory cells are required to trigger T cell activation via CD2-D66 plus CD2-9.6/T11 epitopes. J Immunol 135:1624, 1985.
78. Reinherz EL. Activation of cytolytic T lymphocytes and natural killer cell function through the T11 sheep erythrocyte binding protein. Nature 317:428, 1985.
79. Fox DA, Hussey RE, Fitzgerald KA, Bensussan A, Daley JF, Schlossman SF, Reinherz RL. Activation of human thymocytes via the 50kd T11 sheep erythrocyte binding protein induces the expression of interleukin 2 receptors on both T3-positive and T3-negative populations. J Immunol 134:330, 1985.
80. Tadmori W, Kant JA, Kamoun M. Down regulation of IL2 mRNA by antibody to the 50-kd protein associated with E receptors on human T lymphocytes. J Immunol 136:1155, 1986.
81. Martinez-Maza O, Palacios R. Is the E receptor on human T lymphocytes a "negative signal receptor?" J Immunol 129:2479, 1982.
82. Vollger LW, Tuck DT, Springer TA, Haynes BF, Singer KH. Thymocyte binding to human thymic epithelial cells is inhibited by monoclonal antibodies to CD2 and LFA 3 antigens. J Immunol 138:358, 1987.
83. Womack JE, Yan D, Potier M. Gene for Neuraminidase activity on mouse chromosome 17 near H-2: Pleiotropic effects on multiple hydrolases. Science 212:63, 1981.
84. Bjorn-Rasmussen E. Iron absorption: Present knowledge and controversies. Lancet 1:914, 1983.
85. Van Asbeck, Verbrugh BS, Van Ovst BA, JJM, Imhof HW, Verhoef J. Listeria monocytogenes meningitis and decreased phagocytosis associated with iron overload. Br Med J 284:542, 1982.
86. Bomford A, Walker RJ, Williams R. Treatment of iron overload including results in a personal series of 85 patients with idiopathic haemochromatosis. Q J Med 45:611, 1976.
87. Ammann RW, Muller E, Bansky J, Schuler G, Hacki WH. High incidence of extrahepatic carcinomas in idiopathic hemochromatosis. Scand J Gastroenterol 15:733, 1980.
88. Niederau C, Fisher R, Sonnenberg A, Stremmel W, Trampisch HJ, Strohmeyer G. Survival and causes of death in cirrhotic and in noncirrhotic patients with primary hemochromatosis. N Engl J Med 313:1256, 1985.
89. Constantoulakis M, Trichopoulos D, Avgooustaki O, Economidou J. Serum immunoglobulin concentrations before and after splenectomy in patients with homozygous beta-thalassaemia. J Clin Pathol 31:546, 1978.
90. Mossey RT, Sondheimer J. Listerosis in patients with long-term hemodialysis and transfusional iron overload. Am J Med 79:397, 1985.
91. Boelaert JR, von Landnyt HW, Valcke YJ et al. The role of iron overload in *Yersinia enterocolitica* and *Yersinia pseudotuberculosis* bacteremia in hemodialysis patients. J Infect Dis 156:384, 1987.
92. Robins-Browne RM, Prpic JK. Effect of iron and desferrioxamine on infections with *Yersinia enterocolitica*. Infect Immun 47:774, 1985.

93. Daly AL, Velazquez LA, Bradley SF, Kauffman CA. Mucormycosis: Association with deferoxamine therapy. Am J Med 87:468, 1989.
94. Felton C, Lustbader ED, Mertin C, Blumberg BS. Serum iron levels and response to hepatitis B virus. Proc Natl Acad Sci USA 76:2438, 1979.
95. Edwards CQ, Griffen LM, Kushner JP. Disorders of excess iron. Hosp Pract 26(Suppl 3):30, 1991.
96. Edwards CQ, Skolnick MH, Kushner JP. Hereditary hemochromatosis: Contributions of genetic analysis. Prog Hematol 12:43, 1981.
97. Crosby WH. A history of phlebotomy therapy for hemochromatosis. Am J Med Sci 301:28, 1991.
98. Edwards CQ, Griffen LM, Dadone MM, Skolnick MH, Kushner JP. Mapping the locus for hereditary hemochromatosis: Localization between HLA-B and HLA-A. Am J Hum Genet 38:805, 1986.
99. Coulondre C, Lucotte G. The molecular basis for the association between HLA-A3 and idiopathic haemochromatosis. Exp Clin Immunogenet 1:25, 1984.
100. Cosman D, Khoury G, Jay G. Three classes of mouse H-2 messenger RNA distinguished by analysis of cDNA clones. Nature 295:73, 1982.
101. Bomford AB, Munro HN. Transferrin and its receptor: Their roles in cell function. Hepatology 5:870, 1985.
102. Renswoude J, Bridges KR, Harford JB, Klausner RD. Receptor-mediated endocytosis of transferrin and the uptake of Fe in K562 cells: Identification of a nonlysosomal acidic compartment. Proc Natl Acad Sci USA 79:6186, 1982.
103. Stahl P, Schwartz AL. Receptor-mediated endocytosis. J Clin Invest 77:657, 1986.
104. Brown MS, Goldstein JL. A receptor-mediated pathway for cholesterol homeostasis. Science 232:34, 1986.
105. Neckers LM, Cossman J. Transferrin receptor induction in mitogen-stimulated human T lymphocytes is required for DNA synthesis and cell division and is regulated by interleukin 2. Proc Natl Acad Sci USA 80:3494, 1983.
106. Manger B, Weiss A, Hardy KJ, Stobo JD. A transferrin receptor antibody represents one signal for the induction of IL2 production by a human T cell line. J Immunol 136:532, 1986.
107. Trowbridge IS, Lopez F. Monoclonal antibody to transferrin receptor blocks transferrin binding and inhibits human tumor cell growth in vitro. Proc Natl Acad Sci USA 79:1175, 1982.
108. Lum JB, Infante AJ, Makker DM, Yang F, Bowman BH. Transferrin synthesis by inducer T lymphocytes. J Clin Invest 77:841, 1986.
109. Jacobs A, Summers MR. Iron uptake and ferritin synthesis by peripheral blood leucocytes in patients with primary idiopathic haemochromatosis. Br J Haematol 49:649, 1981.
110. Bassett ML, Halliday JW, Powell LW. Ferritin synthesis in peripheral blood monocytes in idiopathic hemochromatosis. J Lab Clin Med 100:137, 1982.
111. Da Silva B, Fauchat R, Genetet B, Le Mignon L, De Sousa M. Defect of ferritin secretion in HLA-A3 subjects and in idiopathic hemochromatosis. Histocompatibility Testing 1984:661.
112. Pollack MS, Da Silva B, Moshief RD, Groshen S, Bognacki J, Dupont B, De Sousa M. Ferritin secretion by human mononuclear cells: Association with HLA phenotype. Clin Immunol Immunopathol 27:124, 1983.
113. Dorner MH, Silverstone AE, Nishiya K, De Sosta A, Munn CG, De Sousa M. Ferritin synthesis by human T-lymphocytes. Science 209:1019, 1980.
114. Broxmeyer HE, Lu L, Bognacki J. Transferrin, derived from an OKT8-positive subpopulation of T lymphocytes, suppresses the production of granulocyte-macrophage colony-stimulatory factors from mitogen-activated T lymphocytes. Blood 63:37, 1983.

115. Imboden JB, Weiss A, Stobo JD. The antigen receptor on a human T cell line initiates activation by increasing cytoplasmic free calcium. J Immunol 134:663, 1985.
116. Nishizuka Y. The role of protein kinase C in cell surface signal transduction and tumor promotion. Nature 308:693, 1984.
117. Bomford A, Young S, Williams R. Intracellular forms of iron during transferrin iron uptake by mitogen-stimulated human lymphocytes. Br J Haematol 62:487, 1986.
118. Weintraub LR, Goral A, Grasso J, Franzblau C, Sullivan A, Sullivan S. Pathogenesis of hepatic fibrosis in experimental iron overload. Br J Haematol 59:321, 1985.
119. Good MF, Chapman DE, Powell LW, Halliday JW. The effect of iron on the cloning efficiency of human memory $T4^+$ lymphocytes. Clin Exp Immunol (in press).
120. Bentley DP, Cavill I, Ricketts C, Peake S. A method for the investigation of reticuloendothelial iron kinetics in man. Br J Haematol 43:619, 1979.
121. Uchida T, Akitsuki T, Kimura H, Tanaka T, Matsuda S, Kariyone S. Relationship among plasma iron, plasma iron turnover, and reticuloendothelial iron release. Blood 61:799, 1983.
122. Bryan CF, Leech SH, Jumar P, Gaumer B, Bozelka B, Morgan J. The immune system in hereditary hemochromatosis: A quantitative and functional assessment of the cellular arm. Am J Med Sci 301:55, 1991.
123. Bryan CF. The immunogenetics of hereditary hemochromatosis. Am J Med Sci 301:47, 1991.

8
The Role of Metals in the Production of Toxic Oxygen Metabolites by Mononuclear Phagocytes

Joan M. Cook-Mills and Pamela J. Fraker
Michigan State University, East Lansing, Michigan

KNOWN BIOCHEMICAL ROLES FOR ZINC

Zinc is an essential trace element that must be obtained daily in the diet, since there are no significant bodily stores for this metal (1). The major biochemical role for zinc is as a cofactor for over 100 metalloenzymes, including many of the enzymes associated with RNA and DNA synthesis (2). Studies indicate that there are also multiple zinc-binding domains in nucleic acid–binding proteins that may play a role in gene expression (3). This possibility is discussed also in Chapter 9. Membrane integrity and protein synthesis are thought to be zinc dependent; however, definitive evidence is needed (1). Indeed, it is highly probable that there are a variety of reactions and cellular processes yet to be discovered that require zinc. Our subsequent discussion of possible roles for zinc in a single phenomenon, the oxygen burst of the mononuclear phagocytic cells (MNPs), will provide evidence that many potential biochemical roles for zinc remain to be elucidated.

ZINC DEFICIENCY

Deficiencies in zinc are frequently observed in the human population not only in the developing nations, but in the United States as well (4,5). Consumption of diets high in certain grains, cereals, or refined foods can create a marginal dietary deficiency in zinc, especially if consumption of meat and animal products is low (4,5). Deficiencies in zinc can accompany many disease states such as gastrointestinal disorders, renal disease, alcoholism, liver disease, and sickle cell anemia (1,4). Sickle cell anemia is discussed in detail in Chapter 24. The prevalence of zinc deficiency in the human population has fostered a variety of studies to better define the effects of the deficiency on growth, development, and various cellular and tissue functions. A great deal of this work was done with animals, often using rodents as the primary model. In the last decade, a number of laboratories have focused their efforts on defining the effects of zinc deficiency on immune function and host defense of the mouse (6-9). As a result of these efforts, zinc deficiency now represents the best-characterized system with regard to the delineation of the effects of a single-element nutritional deficiency on the immune system.

EFFECT OF ZINC DEFICIENCY ON IMMUNE FUNCTION: A BRIEF REVIEW

Zinc deficiency has a rapid and adverse effect on immune function both in rodents and humankind (6-10). Using the mouse as a model because of its close immunological relationship to humans, extensive information regarding the impact of a moderate period of suboptimal intake of zinc on the host defense system has been generated (6-9). For example, a 30-day period of suboptimal intake of zinc by the young adult mouse reduces antibody-mediated responses to either T-cell-dependent or T-cell-independent antigens 40-60% (6,8,9). Similar depressions in cell-mediated responses were observed when tumor defense or delayed-type hypersensitivity reactions were assessed (8,11). The deficiency caused marked atrophy of the thymus as well as reductions in the size of many lymph nodes (12). As a result, the deficiency was accompanied by a 30-50% reduction in the total numbers of lymphocytes and MNPs (13).

The substantial reduction in the number of leukocytes brought to fore the question of whether the residual cells of the immune system of the zinc-deficient mouse were fully functional. This was, of course, of particular interest given the many enzymes of the cell known to be dependent on zinc for their function. Extensive work by Jardieu and Cook (14,16), who cultured lymphocytes from deficient mice in autologous serum to reduce the opportunity of restoration of zinc-dependent function when cells from deficient mice were placed in culture. This work indicates that the residual lymphocytes of the deficient mice are fully functional (14,16). When proliferative capacity and capacity to produce interleukin 2 was assessed, it was found that splenic T cells from deficient mice performed as well or better than splenic T cells from adequately fed mice regardless of whether the zinc level of the culture system was adequate or limiting (14,16). This included challenges with phytohemagglutinin, concanavalin A, and allogeneic target cells. Likewise, B cells from deficient mice proliferated normally and produced normal levels of antibody when challenged with lipopolysaccharide, dextran sulfate, or actual antigens (14). As before, the outcome was not affected by the level of zinc available to the cells in the culture system. Thus, in the case of lymphocytes, it appeared that the residual cells were capable of performing a variety of functions. It further suggested that a primary effect of zinc deficiency on immunity was to reduce defense capacity via the reduction in the total numbers of lymphocytes available to put into service against an immunogenic challenge. This kind of effect may be responsible for the recent report of Fenwick et al. (15) showing that zinc deficiency impaired explusion of *Trinchinella spiralis* in rats.

Initial tests of macrophage status of the deficient mice indicated that there were significant changes in Fc and complement receptor expression of peripheral blood and splenic MNPs but not of peritoneal MNPs (13). Tests of the ability of the peripheral blood and peritoneal MNPs to phagocytose polystyrene beads revealed no difference among the dietary groups. However, these results were suspect in the light of other experiments to be discussed. In an effort to show the degree to which zinc deficiency could impair host defense, mice fed zinc-adequate, zinc-adequate–restricted-fed, or zinc-deficient diet were challenged at day 10 of the dietary experiment with a sublethal dose of the parasite *Trypanosoma cruzi*. This particular parasite causes Chaga's disease in millions of South Americans each year. Within 12 days of infection, 80% of the zinc-deficient mice had died, exhibiting 20 times greater numbers of *T. cruzi* in their blood than the zinc-adequate or restricted-fed mice (17). At 30 days postinfection, some 85% of the infected zinc-deficient mice were dead (no deaths had occurred in the infected adequately fed mice), whereas the infected restricted-fed mice had experienced 10% mortalities. This experiment dramatically demonstrated the increased vulnerability of the nutritionally deficient mice to pathogenic infections.

Since it is also known that MNPs are a vital first line of defense against *T. cruzi*, the inability of the deficient mice to mount even a minimal defense against the parasite prompted us to look again at MNP function. In this case, peritoneal MNPs were prepared from mice from the deficient, adequate, or restricted-fed dietary groups. The MNPs were then infected in vitro with *T. cruzi* in the presence of ample (10 μg ZnCl$_2$/ml) or limiting quantities of zinc (<0.3 μg Zn/ml). The results of using a natural pathogen were not only extremely interesting, but markedly contrasted to the data obtained with polystyrene beads. As can be seen in Table 1, the degree of association of *T. cruzi* (0 hr) with MNPs from moderately deficient mice (75% the body weight of zinc adequate mice) was moderately reduced from controls. The MNPs from severely deficient mice (67% of the body weight of zinc adequate mice) was reduced by greater than 60%. The data 6 hr postinfection were even more interesting. By then, MNPs from zinc-adequate and restricted-fed mice had killed 40–50%

Table 1 Effect of Pretreatment with Zinc Chloride on the Ability of Peritoneal Macrophages from Various Dietary Treatment Groups to Associate with and Kill *Trypanosoma cruzi*

Dietary treatment group	1-hr pretreatment (10 μg ZnCl$_2$/ml)	Number of *T. cruzi*/100 macrophages	
		0 hr	6 hr
Severely zinc deficient	–	36.2 ± 4.1[a,b]	47.3 ± 3.2
Moderately zinc deficient	–	83.0 ± 1.9[b]	67.7 ± 10.5
Restricted-fed	–	109.7 ± 5.9	58.6 ± 0.5
Control	–	105.3 ± 6.0	56.5 ± 1.3
Severely zinc deficient	+	93.0 ± 9.3	38.5 ± 2.6
Moderately zinc deficient	+	100.5 ± 4.0	53.7 ± 5.1
Restricted-fed	+	89.8 ± 2.4	57.4 ± 7.3
Control	+	111.7 ± 9.7	58.7 ± 4.9

[a]Values are means ±SD of six to eight mice.
[b]The difference between this value and the value of the control at 0 hr is statistically significant at $p < 0.05$ or greater.

of the associated parasites. The MNPs from moderately deficient mice had killed only 18% of associated *T. cruzi* (Table 1). At this point, MNPs from severely deficient mice had not only failed to kill any associated parasites, but there was a modest increase in the number of associated *T. cruzi*, suggesting the parasites were able to proliferate while engulfed in the MNPs. The results indicated that zinc deficiency had significantly impaired the oxygen burst of the MNPs which is essential to the killing of the parasite. More amazingly, preincubation of MNPs from the deficient mice for 1 hr in the presence of zinc chloride at about five times physiological levels completely restored all of these functions (Table 1). The number of associated *T. cruzi* per 100 MNPs was the same for MNPs of deficient mice as those of controls after exposure to zinc. Perhaps more importantly, preincubation with zinc completely restored the capacity of MNPs from deficient mice to kill *T. cruzi* (Table 1). Other metals such as manganese, nickle, and copper were unable to restore these functions (data not shown).

It was evident from these experiments that the MNPs from zinc-deficient mice had functional processes that were impaired owing to the limiting availability of zinc in the host environment. It was intriguing that only a short time of incubation with $ZnCl_2$ was required to restore both the association of and the capacity to kill the parasite by MNPs from deficient mice. As will be discussed, the destruction of *T. cruzi* has been thought to be heavily dependent on the oxygen burst, particularly the production of H_2O_2. In addition, there is increasing evidence that metals may play a greater role than previously thought in the production of toxic oxygen metabolites by cells and tissues (18). Thus, it occurred to us that zinc itself may play an integral role in the respiratory burst of the MNPs. For that reason, we began to search the literature to identify potential roles for zinc in the respiratory burst of the MNPs. What follows is a review of that literature, which we hope the reader will agree indicates that zinc may play a significant role in the production of toxic oxygen metabolites.

PRODUCTION OF TOXIC OXYGEN METABOLITES BY MONONUCLEAR PHAGOCYTES

Contact with a variety of foreign substances, particularly pathogens, initiates the oxygen burst in MNPs. The burst is a critical set of reactions which generate toxic oxygen metabolites responsible for the killing of most pathogens (Fig. 1). Past efforts of immunologists and biochemists have focused heavily on establishing a relationship between the production of H_2O_2 to the killing of pathogens. This continues today because it is feasible to measure H_2O_2 production by MNPs, but it is difficult or impossible to measure other oxygen metabolites. These products may in fact be as important, if not more important, than H_2O_2 in the killing of invading organisms. Furthermore, the production of many of these other oxygen metabolites can be facilitated by metals such as zinc.

The chemical phorbol myristate acetate (PMA) and opsonized zymosan, an antibody-coated yeast cell extract, are frequently used by investigators to activate mononuclear phagocytes for the purpose of initiating the oxygen burst. Actual pathogens such as *Tryponsoma cruzi* are used less frequently because of the past difficulties of obtaining sufficiently high rates of infection in vitro to produce measurable amounts of oxygen metabolites from the respiratory burst. Indeed, much of the evidence which suggests that the killing of *T. cruzi* by mononuclear phagocytes

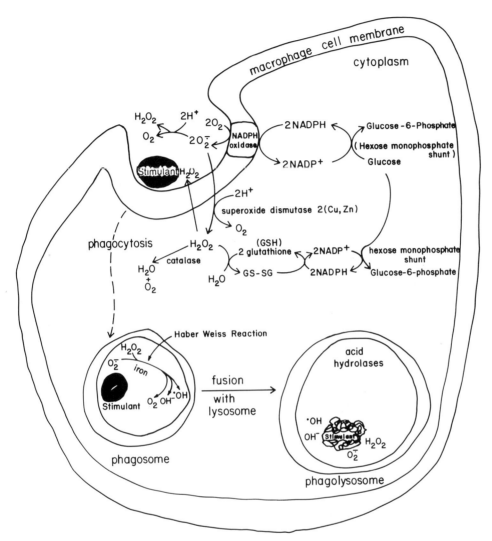

Figure 1 Depiction of the oxygen burst and the production of toxic oxygen metabolites by mononuclear phagocytic cells.

can be correlated to H_2O_2 production was actually obtained by indirect means (19, 20). That is, elicited mononuclear cells were activated by PMA or lipopolysaccharide (LPS), thereby causing production of H_2O_2, which in turn was shown to be able to kill exogenously added *T. cruzi*. Clearly, this field would be enhanced by improvements in the assay systems. This would make it possible to use actual pathogens as stimulants as well as being able to quantitate the production of other oxygen metabolites besides H_2O_2. In the interim, this discussion will necessarily have to revolve around the available experiments which in the main were done with artificial probes.

The oxygen burst as it is currently understood is depicted in Figure 1. Data indicate that PMA and opsonized zymosan promote activation of NADPH oxidase, an enzyme located in the plasma membrane, which catalyzes the production of superoxide (O_2^-) from molecular oxygen. The O_2^- can subsequently be found in the extracellular environment as well as the phagosome/phagolysosome. The reaction requires two NADPH molecules, which are provided by the hexose monophosphate shunt in the cytoplasm. The O_2^-, then, either nonenzymatically dismutates to H_2O_2 or superoxide dismutase catalyzes the dismutation. As O_2^- and H_2O_2 are produced, they can diffuse through the plasma membrane. The O_2^- and H_2O_2 which can be found either in the extracellular fluids or the phagosome/phagolysosome are used to destroy pathogens. Cytoplasmic O_2^- and H_2O_2 are scavenged by superoxide dismutase and catalase, respectively, to protect the macrophage. Glutathione peroxidase also scavenges H_2O_2 while oxidizing glutathione. Within the phagosome/phagolysosome, H_2O_2 reacts with O_2^- to produce O_2, OH^- and $OH^.$. The O_2^-, H_2O_2, and $OH^.$ are known to be toxic to most pathogens.

As an aside, it can be noted that phagolysosomes also contain lysosomal enzymes. Myeloperoxidase, which catalyzes the production of highly reactive hypohalous acids from H_2O_2, is present in phagolysosomes of monocytes, the immature mononuclear phagocytes of the peripheral blood, and polymorphonuclear leukocytes but not macrophages (20). Therefore, the mature macrophage is unable to produce hypohalous acids.

POSSIBLE ROLES FOR ZINC IN THE OXYGEN BURST

Those reactions of the oxygen burst which might be zinc dependent (Fig. 2) will be the focus of this section. The mechanisms of stimulation of NADPH oxidase by PMA and opsonized zymosan are known (Fig. 2). Phorbol myristate acetate stimulates NADPH oxidase by binding to protein kinase C (22,23), which in turn phosphorylates and thus activates NADPH oxidase (22,23). On the other hand, opsonized zymosan stimulates NADPH oxidase via arachidonic acid released from phospholipids (20:4) (24,25,26). In this case, the opsonized zymosan binds to receptors on macrophages for the Fc portion of the antibody (Fig. 2). Suzuki et al. (27) showed that a Fcγ2b-binding protein of macrophage membranes has phospholipase A_2 activity resulting in the cleavage of fatty acids from the C2 position of the glycerol backbone of phosphatidylcholine. The activity of this protein increased fourfold upon binding of complexes to IgG$_{2b}$ (27). Therefore, the binding of opsonized zymosan to Fcγ2b receptors could liberate 20:4 from phospholipids in the macrophage plasma membrane via activation of phospholipase A_2. A considerable amount of the fatty acid (25%) in macrophage phospholipids is 20:4 (28). Once 20:4 is liberated from the plasma membrane phospholipid, it may then stimulate NADPH oxidase. It has been shown that 20:4 and lipoxygenase metabolites of 20:4, such as leukotrienes, 15-HETE, or 15-HPETE, stimulate NADPH oxidase (25,29–31). In contrast, 20:4 metabolites of the cyclooxygenase pathway, the prostaglandins, are not stimulatory for NADPH oxidase (25,29). Thus, upon binding of opsonized zymosan to Fcγ2b receptors, phospholipase A_2 activity of the receptor liberates 20:4 from membrane phospholipids and 20:4 or a lipoxygenase (but not a cyclooxygenase) metabolite of 20:4 stimulates NADPH oxidase for the production of superoxide.

Resident peritoneal macrophages have three phospholipase activities, a phospholipase A_2, which is active at pH 4.5; a Ca^{2+}-dependent phospholipase A_2, which is active at pH 8.5; and a phosphatidylinositol-specific phospholipase C (32–34).

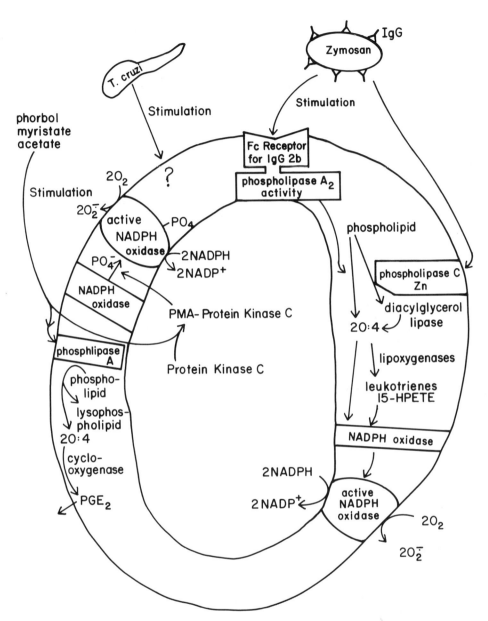

Figure 2 Membrane events associated with initiation of the oxygen burst in mononuclear phagocytes by different stimuli. Examples given here include the chemical, phorbol myristate acetate; the parasite, *Trypanosoma cruzi*; yeast cell wall fragments, zymosan.

The particular phospholipases involved in the degradation of phospholipids apparently varies with the type of stimulant encountered. Zymosan stimulates degradation via both phospholipase A_2 and phospholipase C, whereas PMA stimulates deacylation of phosphatidylinositol via phospholipase A_2 (33). The PMA-stimulated release of 20:4 does not activate NADPH oxidase (Fig. 2), since with this stimulant the 20:4 is converted to prostaglandins (35,36), which are not stimulatory for NADPH oxidase

(25,29). The 20:4 released by phospholipase A_2 and the lipoxygenase metabolites are stimulatory for the oxygen burst (25,29,30). Further evidence for the involvement of phospholipase C in the stimulation of the oxygen burst includes an increase in O_2 uptake and hexose monophosphate shunt activity and a 41% decrease in phospholipid content upon addition of phospholipase C to polymorphonuclear leukocytes (37). Phospholipase C stimulation of the oxygen burst probably involves diacylglycerol lipase catalyzed release of 20:4.

There are several possible roles for zinc in the stimulation of NADPH oxidase by 20:4. Zinc may be important for the release of 20:4 from phospholipids, since phospholipase C is a zinc-dependent enzyme (36,37). This enzyme in conjunction with diacylglycerol lipase can liberate 20:4 from phospholipids (Fig. 2) (39). Phospholipase C has two zinc atoms in the active site, both of which are required for activity (37). Removal of even one zinc atom reduces the enzymatic cleavage of phosphatidylcholine to 3–11% of control and removal of the second zinc atom reduces the activity to less than 1% (39). These zinc atoms are tightly bound to the active site (37). In fact, addition of EDTA does not seem to remove zinc from the enzyme and, therefore, has no effect on enzyme activity (39). Zinc has also been implicated in the regulation of phospholipase A_2 activity (40,41). Phospholipase A_2 liberates fatty acids from the C2 position of the phospholipid glycerol backbone. Manku et al. (41) have suggested that in the presence of physiological levels of zinc, dihomo-γ-linolenic acid (DHGL) is mobilized from plasma membrane phospholipids of the rat superior mesenteric vascular bed. Dihomo-γ-linolenic acid is the immediate precursor to either 20:4 (Fig. 3) or prostaglandins of the one series. If DHGL is converted to 20:4, mobilization of DHGL could play a significant role in stimulating the oxygen burst via

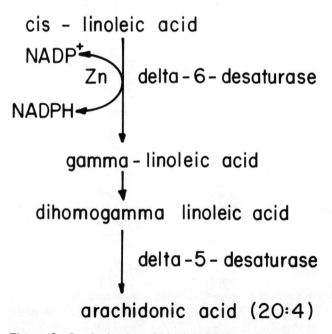

Figure 3 Synthesis of arachidonic acid from *cis*-linoleic acid.

20:4. Zinc mobilization of DHGL for prostaglandin synthesis would not be stimulatory for NADPH oxidase, since, as discussed, prostaglandins do not stimulate NADPH oxidase. However, inhibition of prostaglandin synthesis may allow DHGL or its metabolite, 20:4, to stimulate NADPH oxidase. This is a possibility, since addition of 2 mM zinc in vitro has been shown to inhibit prostaglandin synthesis by polymorphonuclear leukocytes (42). In addition, perhaps DHGL itself could stimulate NADPH oxidase, since shorter chain fatty acids can, albeit to a lesser extent, also stimulate NADPH oxidase (25,29). In contrast to the increased activity of phospholipase A_2 in the presence of zinc reported by Manku et al. (41), Wells (43) has reported that zinc inhibits the calcium-dependent activity of phospholipase A_2 from *Crotalus adamanteus* (snake) venom by binding to the active site and inducing conformational changes in the enzyme. Inhibition of phospholipase A_2 activity by addition of zinc has also been reported by others (44,45). Thus, the effect of zinc on the function of the latter enzyme remains controversial. In summary, zinc may be important in the release of 20:4 from phospholipids via its role in phospholipase C and phospholipase A_2 activity or the release of diacylglycerol.

Zinc may also be important in the stabilization of 20:4 against oxidation and thereby enhance the probability of stimulation of NADPH oxidase. It is known that zinc or iron can complex with 20:4 and oxygen (46,47). Iron catalyzes the oxidation of 20:4, whereas zinc does not (47). Sample reactions are as follows:

$$20:4 + O_2 + Fe^{2+} \rightarrow [20:4, O_2, Fe^{2+}]_{complex} \rightarrow \text{lipid peroxides} + O_2^- + Fe^{3+}$$

$$20:4 + O_2 + Zn^{2+} \rightarrow [20:4, O_2, Zn^{2+}]_{complex}$$

Thus, zinc may compete with iron for formation of this complex (47). Perhaps zinc stabilizes the 20:4, making it unavailable for oxidation by the iron complex and thereby allowing it to act as a stimulant for NADPH oxidase.

Zinc may also play a role in the production of O_2^- by NADPH oxidase, since nucleotides, such as NADPH, are able to complex with zinc. This was determined by examining elution patterns of NADPH from Sephadex G-10 columns equilibrated with zinc ions (48,49). Zinc binds to NADPH in a 2:1 molar ratio (49). The first zinc atom binds between the monophosphate on the C2 of the adenine-ribosyl portion and the diphosphate group (49). The second zinc atom binds to the remaining oxygen of the monophosphate and the diphosphate (49). When zinc complexes with NADPH, it interferes with oxidation of NADPH by making it unavailable as a substrate (49). The activity of the NADPH oxidases derived from liver microsomes and mixed function oxidases from smooth endoplasmic reticulum are inhibited in the presence of zinc ($K_i = 7.22\ \mu M\ Zn^{2+}$) (49). In the presence of physiological levels of zinc, the importance of the possible formation of the Zn_2-NADPH complex in cells is unknown and thus whether such a complex plays any role in the oxygen burst is not known. Conversely, it is also possible that supraphysiological levels of zinc might inhibit NADPH oxidase via complexes formed with NADPH. This might explain the observed inhibition of oxygen consumption and hexose monophosphate shunt activity in polymorphonuclear leukocytes and peritoneal macrophages when high concentrations of zinc were added to such cell preparations in vitro (50).

Superoxide, produced by NADPH oxidase, either nonenzymatically dismutates to H_2O_2, or superoxide dismutase (SOD) catalyzes its dismutation (see Fig. 1). Both the spontaneous and enzymatic dismutation of O_2^- are dependent on metals (51,52). There is a cytoplasmic SOD which contains both copper and zinc, being a dimer of two identical subunits. The mitochondrial SOD contains manganese. Each subunit of the cytoplasmic SOD contains one molecule of copper and one molecule of zinc located at some distance from each other (about 34 Å) (51). The two copper ions are catalytic cofactors, whereas the two zinc ions are structural cofactors (50). Upon removal of zinc from Cu/Zn SOD, the enzyme activity at pH 6 is still 90% of the intact Cu/Zn SOD (52). At pH >7, the copper ion migrates to the zinc-free site (52). It is thought that the role of zinc in SOD is primarily as a structural cofactor (52). The major biological role for Cu/Zn SOD has not been elucidated. It may be important in the production of H_2O_2 for destruction of pathogens or its major role may be scavenging O_2^- to protect the macrophage from O_2^- that has diffused through the membrane into the cytoplasm. Whatever the biological role for SOD in the macrophage, zinc appears to not be crucial for activity of the Cu/Zn SOD. Interestingly, copper supplementation has been noted to cause increased phagocytosis but not killing in sheep (53).

The nonenzymatic dismutation of O_2^- may also be metal dependent. Iron has been shown to react with O_2^- and indirect evidence suggests that zinc may also be involved in related reactions. The reaction known to be facilitated by iron is called the Haber-Weiss reaction (see Fig. 1) (54).

$$Fe^3 + O_2^- \rightarrow Fe^{2+} + O_2$$
$$Fe^{2+} + H_2O_2 \rightarrow Fe^{3+} + OH^- + OH^{\cdot}$$
$$OH^{\cdot} + H_2O_2 \rightarrow H_2O + HO_2^{\cdot}$$
$$HO_2^{\cdot} + H_2O_2 \rightarrow O_2 + H_2O + OH^{\cdot}$$
$$OH^{\cdot} + Fe^{2+} \rightarrow Fe^{3+} + OH^-$$

The resulting oxygen metabolites are OH^- and the toxic $OH^{\cdot}$. These reactions occur at the acidic pHs found in the phagosome/phagolysosome which contain the engulfed pathogen or stimulant (see Fig. 1). These reactions do not occur at the higher pHs found in the cytoplasm, which is important since production of highly reactive oxygen metabolites in areas other than the phagolysosome could destroy the leukocyte itself.

Zinc may also be involved in the nonenzymatic dismutation of O_2^-. There is evidence, albeit inconclusive, that zinc catalyzes reactions with oxygen. In the following reactions, reduction of oxygen in the presence of zinc and bipyridine (bipy) yields highly reactive radicals and zinc peroxides (55).

$$Zn^{II}(bipy)_2^{2+} + O_2 + e^- \xrightarrow{-0.5V} [Zn^{II}(bipy)_3OO^{\cdot}]^+$$
$$[Zn^{II}(bipy)_2OO^{\cdot}]^+ + e^- \rightarrow Zn^{II}(bipy)_2(O_2)$$

These chemical reactions were determined electrochemically under aprotic conditions using dimethylformamide in order to stabilize the superoxide ion so that it would not dismutate to H_2O_2. For this reason, the significance of these reactions for biological systems also remains in doubt. In addition, it has also been observed that oxygen reacts with metal surfaces of zinc at extremely low temperatures (77°K) (56). The molecular steps determined for the dissociative chemisorption of oxygen at the metal surface is as follows: $O_2(g) \rightarrow O_2(a) \rightarrow O^-(a) \rightarrow O^{2-}(a)$ (56). Since these reactions were done at extremely low temperatures, the biological relevance is once again unknown. Other metals (iron, copper, manganese, cobalt) are also known to react with oxygen (57). These metals are more reactive than zinc, since they have unfilled d-shell orbitals. Previously, zinc was thought to be unreactive with oxygen because it has a filled d-shell orbital (d^{10}). However, a zinc metalloporphyrin is reactive with superoxide and forms a superoxo complex (57). These reactions serve to demonstrate nevertheless that zinc, especially a biochemical complex containing zinc, may in the future prove to have biological reactivity with oxygen species essential to the oxygen burst.

CONCLUSIONS

Delineation of the effects of zinc deficiency on immune function now represents a well-characterized nutritional-immunological model. Deficiencies in this essential trace element have been shown to have a rapid and adverse effect on many branches of the host defense system of humankind and rodents. However, when the functional capacity of the residual splenic lymphocytes of the zinc-deficient mouse was examined in vitro using mitogens, their rate of proliferation was found to be normal. Furthermore, lymphocytes from deficient mice produced normal amounts of lymphokines and antibodies even when cultured in autologous sera to reduce the possibility of restoration of zinc-dependent functions. Conversely, mononuclear phagocytes (MNPs) from deficient mice had significantly reduced capacity to associate with and kill the parasite *Trypanosoma cruzi*, which causes Chaga's disease. Nevertheless, a short incubation with $ZnCl_2$ completely restored the capacity of MNPs from deficient mice to take up and kill *T. cruzi*. The dependency of killing of *T. cruzi* on the oxygen burst and the renewed interest in the role of metals in the production of highly reactive oxidants in biological systems suggested that MNPs from zinc-deficient mice might provide a model system for study of such reactions. The possibility that zinc might play an integral role in the oxygen burst seemed evident from the ability of zinc to quickly restore the killing capacity of MNPs from the zinc-deficient mice. To this end, a search was made of the literature to identify enzymes and/or reactions known to be involved in the generation of oxygen radicals or toxic oxygen metabolites that might be zinc dependent. A review of the literature, provided herein, demonstrated that there are indeed many possible roles for zinc in the generation of activated oxygen species in biological systems.

Zinc may participate in a variety of the reactions known to be instrumental to the production of toxic oxygen metabolites by macrophages. Zinc may be involved in the stimulation of NADPH oxidase via its role as a cofactor for phospholipase A_2 or phospholipase C–diacylglycerol lipase–catalyzed release of 20:4 from phospholipids. Zinc may also stabilize 20:4 against oxidation by iron complexes, thereby enhancing the probability that 20:4 will stimulate NADPH oxidase and initiate the oxygen burst. Finally, zinc-containing biological complexes yet to be identified may prove to be extremely reactive with oxygen, thereby generating products highly toxic to pathogens.

ACKNOWLEDGMENTS

This research was supported by a grant from the National Institutes of Health, Bethesda, Maryland (HD10586).

Our appreciation for the technical assistance of Julie Detwiler.

REFERENCES

1. Prasad A. 1979. Clinical, biochemical, and pharmacological role of zinc. Ann Rev Pharmacol 20:393.
2. Vallee B, Galdes A. 1984. The metallobiochemistry of zinc enzymes. Adv Enzymol 56:283.
3. Berg J. 1986. Potential metal-binding domains in nucleic acid binding proteins. Science 232:485.
4. Prasad A. 1984. Discovery and importance of zinc in human nutrition. Fed Proc 43:2829.
5. Sandstead H. 1973. Zinc nutrition in the United States. Am J Clin Nutr 26:1251.
6. Fraker PJ, Gershwin M, Good R, Prasad A. 1986. Interrelationships between zinc and immune function. Fed Proc 45:1474.
7. Gershwin ME, Beach RS, Hurley LS. 1979. Trace elements. *In*: Nutrition and Immunity. New York: Academic Press, pp 190–227.
8. Fernandes G, Nair M, Onoe K, Tanaka T, Floyd R, Good R. 1979. Impairment of cell mediated immunity function by dietary zinc deficiency in mice. Proc Natl Acad Sci USA 76:457.
9. Fraker PJ, Haas SM, Luecke RW. 1977. Effect of zinc deficiency on the immune response. J Nutr 107:1889.
10. Good RA. 1981. Nutrition and immunity. J Clin Immunol 1:3.
11. Fraker PJ, Zwickl CM, Luecke RW. 1982. Delayed type hypersensitivity in zinc deficient adult mice. J Nutr 111:309.
12. Fraker PJ, DePasquale-Jardieu P, Zwickl CM, Luecke RW. 1978. Regeneration of T-cell helper function in zinc deficient adult mice. Proc Natl Acad Sci USA 75:5660.
13. Wirth JJ, Fraker PJ, Kierszenbaum F. 1984. Changes in the levels of marker expression by mononuclear phagocytes in zinc deficient mice. J Nutr 114:1826.
14. Fraker PJ, Jardieu P, Cook JM. 1986. Immunodeficiencies caused by an inadequate intake of zinc. *In*: The Nature, Cellular and Biochemical Basis and Management of Immunodeficiencies. Good, RA, ed., Symposia Medica Hoechst, FK Schattauer Verlag-Stuttgart, 21:453–460.
15. Fenwick PK, Aggett PJ, Macdonald D, Huber C, Wakelin D. 1990. Zinc deficiency and zinc depletion: Effect on the response of rats to infection with Trichinella spiralis. Am J Clin Nutr 52:166–172.
16. Fraker PJ, Jardieu P, Cook-Mills J. 1987. Zinc deficiency and immune function. Arch Dermatol 123:1699.
17. Fraker PJ, Caruso R, Kierszenbaum F. 1982. Alteration of the immune and nutritional status of mice by synergy between zinc deficiency and infection with *Trypanosoma cruzi*. J Nutr 112:1224.
18. Aust SD, Morehouse L, Thomas CE. 1985. Role of metals in oxygen radical reactions. J Free Rad Biol Med 1:3.
19. Nath C, Nogueira N, Juangbhanich C, Ellis J, Cohn Z. 1979. Activation of macrophage in vivo and in vitro: Correlation between hydrogen peroxide release and killing of *Trypanosoma cruzi*. J Exp Med 149:1056.
20. Nathan CF, Siverstein SC, Brukner LH, Cohn Z. 1979. Extracellular cytolysis by activated macrophages and granulocytes II. Hydrogen peroxide as a mediator of cytotoxicity. J Exp Med 149:100.
21. Simmons SR, Karnovsky ML. 1973. Iodinating ability of various leukocytes and their bactericidal activity. J Exp Med 138:44.
22. Castagna M, Takai Y, Kaibuchi K, Sano K, Kikkawa U, Nishizuka Y. 1982. Direct activation of calcium-activated, phospholipid-dependent protein kinase by tumor-promoting phorbol esters. J Biol Chem 257:7847.
23. Nishizuka Y. 1984. The role of protein kinase C in cell surface signal transduction and tumor promotion. Nature 308:693.

24. Hishinuma K, Hosana A, Inaba H, Kimura S. 1990. Effects of intraperitoneally administered dietary fibers on super oxide generation from peritoneal exudate macrophages in mice. Int J Vitam Nutr Res 60:288–293.
25. Bromberg Y, Pick E. 1984. Unsaturated fatty acids stimulate NADPH-dependent superoxide production by cell free system derived from macrophages. Cell Immunol 88:213.
26. Tauber AI, Cox JA, Jeng AY, Blumberg PM. 1986. Sub-cellular activation of the human neutrophil NADPH-oxidase by arachidonic acid and sodium dodecyl sulfate (SDS) is independent of protein kinase C. Clin Res 34:664A.
27. Suzuki T, Saito-Taki T, Sadasivan R, Nitta T. 1982. Biochemical signal transmitted by Fcγ receptors: Phospholipase A_2 activity of Fcγ2b receptor of murine macrophage cell line P388D. Proc Natl Acad Sci USA 79:591.
28. Scott WA, Zrike JM, Hamill AL, Kempe J, Cohn ZA. 1980. Regulation of arachidonic acid metabolites in macrophages. J Exp Med 152:324.
29. Bromberg Y, Pick E. 1983. Unsaturated fatty acids as second messengers of superoxide generation by macrophages. Cell Immunol 79:240.
30. McPhail LC, Shirley PS, Clayton CC, Snyderman R. 1985. Activation of the respiratory burst enzyme from human neutrophils in a cell-free system. J Clin Invest 75:1735.
31. Curnette JT. 1985. Activation of human neutrophil nicotinamide adenine dinucleotide phosphate reduced (triphosphopyridine nucleotide, reduced) oxidase by arachidonic acid in a cell-free system. J Clin Invest 75:1740.
32. Wightman PD, Dahlgren ME, Davies P, Bonney RJ. 1981. The selective release of phospholipase A_2 by resident mouse peritoneal macrophages. Biochem J 200:441.
33. Emilsson A, Sundler R. 1986. Evidence for a catalytic role of phospholipase A in phorbol dister- and zymosan-induced mobilization of arachidonic acid in mouse peritoneal macrophages. Biochim Biophys Acta 876:533.
34. Moscat J, Aracil M, Diez E, Balsinde J, Barreno PG, Municio AM. 1986. Intracellular Ca^{2+} requirements for zymosan-stimulated phosphoinositide hydrolysis in mouse peritoneal macrophages. Biochem Biophys Res Commun 134:367.
35. Brune K. Aehringhaus U, Peskar BA. 1984. Pharmacological control of leukotriene and prostaglandin production from mouse peritoneal macrophages. Agents Actions 14:729.
36. Bonney RJ, Wightman PD, Dahlgren ME, Davies P, Kuehl FA Jr, Humes JL. 1980. Effect of RNA and protein synthesis inhibitors on the release of inflammatory mediators by macrophages responding to phorbol myristate acetate. Biochim Biophys Acta 633:410.
37. Patriarca P, Zatti M, Cramer R, Rossi F. 1970. Stimulation of the respiration of polymorphonuclear leukocytes by phospholipase C. Life Sci 9:841.
38. Ottolenghi AC. 1965. Phospholipase C from *Bacillus cereus*, A zinc-requiring metalloenzyme. Biochim Biophys Acta 106:510.
39. Dennis EA. 1983. Phospholipases. *In*: The Enzymes. Boyer P, ed., New York: Academic Press, p 307.
40. Horrobin DF, Manku MS, Cunnane S, Karmazyn M, Morgan RO, Ally AI, Karmall RA. 1978. Regulation of cytoplasmic calcium: Interactions between prostaglandins, prostacyclin, thromboxane A_2, zinc, copper and taurine. Can J Neurol Sci 5:93.
41. Manku MS, Horrobin DF, Harmazyn M, Cunnane SC. 1979. Prolactin and zinc effects on rat vascular reactivity: Possible relationship to dihomo-γ-linolenic acid and to prostaglandin synthesis. Endocrinology 104:774.
42. Bettger WJ, O'Dell BL. 1981. A critical physiological role of zinc in the structure and function of biomembranes. Life Sci 28:1425.
43. Wells MA. 1973. Spectral perturbations of *Crotalus adamanteus* phospholipase A_2 induced by divalent cation binding. Biochemistry 12:1080.
44. Zor U, Kaneko T, Lowe IP, Bloom G, Field J. 1969. Effect of thyroid-stimulating hormone and prostaglandins on thyroid adenyl cyclase activation and cyclic adenosine 3',5'-monophosphate. J Biol Chem 244:5189.

45. Stossel TP, Murad F, Mason RJ, Vaughan M. 1970. Regulation of glycogen metabolism in polymorphonuclear leukocytes. J Biol Chem 245:6228.
46. Peterson DA, Gerrard JM, Benton MA. 1981. A hypothesis for the mechanism of superoxide production by phagocytic cells. Med Hypoth 7:1389.
47. Peterson DA, Gerrard JM, Peller J, Ras GHR, White JG. 1981. Interactions of zinc and arachidonic acid. Prostaglandins Med 6:91.
48. Chvapil M. 1973. New aspects in the biological role of zinc: A stabilizer of macromolecules and biological membranes. Life Sci 13:1041.
49. Slater TF. 1974. Mechanisms of protection against the damage produced in biological systems by oxygen-derived radicals. *In*: Molecular Mechanisms of Oxygen Activation. Hayaishi Q, ed., New York: Academic Press, pp 143–176.
50. Chvapil M, Stankova L, Berhard DS, Weldy PL, Carlson EC, Campbell JB. 1977. Effect of zinc on peritoneal macrophages in vitro. Infect Immun 16:367.
51. Ricchelli F, Rossi E, Salvato B, Jori G, Bannister JV, Bannister WH. 1983. Fluorescence studies on copper/zinc superoxide dismutase from bovine erythrocytes. *In*: Oxy Radicals and Their Scavenger Systems. Cohen G, Greenwald RA, eds., New York: Elsevier Science, pp 320–323.
52. O'Neill P, Fielden EM, Cocco D, Calabrese L, Rotillo G. 1983. Mechanistic study of superoxide dismutation by "zinc-free" bovine superoxide dismutase. *In*: Oxy Radicals and Their Scavenger Systems. Cohen G, Greenwald RA, eds., New York: Elsevier Science, pp 316–319.
53. Olkowski AA, Gooreratre SR, Christensen DA. 1990. Effects of diets of high sulfur content and varied concentrations of copper, molybdenum and thiamine on in vitro phagocytic and candidacidal activity of neutrophils in sheep. Res Vet Sci 48:82–86.
54. Aust SD, Morehouse LA, Thomas CE. 1985. Role of metals in oxygen radical reactions. Free Rad Biol Med 1:3.
55. Sawyer DT, Roberts JL Jr, Tsuchiya T, Srivatsa GS. Generation of activated oxygen species by electron-transfer reduction of dioxygen in the presence of protons, chlorinated hydrocarbons, methyl viologen and transition metal ions. *In*: Oxygen Radicals in Chemistry and Biology. Bors W, Saran M, Tait D, eds., New York: Walter de Gruyter, pp 25–34.
56. Au CT, Roberts MW. 1986. Specific role of transient O^-(s) at Mg (0001) surfaces in activation of ammonia by dioxygen and nitrous oxide. Nature 319:206.
57. Valentine JS, Tatsuno Y, Nappa M. 1977. Superoxotetraphenylporphinatozinc (1−). J Am Chem Soc 99:3522.

9
Zinc Deficiency, Chromatin Structure, and Gene Expression

C. Elizabeth Castro
University of Hawaii at Manoa, Honolulu, Hawaii

J. Sanders Sevall
Specialty Laboratories, Inc., Santa Monica, California

INTRODUCTION

A key determinant of the interplay between nutrition and immunity is how nutritional factors modify the biological processes of gene expression and subsequent protein synthesis. In view of the complexity of regulated gene expression, transcription of individual or families of genes may be influenced by the nutrient environment on a gene-by-gene case. However, there may be at least some mechanisms by which macro- or micronutrients affect transcriptional processes in a general sense.

One regulatory feature in gene expression is the structural configuration of the DNA template: both fine structure within the gene unit itself and the higher levels of organization of the chromatin surrounding the gene. We have demonstrated under many conditions that nutrient intake directly or indirectly mediates alterations in (a) the higher orders of chromatin structure (Castro et al., 1986b; Castro and Sevall, 1980), and (b) in the fundamental organization of chromatin (Castro, 1983). Weintraub (1985) has suggested that alteration of chromatin may confer a primary, or coarse, level of regulation of gene expression which precedes the processes of fine regulation.

In this chapter, we will first briefly describe how eukaryotic chromatin is organized within the nucleus and how this may be related to gene expression. We will review our findings as well as those of others demonstrating alterations in chromatin structure by a nutritional modulation. We will focus on the micronutrient zinc as a modifier of chromatin structure and demonstrate that zinc deficiency alters histone H1 which is correlated with a coarse level of regulation of gene expression. Zinc deficiency alters the structural features of chromatin and presumably the functional expression as well. In view of the role of zinc in maintaining chromatin structure and as a cofactor for enzymes involved in DNA synthesis and transcription, one may expect zinc to exhibit a major influence over gene expression in many cell types, including those cells which are involved in the immune response.

ARRANGEMENT OF CHROMATIN IN EUCARYOTIC CELLS

Currently, one determinant proposed to have a major role in the primary level of gene regulation is the topology or structure of chromatin. For this reason, a brief description of the various levels of chromatin structure is relevant.

The fundamental packaging unit of eukaryotic chromatin is the nucleosomal core particle consisting of two molecules of histones H2A, H2B, H3, and H4 with 146 base pairs (bp) of DNA. The DNA in core particles is folded on the outside of a histone protein core to form a 1.75 turn of a left-handed solenoid with a radius of 4.3 nm (Richmond et al., 1984). An additional 40–60 bp of DNA associated with a fifth histone, H1, constitute a nucleosome. Nucleosomes can occupy nonrandom locations as dictated by specific DNA elements in yeast. For detailed descriptions of chromatin organization, the reader is directed to reviews by Nelson et al. (1986) and Castro (1987).

The organization of the nucleosomal fiber is affected by core histone variants. For example, chromatin from *Drosophila melanogaster* contains two antigenically distinct H2A histones, H2A.1 and H2A.2. H2A.2 is located specifically in the interbands of chromatin and may be involved in the less compacted structure of chromatin (Donahue et al., 1986). Also, *Tetrahymena* macronuclear DNA, which is transcriptionally inactive, contains a specific histone variant, hv1, which has sequences in common with the H2A family of histones (Allis et al., 1986). Thus, there are a number of different, functionally distinct, nonallelic variants in the H2A histone family which affect the nucleofilament structure and correlate with transcriptional activity. Similarly, H1 consists of a family of molecular subvariants whose differences are due to changes in the amino acid sequences located in the C-terminal half of the molecules (Cole, 1984). Somatic tissue of rodents have at least six different types of H1 (Lennox, 1984). H1 exhibits two structural roles in chromatin: (a) it binds to DNA as the fiber enters and exits the nucleosome (Boulikas et al., 1989), and (b) it is responsible for maintaining the higher-order coiling of nucleosome chains (Thoma and Koller, 1977; Thoma et al., 1979; Butler, 1980). There is evidence that the H1 variants play a major role in aggregation-resistant and aggregation-prone chromatin regions (Jin and Cole, 1985, 1986; Rinsdale and Davis, 1987). The influence of dietary zinc deficiency on the H1 complement from rat liver is discussed below.

Nucleosomal organization condenses chromatin into a fiber that is 10 nm thick (Olins and Olins, 1973; Woodcock, 1973). Continued coiling of the 10-nm fiber results in a 30-nm solenoidal fiber with six nucleosomes per turn (Finch and Klug, 1976). The 30-nm chromatin fiber appears to be organized generally into loops or domains that are defined units of DNA structure in interphase chromatin (Benyajati and Worcel, 1976; Cook and Brazell, 1976; Igo-Kemenes and Zachau, 1977; Volgelstein et al., 1980; Lebkowski and Laemmli, 1982; Mirkovitch et al., 1984) and metaphase chromosomes (Adolph et al., 1977; Paulson and Laemmli, 1977). The DNA loops are approximately 60,000 bp in length (Nelson et al., 1986) and are attached at nonrandom sites to the nuclear matrix, an internal protein network (Marsden and Laemmli, 1979).

The organization of chromatin into loops may have profound consequences on nuclear function. First, the domains could be involved in a modulation of gene expression by allowing different regions to the supercoiled to different extents. Second, different types of attachment could form chromosomal domains with functional attachments being associated with active genes. Third, the RNA or DNA polymerases may progress along the DNA unattached to any larger structure during transcription or replication (Jackson and Cooke, 1985a,b). Fourth, the nucleoskeleton may be part of an active center for replication or transcription organizing the template in close proximity to the polymerization site. However, there is no loop organization corresponding to the banding pattern observed in *Drosophila melanogaster* (Mirkovitch et al., 1986). Direct relation between the nuclear matrix attachment sites and gene activity is not clear, since during development and alteration in transcriptional activity during the cell cycle, the attachment sites do not change, implying a mechanism that selectively turns on specific domains (Cockerill and Garrard, 1986; Dalton et al., 1986; Gasser and Laemmli, 1986).

If structural domains of chromatin remain invariant during alteration of transcription, selectivity of transcription depends on molecular mechanisms that include more than structural attachment of the active gene on the matrix of the nucleus. Generally, selectivity of transcription requires identifying those sequences that act in *cis* to regulate transcription of genes. Second, factors capable of interacting specifically with the *cis* regulatory elements may dictate the selectivity and levels of gene expression (McKnight and Tjian, 1986). To identify *cis* regulatory sequences, methods have been developed whereby expression of a gene can be determined as a function of the DNA region under investigation (Flavell, 1980).

ROLE OF ZINC IN DNA AND CHROMATIN STRUCTURE

Divalent cations are essential for the condensation and the higher-order organization of chromatin. Charge neutralization is required for chromatin condensation. Magnesium ions are required for the maintenance of chromatin conformation (McGhee et al., 1980; Borochov et al., 1984). Calcium ions bind to nucleosome core particles of chicken erythrocytes and result in a significant change of DNA circular dichroism (Hogan et al., 1986). Calcium ions binding to nucleosomes seem to cause sharp bends or kinks in the DNA. Likewise, Ca^{2+} can stabilize metaphase chromosomes, although not as efficiently as Cu^{2+} (Lewis and Laemmli, 1982).

Zinc ions are ubiquitously distributed in biological systems and exhibit critical roles in maintaining the integrity of nucleic acids. As part of an ongoing program aimed at understanding the effects of nutrient intake on genome structure and gene expression, we became interested in the impact of zinc deficiency on chromatin structure. Zinc ligands can bind to alternating purine-pyrimidine sequences (poly[dG-dC]) and cause a shift from a right-handed B form of DNA to a left-handed Z form (Fazakerley, 1984). Circular dichroism (CD) spectra of poly(dG-dC) exhibit the characteristic inversion associated with formation of the left-handed helix upon titration with zinc chloride–diethylenetriamine or zinc chloride *tris*(2-aminoethyl)amine. These zinc complexes are more potent inducers of the Z-form DNA than is Mn(II) or other divalent cations (Zacharias et al., 1982; Russell et al., 1983; Fazakerkey, 1984).

In addition to modifying the structure of poly(dG-dC) DNA, Zn^{2+} can condense chicken erythrocyte chromatin. Other divalent cations (Co^{2+}, Mg^{2+}, Mn^{2+}) among the first period transition metals are capable of condensing chromatin to form the 10-nm fiber to the 30-nm solenoid in a similar manner as Zn^{2+} (Sen and Crothers, 1986a). Electric dichroism indicates only small differences in the concentration of these cations at which chromatin begins to aggregate, a phenomenon which occurs after optimal compaction. The degree of condensation of chromatin conferred by divalent cations, at least for Mg^{2+}, and presumably for others, including zinc, may influence the DNA-binding capability of various drugs (Sen and Crothers, 1986b).

We thought it important to determine whether nutritional zinc deficiency alters the higher-order configuration of rat liver interphase chromatin in intact nuclei. Although zinc concentration affects DNA and chromatin structure in vitro, it is conceivable that homeostatic mechanisms would maintain adequate zinc levels in the nucleus and preclude structural modification of chromatin in rat liver. An enzymatic assay for assessing chromatin structure is based on micrococcal nuclease, MN, (EC 3.1.31.1), which cleaves DNA at accessible internucleosomal sites to yield oligonucleosomes that are subsequently cleaved to smaller fragments that are acid soluble. In eucaryotic chromatin, approximately 50% of DNA in chromatin is accessible to MN and can be hydrolyzed into acid-soluble oligonucleotides (Clark and Felsenfeld, 1974).

Zinc deficiency was established in Sprague-Dawley rats by feeding a diet containing 0.9 ppm zinc for 28 days. A pair-fed group and an ad libitum-fed group consumed a diet containing 40 ppm zinc for the same length of time. Isolated liver nuclei were digested with MN at a constant enzyme:DNA ratio. The perchloric acid–soluble products were measured spectrophotometrically and graphed as a percentage of total chromatin. Figure 1 demonstrates that substantially less chromatin from zinc-deficient rat liver is accessible to MN (34%) than is that of pair-fed (53%) or ad libitum–fed (45%) rats at the saturation point. There are no differences in endogenous nuclease(s) activity among the three groups as shown by the perchloric acid–soluble material generated in the absence of MN (Castro et al., 1986b). The enhanced resistance to micrococcal nuclease shown by chromatin from zinc-deficient rats indicate an alteration in the higher-order organization of the chromatin.

The enhanced nuclease resistance of chromatin from zinc-deficient rats is observed also in the single-celled organism *Euglena gracilis* (Stankiewicz et al., 1983) grown in zinc-depleted (−Zn) medium. Chromatin of *E. gracilis* grown in −Zn medium (0.1 μm) is digested by MN at a rate of 10- to 30-fold less than chromatin from *E. gracilis* grown in zinc-containing (+Zn) medium (10 μM). The differential rates of digestion are not caused by inhibitors because the addition of −Zn chromatin to +Zn chromatin does not alter digestion. The enhanced nuclease resistance of chromatin reflecting an alteration in higher-order chromatin structure observed in zinc-deficient rodents or *Euglena* may underlie an important biological response, since it is evolutionarily conserved.

One determinant of higher-order chromatin structure is histone H1. We investigated whether nutritional zinc deficiency causes alteration to the H1 class of histones. The H1 family of proteins was isolated from liver of zinc-deficient pair-fed or control rats and separated by polyacrylamide sodium–docecyl sulfate gels. The relative amount of one H1 subvariant, H1°, is reduced by zinc deficiency to 50% of the amount from rats pair-fed a zinc-supplemented diet (Castro et al., 1986a). Such a reduction in the relative amount of H1° may be responsible for alterations in the higher-order chromatin structure as observed in the increased resistance to micrococcal nuclease.

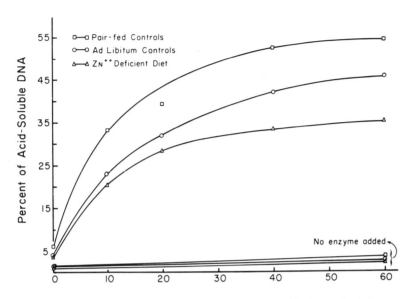

Figure 1 Percent of acid-soluble DNA generated by incubation of rat liver nuclei with micrococcal nuclease. Nuclei were digested with a constant enzyme:DNA ratio. (From Castro et al., 1986b; reprinted with permission from *Federation Proceedings*, Federation of American Societies for Experimental Biology.)

The potential significance of decreased histone H1° caused by zinc deficiency lies in promoting different chromatin structures which may be important in the regulation of gene expression and cell differentiation (Lennox, 1984; Jin and Cole, 1986). Newrock et al. (1978) and Weintraub (1985) have postulated that variable H1 subtypes are a type of coarse control mechanism which may preclude the necessity for fine control in genomic regions that are infrequently or never expressed. The rudimentary controls for gene regulation afforded by H1 subtypes may coexist with precise controlling mechanisms necessary for specific gene expression.

Histones isolated from the liver of zinc-deficient or pair-fed zinc-supplemented rats (Castro et al., 1986a) can be further fractionated by reverse-phase high-performance liquid chromatography (Gurley et al., 1983; Kurokawa and MacLeod, 1985). Using a C-18 column with a pore size of 330 Å and trifluoroacetic acid (0.1%) in the eluting water–acetonitrile solvent, the histone H1 fraction can be resolved into peaks a–d (Fig. 2). The ratio of peak area for b_1 and b_2 shows substantial variation in chromatin isolated from zinc-deficient rat liver compared with that from rats pair-fed a complete diet. The ratio of b_1/b_1+b_2 is reduced 66%, whereas that of b_2/b_1+b_2 is increased twofold after zinc deficiency.

Zinc deficiency alters the pattern of histones, including H1 in *E. gracilis* as well. Log-phase zinc-deficient cells (−Zn) contain H1 and H3, whereas H2A, H2B, and H4 are absent (Mazus et al., 1984). All of the histones are extinguished in stationary-phase −Zn cells. The addition of zinc to stationary-phase −Zn cells reinitiates cell division and all the histones reappear. These results suggest that zinc may affect gene repression and/or activation through the modulation of chromosomal proteins.

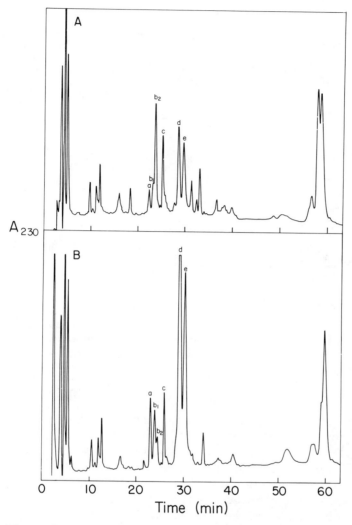

Figure 2 Reverse-phase liquid chromatography fractionation (peaks a–e) of histone H1 from zinc-deficient (panel A) and pair-fed (panel B) rats.

At present, it is unclear as to whether the alterations in chromatin structure and histone H1 complement are directly due to zinc deficiency or are a secondary response related to endocrine status. DePasquale-Jardieu and Fraker (1979) demonstrated that in zinc-deficient mice corticosterone rises fourfold during a 28-day study. In general, zinc deficiency affects thymic hormone function and activates the hypothalamus-pituitary-adrenal cortex axis (Fraker et al., 1986). The determination of the direct cause of chromatin changes in liver associated with zinc deficiency must be accomplished with isolated hepatocytes grown in defined nutrient medium.

ZINC AND GENE EXPRESSION

The element zinc exhibits essential roles in gene expression and regulation (Sandstead, 1985). As described above, zinc affects the structure of both naked DNA and chromatin. Since the topology of DNA and chromatin is fundamental to gene expression, altering the structural conformation is one means by which zinc affects gene expression. Diminished DNA replication associated with zinc deficiency may be the principal cause of the 70% reduction in anti–trinitrophenylated lipopolysaccharide plaque-forming cells in spleen (Fraker et al., 1986).

One aspect of zinc and gene expression involves maintaining the stability and function of DNA-binding proteins. Transcription factor IIIA (TFIIIA) is a 40-K protein in *Xenopus laevis* which facilitates RNA polymerase III transcription of 5S RNA in vitro. Proteolytic digestion of TFIIIA yields intermediate products spaced at 3-K intervals. This characteristic pattern and the presence of 7–11 zinc atoms/molecule suggests that the protein contains repetitive zinc-binding domains (Miller et al., 1985). The linear configuration of these repetitive, independently folding domains, or "fingers," each centered on a zinc ion, explain how this protein binds to a long internal control region of the 5S gene and stays bound during the passage of an RNA polymerase molecule. There is a corresponding repeat in the DNA sequence bound by TFIIIA (Rhodes and Klug, 1986). Transcription factor IIIA interacts with a DNA-binding site that contains a periodicity of 5 bp.

Transcription factor IIIA probably represents a class of structural motifs in other proteins that bind DNA or RNA. Examples include the small RNA-binding protein encoded in the *gag* genes of retroviruses, the adenovirus E1A gene products, and the large T antigens from simian virus 40 and polyoma viruses (Berg, 1986). A single-stranded DNA-binding protein, gene 32 protein (g32P), required for replication, recombination, and translational control in the phage T_4 life cycle contains a zinc-binding sequence (Coleman et al., 1987). Removal of zinc from native g32P renders the molecule sensitive to proteolysis and causes a loss of DNA-binding affinity. In eukaryotic genes, an extensive similarity has been identified between TFIIIA and the product of the *Drosophila* regulatory *Krüppel* locus (Rosenberg et al., 1986). Other eukaryotic DNA-binding proteins have similar structural properties (Vincent, 1986). Thus, zinc is required for newly identified DNA- and RNA-binding proteins which function in gene expression.

The repression of gene expression in the zinc-deficient genome is likely due to multiple factors, including an altered conformation of DNA structure and impaired function of DNA-binding proteins. Interestingly, while genomes in zinc-deficient state are markedly repressed (Falchuk et al., 1975; Eckhert and Hurley, 1979), a discrete number of genes are selectively activated (Mazus et al., 1984; Falchuk et al., 1985). The nature and significance of these latter genes are of particular interest. Preliminary data from our laboratories indicate that the level of hepatic mRNA for a cellular proto-oncogene *c-fms* is induced approximately eightfold in zinc-deficient rats compared with pair-fed rats (C.E. Castro, unpublished data). The *c-fms* proto-oncogene belongs to a class of sequences coding for certain factors and receptor proteins, such as those required for macrophage function. The level of mRNA for a related proto-oncogene, *c-fes*, is unchanged by zinc deficiency, indicating some degree of specific enhancement of *c-fms* mRNA. The confirmation of these results and investigation of the biological consequences are currently in progress.

REFERENCES

Adolph KW, Cheng SM, Laemmli UK. 1977. Role of nonhistone proteins in metaphase chromosome structure. Cell 12:805–816.
Allis CD, Richman R, Gorovsky MA, Ziegler YS, Touchstone B, Bradley WA, Cook RG. 1986. hv1 Is an evolutionarily conserved H2A variant that is preferentially associated with active genes. J Biol Chem 261:1941–1948.
Benyajati C, Worcel A. 1976. Isolation, characterization, and structure of the folded interphase genome of *Drosophila melanogaster*. Cell 9:393–407.
Berg JM. 1986. Potential metal-binding domains in nucleic acid binding proteins. Science 232:485–487.
Borochov N, Ausio J, Eisenberg H. 1984. Interaction and conformational changes of chromatin with divalent ions. Nucleic Acids Res 12:3089–3096.
Boulikas T, Wiseman JM, Garrard WT. 1980. Points of contact between histone H1 and the histone octamer. Proc Natl Acad Sci USA 77:127–131.
Butler PJG, Thomas JO. 1980. Changes in chromatin folding in solution. J Mol Biol 140:505–529.
Castro CE. 1983. Nucleosomal repeat length in rat liver nuclei is decreased by a high carbohydrate, fat-free diet. J Nutr 113:557–565.
Castro CE, Sevall JS. 1980. Alteration of higher order structure of rat liver chromatin by dietary composition. J Nutr 110:105–116.
Castro CE. 1987. Nutrient effects on DNA and chromatin structure. Ann Rev Nutr 7:407–421.
Castro CE, Alvares OF, Sevall JS. 1986a. Zinc deficiency decreases histone H1° in rat liver. Nutr Rep Int 34:67–74.
Castro CE, Armstrong-Major J, Ramirez ME. 1986b. Diet-mediated alteration of chromatin structure. Fed Proc 45:2394–2398.
Clark RJ, Felsenfeld G. 1974. Chemical probes of chromatin structure. Biochemistry 13:3622–3628.
Cockerill PN, Garrard WT. 1986. Chromosomal loop anchorage of the kappa immunoglobulin gene occurs next to the enhancer in a region containing topoisomerase II sites. Cell 44:273–282.
Cole RD. 1984. A minireview of microheterogeneity in H1 histone and its possible significance. Anal Biochem 136:24–30.
Coleman JE, Giedroc DP, Keating KM, Williams KR. 1987. Role of zinc in the structure and function of ssDNA binding proteins. Fed Proc 46:2238 (abstract 1821).
Cook PR, Brazell JA. 1976. Conformational constraints in nuclear DNA. J Cell Sci 22:287–302.
Dalton S, Younghusband HB, Wells JRE. 1986. Chicken histone genes retain nuclear matrix association throughout the cell cycle. Nucleic Acids Res 14:6507–6523.
DePasquale-Jardieu P, Fraker PJ, 1979. The role of corticosterone in the loss in immune function in zinc deficient A/J mouse. J Nutr 109:1847–1855.
Donahue PR, Palmer DK, Condie JM, Sabatini LM, Blumenfeld M. 1986. *Drosophila* histone H2A.2 is associated with the interbands of polytene chromosomes. Proc Natl Acad Sci USA 83:4744–4748.
Eckhert CD, Hurley LS. 1979. Influence of various levels of hypervitaminosis A and zinc deficiency on teratogenesis and DNA synthesis in the rat. Teratology 19:279–284.
Falchuk KH, Fawcett DW, Vallee BL. 1975. Role of zinc in cell division of *Euglena gracilis*. J Cell Sci 17:57–78.
Falchuk KH, Mazus B, Ber E, Ulpino-Lobb L, Vallee BL. 1985. Zinc deficiency and the *Euglena gracilis* chromatin: Formation of an α-amanitin-resistant RNA polymerase II. Biochemistry 24:2576–2580.
Fazakerley GV. 1984. Zinc Z-DNA. Nucleic Acids Res. 12:3643–3648.

Finch JT, Klug A. 1976. Solenoidal model for superstructure in chromatin. Proc Natl Acad Sci USA 73:1897–1901.

Flavell RA. 1980. The transcription of eukaryotic genes. Nature 285:356–357.

Fraker PJ, Jardieu P, Wirth JA. 1986. The immunopathobiological consequences of zinc deficiency. In: Nutritional Diseases: Research Directions in Comparative Pathobiology. D. G. Scarpelli and G. Migaki, eds., New York: Liss, pp 197–213.

Gasser SM, Laemmli UK. 1986. Cohabitation of scaffold binding regions with upstream/enhancer elements of three developmentally regulated genes of *D. melanogaster*. Cell 46:521–530.

Gurley LR, Prentice DA, Valdez JG, Spall WD. 1983. Histone fractionation by high-performance liquid chromatography on cyanoalkylsilane (CN) reverse-phase columns. Anal Biochem 131:465–477.

Hogan ME, Hayes B, Wang NC, Austin RH. 1986. Ion-induced DNA structure change in nucleosomes. Biochemistry 25:5070–5082.

Igo-Kemenes T, Zachau HG. 1977. Domains in chromatin structure. Cold Spring Harbor Symp Q Biol 42:109–118.

Jackson DA, Cook PR. 1985a. A general method for preparing chromatin containing intact DNA. EMBO J 4:913–918.

Jackson DA, Cook PR. 1985b. Transcription occurs at a nucleoskeleton. EMBO J 4:919–925.

Jin Y, Cole D. 1985. Histone H1 is distributed unlike H1 in chromatin aggregation. FEBS Lett 182:455–458.

Jin Y, Cole RD. 1986. H1 histone exchange is limited to particular regions of chromatin that differ in aggregation properties. J Biol Chem 261:3420–3427.

Kurokawa M, MacLeod MC. 1985. Separation of histones by reverse-phase high-performance liquid chromatography: Analysis of the binding of carcinogens to histones. Anal Biochem 144:47–54.

Lebkowski JS, Laemmli UK. 1982. Evidence for two levels of DNA folding in histone-depleted HeLa interphase nuclei. J Mol Biol 156:309–324.

Lennox RW. 1984. Differences in evolutionary stability among mammalian H1 subtypes. Implications for the roles of H1 subtypes in chromatin. J Biol Chem 259:669–672.

Lewis CD, Laemmli UK. 1982. Higher order metaphase chromosome structure: Evidence for metalloprotein interactions. Cell 29:171–181.

Marsden MPF, Laemmli UK. 1979. Metaphase chromosome structure: Evidence for a radical loop model. Cell 17:849–858.

Mazus B, Falchuk KH, Vallee BL. 1984. Histone formation, gene expression, and zinc deficiency in *Euglena gracilis*. Biochemistry 23:42–47.

McGhee JD, Rau DC, Charnay E, Felsenfeld G. 1980. Orientation of the nucleosome within the higher order structure of chromatin. Cell 22:87–96.

McKnight S, Tjian R. 1986. Transcriptional selectivity of viral genes in mammalian cells. Cell 46:795–805.

Miller J, McLachlan AD, Klug A. 1985. Repetitive zinc-binding domains in the protein transcription factor IIIA from *Xenopus* oocytes. EMBO J 4:1609–1614.

Mirkovitch J, Mirault ME, Laemmli U. 1984. Organization of the higher-order chromatin loop: Specific DNA attachment sites on nuclear scaffold. Cell 39:223–232.

Mirkovitch J, Spierer P, Laemmli UK. 1986. Genes and loops in 320,000 base-pairs of the *Drosophila melanogaster* chromosome. J Mol Biol 190:255–258.

Nelson WG, Pienta KJ, Barrack ER, Coffey DS. 1986. The role of the nuclear matrix in the organization and function of DNA. Ann Rev Biophys Biophys Chem 15:457–75.

Newrock KM, Alfageme CR, Nardi RV, Cohen LH. 1978. Histone changes during chromatin remodeling in embryogenesis. Cold Spring Harbor Symp Q Biol 42:421–431.

Olins AL, Olins DE. 1973. Spheroid chromatin units (ν bodies). J Cell Biol 59(2, pt. 2):252a.

Paulson JR, Laemmli UK. 1977. The structure of histone-depleted metaphase chromosome. Cell 12:817–828.

Rhodes D, Klug A. 1986. An underlying repeat in some transcriptional control sequences corresponding to half a double helical turn of DNA. Cell 46:123–132.

Richmond TJ, Finch JT, Rushton B, Rhodes D, Klug A. 1984. Structure of the nucleosome core particle at 7 Å resolution. Nature 311:532–537.

Rinsdale JA, Davie JR. 1987. Selective solubilization of β-globin oligonucleosomes at low ionic strength. Biochemistry 26:290–295.

Rosenberg UB, Schroder C, Preiss A, Kienlin A, Cote S, Riede I, Jackle H. 1986. Structural homology of the product of the *Drosophila Kruppel* gene with *Xenopus* transcription factor IIIA. Nature 319:336–339.

Russell WC, Precious B, Martin SR, Bayley PM. 1983. Differential promotion and suppression of Z leads to B transitions in poly[d(G-C)] by histone subclasses, polyamino acids and polyamines. EMBO J 2:1647–1653.

Sandstead HH. 1985. Zinc: Essentiality for brain development and function. Nutr Rev 43:129–137.

Sen D, Crothers DM. 1986a. Condensation of chromatin: Role of multivalent cations. Biochemistry 25:1495–1503.

Sen D, Crothers DM. 1986b. Influence of DNA-binding drugs on chromatin condensation. Biochemistry 25:1503–1509.

Small D, Nelkin B, Vogelstein B. 1985. The association of transcribed genes with the nuclear matrix of *Drosophila* cells during heat shock. Nucleic Acids Res 13:2413–2431.

Stankiewicz AJ, Falchuk KH, Vallee BL. 1983. Composition and structure of zinc-deficient *Euglena gracilis* chromatin. Biochemistry 22:5150–5156.

Thoma F, Koller T. 1977. Influence of histone H1 on chromatin structure. Cell 12:101–107.

Thoma F, Koller T, Klug A. 1979. Involvement of histone H1 in the organization of the nucleosome and of the salt-dependent superstructures of chromatin. J Cell Biol 83:403–427.

Vincent A. 1986. TFIIIA and homologous genes. The finger proteins. Nucleic Acids Res 14:4385–4391.

Vogelstein B, Pardoll DM, Coffey DS. 1980. Supercoiled loops and eucaryotic DNA replication. Cell 22:79–85.

Weintraub H. 1985. Assembly and propagation of repressed and derepressed chromosomal states. Cell 42:705–711.

Woodcock CLF. 1973. Ultrastructure of inactive chromatin. J Cell Biol 59(2, pt. 2):368a.

Wu FY-H, WU C-H. 1987. Zinc: DNA replication and transcription. Annu Rev Nutr 7:251–272.

Zacharias W, Larson JE, Klysik J, Stirdivant SM, Wells RD. 1982. Conditions which cause the right-handed to left-handed DNA conformational transitions. Evidence for several types of left-handed DNA structures in solution. J Biol Chem 257:2775–2782.

Part II
Effect of Nutritional Conditioning on Immune Response

10
The Influence of Nutrition on Experimental Autoimmune Disease

W. John W. Morrow, Jacques Homsy, and Jay A. Levy
University of California School of Medicine, San Francisco, California

Christian Swanson
University of California School of Medicine, Davis, California

INTRODUCTION

Autoimmune disorders in humans comprise an array of degenerative diseases characterized by tissue injury associated with aberrant and harmful immunological responses. They may be controlled by immunosuppressive or anti-inflammatory drugs, although a number of adjunct therapies may also be employed, including plasmapheresis and total lymphoid irradiation (1). However, such treatment regimens are less than satisfactory, both in terms of their ability to modulate disease and in the number of side effects that they cause.

Over the last decade there has been considerable interest in the effects of nutrition on the development of autoimmunity. Such studies have been aided by the derivation of several murine models in which animals spontaneously develop immunopathological abnormalities similar to human autoimmune syndromes. Thus, the majority of investigations of the effects of dietary manipulation on the progression of autoimmune disease have centered on animal systems because of the obvious difficulties associated with human experimentation. In particular, focus has been on three murine models; namely, the New Zealand Black (NZB) strain, which develops autoimmune hemolytic anemia; the New Zealand Black × White (B/W) F_1 hybrid, in which fatal immune complex nephritis occurs; and the MRL/Mp-lpr/lpr (MRL/lpr) strain, which, like the B/W, develops glomerulonephritis resembling human systemic lupus erythematosus (SLE), but also shows evidence of vasculitis, synovitis, and extensive lymphoproliferation (2).

The basis of nutritional therapeutic approaches to diseases of the immune system stems from the observation that individuals suffering from protein-calorie malnutrition or deficiencies in specific food ingredients have a compromised immune status (see Refs. 3–5 for review). Malnourished individuals have a high frequency of infection, profound depression of both T- and B-cell function, and many serological abnormalities. The recognition of these effects has catalyzed several studies on the influence of nutrition on autoimmune conditions, predominantly in the animal systems described above. In this chapter, we discuss these experiments, examine the possible immunomodulatory mechanisms that may be involved, and consider the potential role of nutrition in the management of human autoimmune disease.

HISTORICAL BACKGROUND

Early work in the field of nutrition and autoimmunity established that changes in any of the major food constituents, proteins, calories, fats, vitamins or minerals, could help preserve normal immune function and markedly prolong the life span of lupus-prone mice. A brief summary of these studies is presented below.

Calorie Restriction

Experiments restricting caloric intake in New Zealand mice were among the first to be conducted in attempts to regulate the autoimmune process by nutritional intervention (6–11). B/W mice fed a low calorie diet had a reduced incidence of immune complex glomerulonephritis and improved immunological parameters, including a reduction in autoantibody production, an increase in cell-mediated cytotoxicity (6–8), and near normal interleukin 2 (IL-2) production and responsiveness (9). In addition, levels of circulating immune complexes (CICs) were decreased (10), and both the expression of retroviral envelope coat glycoprotein gp70 and the formation of anti-gp70 immune complexes (11) were strikingly reduced. The mechanism(s) by which protein-calorie restriction induces such effects is unknown, but it may simply cause an overall downshift in metabolic processes, including immunological function. Recently, James et al. (12) have shown that fractionate exposure to very low-dose ionizing radiation would enhance an immune response in autoimmune mice and the caloric restriction was additive, suggesting that feedback upregulation of the thymic compartment following peripheral cell death induced by both treatments may play a role.

Proteins and Amino Acids

Diets low in protein (13) or containing restricted quantities of selected amino acids (low phenylalanine, low tyrosine) (14) can prevent immune complex nephropathy in New Zealand mice, although the reasons for this effect are uncertain. As with calorie restriction, protein–amino acid deficiencies may not have a selective effect on the immune system, but may induce generalized metabolic retardation. However, the effects of protein on immunological function may be extremely complex, as illustrated in a study by Batsford and colleagues (15). These investigators observed that B/W mice fed a fully synthetic amino acid diet showed a dramatic increase in life span that was accompanied by a decrease in the levels of antinuclear antibodies. Similarly, a diet in which natural proteins were replaced with synthetic L-amino acids conferred a protective effect on Wistar BB rats, a strain in which insulin-dependent autoimmune diabetes develops spontaneously. When the rats were placed on this diet, the incidence of disease was dramatically decreased (16). The inference from these studies is that everyday diets contain allergens (presumably protein or protein complexes that have in some way been rendered antigenic by food-processing techniques) that may trigger or exacerbate the autoimmune cascade. When these substances are removed, autoallergic reactions can be substantially ameliorated.

Trace Elements

Trace metals, particularly zinc, also influence immune responsiveness. In NZB and B/W mice, a reduction of this metal decreased the rate of progression of hemolytic anemia, immune complex glomerulonephritis, and other parameters of autoimmune disease (17,18). In addition, feeding with zinc-deficient diets was associated with lower levels of autoantibodies and serum immunoglobulins and a prolonged life span. Again, the reasons for these effects are unknown, particularly as zinc may be important for the function of approximately 100 metalloenzymes. However, it has been suggested that a paucity of this mineral may impair the production of zinc-dependent thymic hormones which are crucial for normal T-cell differentiation (19).

Thus, virtually any dietary factor can potentially alter the function of the immune system (see Ref. 20 for complete review). While a comprehensive survey of all such studies is beyond the scope of this chapter, we will consider in greater depth the effects of fat on autoimmune disease. Dietary lipid is undoubtedly the best-studied nutritional component known to influence disease in lupus-prone animals. Results obtained from these studies of animal systems may hold true for human immunological diseases, and may be especially timely with the growing public awareness of the potentially harmful effects of increased fat intake. Thus, in our opinion, the greatest advances in public health in terms of controlling, to some extent, autoimmune disorders such as rheumatoid arthritis, SLE, Sjögren's syndrome, and diabetes, could be made by changing the fat content of the current "western" diet.

EFFECTS OF DIETARY LIPID ON PATHOLOGY AND IMMUNE FUNCTION

The dramatic effects of fats on the immune system were first described by Fernandes and colleagues (21) using NZB mice. Two commercial diets differing in protein and fat content were found to influence longevity and appearance of autoimmune symptoms in these animals. Groups fed the high-fat/low-protein diet had a more severe anemia and decreased life span than those fed the low-fat/high-protein diet. Follow-up studies revealed that immunopathological parameters, including autoantibody production and cell-mediated immune responses, were similarly affected by these diets. Unfortunately, the caloric content of the diets was not controlled in these experiments, thus making the task of correlating immune function with fat content difficult.

More recently, investigators have attempted to isolate the influence of fat on the progression of spontaneous murine autoimmune disease by utilizing diets of highly specific composition. In our laboratory, we have used diets that have differed only in the type and amount of fat but calorically varied by no more than 10% (22–24). Female B/W mice fed a diet low in fat (1.2% corn oil) exhibited a dramatic reduction in the appearance of autoimmune symptoms and a significant increase in life span when compared with littermates fed a diet high in saturated (9–18% lard) or unsaturated (9% corn oil) fat. These high-fat diets were also associated with more severe immune complex glomerulonephritis, and significantly shortened the life span and decreased immune function. The salient features of these data are summarized in Table 1.

Similar results have been obtained with MRL/lpr mice (25). Females fed near-isocaloric diets high in saturated or unsaturated fat exhibited impaired immunological capabilities, including decreased natural killer (NK) cell activity, reduced macrophage phagocytosis, and impaired IL-2 production. Those counterparts fed the diet low in fat had preserved immune function approximating a nonautoimmune mouse.

The importance of differentiating between the effects of saturated and unsaturated fats was indicated by one of our earlier studies (22). In this investigation, autoantibody production in female B/W mice appeared to be selectively influenced by the degree of fat saturation. Those animals fed a diet high in saturated fat exhibited increased titers of natural thymocytotoxic antibody, an IgM autoantibody. Mice fed the diet high in unsaturated fat had increased levels of anti-DNA autoantibodies, primarily of the IgG class. These results suggest that different fatty acids may influence

Table 1 Results of Immune Studies of 7-Month-Old Female B/W Receiving Diets Varying in Fat Content

Immune parameter	High saturated fat	High unsaturated fat	Low fat	Conventional rodent pellet
T-cell mitogenesis	−	(−)	+	−
B-cell mitogenesis	+	+	−	−
Bromelain plaque assay	N	+ + T helper	N	+ T helper
Macrophage phagocytosis	−	−	N	(−)
NK cell activity	−	−	N	(−)
Interferon production	−	−	N	−
Response to IgG	−	+	−	+
IP SRBC IgM	NE	NE	NE	NE
Serum IgG, IgM	NE	NE	NE	NE
Autoantibody production	+NTA [IgM]	+dsDNA [IgG]	−	+dsDNA
Circulating ICs	N	+	N	+
IC nephritis	+glom	+glom	(+) meseng	(+) mesang
Sjögren's syndrome	+ +	+ +	N	+
Hemolytic anemia	+	+	N	(+)
Skin hypersensitivity to DNFB	NE	NE	NE	NE

Abbreviations: glom, glomerular; N, normal; mesang, mesangial deposits; NE, no substantial effect; NK cell, natural killer cell; NTA, natural thymocytotoxic antibody; +, increased; SRBC, sheep red blood cell; −, decreased; IC, immune complex; ( ), mild effect; IP, intra-peritoneal; DNFB, dinitrofluorobenzene.
Source: Adapted from Ref. 20; used with permission.

various aspects of the immune response, including antibody production from certain B-cell subpopulations and/or T-cell help. This hypothesis was further substantiated in a subsequent study in which the number of antibody-secreting indirect (immunoglobulin G) plaque-forming cells, made in response to challenge from sheep erythrocytes, was greater in a group of 7-month-old B/W mice fed unsaturated fat (23) than in animals fed a high–saturated fat regimen. The number of lipopolysaccharide (LPS)–stimulated peritoneal lymphocytes making antibodies to autologous, bromelain-treated red cells was also greatest in the group maintained on unsaturated fat. The response to bromelain-treated autologous erythrocytes is normally regarded as being independent of T-cell help, but under the control of suppressor cells, and treatment of the LPS-stimulated cultures with anti–Thy-1 antiserum and complement (to remove T lymphocytes) increases the magnitude of the response. In our hands, however, the response was significantly decreased in animals fed high levels of unsaturated but not saturated fat, suggesting that ingestion of these particular lipids influences immune reactivity and changes the requirement for T-cell help in the bromelain system (23).

We observed further differences with macrophage phagocytosis and natural killer cell activity (23). Both of these functions were most seriously impaired in cells from animals fed high levels of saturated fat, and we believe that this lipid may cause abnormalities in immune cells that require membrane contact to function normally. Analysis of membrane fatty acid content may elucidate the mechanism underlying this finding (see also below).

In addition to the serological and cellular changes induced by alterations in dietary lipid, the pathological abnormalities associated with murine lupus are also influenced. When examining the extent of nephritis in mice fed diets varying in lipid content, Yumura et al. (24) demonstrated that B/W mice maintained on a diet low in fat (1.2% corn oil) were conspicuously protected from the development of severe immune complex glomerulonephritis. Furthermore, analysis of the deposition site revealed that in those mice fed diets containing high (9%) concentrations of either saturated or unsaturated lipid, immune complexes were concentrated in the glomerular capillary walls. In contrast, those animals fed the low-fat diet exhibited primarily mesangial deposits, which are typical of mild nephritis in humans. While there were no obvious differences in the pattern of immune deposition or the incidence of mortality in either the groups fed high saturated or unsaturated fat, levels of CICs, as measured by the polyethylene glycol precipitation test, were greatest in the group fed high unsaturated fat. This finding suggests that although unsaturated fat may "drive" antibody responses and result in the production of high levels of autoantibodies and immune complexes, other factors regulate their deposition and the inflammation seen in the glomeruli.

Kelley and Izui (26) also reported that a diet containing very high levels of saturated fat (50%) led to a higher incidence of severe vascular injury and accelerated development of glomerulonephritis, although in this case the pathology appeared to result from a synergy between immune complexes and increased lipid deposition in the glomerulus. Not surprisingly, diets rich in saturated fat (20%) have been found to cause a high incidence of aortic and renal arteritis as well as atherosclerotic lesions in B/W mice (27).

Other effects of fat on the immunopathology of B/W mice have been concerned with Sjögren's syndrome and hemolytic anemia. New Zealand mice serve as good models of human Sjögren's syndrome, and we have also demonstrated that levels of dietary lipids influence lymphocytic infiltration in the exocrine glands of these animals (28). Those animals fed a diet low in fat were found to have substantially reduced infiltration of mononuclear cells and normal tear production in comparison with their high fat–fed counterparts. B/W mice exhibit a mild form of hemolytic anemia, and the manifestation of this symptom was greatest in animals fed the high-fat diets: mice maintained on high levels of dietary lipid had decreased hematocrit levels and reticulocytosis was evident. Mice fed a low-fat diet were partially protected against this hematological disorder (28).

Overall, it is clear that alterations in dietary lipid can dramatically alter the immunological and pathological abnormalities associated with murine autoimmune disease. Despite substantial progress, the mechanisms by which lipids influence immune function remain unclear. Some of the possibilities are considered below.

MECHANISMS OF IMMUNE MODULATION BY LIPIDS

Cyclo- and Lipooxygenase Pathways

In 1976, Mertin and Hunt (29) proposed that lipids may influence immune responsiveness via alterations in the synthesis of prostaglandins (PGs) and leukotrienes (LTs). Prostaglandins and LTs form a family of biological compounds that are active at very low concentrations, and which are believed to play a critical role in the development and regulation of inflammatory and immune responses. The major biochemical precursor of PGs and LTs is the polyunsaturated fatty acid (PUFA) arachidonic acid (ArAc). Through cyclooxygenase and lipooxygenase oxidation, ArAc leads to the formation of PGs and LTs, respectively. In mammals, the essential fatty acid (EFA) linoleic acid is a necessary precursor for the biosynthesis of ArAc. Although substantial quantities of ArAc are not found in any type of dietary fat, the linoleic acid precursor is an important constituent of most unsaturated vegetable oils, particularly corn oil. A simplified scheme of the biosynthetic pathways is presented in Figure 1.

At present, the precise role of PGs is uncertain in terms of both their stimulating and suppressing immune mechanisms. Both PGE_1 and PGE_2 have been found to reduce the ability of the mitogens phytohemagglutinin and concanavalin A to stimulate T lymphocytes, as well as to inhibit the function of interferon-activated murine macrophages (30). Similarly, PGE_1 injections reduced the manifestations of lupus in B/W (31,32) and MRL/lpr mice (33). In contrast, Mertin and Stackpoole (34) have shown that antibodies against PGE_1 can suppress cell-mediated immunity in Lewis rats. Suppression was greatest when the antiserum was given early in the development of the immune response, suggesting that this PG functions as an augmentative mediator during the initial stages of cell-mediated immunity. In addition, our group has reported that PGE_2 production by mononuclear cells did not differ in B/W mice fed a diet low in fat or high in saturated or unsaturated fats, although the disease was markedly accelerated and the mitogenic response of T cells was much reduced in animals fed the high-fat diets (22). Finally, B/W mice fed a diet high in saturated fat but deficient in EFA exhibited a significant increase in survival and reduced symptoms (35), whereas a diet of safflower oil containing 78% linoleic acid did not exacerbate the disease as would be expected (36). These apparent contradictions probably

Influence of Nutrition on Autoimmune Disease

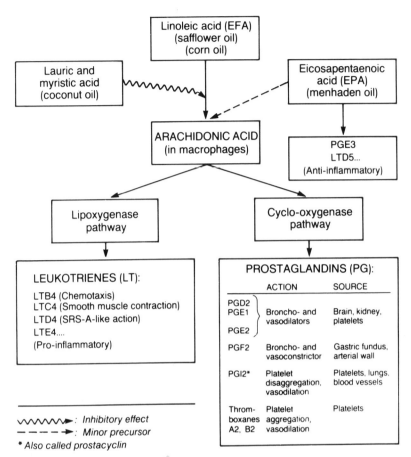

Figure 1 Biosynthesis of inflammatory mediators. Schematic diagram of prostaglandin and leukotriene synthesis from polyunsaturated fatty acids. The major biological effects of prostaglandin products are indicated. Linoleic acid, an essential fatty acid found in most vegetable oils, particularly corn oil, is in mammals a primary precursor for arachidonic acid which leads to the synthesis of leukotrienes through the lipooxygenase pathway, and to prostaglandins via the cyclooxygenase pathway. Eicosapentaenoic acid, a component of fish oil, is a minor precursor of arachidonic acid and induces preferentially the formation of the anti-inflammatory compounds PGE_5 and LTD_3, which suppress the synthesis of inflammatory products of arachidonic acid metabolism. Lauric and myristic acids are found in coconut oil and are antagonists of the transformation of linoleic acid into arachidonic acid. (Adapted from Ref. 20; used with permission.)

reflect the wide variety of actions of PG, not only in different animal systems in vivo, but also in vitro. Moreover, the importance of PG and LT ratios is not well understood, and immune regulation may to a great extent rely upon local rather than systemic levels of these mediators.

It has been suggested that lipooxygenase products, primarily the LTs, are important in generating the initial immune response and PGs of the E series downregulate the extent of the response (37). The possible importance of LTs in exacerbating autoimmune disease is reflected in the effectiveness of both steroidal and nonsteroidal anti-inflammatory drugs in controlling these diseases. Steroidal preparations prevent the release of ArAc substrates from phospholipids, thus blocking both the cyclooxygenase and lipooxygenase pathways. Nonsteroidal anti-inflammatory drugs inhibit only PG synthesis. Indeed, B/W female mice given daily injections of ibuprofen, an inhibitor of the cyclooxygenase pathway, did not exhibit an increase in survival or a decrease in the manifestations of the diseases (38). Figure 2 depicts the immunopathological events that may occur in autoimmune disease and indicates the points at which these mediators probably exert the greatest effect.

Eicosapentaenoic acid (EPA) is one of the three EFA involved in PG and LT synthesis and is found in high concentrations in fish oil. Unlike ArAc, which is transformed into the dienoic PG and LT4, EPA forms the trienoic PG and LT_5. It has been suggested that PGs and LTs synthesized from EPA may have an immunoinhibitory effect. Indeed, B/W mice placed on an EPA-rich fish oil diet were protected from the autoimmune nephritis, even when this diet was instigated late in life (5 months of age) (39). Interestingly, Alexander et al. (40) found that B/W mice fed a diet containing ω-3 fatty acids (fish oil) had lower levels of anti–double stranded DNA antibodies and CICs than their littermates fed near-isocaloric diets high in saturated (lard) or unsaturated fat (corn oil). A fish oil diet was also able to suppress the autoimmune sequelae in MRL/lpr mice (41–42). When compared with a safflower oil–fed group, the fish oil–fed mice had decreased T-cell lymphoproliferation and expression of Ia antigen on peritoneal macrophages. The fish oil diet was associated with reduced PGE, thromboxane B2, and prostacyclin levels in the lungs and kidneys, increased formation of circulating retroviral gp70 immune complexes, and delayed development of immune nephritis in MRL/lpr mice (41). In a recent study (43), suppression of immune nephritis in MRL/lpr mice appeared to be dependent upon a high concentration of EPA in the diet (4% by weight). Diets containing lower concentrations of EPA had little effect upon the development of kidney pathology. Interestingly, in this study it was noted that anti-DNA antibody levels were not influenced by the amount of dietary EPA. There were, however, marked weight differences noted between animal groups.

Early evidence suggested that in Sprague-Dawley rats, which develop a polyarthritis following injection of type II collagen in complete Freund's adjuvant, had a higher incidence of disease when fed a fish oil diet rather than a safflower oil or beef tallow diet (44). It may be possible that PGE_2 (produced from the high levels of linoleic acid in the safflower diet) limits the induction of arthritis in this particular animal model, and that the fish oil diet amplifies this disease by reducing the production of this PG. Most recently, Tate et al. (45) demonstrated that both the acute and chronic inflammatory processes, assessed in the rat by subcutaneous air pouch and adjuvant-induced arthritis, respectively, can be suppressed by a diet enriched with borage seed oil, which contains 23% γ-linolenic acid (GLA). Metabolically, GLA can be converted to dihomo-γ-linolenic acid (the fatty acid precursor of monoenoic prostaglandins) and compete for arachidonate-binding sites on oxidative enzymes. Animals given the GLA-enriched diet demonstrated reduced production of the inflammatory mediators PGE_2 and LTB_4 when compared to those animals placed on a diet enriched with safflower oil (<1% GLA) (45).

From these studies, it is clear that PG and LT regulation of immune responsiveness is very complex and most likely differs from one animal model to another. Al-

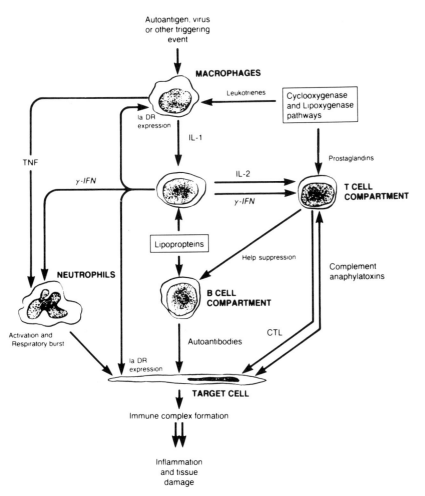

Figure 2 Pathological mechanisms in autoimmune disease. A representation of some of the inflammatory circuits that occur in autoimmune disease. Macrophages may be initially triggered to release IL-1 by either abnormal presentation of an autoantigen, a microorganism that perhaps has antigenic determinants with self-tissues or similarly cross-reacting food antigens. Proinflammatory leukotrienes may also influence this release. As a result of this event, the T-cell compartment becomes activated and releases other lymphokines, primarily IL-2 and γ interferon. In consequence, the entire immune system becomes highly activated and class II MHC molecules (Ia/DR) are expressed on T cells and the target cells of the autoimmune attack as well as B cells and macrophages. Inflammatory cyclooxygenase products may drive the T-cell response more aggressively, especially in terms of helper function. Serum lipoproteins may exacerbate the process by causing selective dysfunction in both T- and B-cell populations. Thus, target cell damage occurs through the production of autoantibodies and the generation of cytotoxic T cells. The inflammatory cascade is enhanced further by the release of tumor necrosis factor from macrophages, which in turn triggers neutrophil activation. Antigen-antibody immune complexes fix complement and cause the release of biologically active kinins, which also amplify the tissue damage. CTL = cytotoxic T lymphocytes; IFN-γ = gamma interferon; IL = interleukin; MHC = major histocompatibility complex; TNF = tumor necrosis factor.

though the presence of linoleic acid did not always result in enhancing the autoimmune symptomology in the different animals tested, the absence of ArAc precursors in the diet as well as supplementation with EPA resulted in significant improvement of the animals' survival and pathology.

It has been reported that the anti-inflammatory properties of a fish oil diet in autoimmune mice may be the indirect effect of ω-3 fatty acids. Fish oil contains high quantities of ω-3 fatty acids, which recently have been found to be extensively incorporated into several classes of lipids in the spleens of autoimmune mice placed on a fish oil diet (46). This lipid substitution could result in altered production of platelet-activating factor and synthesis of arachidonic acid–derived eicosanoids, thus exerting anti-inflammatory effects. Additionally, EPA has been believed to induce the production of trienoic PG and LT_5, which have immunoinhibitory effects (47,48).

Although much of the current interest in the potential use of fish oil supplements in humans has been based on the low cardiovascular mortality rate seen in people such as the Eskimos whose diet contains a large portion of fish, few human trials have been performed. Several years ago, Kremer et al. (49) examined the possible immunoinhibitory effects of EPA supplements on the clinical manifestations of human rheumatoid arthritis. Individuals with established rheumatoid arthritis were placed on a diet high in polyunsaturated fat and low in saturated fat, supplemented with EPA (1.8 g daily). Over a 12-week period, this group demonstrated some improvement in clinical manifestations, including morning stiffness and a reduction in the number of tender joints, compared to a control group who consumed an "American diet" high in saturated fat. Several clinical trials investigating dietary manipulation of autoimmune disease are currently underway in Europe; encouraging results with fish oil supplements have been demonstrated in ameliorating other human autoimmune disorders such as SLE (50), psoriasis, and atopic dermatitis (51). In addition, reduced intake of PUFA appears to be promising for the management of patients with SLE (52). Nevertheless, further investigation with special emphasis on double-blind clinical trials is needed.

Lipoproteins

The mechanism by which fats modulate immune responses may also involve production of immunoregulatory lipoproteins (LPs). For example, in mice, diets high in fat have been associated with greatly increased levels of a serum factor that specifically neutralizes the xenotropic (but not ecotropic) type C retroviruses (53). These viruses are found in all mice, but are expressed in very high titers in the New Zealand strains; although they are no longer thought to be the etiological agent responsible for the autoimmune disease, they probably play an important part in the immunopathological process (54). Neutralizing factor (NF) is an LP, and its discovery has led to the hypothesis that if some interaction between NF and xenotropic retroviral antigens budding from the lymphocyte membrane occurs, this reaction could interfere with immunological function and thereby contribute to the pathology seen in these mice (55). It should be emphasized, however, that an endogenous human retrovirus has yet to be isolated, and thus no equivalent of NF in humans can be identified. Thus, for the time being, the role of this particular LP can only be considered in the context of murine disease.

Lipoproteins per se have an immunoregulatory role, although how these nutritionally important substances relate to the effect of high-fat diets on lymphocyte responses in lupus-prone mice has not been well explored. Lymphocytes of several mouse strains, including the NZB, are inhibited by high-, low-, and very low-density lipids (HDL, LDL and VLDL) (56). However, the role played by NF, if any, in these reactions is unknown.

Most of the available data on the interaction of lipoproteins with immune cells originate from studies on human lymphocytes. Low-density lipoproteins have the capacity to either inhibit or enhance lymphocyte proliferation. For example, in vitro, high concentrations of a certain fraction of LDL exert an inhibitory effect on human T-cell stimulation by mitogens or allogeneic cells (57,58). The immunoregulatory properties of LPs appear to be linked to the apoprotein moiety of the molecule. These apoproteins solubilize the highly hydrophobic lipids as well as regulate the entry and exit of particular lipids at specific sites. Apoprotein E (apo-E), which is found in both LDLs and phospholipid and cholesterol-transporting HDLs and, to a lesser extent, apo-B, which is found only in the LDL fraction, exhibit the strongest interfering immunosuppressive capabilities on lymphocyte proliferation. This effect has been measured by calcium incorporation, phospholipid turnover, and DNA synthesis (59,60). More recently, addition of transferrin to the culture medium has been found to completely reverse the suppression of the mitogenic response of human lymphocytes induced by high concentrations of LDLs, whether the lymphocytes were normal or lacking their LDL receptor (61,62). Transferrin is a transport protein for iron, an essential micronutrient and, like LDL, binds to a specific cell surface receptor. Since neither LDL nor transferrin appear to prevent each other from binding to its specific receptor, LDLs must inhibit lymphocyte responses in a non-LDL receptor-mediated way by interfering with transferrin metabolism.

In contrast, in other experiments studying the regulatory role of LDLs on lymphocyte function, LDL receptor–lacking lymphocytes were cultured in transferrin-supplemented medium. Under these conditions, they did not respond to the low concentrations of LDLs that generally stimulate normal lymphocytes. Therefore, enhancement of lymphocyte responses could be mediated by lymphocyte LDL receptors (62).

Thus, various factors, possibly interacting with each other, influence the LP-mediated immunoregulation. In humans, for instance, diets rich in PUFA markedly reduce apo-B VLDLs and, to a lesser extent, HDL serum concentrations (63). These changes, by affecting LPs, could alter lymphocyte responses substantially. The influence of lipoproteins on the autoimmune process is depicted in Figure 2.

Membrane Fluidity

Besides their possible influence on PG synthesis and LPs, dietary fats may affect immune responsiveness via alterations in membrane structure and fluidity. Membrane fluidity is an important factor when considering the interactions between receptor and antigen. Altered communication between surface antigens and receptors on lymphocytes and macrophages could lead to a modulation in immune responsiveness.

Arachidonic acid constitutes a large proportion of cytoplasmic and membrane phospholipids of lymphocytes and macrophages (64). Indeed, data from in vitro studies has demonstrated that macrophage phagocytosis of radiolabeled bacteria was altered significantly by the presence of *cis*-unsaturated fatty acids (65). Thus, it is easy to imagine that an inappropriate intake of dietary fat could alter the function of these immune cells, although there is a general dearth of information regarding the membrane fatty acid composition and the function of mononuclear cells.

The cholesterol content of membranes is also important for the structure and function of the cell but, to date, this parameter has been largely ignored in relation to immune function (see Ref. 5 for review).

CONCLUSIONS

As is evident from the studies discussed above, the fact that diets can have a major influence on the manifestation and progression of spontaneous autoimmune disease in several animal systems, particularly those representing human rheumatic disorders, must now be considered unequivocal. Fat in particular seems to influence the course of these diseases profoundly, with both qualitative and quantitative variations exerting quite different effects.

Research in this area is still in its infancy, and much work needs to be carried out in order to elucidate the mechanisms by which dietary components cause immunoregulatory effects. In particular, we envisage investigations being focused on the ways in which lipid can influence inflammatory mediators such as the products of the cyclooxygenase and lipooxygenase pathways and the various classes of serum LPs. The relationship between dietary fat, cell membrane composition, and immune function also needs to be examined in depth.

Sufficient data from experimental models now exist to support the use of diet therapy (we believe that modification of lipid intake in some way is the most practical to implement and the most acceptable to the patient) in preliminary trials for human autoimmune disease.

It is now recognized that many of the most common diseases of our society, such as cancer and heart disease, are influenced by diet, and in many cases are avoidable. Autoimmune disorders should most likely be placed in this category, although this hypothesis can only be substantiated by continued research efforts. It is our hope that such investigations will yield valuable information regarding the underlying etiopathogenesis of these diseases and, when combined with suitable public education, may lead to changes in dietary habits that will reduce their incidence.

ACKNOWLEDGMENTS

W.J.W.M. was supported by a grant from the Muir-Hambro Trust/Royal College of Physicians, London.

The authors wish to thank Ms Liz Carr for helping to prepare the manuscript.

REFERENCES

1. Morrow WJW, Isenberg DA. Autoimmune Rheumatic Disease. Blackwell Scientific, Oxford, England, 1987.
2. Theofilopoulos AN, Dixon FJ. Murine models of systemic lupus erythematosus. Adv Immunol 1985, 37:269.
3. Beisel WR. Single nutrients and immunity. Am J Clin Nutr (Suppl) 1982, 35:(Suppl):417.
4. Stinnett JD. Nutrition and the Immune Response. CRC Press, Boca Raton, Florida, 1983.
5. Gershwin ME, Beach RS, Hurley LS. Nutrition and immunity. Academic Press, New York, 1985.
6. Dubois EL, Strain L. Effect of diet on survival and nephropathology of NZB-NZW hybrid mice. Biochem Med 1973, 7:336.

7. Fernandes G, Yunis EJ, Jose DG, Good RA. Dietary influence on antinuclear antibodies and cell-mediated immunity in NZB mice. Int Arch Allergy Appl Immunol 1973, 44:770.
8. Fernandes G, Friend P, Yunis EJ, Good RA. Influence of dietary restriction on immunologic function and renal disease in (NZB × NZW)F_1 mice. Proc Natl Acad Sci USA 1978; 75:1500.
9. Jung LKL, Palladino MA, Calvano S, Mark DA, Good RA, Fernandes G. Effect of calorie restriction on the production and responsiveness to interleukin-2 in (NZB × NZW)F_1 mice. Clin Immunol Immunopathol 1982, 25:295.
10. Safai-Kutti S, Fernandes G, Wang Y, Safai B, Good RA, Day NK. Reduction of circulating immune complexes by calorie restriction in (B/W)F_1 mice. Clin Immunol Immunopathol 1980, 15:293.
11. Izui S, Fernandes G, Hara I, McConahey PJ, Jensen FC, Dixon FJ, Good RA. Low-calorie diet selectively reduces expression of retroviral envelope glycoprotein gp70 in sera of NZB × NZW F_1 hybrid mice. J Exp Med 1981, 154:1116.
12. James SJ, Enger SM, Peterson WJ, Makinodan T. Immune potentiation after fractionated exposure to very low doses of ionizing radiation and/or caloric restriction in autoimmune prone and normal C57/Bl6 mice. Clin Immunol Immunopathol 1990; 55:427.
13. Fernandes G, Yunis EJ, Good RA. Influence of protein restriction on immune function in NZB mice. J Immunol 1976, 116:782.
14. Gardner MB, Ihle JN, Pillarisetty RJ, Talal N, Dubois EL, Levy JA. Type C virus expression and host response in diet-cured NZB/W mice. Nature 1977, 268:341.
15. Batsford S, Schwerdtfeger M, Rohrbach R, Cambiaso C, Kluthe R. Synthetic amino acid diet prolongs survival in autoimmune murine disease. Clin Nephrol 1984, 21:60.
16. Elliot RB, Martin JM, Dietary protein: A trigger of insulin-dependent diabetes in the BB rat? Diabetologia 1984, 26:297.
17. Beach RS, Gershwin ME, Hurley LS. Nutritional factors and autoimmunity. I. Immunopathology of zinc deprivation in New Zealand mice. J Immunol 1981, 126:1999.
18. Beach RS, Gershwin ME, Hurley LS. Nutritional factors and autoimmunity. II. Prolongation of survival in zinc-deprived B/W mice. J Immunol 1982, 128:308.
19. Bach JF. The multi-faceted zinc dependency of the immune system. Immunol Today 1981, 2:225.
20. Homsy J, Morrow WJW, Levy JA. Nutrition and autoimmunity: A review. Clin Exp Immunol 1986, 65:473.
21. Fernandes G, Yunis EJ, Smith J, Good RA. Dietary influence on breeding behaviour, hemolytic anemia and longevity in NZB mice. Proc Soc Exp Biol Med 1972, 139:1189.
22. Levy JA, Ibrahim AB, Shirai T, Ohta K, Nagasawa R, Yoshida H, Estes J, Gardner M. Dietary fat affects immune response and production of antiviral factors and immune complex disease in NZB/NZW mice. Proc Natl Acad Sci USA 1983, 79:1974.
23. Morrow WJW, Ohashi Y, Hall J, Pribnow J, Hirose S, Shirai T, Levy JA. Dietary fat and immune function. I. Antibody responses, lymphocyte and accessory cell function in (NZB × NZW)F_1 mice. J Immunol 1985, 135:3857.
24. Yumura W, Hattori S, Morrow WJW, Mayes DC, Levy JA, Shirai T. Dietary fat and immune function. II. Effects on immune complex nephritis in (NZB × NZW) F_1 mice. J Immunol 1985, 135:3864.
25. Morrow WJW, Homsy J, Swanson CA, Estes J, Levy JA. Dietary fat influences the expression of autoimmune disease in MRL/*lpr/lpr* mice. Immunology 1986, 59:439.
26. Kelley VE, Izui S. Enriched lipid accelerates lupus nephritis in NZB × NZW mice. Synergistic action of immune complexes and lipid in glomerular injury. Am J Pathol 1983, 111:288.
27. Fernandes G, Alonso DR, Tanaka T, Thaler HT, Yunis EJ, Good RA. Influence of diet on vascular lesions in autoimmune-prone B/W mice. Proc Natl Acad Sci USA 1983, 80:874.

28. Swanson CA, Levy JA, Morrow WJW. Effect of low dietary lipid on the development of Sjögren's syndrome in (NZB × NZW) f1 mice. Ann Rheum Dis 1989, 48:765.
29. Mertin J, Hunt R. Influence of polyunsaturated fatty acids on survival of skin allografts and tumor incidence in mice. Proc Natl Acad Sci USA 1976, 73:928.
30. Schultz RM, Pavlidis NA, Stylos WA, Chirigos MA. Regulation of macrophage tumoricidal function: A regulatory role for prostaglandins of the E series. Science 1978; 202:320.
31. Izui S, Kelley VE, McConahey PJ, Dixon FJ. Selective suppression of retroviral gp70-anti-gp70 immune complex formation by prostaglandin E1 in murine SLE. J Exp Med 1980; 152:1645.
32. Winkelstein A, Kelley VE. Effects of prostaglandin E1 in murine models of SLE: Changes in circulating immune complexes. Clin Immunol Immunopathol 1981, 20:188.
33. Kelley VE, Winklestein A, Izui S, Dixon FJ. Prostaglandin E1 inhibits T cell proliferation and renal disease in MRL/l mice. Clin Immunol Immunopathol 1981, 21:190.
34. Mertin J, Stackpoole A. Anti-PGE antibodies inhibit *in vivo* development of cell-mediated immunity. Nature 1981, 62:293.
35. Hurd ER, Gilliam JN. Beneficial effect of an essential fatty acid deficient diet in NZB/NZW F_1 mice. J Invest Derm 1981, 77:381.
36. Hurd ER, Johnston JM, Okita JR, MacDonald PC, Ziff M, Gilliam JN. Prevention of glomerulonephritis and prolonged survival in NZB/NZW F_1 hybrid mice fed an essential fatty acid-deficient diet. J Clin Invest 1981, 67:476.
37. Ninnemann JL. Prostaglandins and immunity. Immunol Today 1984, 5:170.
38. Kelley VE, Izui S, Halushka PV. Effect of ibuprofen, a fatty acid cyclooxygenase inhibitor, on murine lupus. Clin Immunol Immunopathol 1982, 25:223.
39. Prickett JD, Robinson DR, Steinberg AD. Dietary enrichment with the polyunsaturated fatty acid eicosapentaenoic acid prevents proteinuria and prolongs survival in B/W mice. J Clin Invest 1981; 68:556.
40. Alexander NJ, Smythe NL, Jokinen MP. The type of dietary fat affects the severity of autoimmune disease in NZB/NZW mice. Am J Pathol 1987, 127:106.
41. Kelley VE, Ferreti A, Izui S, Strom TB. A fish oil diet rich in eicosapentaenoic acid reduces cyclooxygenase metabolites and suppresses lupus in MRL/*lpr* mice. J Immunol 1985, 134:1914.
42. Watson J, Godfrey D, Stimson WH, Belch JJ, Sturrock RD. The therapeutic effects of dietary fatty acid supplementation in the autoimmune disease of the MRL-mp-*lpr/lpr* mouse. Int J Immunopharmacol 1988, 10:467.
43. Westberg G, Tarkowski A, Svalander C. Effect of eicosapentaenoic acid on the autoimmune disease of MRL/l mice. Int Arch Allergy Applied Immunol 1989, 88:454.
44. Prickett JD, Trentham DE, Robinson DR. Dietary fish oil augments the induction of arthritis in rats immunized with type II collagen. J Immunol 1984, 132:725.
45. Tate G, Mandell BF, Lapostat M, Ohliger D, Baker DG, Schumacher HR, Zurier RB. Suppression of acute and chronic inflammation by dietary linolenic acid. J Rheum 1989, 16:729.
46. Robinson DR, Tateno S, Knoell C, Olesiak W, Xu I, Hirai A, Guo M, Colvin RB. Dietary marine lipids suppress murine autoimmune disease. J Int Med 1989, 225:211.
47. Needleman P, Raz A, Minkes MS, Ferendelli JA, Sprecher H. Triene prostaglandins: PG1 and thromboxane biosynthesis and unique biological properties. Proc Natl Acad Sci USA 1979, 76:944.
48. Hammarstrom S. Leukotriene C5: A slow reacting substance derived from eicosapentaenoic acid. J Biol Chem 1980, 255:7093.
49. Kremer JM, Bigauoette J, Michalek AV, Timchalk MA, Lininger L, Rynes RI, Huyck C, Zieminski J, Bartholomew LE. Effects of manipulation of dietary fatty acids on clinical manifestations of rheumatoid arthritis. Lancet 1985, 1:184.
50. Walton AJE, Snaith ML, Locniskar M, Morrow WJW, Isenberg DA. Dietary fish oil reduces the severity of symptoms in patients with systemic lupus erythematosus. Ann Rheum Dis 1991, 50:463.

51. Yetiv JZ. Clinical applications of fish oils. JAMA 1989, 260:665.
52. Thörner Å, Walldius G, Nilsson E, Hådell K, Gullberg G. Beneficial effects of reduced intake of polyunsaturated fatty acids in the diet for one year in patients with systemic lupus erythematosus. Ann Rheum Dis 1990, 49:134.
53. Levy JA, Ihle JN, Oleszko O, Barnes RD. Virus-specific neutralization by a soluble, non-immunoglobulin factor found naturally in normal mouse sera. Proc Natl Acad Sci USA 1975, 72:5071.
54. Levy JA. C-Type RNA viruses and autoimmune disease. *In*: Autoimmunity. Genetic, Immunologic, Virologic, and Clinical Aspects. Talal N, ed. Academic Press, New York, 1977, p 404.
55. Levy JA. Viral, anti-viral, cellular and nutritional factors associated with autoimmunity in mice. *In*: Immunoregulation and Autoimmunity. Krakauer R, Cathcart MK, eds. Elsevier/North-Holland, Amsterdam, 1980, p 117.
56. Hsu KHL, Ghanta VK, Hiramoto RN. Immunosuppressive effect of mouse serum lipoproteins. I. *In vitro* studies. J Immunol 1981, 126:1909.
57. Curtiss LK, Edgington TS. Regulatory serum lipoproteins: Regulation of lymphocyte stimulation by a species of low density lipoprotein. J Immunol 1976, 116:1452.
58. Fujii DK, Edgington TS. Direct suppression of lymphocyte induction by the immunoregulatory human serum low density lipoprotein, LDL-In. J Immunol 1980, 124:156.
59. Hui DY, Harmony JAK, Innerarity TL, Mahley RW. Immunoregulatory plasma lipoproteins: Role of apoprotein E and apoprotein B. J Biol Chem 1980, 225:1775.
60. Macy M, Okano Y, Cardin AD, Avila EM, Harmony JAK. Suppression of lymphocyte activation by plasma lipoproteins. Cancer Res 1983, 43(Suppl):2496s.
61. Cuthbert JA, Lipsky PE. Immunoregulation by low density lipoproteins in man. J Clin Invest 1984, 73:992.
62. Cuthbert JA, Lipsky PE. Modulation of human lymphocyte responses by low density lipoproteins. Proc Natl Acad Sci USA 1984, 81:4539.
63. Nestel PJ, Connor WE, Reardon MF, Connor S, Wong S, Boston R. Suppression by diets rich in fish oil of very low density lipoprotein production in man. J Clin Invest 1984, 74:82.
64. Meade CJ, Mertin J. Fatty acids and immunity. Adv Lipid Res 1978, 16:127.
65. Schroit AJ, Gallily R. Macrophage fatty acid composition and phagocytosis: Effect of unsaturation on cellular phagocytic activity. Immunology 1979, 36:199.

11
Cholesterol, Apolipoprotein E, and Immune Cell Function

Linda K. Curtiss
The Scripps Research Institute, La Jolla, California

INTRODUCTION

The concept that plasma lipoproteins can regulate cellular activation and proliferation is well established. Among the numerous regulatory phenomena that are mediated by either native or modified lipoproteins is the suppression of lymphocyte function. A biologically active moiety of the immunosuppressive lipoprotein, LDL-In, that possesses regulatory activity characteristic of the native lipoprotein, has been identified as apolipoprotein (apo) E. Apoprotein E is also one of the major proteins synthesized and secreted by macrophages. Macrophage synthesis of apo E is enhanced by plasma lipoprotein–induced cholesteryl ester loading and inhibited by immunological activation of the cells. An essential biological theme of the immune response is the use of cellular collaboration via the synthesis of soluble effector molecules to regulate specific responses to relevant stimuli. Thus, it is hypothesized that plasma cholesterol via its effect on intracellular macrophage cholesterol can influence the levels of the immunosuppressive protein, apo E. The data are consistent with the existence of a regulatory network between lymphocytes and monocytes involving monocyte-macrophage–produced apo E, which is influenced by dietary fats.

PLASMA LIPOPROTEINS AND THE IMMUNE SYSTEM

The immune system is composed of a variety of cells (e.g., T cells, B cells, natural killer [NK] cells, antibody-dependent cell-mediated cytoxic [ADCC] cells, monocyte-macrophages) and soluble factors (e.g., immunoglobulins, complement, lymphokines, monokines), all of which play an important role in the maintenance and the proper functioning of the immune system. To thoroughly understand how the immune system functions, one must understand the cellular events involved in the activation of each of the cells of the immune system, characterize the various cellular regulatory circuits and collaborative interactions, and identify factors present in plasma and other biological fluids that promote or suppress the function of each of the cells of the immune system. In the last decade, a specific group of plasma proteins, called plasma lipoproteins, that possess immunoregulatory activity both in vitro and in vivo (1–4) has been identified. Furthermore, a specific low-density plasma lipoprotein (LDL) that is enriched in apo E, termed low-density lipoprotein inhibitor (LDL-In), has been described that has potent inhibitory activity for primary lymphocyte stimulation (1–3).

In addition to genetic factors, a number of external factors, including diet, exercise, emotional state, disease, and drugs, determine the types and amounts of the various circulating lipoproteins in plasma (5–12). Because lipoproteins can alter immune function, it follows that some of these externally or environmentally controlled factors could influence immune function as well. The effect of diet on host immunocompetence has been documented (13,14), and investigators have described the influences of dietary lipids on the immune system. A depression of reticuloendothelial phagocytic function by ingested lipids has been reported (15), and inhibition of host resistance to viral, bacterial, and tumor challenge can be induced by nutritional hypercholesterolemia (6). A positive correlation between high-fat diets and mammary tumor

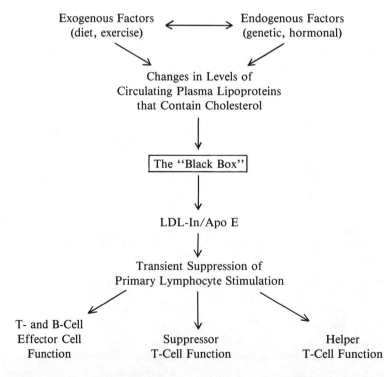

Figure 1 Schematic representation of the relationship between dietary fats and immune cell function mediated by plasma lipoproteins and apo E.

incidence is observed in rodents (16,17) and humans (18), and one of the contributing factors to this heightened tumor incidence is impaired immune responsiveness that can be attributed in part to the lipoprotein fraction of plasma (18). Thus, there is reasonable evidence to suggest that a link exists between dietary fats and immune function. However, most of the research performed to date has dealt with this issue on only a phenomenological level. There is now a very real need to understand the participants and the mechanisms involved.

As will be discussed in detail later, plasma lipoproteins that contain apo E have significant immunoregulatory properties both in vitro and in vivo (Fig. 1). Various exogenous factors (e.g., diet and exercise) as well as endogenous factors (e.g., genetic and hormonal) influence the levels of circulating plasma lipoproteins. If these phenomena are related, various exogenous factors such as diet and exercise can influence immune cell function. Thus, investigations directed toward the "black box" of Figure 1 may reveal how this is accomplished.

Plasma lipoproteins and the cholesterol that they carry may be the critical "link" between dietary fat and immune cell function. Thus, a direct regulatory relationship appears to exist between changes in the circulating levels of certain diet-induced, cholesterol-rich plasma lipoproteins and changes in a specific immunoregulatory lipoprotein; i.e., LDL-In or its biologically important constituent apo E. Our working concept of the "black box" is illustrated in Figure 2, where monocyte-macrophages and apo E occupy important places. The black box consists of a regulatory network whereby monocytes inhibit lymphocyte proliferation by increasing their production and secretion of the soluble suppressive mediator epo E. In turn, lymphocytes feedback and complete this regulatory loop by producing and secreting certain lymphokines which regulate apo E production by the monocyte-macrophage. The dietary link to this regulatory network rests in the fact that monocyte-macrophage epo E production is readily influenced by a number of diverse factors that include in addition to numerous immunological signals plasma cholesterol and/or plasma lipoprotein-induced cholesteryl ester loading of the monocytes.

LDL-In, AN IMMUNOREGULATORY PLASMA LIPOPROTEIN

In 1976, it was reported that a discrete lipoprotein fraction isolated from normal human plasma inhibited mitogen- and allogenic cell–stimulated human lymphocyte proliferation in vitro (1). This inhibitory plasma lipoprotein was termed low-density lipoprotein inhibitor because the active fraction is localized to a less dense subfraction of total LDLs of density 1.006–1.063 g/ml. The characteristics of LDL-In–mediated inhibition in vitro are as follows: LDL-In has comparable inhibitory activity for phytohemagglutinin (PHA), pokeweed mitogen (PWM), and allogenic cell–stimulated human lymphocyte proliferation. The inhibitory activity of LDL-In is nontoxic and independent of mitogen concentration. Suppression by LDL-In is time dependent and approximately 18 hr of exposure of the lipoprotein to the lymphocytes before stimulation is required for maximum induction of a stable suppressed state. [^{3}H]Thymidine uptake is not inhibited by LDL-In when it is added to the cultures 18–20 hr after stimulation, suggesting that this lipoprotein influences metabolic events associated with an early inductive phase of lymphocyte activation.

The immunosuppressive activity of LDL-In has been studied in a number of systems both in vitro and in vivo. To summarize, in vitro activities of LDL-In include

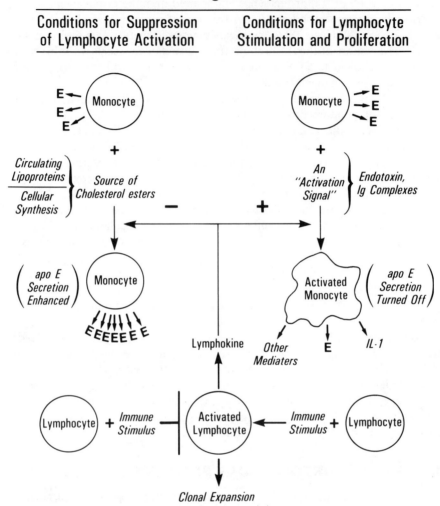

Figure 2 The Apo E immunoregulatory network. Production of apo E by monocytes/macrophages is increased by cholesterol loading and decreased by "activation." High levels of locally produced apo E will prevent lymphocyte activation, whereas low levels of apo E will permit activation to occur. Activated lymphocytes in turn can regulate monocyte apo E synthesis via the release of soluble lymphokine(s). The dietary link to this immunoregulatory network is represented by the fact that dietary fats and cholesterol have a direct influence on the types and amounts of cholesterol-rich plasma lipoproteins in the circulation, the same lipoproteins that cause cholesterol loading of the monocyte.

suppression of (a) mitogen-stimulated [^{3}H]thymidine uptake (1), (b) allogenic cell-stimulated [^{3}H]thymidine uptake (1,19), (c) the primary generation of cytotoxic T cells (20), (d) pokeweed mitogen–stimulated immunoglobulin synthesis (21), and (e) B-cell Epstein Barr virus transformation (22). In vivo, LDL-In has been shown to inhibit (a) the primary humoral immune response to sheep red blood cells (2,23,24),

(b) the primary generation of cytotoxic T cells (20), and (c) immunological attenuation of tumor growth (25,26).

The effects of lipoproteins on immune cell function in vivo are exceedingly complex. A major finding of the investigation of the physiological implications of immunosuppression by LDL-In in vivo is that the observed functional outcome is strikingly dose dependent. This important concept is best illustrated by describing in more detail studies of the effects of LDL-In on the survival of experimental animals challenged with syngeneic tumors (25,26). Seemingly divergent effects of LDL-In are observed on the growth of the syngeneic SaD2 fibrosarcoma in DBA/2 mice. The growth of 1 × 10^5 viable tumor cells in control mice without immunoprotection (i.e., 10-day prior immunization with 10^{-6} irradiated tumor cells) is detectable at 25 days and proceeds rapidly until death at about 45 days. In contrast, tumor growth is slower in immunoprotected mice. This tumor growth is characterized by a reduction in tumor mass of at least a half and no deaths by day 60. Intravenous administration of high doses of LDL-In 24 hr before immunoprotection with killed tumor cells abolishes the protective effect of immunization. This dose corresponds to a dose that is required to abolish both B-cell and T-cell effector cell functions. The administration of an intermediate dose of LDL-In before immunoprotection with the killed tumor cells has no discernible effect on the subsequent growth of the viable tumor cell challenge. In contrast, intravenous administration of even lower doses of LDL-In 24 hr before immunoprotection with killed tumor cells results in the enhancement of tumor rejection and host survival. This dose of LDL-In is concordant with the dose required for selective inhibition of suppressor cell function in vitro (21). Thus, depending upon the amount of immunoregulatory lipoprotein that a particular lymphocyte population is exposed to in vivo, very different functional outcomes will result.

THE BIOLOGICALLY ACTIVE COMPONENT OF LDL-In

Plasma lipoproteins differ from most humoral immunoregulatory molecules in that they are large heterogenous noncovalent complexes of lipid and protein. An important step to understanding the mechanism of lipoprotein regulation of cell function is an identification of the constituent(s) of the lipoprotein particle that mediate the observed biological effects. Plasma lipoproteins contain various amounts of apoproteins, glyceride, free and esterified cholesterol, phospholipid, glycolipid, and free fatty acid. Many of these constituents of lipoproteins can by themselves influence immune cell function; therefore, it is important to relate the characteristics of the inhibition observed with individual constituents to the characteristics of inhibition observed with the native lipoprotein, LDL-In.

Cholesterol

Low-density lipoprotein inhibitor contains cholesterol. It has been suggested that the suppression of lymphocyte function might result from either interruption of cellular cholesterol biosynthesis or alteration of membrane integrity by cholesterol or its oxygenated derivatives. However, it was determined that LDL-In does not inhibit mitogen stimulation in a manner comparable to the inhibition obtained with oxygenated sterols (27), discussed in Chapter 12. Furthermore, full biological activity is retained in a neutral lipid-depleted LDL-In preparation (28). Therefore, mechanisms other than suppression of sterol synthesis and cholesterol loading of the plasma membrane must be operative.

Free Fatty Acids

Because the biological activity of LDL-In is retained within a neutral lipid-depleted particle and because the recovery of protein, phospholipid, and free fatty acids (FFAs) is quantitative (28), the FFAs remain potentially important constituents. However, there is no evidence that the endogenous FFAs of LDL-In are biologically active. First, the concentration of endogenous FFAs of LDL-In is less than that amount required for suppression of mitogen stimulation by any individual FFA added to lymphocyte cultures (29). Second, the temporal characteristics of FFA suppression, typified in all cases by their ability to inhibit lymphocyte [^{3}H]thymidine uptake even when they are added many hours after mitogen stimulation, differs from that of LDL-In (29). Third, FFA-depleted LDL-In retains full suppressive activity for PHA-stimulated [^{3}H]thymidine uptake. Therefore, the endogenous FFAs of LDL-In are not biologically active and the inhibitory activity of LDL-In must reside with one or all of the remaining structural entities of the native lipoprotein particle, including the apoproteins, phospholipids, and/or trace glycolipids (29).

Apoproteins

The heterogeneity of apoproteins in terms of structure, exposure, and function make them likely candidates as biologically important constituents of LDL-In, and the contribution of the apoproteins to biological activity has been extensively studied. Low-density lipoprotein inhibitor contains apo B, apo E, and each of the C apoproteins. The specific role played by apo B and apo E in LDL-In was investigated immunochemically using apo B-specific and apo E-specific monoclonal antibodies (30–33). Some, but not all, of the apo B antibodies and each of the apo E-specific antibodies bind and facilitate the indirect precipitation and removal of the inhibitory activity of LDL-In from a lipoprotein fraction. These results indicate that LDL-In contains both apoproteins B and E, but they do not identify which apoprotein is important to or required for activity.

Further substantiation that apo E– and apo E–containing lipoproteins are important regulators of lymphocyte function has come from studies of the inhibitory properties of fetal cord blood plasma lipoproteins (34). In these studies, a direct correlation between apo E and inhibition was established. Cord blood lipoprotein concentrations are lower than those of the adult; i.e., the low-density lipoprotein level in cord blood is 30% that of adult, whereas the high-density lipoprotein (HDL) level is 50% of adult levels. In contrast, the apo E concentration in fetal cord blood is twofold higher than in the adult (34). Therefore, the capacity of LDL and HDL to inhibit mitogen-stimulated [^{3}H]thymidine uptake in adult peripheral blood mononuclear cells was used as an in vitro system to study immunosuppression. Relative to adult lipoproteins, cord blood LDL and HDL are two to four times more potent in inhibiting cellular proliferation. Radioimmunoassay shows a strong correlation between the amount of apo E in cord blood LDL and HDL and the inhibition of cell proliferation. Furthermore, selective removal of apo E–containing lipoproteins decreases the inhibitory capacity of cord blood LDL and eliminates almost completely inhibition by

HDL. The results indicate that cord blood lipoproteins containing apo E in association with either LDL or HDL can suppress the immune response (34). The fetus is an allograft to its mother. Therefore, the relatively high fetal levels of apo E may have functional significance in the establishment of self as well as maintenance of the fetus in utero.

More recently, the inhibitory activity of isolated (lipid-free) apo E has been studied. Immunosuppression was measured as inhibition of [^{3}H]thymidine uptake by peripheral blood mononuclear cells (PBMs) with phytohemagglutinin (PHA). Apoprotein E isolated from lipoproteins had good activity (i.e., approximately 15 μg/ml was required for 50% inhibition, and maximal inhibition occurred at 20 μg/ml), whereas fractions containing the lipid-free C apoproteins were not inhibitory at >20 μg/ml (35). Suppression of lymphocyte proliferation by the native lipoprotein LDL-In is irreversible and has distinguishable temporal requirements (1,19). Suppression by the isolated apo E is identical. That is, cells exposed to isolated apo E for 24 hr and washed free of non-cell associated apo E before mitogen stimulation remain fully suppressed. Maximal inhibition is obtained with either LDL-In or apo E only after a 24-hr exposure of the cells before the addition of mitogen. Exposure periods of 18 hr or less result in little or no suppression by either inhibitor. Furthermore, cels receiving inhibitors or PHA simultaneously, or cells receiving either inhibitor after PHA exposure, are fully capable of responding to mitogen induction, suggesting that neither LDL-In nor apo E is directly toxic. The irreversibility and temporal requirements of suppression confirm that apo E isolated from lipoproteins has the same characteristics of immunosuppression as LDL-In and that an active moiety of LDL-In is apo E (35,36). Thus, apo E is an important participant in the link between dietary fat and immune function.

MONOCYTE-MACROPHAGES SYNTHESIZE APO E

Apo E is a 34,000 molecular weight glycoprotein that serves as a major protein component of several plasma lipoproteins (37). Metabolic studies have demonstrated that apo E is involved directly in the transport and cellular uptake of cholesterol-rich plasma lipoproteins. Lipoproteins containing apo E deliver cholesterol to cells via interaction with a number of distinct receptors, including the apo B/E or LDL receptors, hepatic apo E receptors, and immunoregulatory receptors on lymphocytes (38). Plasma apo E levels are increased in hyperlipidemic patients, hypothyroidism, and diabetes (39), and more importantly plasma apo E is a major component of the cholesterol-rich lipoproteins that accumulate during cholesterol feeding in both humans and experimental animals (40). Biochemical and genetic analyses have shown the existence of multiple apo E isoforms arising from three common alleles and additional posttranslational modifications (41,42). The structural basis for these isoforms has been established and correlated with receptor binding activity (37).

What is the synthetic source of plasma apo E? Major sites of synthesis of apo E are the liver and intestine. However, more recently, numerous other tissues have been shown to possess significant quantities of the mRNA for apo E. These tissues include the brain, adrenal, spleen, ovary, testes, kidney, lung, and muscle (43–45). Furthermore, cultured mouse macrophages and human monocytes-macrophages are important sources of apo E (46), and this production is strongly enhanced by platelets (47). Whereas all other apoproteins are made only by the liver and/or intestine, it is estimated that 10–20% of the circulating apo E can be derived from synthesis by the other peripheral tissues. Why is apo E unique among all the apoproteins and why do so many tissues produce apo E? The fact that apo E is an immunoregulatory molecule may be key to answering these questions.

Cholesterol Loading Increases Apo E Production

Apoprotein E production by monocytes-macrophages is regulated by a complex set of stimuli. The cholesteryl ester–loaded mouse peritoneal macrophage or human peripheral blood monocyte produce large amounts of apo E (46). Both of these cells have surface receptors that allow them to take up and degrade large amounts of abnormal, chemically modified, or oxidized plasma lipoproteins (48–53). Large amounts of cholesterol obtained from these lipoproteins are stored in the cytoplasm as visible cholesteryl ester droplets (54). Under appropriate conditions, macrophages will release the stored cholesterol upon intracellular hydrolysis of the ester. At the same time, the secretion of apo E is stimulated (up to 10-fold in macrophages and twofold in human monocytes) (55,56). Apoprotein E production by these cells can represent as much as 5–10% of total secreted proteins. Thus, under the proper conditions, cholesterol-loaded monocytes-macrophages will secrete large amounts of both cholesterol and apo E, although these two functions can occur independently. Whereas reasons for the independent but coordinate control of these two processes is not yet known, it has been hypothesized that . . . "apo E secretion does not function to remove cholesterol from macrophages, but rather to participate in reverse cholesterol transport" (i.e., transport of cholesterol from peripheral tissues back to the liver) (56). But because apo E also can inhibit cellular and in particular lymphocyte proliferation, apo E may function as a more general chalone or antiproliferative agent as well.

Although cholesterol-loading is often achieved with modified plasma lipoproteins, macrophages can be loaded also by coculture with other cholesterol-rich particles, including platelets (47,57). The relationship between platelet-mediated cholesteryl ester (CE) accumulation and apo E secretion has been described (57), and it has been demonstrated that platelet-mediated monocyte apo E secretion is consistently greater than that obtained by culture with modified cholesterol-rich lipoproteins. In all cases, platelet-induced secretion of apo E paralleled the capacity of the platelets to induce macrophage cholesteryl ester accumulation (58), indicating again that macrophage apo E secretion is readily influenced by the cellular content of esterified cholesterol.

In additional studies, the chemical nature of the monocyte-macrophage–synthesized apo E has been studied (46). The apo E emerges from macrophages associated with phospholipid and appears as a lipoprotein particle with a mean density of 1.075 g/ml. By electron microscopy, the lipoproteins appear as bilayer disks. The secreted protein apparently has more sialic acid residues than the circulating plasma form of apo E from the same individual; however, both forms of apo E appear to be products of the same gene (46). Recent studies to determine the fate of monocyte-secreted apo E have suggested that the apo E can form stable complexes with plasma HDL. That is, monocyte apo E incubated with HDL will remain with HDL by either coelectrophoresis under nondenaturing conditions or coprecipitation with an HDL antibody. The association of apo E with numerous lipoprotein subclasses has been reported

(60,61). Thus, the apo E of LDL-In, the immunoregulatory lipoprotein, could be derived from monocyte-macrophage–derived apo E which is transferred to circulating LDL. Furthermore, we have recently demonstrated that human monocyte-secreted apo E has comparable potent inhibitory activity for lymphocyte stimulation, suggesting that the two molecules are functionally similar, if not identical.

"Activation" Decreases Apo E Production

In separate studies to identify the various functional and morphological states of the macrophage (62–64), apo E secretion was shown also to be closely regulated by the functional state of the cell. In these studies it was demonstrated that apo E is synthesized and secreted by both resident and thioglycollate-elicited mouse macrophages, such as macrophages exposed in vitro or in vivo to BCG, pyran copolymer, *Corynebacterium parvum*, or endotoxin (62,63). However, apo E secretion, which appears to be a constitutive property of resident macrophages, is suppressed by the exposure of macrophages to agents which are known to activate the cells for antimicrobial and antitumor functions and then returns upon loss of the activated state. Thus, monocyte synthesis of apo E is reduced under conditions that favor lymphocyte proliferation (i.e., monocyte activation). Similar results have recently been obtained in this laboratory, where it has been demonstrated that both lipopolysaccharide and urate crystals will decrease apo E production by cultured human monocytes (57). Urate crystal activation of inflammatory cells is blocked by LDL, which saturably and reversibly binds to urate crystals with high affinity (65,66).

The immune response is made up of a complex system of multiple regulatory networks involving cellular communication not only between lymphocyte subpopulations, but also between lymphocytes and monocytes. Monocytes "talking" to lymphocytes via apo E would be one more connection in this communication network (see Fig. 2). Interestingly, there is evidence that this could be a circular communication network. Fogelman et al. (67,68) have reported that lymphokines obtained from the supernatants of concanavalin A–stimulated human lymphocytes (or an established T-cell line) markedly reduced both the influx of exogenous cholesterol and cellular cholesterol synthesis in cultured human monocytes. In these studies, the reduction of monocyte-macrophage cholesterol influx appeared to result from a dramatic decrease in receptor-mediated uptake and degradation of the modified lipoproteins that lead to cholesteryl ester loading. As pointed out earlier, monocyte apo E synthesis is readily influenced by both the cholesteryl ester content of the cell (56) and the functional state of "activation" of the cell (62,63). Thus, the effect of the lymphokine(s) on monocyte cholesteryl ester accumulation could very well be an indirect result of monocyte "activation," activation which has already been characterized as resulting in a "shutdown" of apo E secretion. Further studies will be required to identify if lymphokines can also directly regulate monocyte apo E synthesis. Since we have observed that androgen synthesis can be directly affected by apo E-rich LDL, and apo E, there is reason to consider a broad role for apo E in immune networks (36,69).

CONCLUSIONS

The significance of either activation-mediated suppression of monocyte apo E secretion or cholesterol loading–mediated enhancement of monocyte apo E secretion remains unsolved. However, because apo E is a soluble mediator of T-cell and B-cell activation and proliferation, decreased synthesis of apo E by macrophages-monocytes during immunological activation may promote or enhance immune responsiveness. The work discussed here provides a framework for understanding how dietary fat and cholesterol could influence the immune response and it furthers our understanding of both the physiology and the mechanism of plasma lipoprotein–mediated suppression of immune cell function. Furthermore, the studies identify key elements (such as macrophages and apo E) in an immunoregulatory network by which circulating levels of plasma cholesterol can influence the immune response.

ACKNOWLEDGMENTS

This is publication number 4685-IMM from the Department of Immunology of The Scripps Research Institute, La Jolla, California 92037. Portions of this work were supported by grants from the National Institutes of Health, Bethesda, Maryland (HL-35297 and HL-32108).

REFERENCES

1. Curtiss LK, Edgington TS (1976). Immunoregulatory serum lipoproteins. Regulation of lymphocyte stimulation by a species of low density lipoproteins. J Immunol 116:1452.
2. Curtiss LK, DeHeer DH, Edgington TS (1977). In vivo suppression of the primary immune response by a species of low density lipoprotein. J Immunol 118:648.
3. Edgington TS, Curtiss LK (1983). Lipoprotein regulation of immune cell function. *In*: Dietary Fats and Health. J Am Oil Chem Soc, p 901.
4. Stenback EI (1984). The influence of human plasma lipoproteins and fatty acids in immunological reactions. A review. Allergy 39:1.
5. Mistry P, Miller NE, Laker M, Hazzard WR, Lewis B (1981). Individual variation in the effects of dietary cholesterol on plasma lipoproteins and cellular cholesterol hemostasis in man. J Clin Invest 67:493.
6. Kos WL, Loria RM, Snodgrass MJ, Cohen D, Thorpe TG, Kaplan AM (1979). Inhibition of host resistance by nutritional hypercholesterolemia. Infect Immun 26:658.
7. Klurfeld DM, Allison MJ, Gerszten E, Dalton HP (1979). Alterations of host defenses parallel cholesterol-induced atherogenesis. I. Interactions of prolonged experimental hypercholesterolemia and infections. J Med 10:35.
8. Nerem RM, Levesque MJ, Cornhill JF (1980). Social environment as a factor in diet-induced atherosclerosis. Science 208:1475.
9. Bostofte E, Hemmingsen L, Alling-Moller KJ, Serup J, Weber T (1978). Serum lipids and lipoproteins during treatment with oral contraceptives containing natural and synthetic aestrogens. Acta Endocrinol 87:855.
10. Nydegger UE, Butler RE (1972). Serum lipoprotein levels in patients with cancer. Cancer Res 32:1756.
11. Barclay M, Skipski UP, Terebus-Kekish O, Green EM, Kaufman RJ, Stock CC (1970). Effects of cancer upon high density and other lipoproteins. Cancer Res 30:2420.
12. Day CE (1978). Pharmacologic regulation of serum lipoproteins. Am Rep Med Chem 13:184.
13. Suskind RM (1977). Malnutrition and the Immune Response. Kroc Foundation Series. Vol. 7, Raven Press, New York.

14. Chandra RK (1980). Cell mediated immunity in nutritional imbalance. Fed Proc 39:3088.
15. Berken A, Benacerraf B (1968). Depression of reticuloendothelial system phagocytic function by ingested lipids. Proc Soc Exp Biol Med 128:793.
16. Carroll KK, Khor HT (1971). Effects of level and type of dietary fat on incidence of mammary tumors induced in female Sprague-Dawley. Lipids 6:415.
17. Chan PC, Dao TL (1981). Enhancement of mammary carcinogenesis by a high fat diet in Fischer, Long-Evans, and Sprague-Dawley rats. Cancer Res 41:164.
18. Carroll KK, Gammal EB, Plunkett ER (1986). Dietary fat and mammary cancer. Can Med Assoc J 98:590.
19. Curtiss LK, Edgington TS (1977). Effect of LDL-In, a normal immunoregulatory human serum low density lipoprotein, on the interaction of macrophages with lymphocytes proliferating in response to mitogen and alogeneic stimulation. J Immunol 118:1966.
20. Edgington TS, Henney CS, Curtiss LK (1977). The bioregulatory properties of low density lipoprotein inhibitor (LDL-In) on the generation of killer T cells. *In*: Regulatory Mechanisms in Lymphocyte Activation: Proceedings of the Eleventh Leukocyte Culture Conference. D.O. Lucas, ed. Academic Press, New York, p 736.
21. Curtiss LK, Edgington TS (1979). Differential sensitivity of lymphocyte subpopulations to suppression by LDL-In, an immunoregulatory human serum low density lipoprotein. J Clin Invest 63:193.
22. Chisari FV, Curtiss LK, Jensen FC (1981). Physiologic concentrations of normal human plasma lipoproteins inhibit the immortalization of peripheral B lymphocytes by the Epstein-Barr virus. J Clin Invest 68:329.
23. DeHeer DH, Curtiss LK, Edgington TS (1979). The influence of antigen on a model for analysis of multiple coordinate events associated with the primary immune response. Immunopharmacology 2:9.
24. Curtiss LK, DeHeer DH, Edgington TS (1980). Influence of an immunoregulatory serum lipoprotein (LDL-In) on the in vivo differentiation and proliferation of antigen-binding and antibody-secreting lymphocytes during a primary immune response. Cell Immunol 49:1.
25. Edgington TS, Curtiss LK (1981). Plasma lipoproteins with bioregulatory properties including the capacity to regulate lymphocyte function and the immune response. Cancer Res 41:3786.
26. Edgington TS, Curtiss LK (1983). Lipoprotein regulation of immune cell function. *In*: Dietary Fats and Health. ACOS Monograph No. 10, Perkins and Visek, eds. p 901.
27. Curtiss LK, Edgington TS (1980). Differences in the characteristics of inhibition of lymphocyte stimulation by 25-hydroxycholesterol and by the immunoregulatory serum lipoprotein LDL-In. J Immunol 125:1470.
28. Curtiss LK, Edgington TS (1981). Immunoregulatory plasma low density lipoprotein. The biological activity and receptor specificity is independent of neutral lipids. J Immunol 126:1008.
29. Curtiss LK, Edgington TS (1981). The biological activity of the immunoregulatory lipoprotein, LDL-In, is independent of its free fatty acid content. J Immunol 126:1382.
30. Curtiss LK, Edgington TS (1981). The immunoregulatory plasma lipoprotein, LDL-In, is a subset of intermediate density lipoprotein: Immunochemical evidence using monoclonal antibodies. Fed Proc 40:348.
31. Curtiss LK, Via DP, Voyta JS, Smith LC, Edgington TS (1982). The immunoregulatory plasma lipoprotein, LDL-In, is a minor subset of intermediate density lipoprotein that contains apoproteins B and E. Atherosclerosis 2(5):A111.
32. Palinski W, Herttuala S, Rosenfeld ME, Buller SW, Socher SA, Parthasarathy S, Curtiss LK, Witztum JL (1990). Antisera and monoclonal antibodies specific for epitopes generated during oxidative modification of low density lipoprotein. Arteriosclerosis 10:325.

33. Albers JJ, Lodge MS, Curtiss LK (1989). Evaluation of a monoclonal antibody based enzyme-linked immunosorbant assay as a candidate reference method for the measurement of apolipoprotein B-100. J Lipid Res 30:1445.
34. Curtiss LK, Forte TM, Davis PA (1984). Immunosuppressive lipoproteins in cord blood. J Immunol 133:1379.
35. Pepe MG, Curtiss LK (1986). Apolipoprotein E is a biologically active constituent of the normal immunoregulatory lipoprotein, LDL-In. J Immunol 136:3716.
36. Dyer CA, Smith RS, Curtiss LK (1991). Only multimers of a synthetic peptide of human apolipoprotein E are biologically active. J Biol Chem 266:15009.
37. Mahley RW, Innerarity TL, Rall SC Jr, Weisgraber KH (1984). Plasma lipoproteins: Apolipoprotein structure and function. J Lipid Res 25:1277.
38. Mahley RW, Innerarity TL (1983). Lipoprotein receptors and cholesterol homeostasis. Biochem Biophys Acta 737:197.
39. Mahley RW (1978). Alterations in plasma lipoproteins induced by cholesterol feeding. In: Disturbances in Lipid and Lipoprotein Metabolism. JM Dietsch, ed. American Physiological Society, Bethesda, Maryland, p 181.
40. Mahley RW, Weisgraber KH, Innerarity T (1976). Atherogenic hyperlipoproteinemia induced by cholesterol feeding in the Patas monkey. Biochemistry 15:2979.
41. Zannis VI, Breslow JL (1981). Human very low density lipoprotein apolipoprotein E isoprotein polymorphism is explained by genetic variation and posttranslational modification. Biochemistry 20:1033.
42. Weisgraber KH, Rall SC Jr, Mahley RW (1981). Human E apoprotein heterogeneity cysteine-arginine interchanges in the amino acid sequence of the apo E isoforms. J Biol Chem 256:9077.
43. Blue M, Williams DC, Zucker S, Khan SA, Blum CB (1983). Apolipoprotein E synthesis in human kidney, adrenal gland and liver. Proc Natl Acad Sci USA 80:283.
44. Driscoll DM, Getz GS (1984). Extrahepatic synthesis of apolipoprotein E. J Lipid Res 25:1368.
45. Elshourbagy NA, Liau WS, Mahley RW, Taylor JM (1985). Apolipoprotein E mRNA is abundant in the brain and adrenals as well as in the liver, and is present in other peripheral tissues of rats and marmosets. Proc Natl Acad Sci USA 82:203.
46. Basu SK, Ho YK, Brown MS, Bilheimer DW, Anderson RGW, Goldstein JL (1982). Biochemical and genetic studies of the apoprotein E secreted by mouse macrophages and human monocytes. J Biol Chem 257:9788.
47. Takagi Y, Dyer CA, Curtiss LK (1988). Platelet enhanced apolipoprotein E production by human macrophages: A possible role in atherosclerosis. J Lipid Res 29:859.
48. Ho YK, Brown MS, Goldstein JL (1981). Hydrolysis and secretion of cytoplasmic cholesteryl esters by macrophages: Stimulation by high density lipoproteins as other agents. J Lipid Res 21:391.
49. Mahley RW, Innerarity TL, Brown MS, Ho YK, Goldstein JL (1980). Cholesteryl ester synthesis in macrophages: Stimulation by β-very low density lipoproteins from cholesterol-fed animals of several species. J Lipid Res 21:970.
50. Fogelman AM, Shechter I, Seager J, Hokom M, Child JS, Edwards PA (1980). Malondialdehyde alteration of low density lipoproteins leads to cholesteryl ester accumulation in human monocyte-macrophages. Proc Natl Acad Sci USA 77:2214.
51. Henrikson T, Mahoney EM, Steinberg D (1981). Enhanced macrophage degradation of low density lipoprotein previously incubated with cultured endothelial cells: Recognition by receptors for acetylated low density lipoproteins. Proc Natl Acad Sci USA 78:6499.
52. Fogelman AM, Haberland ME, Seager J, Hokom M, Edwards PA (1981). Factors regulating the activities of the low density lipoprotein receptor and the scavenger receptor on human monocyte-macrophages. J Lipid Res 22:1131.

53. Fogelman AM, Hokom MM, Haberland ME, Tanaka RD, Edwards PA (1982). Lipoprotein regulation of cholesterol metabolism in macrophages-derives from human monocytes. J Biol Chem 257:14081.
54. McGooley DJ, Anderson RGW (1983). Morphological characterization of the cholesteryl ester cycle in cultured mouse macrophage foam cells. J Cell Biol 97:1156.
55. Basu SK, Brown MS, Ho YK, Havel RJ, Goldstein JL (1981). Mouse macrophages synthesize and secrete a protein resembling apolipoprotein E. Proc Natl Acad Sci USA 78: 7545.
56. Basu SK, Goldstein JL, Brown MS (1983). Independent pathways for secretion of cholesterol and apolipoprotein E by macrophages. Science 219:871.
57. Curtiss LK, Black AS, Takagi Y, Plow EF (1987). A new mechanism for foam cell generation in atherosclerotic lesions. J Clin Invest 80:367.
58. Banka CL, Black AS, Dyer CA, Curtiss LK (1991). THP-1 cells form foam cells in response to coculture with lipoproteins but not platelets. J Lipid Res 32:35.
59. Curtiss LK, Dyer CA, Banka CL, Black AS (1990). Platelet mediated foam cell formation in atherosclerosis. Clin Invest Med 13:189.
60. Gibson JC, Rubinstein A, Bukberg PR, Brown WV (1983). Apolipoprotein E-enriched lipoprotein subclasses in normolipidemic subjects. J Lipid Res 24:886.
61. Gordon V, Innerarity TL, Mahley RW (1983). Formation of cholesterol and apoprotein E-enriched high density lipoproteins in vitro. J Biol Chem 258:6202.
62. Werb Z, Chin JR (1983). Apoprotein E is synthesized and secreted by resident and thioglycollate-elicited macrophages but not by pyran eopolymer- or bacillus calmette-guerin-activated macrophages. J Exp Med 158:1272.
63. Werb Z, Chin JR (1983). Endotoxin suppresses expression of apoprotein E by mouse macrophage in vivo and in culture. A biochemical and genetic study. J Biol Chem 258: 10642.
64. Werb Z, Chin JR (1983). Onset of apoprotein E secretion during differentiation of mouse bone marrow-derived mononuclear phagocytes. J Cell Biol 97:1113.
65. Terkeltaub R, Martin J, Curtiss LK, Ginsberg MH (1990). Glycosaminoglycans alter the capacity of low density lipoproteins to bind to monosodium urate crystals. J Rheumatol 17:1211.
66. Terkeltaub RA, Dyer CA, Martin J, Curtiss LK (1991). Apolipoprotein E inhibits the capacity of monosodium urate crystals to stimulate neutrophils. J Clin Invest 87:20.
67. Fogelman AM, Seager J, Haberland ME, Hokam M, Tanaka R, Edwards PA (1982). Lymphocyte-conditioned medium protects human monocyte-macrophages from cholesteryl ester accumulation. Proc Natl Acad Sci USA 79:922.
68. Fogelman AM, Seager J, Groopman JE, Berlinger JA, Haberland ME, Edwards PA, Golde DW (1983). Lymphokines secreted by an established lymphocyte line modulate receptor-mediated endocytosis in macrophages derived from human monocytes. J Immunol 131:2368.
69. Dyer CA, Curtiss LK (1988). Apoprotein E-rich high density lipoproteins inhibit ovarian androgen synthesis. J Biol Chem 263:10965.

12
Oxygenated Derivatives of Cholesterol: Their Possible Role in Lymphocyte Activation and Differentiation

Hans-Jörg Heiniger
Swiss Red Cross, Bern, Switzerland

Harry W. Chen
Du Pont Merck Pharmaceutical Company, Wilmington, Delaware

INTRODUCTION

Many excellent reviews have been written about plasma membrane structure and cholesterol biosynthesis. Therefore, this chapter limits its focus to a brief synopsis of the role of cholesterol in mammalian plasma membranes and a more thorough overview of the effects of cholesterol and its oxygenated derivatives on certain specific lymphocyte functions. The last section contains speculations in the context of the central question raised by this text: Are cholesterol and oxysterols involved in the overall outcome of immune reactions in vivo? These speculations, many of which are based on preliminary evidence, are intended to provoke new working hypotheses aimed at a better understanding of how the nutritional status can modify immune response. (It should be noted that unless otherwise referenced, all research mentioned in the chapter has been performed by the authors in their laboratories at The Jackson Laboratory, Bar Harbor, Maine.)

With the proposal of the modern models of fluid-mosaic membrane structure, significant interest emerged concerning the function of plasma membrane lipids (1, 2). At about that time, the regulatory role of oxygenated derivatives of cholesterol in sterol biosynthesis was proposed (3,4). It was then demonstrated that cholesterol itself is not involved in the regulation of 3-hydroxy-3-methylglutaryl-CoA reductase (HMG-CoA reductase, EC 1.1.1.34), the rate-limiting enzyme in the pathway which generates isoprenoid compounds such as cholesterol, dolichol, ubiquinone, and, in tRNA, isopentenyl adenosine (IPA).

For the purposes of this chapter, the assumption has been made that cholesterol is not only an important cellular metabolite, but also a significant component of many human diets. Its oxygenated derivatives are spontaneously generated by autoxidation in the presence of oxygen. Inevitably, many of these derivatives are minor components in a variety of foodstuffs. Hence, both cholesterol and oxysterols may play a role in the immune response in vivo.

FUNCTION OF CHOLESTEROL IN MAMMALIAN PLASMA MEMBRANES

Cholesterol is the primary, if not the only, membrane sterol in most mammalian cell membranes. Its physiochemical role has been investigated intensively and is well understood (5-13). Lymphocyte plasma membrane as well as plasma membrane of many other cell types contains approximately 50% lipid and 50% protein. Membrane lipid is composed of equal molar concentrations of cholesterol and phospholipids. The ratio of cholesterol to phospholipid (CPR) appears to be lower in cultured, transformed, and cancerous cells (14).

The phospholipid bilayers found in cell membranes undergo characteristic crystalline to liquid-crystalline phase transitions (15). If cholesterol is added to such bilayers at concentrations of more than 33 mol percent, these phase transitions are abolished (9,15-17). This indicates that cell membranes containing cholesterol and phospholipid are most likely in a state of intermediate fluidity, or "gel state" (9).

The gel state concept of plasma membrane originated some 30 years ago (18). It has since been substantiated by a number of sophisticated experimental approaches (9,19,20), most elegantly by Drake et al. and Stoffels et al. using nuclear magnetic resonance analyses (22,23). Based on these findings, it was postulated that the modulation of fluidity in mammalian membrane occurs by chemotrophic (specific molecule interaction) rather than thermotropic (temperature-dependent phase transition) means (14). Changes in membrane cholesterol concentration can alter the fluidity of membrane lipids. Since membrane cholesterol derives from endogenous synthesis and/or exogenous supply, dietary uptake of cholesterol and oxysterols may also affect modulations of membrane fluidity.

Membrane lipids are predominantly composed of interacting phospholipids and cholesterol that serve as a support matrix for a variety of complex proteins. The proteins in turn interact with the lipids as well as with each other. These cooperative interactions between complex membrane components appear to be highly specific, though as yet poorly characterized. However, they are critical for successful functioning of membrane-found proteins such as membrane-associated enzymes and cell surface receptors.

Microdomains in plasma membranes are also in a highly dynamic state and may constantly undergo changes dependent on the stage of the cell cycle and the state of the cellular differentiation. The short duration of cooperative lipid-lipid and lipid-protein interactions causes lateral diffusion of proteins through entire membrane domains to occur at speeds determined by the specific proteins in question. Available experimental data for a number of different proteins suggests that their mobilities differ from each other by a factor of more than 10,000 (13,24-26).

It is not surprising that many of a cell's functional aspects are altered when the concentration of one molecular species in the plasma membrane, such as cholesterol, changes. These changes presumably bring about perturbations of the membrane fluidity (1,14,24). Alteration of the cholesterol concentration in plasma membrane results in changes in the stability and osmotic fragility of cells and in cellular attachment and cell shape (14,27-32). Depletion of cholesterol affects membrane permeability to ionic and nonionic solutes, active transport of sugars, and the activities of membrane-associated enzymes. Blocking cholesterol synthesis alters the rate of pinocytosis of fibroblasts, fusion of myogenic cells, differentiation of neuronal cells, and specific immune responses of lymphocytes to various antigens (14,27,28). The binding affinity of ligands and receptors (21) and lateral diffusion of receptors (33) are also affected when the membrane lipid composition is modified. Malnutrition, particularly with associated parasitism, e.g., malaria, has been associated with reduced plasma cholesterol (34).

Cholesterol is found in many foods in significant concentrations. Since cholesterol is easily auto-oxidized in air (35), its oxygenated derivatives must also be present in food. It is known that cellular cholesterol may be exogenously supplied. Thus, the dietary intake of cholesterol and its oxysterols could presumably affect the rapid changes of a cell's surface-related events. For example, in lymphocytes, the cellular processes of capping, display of membrane antigens, antibody secretion, and specific effector-target cell interactions may be altered by cholesterol. The implications of oxysterols in immune functions are discussed below. Although many of their effects have been attributed to inhibition of cholesterol synthesis of HMG-CoA reductase, other effects, as described below, and even the results of insertion into membranes (36) have been postulated.

STEROL BIOSYNTHESIS AND REGULATION IN LYMPHOCYTES

Lymphoid cells appear to regulate their de novo synthesis of cellular cholesterol by mechanisms similar to those identified in other cells. It is well established that the major rate-limiting step in the cholesterol biosynthetic pathway is the formation of mevalonate, catalyzed by HMG-CoA reductase. A small percentage of endogenously produced mevalonate also serves as an obligatory precursor for dolichol, the side chain of ubiquinone, and isopentenyl adenosine (IPA). Dolichol serves as an important sugar carrier for the assembly of N-linked glycoproteins (37-39). Ubiquinone is engaged in electron transfer in oxidative phosphorylation (40). The function of IPA, found in certain tRNA species, remains poorly understood in mammalian cells.

Based on feeding experiments, it was originally believed that cholesterol itself regulates its biosynthesis via suppression of HMG-CoA reductase. However, it was then discovered that chemically pure cholesterol has no effect of HMG-CoA reductase activity in cultured cells, whereas oxygenated derivatives of cholesterol (diols) are powerful inhibitors of the enzyme even in nanomolar concentrations (3,4). These oxysterols occur spontaneously as a result of auto-oxidation. They are also produced as obligatory intermediates in the biosynthesis of cholesterol, bile acid (7α-hydroxycholesterol), and steroid hormones (20α-hydroxycholesterol, 22-hydroxycholesterol) (27,41,42). A possible regulatory oxysterol, 24S-epoxycholesterol, has been detected in cultured fibroblasts (43).

The exact mechanism by which oxysterols regulate transcription of the HMG-CoA reductase gene and thus cholesterol biosynthesis is not yet clear. However, experimental data obtained in mutant Chinese hamster cell lines suggest that all oxysterols inhibit sterol biosynthesis through a common mechanism (44-46). Furthermore, a 7.5S cytosolic binding protein has been detected in several mammalian cells and tissues (27,47,50). This protein binds oxysterols with high affinity and specificity. It is possible that formation of an oxysterol and binding protein complex could lead to suppression of transcription of the HMG-CoA reductase gene analogous to the action of certain steroid hormones. Most, if not all, of the oxysterols identified as potential regulatory compounds could be minor components of the human diet, and could, therefore, have an effect on the synthesis of sterols and other isoprenoid-containing metabolites.

Lymphocytes display certain unique features which may be related to their specific physiological functions. As a result of recirculation, they are constantly exposed to different environments, including the serum and interstitial space in various organs and tissues. Quiescent lymphocytes synthesize cholesterol at a very low rate (51-54). The significance of this low rate of endogenous synthesis, also observed in vivo, remains obscure. Yet, it appears that endogenous sterol synthesis is critical for quiescent cells, which apparently cannot satisfy their needs from an exogenous supply. Further investigation of this particular lymphocyte metabolic behavior is required to address whether or not a minimal rate of sterol synthesis is necessary for the functional maintenance of some specific cell surface structures, e.g., receptors. Interestingly, oxidation of cholesteryl linoleate by human monocyle macrophages in vitro appears to show correlation with age of the cell donor and to be higher when test monocytes were isolated from men (55).

The preceding question is of particular interest in memory cells which have undergone primary stimulation but are temporarily in an inactive state. Preliminary data from spleen cells indicate that the ratio of endogenously synthesized cholesterol to cholesterol uptake from exogenous sources increases constantly over time independent of the concentration of serum in the medium. This relative refractiveness of lymphocytes to exogenous sterol concentrations is in contrast to results obtained in established tissue culture cells which readily take up exogenous serum cholesterol (14,56).

In contrast, activated lymphocytes, stimulated either by lectins (54,57-60), antigens (61,62), or mixed lymphocyte culture (MLC) (63), synthesize cholesterol at a high rate. In PHA- and concanavalin A-stimulated lymphocytes, a discrete cycle of sterol synthesis precedes the cycle of DNA synthesis (54,64), and these cells appear to be more sensitive to oxysterols than other cell types (unpublished results). The biological effects of oxysterols on these cells and the implication of this particular feature of immunological phenomena is discussed below.

Leukemic cells from mice, guinea pigs, and humans display an excessively high rate of sterol synthesis, elevated up to 150-fold in the paraplasts of acute lymphocytic leukemia in comparison to normal lymphocytes (51,65-67). This high rate can be further enhanced by small doses of PHA in leukemic cells of AKR/J mice (68). Unfortunately, to date, the mechanisms and causes of this excessive synthesis is not yet known. It does not appear to be correlated with serum sterol concentration. Further, it is not a result of a loss in feedback regulation, since these cells' sterol synthesis can be suppressed by oxysterols, although not as efficiently as in normal cells. At present, one can only speculate that exaggerated synthesis may be the result of altered molecular mechanisms involved in the synthesis and degradation of HMG-CoA reductase in these malignant cells (14). Interestingly, some synthetic oxysterols can inhibit tumor growth (69).

Owing to cellular heterogeneity in lymphoid tissues, in vivo studies on the regulation of lymphocytic sterol synthesis are difficult to carry out. In the steady state, lymphoid organs such as the spleen synthesize little cholesterol compared to other tissues

(70). Future experimentation will have to rely on specifically stimulated animals and sophisticated cell separation techniques to be able to characterize a relevant cell population; i.e., lymphoid cells in a state of activation and specific differentiation. Recent studies (71) indicate that both mitogenic stimuli and exogenous sterol level regulate lipoprotein receptor expression at the gene level.

In summary, currently available evidence supports the hypothesis that the biosynthesis of cholesterol represents a crucial metabolic activity of lymphocytes. The data further indicate that cholesterol biosynthesis is essential if lymphocytes are to perform their complex task of interacting with the environment. The recent characterization of a human monocytelike cell line, 4937, which is a cholesterol auxotroph (72), may be useful in future studies of this type.

IN VITRO INVESTIGATIONS OF THE BIOLOGICAL EFFECTS OF CHOLESTEROL AND OXYSTEROLS IN LYMPHOCYTE FUNCTIONS

Sterol biosynthesis has been investigated for some time in normal and malignant lymphoid cells (14,65). However, its significance for lymphocytic functions was poorly understood until it was discovered by the authors that a distinct cycle of sterol synthesis precedes the cycle of DNA synthesis in PHA-stimulated lymphocytes (64) (Fig. 1). When these cells are incubated with oxysterols, e.g., 25-hydroxycholesterol or 20α-hydroxycholesterol, their endogenous supply of cholesterol is interrupted as a result of suppression of its biosynthesis, whereas normally, mitogen stimulation increases cholesterol synthesis within 4 hr (73).

The dose of oxysterol required to completely abolish sterol synthesis (as detected by [^{14}C]acetate incorporation into a digitonin-precipitable sterol fraction) is as low as 0.75 µg/ml medium, or 1.8 µM. Under these conditions, DNA synthesis is inhibited by 80% or more, whereas fatty acid synthesis and CO_2 production (cellular respiration) are unaffected. Most importantly, DNA synthesis is only inhibited when the oxysterols are present in the medium before or during the peak of sterol synthesis. When oxysterols are added at a later time interval, there is no effect on DNA synthesis. These observations have been confirmed by several laboratories using lymphocytes from various species, including humans (54,58,63,68,74). On the other hand, Cutnbert and Lipsky (73) have shown that blocking sterol synthesis by suppressing HMG-CoA reductase did not prevent entry of cells into S phase, suggesting a discrete inhibitory role for oxysterol inhibition. We have now found (75) that the oxysterol effect requires protein synthesis.

Hence it has been established that inhibition of sterol synthesis by oxysterols prevents the initiation of DNA synthesis; whereas hydroxyurea, which inhibits DNA synthesis, does not affect sterol synthesis and inhibition of HMG-CoA reductase blocks proliferation but not at the point of entry into a phase (73). Of particular interest are the observations that some serum batches also inhibit sterol synthesis and DNA synthesis in lectin-stimulated lymphocytes (64), as did the addition of low-density lipoprotein (LDL) (76,77). It is suspected that the inhibitory components in these serum and lipoprotein preparations may prove to be oxysterols. Schuh et al. have provided good evidence that an oxidized lipid is one agent in lipoprotein that inhibits lymphocyte mitogenesis (78).

The relationship between the synthesis of sterols and DNA has been further analyzed in mixed lymphocyte reactions (MLRs) involving an allogenic difference at the

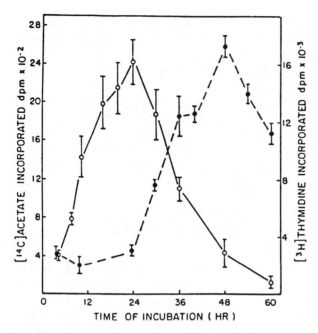

Figure 1 Time course of PHA stimulation of the syntheses of sterol and DNA. PHA was added at the beginning of the experiment and radio-active acetate or thymidine was added 2 hr before the end of the experiments. In experiments concerned with sterol synthesis (0—0) 0.5 ml of blood was cultured in a total volume of 5 ml. In those concerned with DNA synthesis (●—●), 0.05 ml of blood was cultured in a total volume of 0.5 ml. Triplicate samples were analyzed; points and range represent mean + SEM. Data for control cultures without PHA are not shown; however, both sterol and DNA radioactivity counts were very low and were linear over the entire incubation period. (From Ref. 64; used with permission.)

major histocompatibility locus H-2 (H-2^b versus H-2^d). The time course for lymphocytic sterol and DNA synthesis was found to be somewhat different than those in lectin-stimulated cultures. In MLR primary cultures the onset of sterol synthesis precedes DNA synthesis, but continues to increase up to day 5 after DNA has peaked. Cytotoxic titers in these cultures peak between days 5 and 7 and then decline steadily (79,80).

The difference in the time course of sterol and DNA synthesis between lectin-stimulated lymphocytes and MLR may be attributed to several factors. One of them may relates to the fact that while lectin induces a somewhat synchronous population of various activated T cells, MLRs may produce an asynchronous population of cells exhibiting either helper function or cytotoxic capacity (81). The observed rates of sterol and DNA synthesis in MLRs over time thus reflect average synthetic activity at a given time rather than activity at distinct phases of the cell cycle of a single cell population. However, the initial increase in sterol synthesis preceding DNA synthesis may be directly related to the first proliferative wave of cell populations which respond to the allogenic stimulation analogous to the circumstances observed in lectin-stimulated lymphocytes. The continuing elevated rate of sterol biosynthesis observed between days 4 and 8 is probably related to the actual maintenance of the cytotoxic state of effector cells.

Mixed lymphocyte cultures, like lectin-stimulated lymphocytes, are very susceptible to inhibition of sterol and DNA synthesis by oxysterols. When mevalonic acid (MVA, the product of HMG-CoA reductase) was simultaneously added with the oxysterols, DNA synthesis remained intact for a minimum of 24-48 hr. This indicates a specificity of oxysterol for depletion of MVA as well as a requirement of MVA for DNA synthesis. The possibility that some cellular activation may be regulated by a putative endogenous regulatory oxysterol is suggested. We have recently described a Chinese hamster ovary cell mutant which lacks lanosterol-14-α-methyldemethylase activity, and is thus a cholesterol auxotroph where we hope to study cell activation further (82).

It seems that few studies on the role of sterol biosynthesis and the function of membrane lipids have been conducted on B cells. Humphries and McConnell exposed B-cell precursors during the phase of antigenic stimulation (activation) to oxysterols and found a very significant reduction in the number of plaques formed (67). They have interpreted their findings as being the result of inhibited proliferation; i.e., the inability of B-cell clones to expand.

There are several explanations for the need for increased sterol synthesis preceding DNA synthesis and cell division in stimulated lymphocytes: (a) the cell requires cholesterol to synthesize new plasma membrane, even in the presence of extracellular serum cholesterol; and (b) modulation of membrane fluidity may be necessary during certain periods of the cell cycle as a mechanism for altering ion transport and other membrane-related biochemical events. Modulation of fluidity may be accomplished by changing the rate of sterol synthesis. Additionally, the possibility cannot be excluded that the availability of mevalonate as a precursor to IPA, ubiquinone, dolichol, or other metabolites may be critical for DNA synthesis (83). For example, IPA has been postulated to be required for DNA synthesis and progression of the cell cycle in cultured cells (84,85). One group has reported that IPA exhibits a stimulatory action on lymphocytes similar to the mitogenic effect of lectins (86). The authors have not been able to reproduce these observations consistently. So although the possibility that nonsteroidal mevalonate metabolites play a role in regulating DNA synthesis is an interesting one, it remains to be proven.

All the preceding interpretations, even if proven to be correct, address only a portion of the issue, as they are simplifications, focusing on proliferation alone. It is important to point out that when these cells divide, they also simultaneously differentiate from immunologically inactive state into mature immunocytes. It is well established that T-cell precursors will develop into interacting cytokine-producing cells and into differentiated cells such as cytotoxic effector cells, whereas B-cell precursors will become antibody-producing cells.

EFFECTS OF OXYSTEROLS IN LYMPHOCYTE DIFFERENTIATION IN VITRO

Two experimental systems were used to analyze the role of cholesterol biosynthesis and the effect of oxysterols on lymphocyte differentiation: the allogenic mixed lymphocyte reaction (MLR) and the polyclonal induction of cytotoxic T-cells by concanavalin (Con A).

When exposed to micromolar concentrations of the oxysterols 25-hydroxysterol and 7-ketocholesterol, MLCs (H-2^b versus H-2^d) were unable to generate or maintain cytotoxic activity (63). Interestingly, these oxysterols had to be present at least 12-24 hr before the cytotoxic assay to exhibit any effect. Addition of even high concentrations of oxysterols shortly before or during the assay did not affect cytotoxic activity. Furthermore, the oxysterols did not seem to interfere with initial lymphocyte-target binding (conjugate formation) and addition of PHA did not restore the capability of effector cells to lyse target cells. This conclusion is based on the observation that addition of PHA to these cells will normally form artifactual doublets, even under conditions of allogenic mismatching. These results raise the question of how oxysterols affect cytotoxic effector cells: Do they simply inhibit cellular proliferation (i.e., expansion of specific clones of T-cell precursors) through blockade of cytokine production, or do they also suppress the differentiation of these cells? The following experiments were performed to investigate these hypotheses.

Eleven-day-old primary MLCs exhibiting low residual cytotoxicity titer were restimulated either by allogenic cells or by supernatants from secondary MLCs (63). Other investigators had established that cytotoxic activity in these cultures could rise 10-fold within 24 hrs following restimulation (87,88). The increase in cytotoxic activity occurred even in the presence of potent inhibitors of DNA synthesis, such as cytosine arabinoside (Ara-C). Our studies indicated that in secondary MLCs, sterol synthesis increases dramatically within hours after restimulation and the rise closely parallels an increase in cytotoxic function (63). After 24 hr, sterol synthesis had increased 20-fold while cytotoxic activity was enhanced 10-fold.

Oxysterols such as 25-hydroxycholesterol were added to cultures in doses of 0.5-3.0 µg/ml at the time of restimulation. With this treatment, not only were cytotoxic titers prevented from increasing, but even the residual 11-day titers were eliminated (Fig. 2). The effects of oxysterols could be partially prevented by simultaneously adding large doses of cholesterol purified by recrystallization or MVA along with the oxysterols. Dabrowsky et al. reported similar results in human lymphocytes (89).

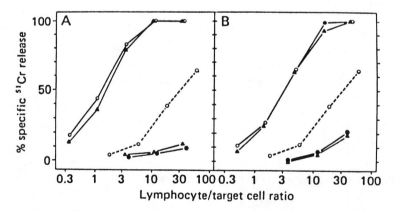

Figure 2 Effect of inhibitor (25-OH-cholesterol) on induction of CTLs. Cells recovered from C57BL/6 anti-DNA/2 long-term primary MLC (days 11-12) were restimulated with irradiated allogeneic (DBA/2) spleen cells (A) or with secondary MLC supernatants (B), alone (control) (O), in the presence of Ara-C (10 µg/ml) (▲), in the presence of 25-OH-cholesterol (2 µg/ml) (●), or in the presence of 25-OH-cholesterol (2 µg/ml) and Ara-C (10 µg/ml) (▲). Additional cultures were left unstimulated (O—O). After 24 hr of incubation, viable cell recoveries were determined, and cytolytic activities were assayed. (From Ref. 63; used with permission.)

Hence, an adequate supply of cholesterol appears to be critical for T cells to acquire and maintain their cytotoxic function. This may be independent of cholesterol requirements for DNA synthesis and cellular proliferation. De novo sterol synthesis seems to be a necessity as an exogenous supply of MVA or cholesterol could not completely overcome the adverse effects of oxysterols. Although prostaglandin E_2 production is stimulated by oxysterols (90), recent studies by Moog et al. (91) using a synthetic (7,25-dihydroxycholesterol) oxysterol show that in vivo suppression is not blocked by inhibiting PGE_2 synthesis. Furthermore, the in vitro suppression was not abrograted.

Immunologists have documented that certain batches of fetal calf and bovine serum cannot sustain MLC growth, which is why each serum batch should be tested before use. Serum acquires inhibitory potential during prolonged storage at 4-8 °C. However, its capacity to sustain MLC growth can be restored by delipidation (Fig. 3). This correlates with the observation that oxysterols, which would naturally occur over time, can inhibit cell growth by preventing cholesterol synthesis and, quite probably, through direct effects on cytokine interaction. As mentioned above, oxidized lipids found in serum have been reported to be the active components inhibiting lectin-stimulated lymphocyte mitogenesis (78). It is speculated that these oxidized lipids may be oxysterols generated by auto-oxidation of cholesterol in the serum during prolonged storage. Positive proof for this has yet to be established; however, several potent oxysterols, including 25-hydroxycholesterol and 26-hydroxycholesterol, have

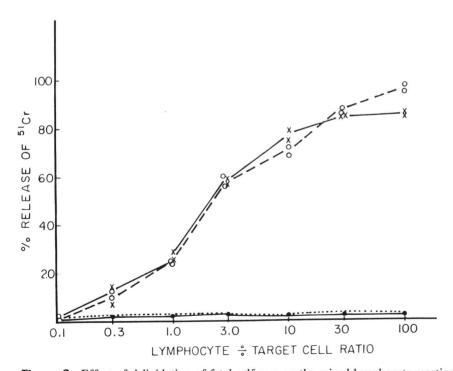

Figure 3 Effect of delipidation of fetal calf sera on the mixed lymphocyte reaction. Sera stored for prolonged time (●——●), (● . . . . ●) can completely inhibit cytotoxic titers in MLR, i.e., inhibit the growth and differentiation of cytotoxic effector cells. After delipidation (0——0) the serum has lost its inhibitory activity and is able to support fully the growth of cytotoxic T cells. As a control fresh calf serum (not delipidized) was used (X——X).

been detected in human tissues, circulating human plasma lipoproteins, and in bovine serum preparations (56,92,93).

The results obtained from MLRs have been further corroborated in lymphocyte cultures where lectins are used to produce polyclonally activated cytotoxic T cells (60,89). It has been demonstrated that in lymphocyte cultures, if the cells are permitted to go through a normal cycle of sterol synthesis, they will differentiate, even in the absence of proliferation (as seen in secondary MLCs) (60). Addition of oxysterols to these cultures abolished sterol synthesis and cellular differentiation. The specific function of cholesterol in the plasma membrane of cytotoxic T cells must be further investigated to characterize the molecular mechanism of T-cell killing, which remains poorly understood (94). Their role in the natural regulation of immune response perhaps through effects at the receptor level need to be studied. Since oxysterols affect primarily activated rather than quiescent lymphocytes and nenocytes and reduction of interleukin production has been reported (95), it seems likely that oxysterols might regulate receptor expression.

The role of cholesterol and its biosynthesis in B cells has not been extensively investigated. Humphries and McConnell's studies suggest that oxysterols affect the production of antibody mainly by preventing the relevant clones from proliferating (61,67). Preliminary experiments using mouse hybridoma cells suggest that secretion of the antibody molecules may be suppressed if endogenous sterol synthesis is inhibited by oxysterols. If these findings are confirmed, it will be important to determine precisely what B-cells' membrane lipid requirements are in relation to their receptor functions and secretion of humoral antibodies.

EFFECTS OF CHOLESTEROL AND OXYSTEROLS ON IMMUNE REACTIONS IN VIVO: PRELIMINARY FINDINGS, HYPOTHESES, AND SPECULATIONS

Human diets, particularly in Western societies, contain a significant amount of cholesterol (Table 1). The average cholesterol uptake in the United States is approximately 500 mg per person per day, but in many cases it can easily be as high as 1 g daily. Dietary cholesterol is easily oxidized into a variety of oxygenated compounds both before and during food processing, any time it is heated in the presence of air: cooking, frying, roasting (35).

It may be assumed up to 50% of the "cholesterol" present in processed food is oxidized in certain cases, as even higher relative amounts of oxysterols have been found in "cholesterol" samples (96). Hence, individuals potentially can be exposed to 250-500 mg, or 4-8 mg/kg body weight, of oxysterols each day. As previously discussed, many of these oxysterols are potent suppressors of HMG-CoA reductase and de novo synthesis of cholesterol. The biological effects of these dietary oxysterols in vivo have not been extensively studied.

Oxygenated sterols suppress sterol biosynthesis in vivo just as they do in cell cultures. In mice, dietary 7-ketocholesterol and 25-hydroxycholesterol suppress sterol synthesis in the intestine but not significantly in the liver (97). In rats, 7-ketocholesterol causes a transient inhibition of hepatic sterol synthesis (98). The inhibitory effect of some oxysterols in vivo appears to be limited by their rapid metabolism and their ability to induce as yet unidentified enzyme systems resulting in their inactivation by the liver (98). Preliminary experiments also revealed that the oxysterols cause

Table 1 Fat and Cholesterol[a] Content per 100 g of Foodstuff Used for Human Consumption

Foodstuff	Total fat (g)	Cholesterol (mg)
Raw eggs (large)	11.5	500
Egg powder	41.2	1900
Milk (cow, fresh)	3.7	13
Buttermilk	0.5	4
Milkpowder (decreamed)	1.0	20
Ice cream	12.5	40
Cheese		
Cream Cheese	30.5	110
Emmenthal	30.5	90
Blue Cheese	32.0	80
Meat		
Chicken	5.2	90
Chicken liver	3.7	560
Beef, sirloin	19.2	120
Pork, roast	32.0	100
Ham, cooked	20.6	70
Bacon	65.0	90
Hotdogs	27.6	70
Oysters	1.2	110-330

[a]The term *cholesterol* used in this table refers to total sterols reacting in the routine assays used including oxysterols.
Source: Data obtained from Scientific Tables, Geigy, 1977, 8th edition.

a dramatic change in the morphology of intestinal mucosa, suggesting a decreased number of differentiated cells in the villi and sudden exposure to oxysterols can produce a strong inflammatory response (91).

In all of the oxysterols tested thus far, a moderate loss of body weight in mature animals and suppressed growth in juvenile mice has been noted (97-99). This effect appears to be due to reduced food intake, although the appetite suppression was not a result of any unpalatable flavor from the sterols (97). Experiments indicate that mice on a diet containing 0.25% 7-ketocholesterol exhibited an impaired secondary response to tetanus toxoid, although their primary response was not affected (100).

It would be of great interest to know the impact of these complex biological effects of cholesterol and its oxysterols on the immune system in vivo. As rapidly circulating cells, lymphocytes are directly exposed to sterols in the serum and interstitium. The effect on appetite and other metabolic functions of the body may indirectly affect the optimal functioning of the immune system. To date, relatively few investigations have been conducted in this area.

IMPORTANT ISSUES TO BE ADDRESSED IN FUTURE STUDIES

1. Oxysterols spontaneously arise in cholesterol-containing diets. To what extent do dietary oxysterols destabilize the immune system by modifying cellular proliferation and differentiation? How does this affect the outcome of a primary or secondary immune response? Specific questions that must be addressed include the

type of effect on cytokine production such as gamma interferon and transforming growth factor β and on membrane-signaling systems such as protein kinase C.

2. Are oxysterols present in vivo in the serum? Present evidence seems to indicate that it is (35,93,101). Peng et al. demonstrated that VLDL (very low-density lipoprotein) and LDL (low-density lipoprotein) have a significantly higher affinity for oxysterols than for cholesterol (102). The reason for this is unclear, but it may be related to oxysterols having a more hydrophilic structure than cholesterol. Hagmann et al. showed that LDL is a potent suppressor of lymphocyte stimulation (76), and this is discussed in detail in Chapter 11. Again, the possibility is raised that the active ingredients in the LDL preparation are oxysterols. However, since biological activity (inhibitory capacity) is retained in neutral lipid-depleted, LDL, this is unlikely. On the other hand, the cholesterol-ester-loaded mouse peritoneal macrophage or human peripheral blood monocyte produces large amounts of the active moeity of LDL, apaprotein E.

3. In conditions of hypercholesterolemia, is the immune system compromised by a constant exposure to abnormally high physiological concentrations of oxysterols? Detailed and specific studies addressing this issue in human populations have not been conducted. If this suspicion is substantiated, then does an inefficient overall immune response contribute to the complexity of clinical symptoms manifested, particularly in more severe cases of hypercholesterolemia? Such studies would facilitate detailed understanding of atherosclerosis and its related diseases. Recent studies show that atherosclerotic plaques contain significant numbers of activated T cells and macrophages forming foam cell-rich lesions and that this process is strongly affected by dietary cholesterol (103).

4. Finally, do dietary cholesterol and products of its auto-oxidation affect the interactions of the immune systems with tumor cells? Since interactions between tumors and lymphoid cells are a somewhat controversial issue, the suggestion of sterol involvement will remain speculative. However, as discussed above, effector cells exposed in vitro to small amounts of oxysterols are unable to kill target cells. If cellular cytotoxicity is an important immune defense mechanism against tumor cells, then dietary oxysterols may significantly affect the clinical progression of a malignant process. Future experimental and clinical investigations should focus on establishing whether or not naturally prevailing dietary oxygenated derivatives of cholesterol contribute to debilitating the immune system to such an extent that an adequate immune surveillance required for a concerted defense against spontaneous tumors and their metastases is affected. On the other hand, certain hydroxysteroids such as 7β-hydroxysterol appear to have significant antitumor potential (90).

Although specific studies approaching such complex biological phenomena will be difficult to undertake, it is encouraging that the Division of Nutrition of the U.S. Food and Drug Administration has recognized the potential hazard of oxysterols as a public health issue and has called for determination of the impact of cholesterol oxides on human health (104). This awareness should promote future research in these areas.

ACKNOWLEDGMENT

The writing of this article was made possible by an institutional grant from the Jackson Laboratory, Bar Harbor, Maine.

We thank the New York Academy of Sciences in allowing us to use some material discussed in one of our reviews in their *Annuals* (100).

We also gratefully acknowledge the technical assistance of Jan Marshall and Oral Applegate, Jr. Editorial review of the article by Tiiu Lutter is greatly appreciated.

REFERENCES

1. Nicholson GL, Poste G, Ji TH (1977). The dynamics of cell membrane organization. In: Dynamic Aspects of Cell Surface Organization. G. Poste and G. L. Nicholson, eds. Elsevier/North-Holland Biomedical Press, Amsterdam, 1.
2. Singer SJ, Nicolson GL (1972). The fluid mosaic model of the structure of cell membranes. Science 175:720.
3. Kandutsch AA, Chen HW (1973). Inhibition of sterol synthesis in cultured mouse cells by 7-hydroxycholesterol 7-hydroxycholesterol, and 7-ketocholesterol. J Biol Chem 248:8403.
4. Kandutsch AA, Chen HW (1974). Inhibition of sterol synthesis in cultured mouse cells by cholesterol derivatives oxygenated in the side chain. J Biol Chem 249:6057.
5. Bretscher MS (1973). Membrane structure: some general principles. Science 181:622.
6. Chapman D (1968). Biological Membranes, Physical Fact and Function. Academic Press, New York.
7. Chapman D. (1973). Some Recent Studies of Lipids, Lipid-Cholesterol and Membrane Systems in Biological Membranes. Vol 2. D. Chapman and D. Wallach, eds. Academic Press, New York, 91.
8. Cronan JE, Gelmann EP (1975). Physical properties of membrane lipids: biological relevance and regulation. Bacteriol Rev 39:232.
9. Demel RA, de Kruyff B (1976). The functions of sterols in membranes. Biochim Biophys Acta 457:109.
10. Green DE (1972). Membrane structure and its biological applications. Ann NY Acad Sci 195:5.
11. McConnell HM (1975). Role of lipid in membrane structure and function. In: Cellular Membranes and Tumor Cell Behavior. A collection of papers presented at the 28th Annual Symposium of Fundamental Cancer Research Williams & Wilkins, Baltimore.
12. Brockenhoff H. (1974). Model of interaction of polar lipids, cholesterol, and proteins in biological membranes. Lipids 9:645.
13. Shamoo AE (1975). Carriers and channels in biological systems. Ann NY Acad Sci 264:1.
14. Chen HW, Kandutsch AA, Heiniger H-J (1978). The role of cholesterol in malignancy. In: Progress in Experimental Tumor Research. Vol. 22. F. Homburger, ed. Karger, Basel, 275.
15. Chapman D (1975). Phase transitions and fluidity characteristics of lipids and cell membranes. Q Rev Biophys 9:195.
16. Kroes J, Ostward R, Keith A (1972). Erythrocyte membranes: Compression of lipid phases by increased cholesterol content. Biochim Biophys Acta 274:71.
17. Ladbroke BD, Williams RM, Chapman D (1968). Studies on lecithin-cholesterol-water interactions by differential scanning calorimetry and x-ray differentiation. Biochim Biophys Acta 150:333.
18. Finean JB (1953). Phospholipid-cholesterol complex in the structure of myelin. Experimentia 9:17.
19. Huang C-H (1976). Roles of carbonyl oxygens at the bilayer interface in phospholipid-sterol interaction. Nature 259:242.

20. Lucy JA (1968). Theoretical and experimental models for biological membranes. In: Biological Membranes. D. Chapman, ed. Academic Press, New York, 233.
21. Marshall JD, Heiniger H-J (1979). High affinity concanavalin A binding to sterol-depleted L-cells. J Cell Physiol 100:539.
22. Drake A, Finer EG, Flook AG, Phillips MC (1972). Nuclear magnetic resonance of lecithin-cholesterol interactions. J Mol Biol 63:265.
23. Stoffel W, Tunggal BC, Zierenberg O, Schreiber E, Binczek E (1974). ^{13}C-nuclear magnetic resonance studies of lipid interactions in single and multicomponent lipid vesicles. Hoppe-Seyler's Z Physiol Chem 355:1367.
24. Cherry RJ (1976). Protein and lipid mobility in biological and model membranes. In: Biological Membranes. Vol. 3. D. Chapman and D. Wallach, eds. Academic Press, New York, 47.
25. Hynes RO 1976. Cell surface proteins and malignant transformation. Biochim Biophys Acta 458:73.
26. Kleeman W, McConnell HM (1976). Interactions of proteins and cholesterol with lipids in bilayer membranes. Biochim Biophys Acta 419:206.
27. Kandutsch AA, Chen HW, Heiniger H-J (1978). Biological activity of some oxygenated sterols. Science 201:498.
28. Chen HW (1984). The role of cholesterol metabolism in cell growth. Fed Proc 43:126.
29. Chen HW, Heiniger H-J, Kandutsch AA (1978). Alteration of ^{86}Rb$^+$ influx and efflux following depletion of membrane sterol in L cells. J Biol Chem 253:3180.
30. Cavanee WK, Chen HW, Kandutsch AA (1981). Cell-substratum and cell monolayer adhesion are dependent upon cellular cholesterol biosynthesis. Exp Cell Res 131:31.
31. Cohen DC, Massoglia SL, Gospodarowicz D (1982). Feedback regulation of 3-hydroxy-3-methylglutaryl coenzyme A reductase in vascular endothelial cells, separate sterol and non-sterol components. J Biol Chem 257:11106.
32. Schmidt RA, Glomset JA, Wight TN, Habenicht AJR, Ross R (1982). A study of the influence of mevalonic acid and its metabolites on the morphology of Swiss 3T3 cells. J Cell Biol 995:144.
33. Fahey PF, Koppel DE, Barak LS, Wolf DE, Elson EL, Webb WW (1977). Lateral diffusion in planar lipid bilayers. Science 195:305.
34. Agbedana EO, Salimonu LS, Taylor GO, Williams AIO (1990). Studies of total and high density lipoprotein cholesterol in childhood malaria: A preliminary study. Ann Trop Med Parasitol 84(5):529.
35. Smith LL (1981). Cholesterol Autoxidation. Plenum Press, NY and London.
36. Lelong I, Luu B, Mersel M, Rottem S (1988). Effects of 7B-hydroxycholesterol on grown and membrane composition of mycoplasma capricolum. FEBS Lett 232:354.
37. James MJ, Kandutsch AA (1979). Interrelationship between dolichol and sterol synthesis in mammalian cell cultures. J Biol Chem 254:8442.
38. James MJ, Kandutsch AA (1980). Evidence for independent regulation of dolichol and cholesterol synthesis in developing mouse brain. Biochim Biophys Acta 619:432.
39. James MJ, Kandutsch AA (1980). Elevated dolichol synthesis in mouse testes during spermatogenesis. J Biol Chem 255:16.
40. Gold PH, Olson RE (1966). Studies on coenzyme Q. The biosynthesis of coenzyme Q in rat tissue slices. J Biol Chem 241:3501.
41. Gibbons GF, Pullinger CR, Chen HW, Cavanee WK, Kandutsch AA (1980). Suppression of cholesterol biosynthesis in cultured cells by probable precursor sterols. J Biol Chem 255:295.
42. Tabacik C, Altan S, Serrou B, Crastes de Paulet A (1981). Post HMG CoA reductase regulation of cholesterol biosynthesis in normal human lymphocytes: Lanosten-3-β-ol-32-al, a natural inhibitor. Biochem Biophys Res Comm 101:1087.

43. Saucier SE, Kandutsch AA, Taylor FR, Spencer TS, Phirwa S, Gayen AK (1985). Identification of regulatory oxysterols, 24(S), 25-epoxycholesterol, and 25-hydroxy-cholesterol, in cultured fibroblasts. J Biol Chem 260:13391.
44. Cavanee WK, Gibbons GF, Chen HW, Kandutsch AA (1979). Effects of various oxygenated sterols and cellular sterol biosynthesis in Chinese hamster lung cells resistant to 25-hydroxycholesterol. Biochim Biophys Acta 575:255.
45. Chen HW, Cavanee WK, Kandutsch AA (1979). Variant Chinese hamster lung cells selected for resistance to 25-hydroxycholesterol: cross resistance to 7-ketocholesterol, 20α-hydroxycholesterol, and serum. J Biol Chem 254:715.
46. Sinensky M, Duwe G, Pinkerton F. (1979). Defective regulation of 3-hydroxy-3-methylglutaryl coenzyme A reductase in a somatic cell mutant. J Biol Chem 254:4482.
47. Kandutsch AA, Chen HW, Shown EP (1977). Binding of 25-hydroxycholesterol and cholesterol to different cytoplasmic proteins. Proc Natl Acad Sci USA 74:2500.
48. Kandutsch AA, Thompson EB (1980). Cytosolic proteins that bind oxygenated sterols: Cellular distribution, specificity and some properties. J Biol Chem 255:10813.
49. Kandutsch AA, Shown EP (1981). Assays of oxysterol-binding protein in a mouse fibroblast, cell free system: Dissociation constant and other properties of the system. J Biol Chem 256:13068.
50. Taylor FR, Saucier SE, Shown EP, Parish EJ, Kandutsch AA (1984). Correlation between oxysterol binding to a cytosolic binding protein and potency in the repression of hydroxymethylglutaryl Coenzyme A reductase. J Biol Chem 259:12382.
51. Chen HW, Heiniger H-J (1974). Stimulation of sterol synthesis in peripheral leukocytes of leukemic mice. Cancer Res 34:1304.
52. Fogelman AM, Seager J, Hokum M, Edwards PA (1979). Separation of and cholesterol synthesis by human lymphocytes and monocytes. J Lipid Res 20:379.
53. O'Donnell VJ, Ottolenghi P, Malkin A, Denstedt OF, Heard RDH (1958). The biosynthesis from acetate-1-14C of fatty acids and cholesterol in formed blood elements. Can J Biochem 36:1125.
54. Pratt HPM, Fitzgerald PA, Saxon A (1977). Synthesis of sterol and phospholipid induced by the interaction of phytohemagglutinin and other mitogens—with human lymphocytes and their relation to blastogenesis and DNA synthesis. Cell Immunol 32:160.
55. Carpenter KL, Ballantine JA, Fussell B, Enright JH, Mitchinson MJ (1990). Oxidation of cholesteryl linoleate by human monocyte-macrophages in vitro. Atherosclerosis 83 (2-3):217.
56. Chen HW, Kandutsch AA (1981). Cholesterol requirement for cell growth: Endogenous synthesis vs. exogenous sources. In: The Nutritional Requirements of Vertebrate Cells in Vitro. R. G. Ham and C. Waymouth, eds. University of Cambridge Press, New York London, 327.
57. Respess JG, Stubbs JD, Chambers DA (1978). The effects of dibutyryl cyclic adenosine 3'-5'-monophosphate on concana valin A-stimulated sterol and fatty acid synthesis in mouse spleen lymphocytes. Biochim Biophys Acta 529:38.
58. Chen SSH (1979). Enhanced sterol synthesis in concanavalin A-stimulated lymphocytes: Correlation with phospholipid synthesis and DNA synthesis. J Cell Physiol 100:147.
59. Cuthbert JA, Lipsky PE (1980). Sterol metabolism and lymphocyte functions inhibition of endogenous sterol biosynthesis does not prevent mitogen-induced human T-lymphocyte activation. J Immunol 124:2240.
60. Heiniger H-J, Marshall JD (1982). Oxygenated derivatives of cholesterol and lymphocyte function: Cholesterol synthesis in polyclonally activated cytotoxic lymphocytes and its requirement for differentiation and proliferation. Proc Natl Acad Sci USA 79:3823.
61. Humphries HMK (1981). Compactin and oxidized cholesterol, both known to inhibit cholesterol biosynthesis, differ in their ability to suppress in vitro immune responses. Cancer Res 41:3789.

62. Humphries GMK, McConnell HM (1979). Potent immunosuppression by oxidized cholesterol. J Immunol 122:121.
63. Heiniger H-J, Brunner KT, Cerottini J-C (1978). Cholesterol is a critical cellular component for T-lymphocyte cytotoxicity. Proc Natl Acad Sci USA 75:5683.
64. Chen HW, Heiniger H-J, Kandutsch AA (1975). Relationship between sterol synthesis and DNA synthesis in phytohemagglutin-stimulated mouse lymphocytes. Proc Natl Acad Sci USA 72:1950.
65. Chen HW, Kandutsch AA, Heiniger H-J, Meier H (1973). Elevated sterol synthesis in lymphatic leukemia cells from two inbred strains of mice. Cancer Res 33:2774.
66. Heiniger H-J, Chen HW, Applegate OL, Schacter LP, Schacter BZ, Anderson PN (1976). Elevated synthesis of cholesterol in human leukemic cells. J Molec Med 1:109.
67. Philippot JR, Cooper AG, Wallach DFH (1976). 25-Hydroxycholesterol and 1,25-dihydroxycholecalciferol are potent inhibitors of cholesterol biosynthesis by normal and leukemic (L2C) guinea pig lymphocytes. Biochim Biophys Acta 72:1035.
68. Chen HW, Heiniger H-J, Kandutsch AA (1977). Stimulation of sterol and DNA synthesis in leukemic blood cells by a low concentration of phytohemagglutinin. Exp Cell Res 109:253.
69. Hietter H, Mogg T, Luu B, Beck JP, Bischoff P (1986). Effect of 7-B-hydroxycholesterol and t,25-dihydroxycholesterol towards cultured murine lymphama cells: Conditions for cytotoxic expression Eur J Cell Biol 42 (Suppl.) 15:41.
70. Turley SD, Anderson JM, Dietschy JM (1981). Rates of sterol synthesis and uptake in the major organs of the rat in vivo. J Lipid Res 22:551.
71. Cuthbert JA, Lipsky PE (1989). Regulation of LDL receptor mRNA levels in human lymphocytes by functional demand and ambient sterols. Trans Assoc Am Physicians 102:68.
72. Billheimer JT, Chamoun D, Esfahani M (1987). Defective 3-ketosteroid reductase activity in a human monocyte-like cell line. J Lipid Res 28(6):704.
73. Cuthbert JA, Lipsky PE (1987). Regulation of lymphocyte proliferation by cholesterol: The role of endogenous sterol metabolism and low density lipoprotein receptors. International J Tiss React 9(6):447.
75. Trzaskos JM, Jonas M, Chen HW (1989). Sterol-mediated suppression of HMG-CoA reductase mRNA levels in cultured cells requires protein synthesis. Biochem Biophys Res Commun 161(1):267.
76. Hagmann J, Weiler I, Waelti E (1979). Effects of low density lipoproteins on lymphocyte stimulation. FEBS Lett. 97:230.
77. Morse JH, Witte LD, Goodman PS (1977). Inhibition of lymphocyte proliferation stimulated by lectins and allogenic cells by normal lipoproteins. J Exp Med 146:1791.
78. Schuh J, Novogrodsky A, Haschemeyer RH (1978). Inhibition of lymphocyte mytogenesis by autooxidized low density lipoprotein. Biochim Biophys Acta 84:763.
79. Cerottini J-C, Engers HD, MacDonald HR, Brunner KT. Generation of cytotoxic T-lymphocytes in vitro. I. Response of normal and immune mouse spleen cells in mixed leukocyte culture. J Exp Med 140:703.
80. Engers HD, MacDonald HR (1976). Generation of cytolitic T-lymphocytes in vitro. In: Contemporary Topics in Immunobiology. Vol. 5. W. Weigle, ed. 145.
81. Ryser JE, MacDonald HR (1979). Limiting dilution analysis of alloantigen-reactive T-lymphocytes. I. Comparison of precursor frequencies for proliferative and cytolytic responses. J Immunol 122:1691.
82. Chen, HW, Leonard DA, Fischer RT, Trzaskos JM (1988). A mammalian mutant cell lacking detectable lanosterol 14 alpha-methyl demethylase activity. J Biol Chem 263(3):1248.
83. Habenicht AJR, Glomset JA, Ross R (1980). Relation of cholesterol and mevalonic acid to the cell cycle in smooth muscle and Swiss 3T3 cells stimulated to divide by platelet-derived growth factor. J Biol Chem 255:5134.

84. Quesney-Huneeus V, Wiley MH, Siperstein MD (1979). Essential role for mevalonate synthesis in DNA replication. Proc Natl Acad Sci USA 76:5056.
85. Quesney-Huneeus V, Wiley MH, Siperstein MD (1980). Isopentenyl adenesine as a mediator of mevalonate-regulated DNA replication. Proc Natl Acad Sci USA 77:5842.
86. Gallo RC, Wang-Peng J, Perry S (1969). Isopentenyl adensin stimulates and inhibits mitosis of human lymphocytes treated with phytohemagglutinin. Science 165:400.
87. MacDonald HR, Engers HD, Cerottini J-C, Brunner KT (1974). Generation of cytotoxic T-lymphocytes in vitro. J Exp Med 140:718.
88. MacDonald HR, Engers HD, Cerottini J-C, Brenner KT (1975). Generation of cytotoxic T-lymphocytes in vitro. J Exp Med 142:622.
89. Dabrowski MP, Peel WE, Thompson AER (1980). Plasma membrane cholesterol regulates human lymphocyte cytotoxic function. Eur J Immunol 10:821.
90. Lahoua Z, Astruc ME, Crastes De Paulet A (1988). Effect of oxysterols on the activity of phospholipase A in NRK cells. Biol Activ Oxygen Sterols 166:57.
91. Moog C, Ji YH, Waltzinger C, Luu B, Bischoff P (1990). Studies on the immunological properties of oxysterols: In vivo actions of 7,25-dihydroxycholesterol upon murine peritoneal cells. Immunology 70:344.
92. Smith LL, Teng JI, Lin YY, Seitz PK, McGehee MF (1981). Sterol metabolism-XLVIII. Oxidized cholesterol esters in human tissues. J Biol Chem 14:889.
93. Javitt NB, Kok E, Burnstein S, Cohen B, Kutscher J (1981). 26-Hydroxycholesterol, identification and quantitation in human serum. J Biol Chem 256:12644.
94. Berke G (1980). Interaction of cytotoxic T-lymphocytes and target cells. Prog Allergy 27:133.
95. Moog C, Luu B, Beck JP, Italiano L, Bischoff P (1988). Studies on the immunosuppressive properties of 7,25-dihydroxycholesterol. 1. Reduction of interleukin production by treated lymphocytes. Int J Immunopharmacol 10:511.
96. Peng SK, Taylor CB, Thau P, Werthessen NT, Mikkelson B (1978). Effect of autooxidation products from cholesterol on aortic smooth muscle cells. Arch Pathol Lab Med 102:57.
97. Kandutsch AA, Heiniger H-J, Chen HW (1977). Effects of 25-hydroxycholesterol and 7-ketocholesterol inhibitors of sterol synthesis, administered orally to mice. Biochim Biophys Acta 486:260.
98. Erickson SK, Cooper AD, Matsui SM, Gould RG (1977). 7-Ketocholesterol. Its effects on hepatic cholesterogenesis and its hepatic metabolism in vivo and in vitro. J Biol Chem 252:5186.
99. Kisic A, Taylor AS, Champerlain JS, Parish EJ, Schroepfer GJ (1978). Inhibitors of sterol synthesis. Further studies of the effect of 5α choles-8(14)-en-3β-ol-15-one on serum cholesterol levels of rats. Fed Proc Fed Am Soc Exp Biol 37:1663.
100. Heiniger H-J, Chen HW, Boissonneault GA, Hess M, Cottier H, Stoner RD (1985). The role of cholesterol and oxysterols in lymphocyte proliferation and differentiation. Ann NY Acad Sci 459:111.
101. Kandutsch A, A. Apo B dependent and independent cellular cholesterol homeostasis. In: Biochemistry and Biology of Plasma Proteins. A. M. Scann and A. Spector, eds. Marcel Dekker, New York.
102. Peng SK, Taylor CB, Mosbach EH, Huang WY, Hill J, Mikkelson B (1982). Distribution of 25-hydroxycholesterol in plasma lipoproteins and its role in atherogenesis. A study in squirrel monkeys. J. Atherosclerosis 41:395.
103. Hansson GK, Seifert PS, Olsson G, Bondjers G (1991). Immunohistochemical detection of macrophages 2nd T lymphocytes in atherosclerotic lesions of cholesterol-fed rabbits. Arteriosclerosis thrombosis 11(3):745.
104. Sheppard AJ, Shen CJ (1980). Activities of FDA's Division of Nutrition regarding cholesterol oxides. In: Autoxoidation in Food and Biological Systems. M. G. Simic and M. Kavel, eds. Plenum Press, New York, London, 119.

13
Prostaglandins, Fatty Acids, and Arthritis

Robert B. Zurier
University of Massachusetts Medical Center
Worcester, Massachusetts

INTRODUCTION

Abundant experimental evidence supports the view that prostaglandins, thromboxanes, and leukotrienes, collectively termed eicosanoids, participate in the development and regulation of immunological and inflammatory responses. Because essential fatty acids are precursors to eicosanoids, and because essential fatty acids are important determinants of cell membrane structure and function, they have an important influence on the course of an immune response. Diseases such as rheumatoid arthritis (RA), characterized by abnormal immune responses, persistent inflammation, and tissue injury, may therefore be amenable to control by dietary means. Indeed, considerable public interest has been provoked recently by the treatment of a variety of disorders, including RA, with plant seed and fish oils.

The regulation of inflammation and immune responses by eicosanoids, with special attention to studies done in vivo is reviewed in this chapter. In addition, the potential use of dietary fatty acid supplementation in the treatment of RA is considered.

EICOSANOIDS AS REGULATORS OF INFLAMMATION AND IMMUNE RESPONSES
Mediators of Inflammation

Although the precise role of eicosanoids in inflammation and immune responses is not clear, abundant experimental evidence supports the view that eicosanoids participate in the development of the inflammatory reaction (1) and in the regulation of immune responses (2). All the criteria presented by Dale (3) which must be met before a compound may be classified as a mediator of inflammation have been satisfied by prostaglandins and leukotrienes. Critical in this regard are the increased concentrations of eicosanoids at sites of inflammation and the demonstration that aspirin and other anti-inflammatory drugs inhibit prostaglandin synthesis. The proinflammatory effects of eicosanoids have been ascribed to their vasoactivity, to increases in the transudation of plasma at sites of inflammation, and to their ability to potentiate the action of other mediators of inflammation (4).

Regulators of Inflammation

Although eicosanoids are clearly local mediators of inflammation, evidence from both in vitro and in vivo experiments indicates they can also suppress diverse effector systems of inflammation (5). In addition, eicosanoids can both enhance and diminish cellular and humoral immune responses, observations which reinforce a view of these compounds as *regulators* of cell function.

Defective regulation of inflammatory responses or disordered immune mechanisms, or both, are probably central to the pathological processes encountered in rheumatic diseases such as rheumatoid arthritis and systemic lupus erythematosus (SLE). Eicosanoids, largely by virtue of their ability to influence celluilar cyclic nucleotides, appear to be important regulators of cell function and, therefore, are potentially able to influence the function of those cells that participate in tissue injury in these diseases. A regulatory effect of eicosanoids is not without precedent. For example, prostaglandin E (PGE) inhibits the release of norepinephrine from the spleen in response to sympathetic nerve stimulation (6) and PGE is released from spleen when it contracts in response to sympathetic nerve stimulation. Thus, by a feedback mechanism the contracting smooth muscle can reduce the stimulus that leads to its contraction. The release of PGE may therefore be a defense mechanism aimed at minimizing potential injury. It is also clear that the protection by PGE compounds of the gastric mucosa is a direct cellular effect (7). It is this view of eicosanoids as modulators of host defenses as well as mediators of inflammation—as protective agents—that led to studies using PGE to restrain inflammation and tissue injury.

Regulation by Prostaglandins of Acute Inflammatory Reactions

Studies In Vitro

The observation of Kloeze (8) that PGE inhibits platelet aggregation led to the notion that products of arachidonic acid metabolism might have anti-inflammatory activity. These potential beneficial effects were overlooked because of studies which indicated that eicosanoids are "proinflammatory" agents. However, subsequent in vitro studies demonstrated the ability of PGE and prostacyclin (PGI_2) to suppress the functional response of a variety of inflammatory cells besides platelets. These include mast cells and basophils (9,10), polymorphonuclear leukocytes (PMNs) (11—13) monocytes and macrophages (14), lymphocytes (15), and natural killer (NK) cells (16,17).

The capacity of PGE and PGI_2 to suppress function of inflammatory cells appears to reside in large part in their capacity to increase intracellular cyclic AMP, although a cause and effect relationship has not been established definitely in each cell type. The ability of PGE to suppress the production of leukotriene B_4 (LTB_4) may also help explain the potential antiinflammatory effects of PGE (18). Leukotrienes were first described in PMNs (19) and are potent mediators of inflammation at nanamolar concentrations. Leukotriene enhances the adherence of PMNs to endothelial cells, a process blocked by PGE and PGI_2 (20,21). In addition, LTB_4 "activates" PMNs to migrate, degranulate (release enzymes), and generate superoxide anion (22). Thus, PGE or PGI_2 made by vascular endothelial cells could by virtue of inhibiting LTB_4 production reduce PMN egress from the circulation, migration to a site of inflammation, and degranulation. Increases in LTB_4 induced in vitro by nonsteroidal anti-inflammatory agents are as likely due to the removal of PGE as a restraint to LTB_4 synthesis as they are to "shunting" of arachidonate from the cyclooxygenase to the lipoxygenase pathway.

Studies In Vivo

VASOACTIVE MEDIATOR-INDUCED VASCULAR PERMEABILITY. The central role of changes in venules during the immediate phase of increased vascular permeability has been demonstrated by several investigators. Ultrastructural studies suggest that increases in vascular permeability may result from the contraction of juxtaposed venular endothelial or periendothelial cells with the subsequent widening of intercellular junctions (23). Apart from direct endothelial damage, the most important inducers of vasopermeability appear to be vasoactive chemical mediators that initiate inflammatory reactions. These include histamine, serotonin, bradykinin, and the classic anaphylatoxins. An early step in the degradation of PGE is oxidation by 15-hydroxydehydrogenase. Thus, methylation of PGE_1 at the carbon-15 position results in a far more stable analog: 15S-15-methyl-PGE_1 ($15MPGE_1$), which can be administered subcutaneously at 0.02 the dose of PGE_1. Further, $15MPGE_1$ is biologically active after oral administration. The effects of PGE_1 and its 15-methyl derivative on the initial permeability changes mediated by humoral and cell-derived vasoactive mediators were examined. Systemic treatment (subcutaneous or oral administration) of rats with PGE_1 or $15MPGE_1$ markedly attenuates vasopermeability increases (monitored by extravasation of $[^{125}I]$albumin) induced by intradermal injection of histamine, serotonin, bradykinin, and the mast cell degranulating substances C3a and compound 48/80 (24). Inhibition is dependent on the dose of permeability factor and the time between its injection and PGE treatment. This is a long-lasting effect, since significantly reduced permeability was observed for 48 hr after *oral* administration of $15 MPGE_1$. Inhibition of vascular permeability by systemic PGE_1 treatment is in marked contrast to the local effects of PGE_1; namely, the potentiation of the leakage of plasma proteins induced by bradykinin in rat skin and bradykinin and histamine in dog knee joints. The structure-function relationships which influence the ability of PGE to inhibit mediator-induced permeability changes are demonstrated by the observations that PGA_2 (vasodilator) and PGF_2 (vasoconstrictor) fail to reduce permeability. Electron microscopic studies indicate that PGE_1 treatment preserves the tight junctions of endothelial cells and prevents the endothelial cell gap formation that usually follows injection of a vasopermeability mediator.

Carrageenin-Induced Vascular Permeability Change

The acute inflammatory response associated with carrageenin administration in the skin is enhanced by *local* administration of PGE_1. The reaction represents a complex of inflammatory events during which three distinct phases of mediator-induced vascular permeability changes are observed (25). The initial phase during the first 30 min after injection results from the release of histamine and serotonin from mast cells and is inhibited by antihistamines. The second phase, which occurs between 1.0 and 2.5 hr after injection, is attributed to the reaction of bradykinin, since pretreatment of rats with cellulose sulfate reduces edema. The third phase of persistent edema is complement dependent and has been attributed to the local production by inflammatory cells of eicosanoids, especially prostaglandins of the E series. This phase of edema formation is inhibited by indomethacin and aspirin and is potentiated by local injection of vasodilatory eicosanoids such as PGE_2 (26). However, it has been suggested (27) that the systemic administration of PGE and the stimulation of PGE production (28) may reduce carrageenin-induced edema formation. The systemic treatment of rats with 15-methyl-PGE_1 exhibits a dose-dependent inhibition of all three phases of carrageenin-induced edema formation (29). Consistent with the above findings, there is up to a 30% decrease in footpad thickness 1 hr after injection of carrageenin into the footpad. Whereas control animals showed a progressive increase in footpad swelling over the next 5 hr, the systemic administration of 15-methyl-PGE_1 (1 mg/kg S.C.) completely suppressed the second and third phases of edema formation. These findings emphasize the marked differences between the *local* and *systemic* effects of PGE on acute inflammatory reactions. The ability of PGE_1 to inhibit the later phase of carrageenin-induced edema formation, which is in part dependent upon the recruitment of PMNs to the inflammatory site, is consistent with in vitro studies demonstrating the ability of PGE to inhibit neutrophil chemotaxis, superoxide anion production, and lysosomal enzyme release. Although PGE_2 concentrations at sites of acute inflammation are increased, it is possible that the delayed permeability changes induced by carrageenin are not secondary to PGE_2 as previously described, but are the results of the local production of lipoxygenase products and other secretory products of stimulated neutrophils. Increased PGE concentrations associated with inflammatory reactions may in fact represent a modulating system that limits the extent of the inflammatory response.

Immune Complex-Induced Tissue Injury

Immune complex-induced vasculitis appears to be an early event at sites of inflammation (i.e., skin, kidney) in SLE patients and in subsynovial vessels in rheumatoid arthritis patients. The effect of PGE_1 was therefore investigated in vivo on experimental models of tissue injury which share features of immune complex-induced nephritis. The reversed passive Arthus reaction is induced in rat skin by the intravenous administration of antigen and the intradermal injection of antibody. The formation of immune complexes in vessel walls leads to the activation of complement and the local generation of C5-derived chemotactic peptides. Neutrophils respond to the chemotactic products, infiltrate the skin site, ingest the immune complexes, and then release lysosomal enzymes and other mediators of inflammation and tissue injury. Injury to vessels can be measured by an increase in vascular permeability (leakage into tissue of [^{125}I]albumin) and the development of hemorrhage. Treatment of rats with PGE_1 or its more stable analog $15MPGE_1$ inhibits increased vascular permeability and tissue injury even though vascular and perivascular deposition of antigens and complement are not prevented (30). Immunofluorescence microscopic studies suggest that in PGE-treated animals immune complexes form and the complement sequence is activated. However, the egress of leukocytes from blood vessels appears to be impaired in these animals. Electron microscopic studies indicate that neutrophils that leave the circulation and find their way to the reaction site do not ingest immune complexes. Biochemical studies indicate that peripheral blood neutrophils from PGE-treated animals have a reduced response to a chemotactic peptide and do not release lysosomal enzymes when they are treated in vitro with cytochalasin B and exposed to the peptide. Thus, the cytoprotective effects of PGE demonstrated in this model appear to be in part due to interference with the directed motion of neutrophils and degranulation of these cells. Of interest in these studies is the finding that 15MPGE$_1$ exhibits potent anti-inflammatory activity even after oral administration.

In a second model of immune complex-mediated tissue injury (the nephrotoxic serum nephritis model), the systemic treatment of animals with 15-methyl-PGE$_1$ suppressed both the glomerular hypercellularity and the proteinuria associated with a single intravenous injection of antibodies directed against rat glomerular basement membrane, without altering binding of specific antibody to the glomerular basement membrane (31). In this model of tissue injury, local activation of complement components and sequestration of PMNs within the capillary lumens of glomeruli are thought to be critical to the development of tissue injury. These studies provide additional support for the hypothesis that systemic PGE$_1$ treatment will inhibit immune complex-induced inflammatory reactions, and that certain eicosanoids may play an important role in the regulation of type II immune reactions.

Further evidence for the ability of PGE to modulate vascular injury and edema formation is provided by studies examining the effects of these agents on the development of passive cutaneous anaphylaxis in rabbits (32). Intravenously administered PGE$_1$ inhibited the transudation of proteins in the skin of rabbits at sites of initiation of the anaphylactic response. Inhibition of passive cutaneous anaphylactic reactions in rabbits was observed with other pharmacological agents known to increase intracellular levels of cyclic AMP. The studies suggest that PGE$_1$ may modulate acute inflammatory reactions by increasing the levels of cAMP in inflammatory cells.

Circulating Phlogistic Agents

The systemic treatment of rabbits with PGI$_2$ inhibits the neutropenia and thrombocytopenia associated with the infusion of immune complexes (33). Prostaglandin did not alter the interaction of immune complexes with PMN membrane receptors in vitro, but did inhibit platelet aggregation and secretion of platelet-activating factor (PAF) induced by immune complexes. In a separate study, the intravenous infusion of prostacyclin (10-50 ng/kg/min) in rabbits inhibited PAF-induced neutropenia, thrombocytopenia, and sequestration of PMNs in the pulmonary capillary bed (34). These observations support the hypothesis that PGI$_2$ has anti-inflammatory activity, and suggest a physiological role for PGI$_2$ in modulating the interaction between immune complexes and neutrophils. Additional studies in mongrel dogs indicate that prostacyclin infusion inhibits an increase in filtration coefficient and in lung vascular permeability changes following microembolization (35). Since microembolization in the lung is associated with acute lung injury and is dependent on the presence of circulating neutrophils (36), the data support the view that PGI$_2$ may be an important regulator of neutrophil activation within the vascular compartment. In addition, the data support previous observations implicating PGI$_2$ as an important modulator of vascular tone, and suggest a critical role for PGI$_2$ in the development of acute pulmonary hypertension.

Systemic prostacyclin treatment prolongs survival and inhibits pulmonary vascular changes associated with the intravenous infusion of endotoxin (37). Endotoxin-mediated lung injury depends upon neutrophil and platelet activation as well as the activation of the clotting system and fibrin deposition. After infusion of PGI_2 there is not only an improvement in the pulmonary hemodynamic parameters associated with endotoxin administration, there is also an increase in the numbers of circulating platelets and a decrease in fibrin degradation products. In view of these observations, it is of interest that the intravascular infusion of prostacyclin reduces some of the clinical changes associated with pulmonary embolism. Although the mechanisms whereby PGI_2 inhibit the tissue injury associated with endotoxemia are not clear, several mechanisms are possible, including the inhibition of platelet aggregation, the inhibition of neutrophil functional responses, and vasodilation. Similar findings were observed in rats in that intravenous infusion of prostacyclin inhibited the development of the generalized Schartzman reaction (38). The infusion of prostacyclin to a mean dose of 57 ng/kg/min before and after the administration of endotoxin inhibited the development of fibrin and platelet thrombi within capillaries. There was also an attenuation of endotoxin-induced decreases in renal blood flow and glomerular filtration. Prostacyclin treatment also inhibited completely the endotoxin-induced decrease in circulating platelet counts.

REGULATION BY PROSTAGLANDINS OF CHRONIC INFLAMMATORY REACTIONS

The term *inflammation* of course includes both acute and chronic conditions. Emphasis in eicosanoid research has been on their role in *acute* inflammatory responses. However, eicosanoids may also help modulate the chronic phase of inflammation. Thus, it is worthwhile to review the ability of these compounds to influence the development and progression of some chronic immune reactions.

Studies In Vitro

Current experimental evidence indicates that the addition of arachidonate products profoundly influences lymphocyte transformation (2), cell-mediated cytotoxicity (39), and the production of soluble mediators involved in the initiation and maintenance of cell-mediated immune responses. With regard to the production of inflammatory mediators, Gordon et al. (40) and Bray et al. (41) demonstrated that prostaglandins of the E series suppress lymphokine production, as monitored by macrophage migration inhibition. Rappaport and Dodge (42) and Baker et al. (43) have demonstrated that exogenous PGE inhibits another lymphocyte product, interleukin 2 (IL-2). Prostaglandin E was the only classic eicosanoid shown to suppress IL-2 production, as PGF and PGA were both ineffective. Cyclooxygenase inhibitors increased the production of IL-2 above normal levels, supporting the view that endogenous PGE might modulate the production of IL-2. Prostaglandin also inhibits macrophage IL-1 production (44), probably by interfering with IL-1 expression at a posttranscriptional site (45). Since lymphocyte products are intimately associated with macrophage activation and the initiation of cell-mediated immune mechanisms, regulation of these mononuclear cell-derived mediators might be an important way to regulate chronic inflammation.

Although conventional wisdom has it that increases in cAMP inhibit the mitogen-induced proliferation of lymphocytes (46), it seems clear that cAMP is one of several signals that help *regulate* (47) cell proliferation. Thus, both an increase and subsequent decrease of cAMP are necessary for the initiation of proliferation by lymphocytes exposed to concanavalin A (48). Artificial maintenance of cAMP concentrations (by addition of theophylline) prevents cell proliferation. Further, addition to Swiss 3T3 cells of cAMP or compounds which enhance cellular cAMP induces the proliferation of cells exposed to appropriate stimuli (49). Yoneda and Mundy demonstrated (50) that PGE_1 enhances the mitogen-induced production of osteoclast activation factor by T cells. Stobo and colleagues showed (51) that a population of low-density T lymphocytes exhibit enhanced blastogenic responses to phytohemagglutinin when treated in vitro with PGE. Moreover, the ability of T lymphocytes to adhere to virus-infected cells is enhanced by the addition of PGE_1 in vitro (52) and by the oral administration of PGE to humans (53). Further evidence for a *regulatory* role of PGE on immune responses is supplied by the results of studies which document the selective effects of physiologically relevant concentrations of PGE_2 on human B-cell responses. Thus, PGE_2 suppresses B-cell DNA synthesis and proliferation stimulated by *Staphylococcus aureus*, but has minimal effect on pokeweek mitogen-stimulated B-cell DNA synthesis (54). Further, PGE_2 causes concentration-dependent inhibition of the generation of immunoglobulin-secreting cells from B cells stimulated with *S. aureus* (55).

Several arachidonate metabolites have also been associated with the modulation of macrophage activation and the subsequent expression and/or release of macrophage-derived products. Snyder et al. (56) suggested that eicosanoids can regulate lymphokine-induced expression of I-region associated (Ia) antigens on macrophages. Both PGE_1 and PGE_2 (10^{-9} to 10^{-10} M) reduced by 50% the number of Ia-positive macrophages normally induced by conditioned T-cell media. Addition of thromboxane B_2 antagonized the effect of PGE compounds. The stable analog of PGE_1, 15-methyl-PGE_1, completely suppressed the ability of lymphokine-stimulated cultured granuloma macrophages isolated from pulmonary granulomas to reexpress Ia antigen (57). The same concentration of $PGF_{2\alpha}$ (10^{-7}M) failed to influence reexpression of Ia antigen. Similarly, Steeg et al. (58) demonstrated that partially purified gamma interferon could induce cultured P388D cell line macrophages and thioglycollate-elicited peritoneal macrophages to express Ia antigen and that this expression could be abrogated in a dose-dependent manner by 10^{-10} to 10^{-6} M PGE_2. Whereas PGE compounds suppress macrophage Ia antigen expression, lipoxygenase products, especially the monohydroxyeicosatetraenoic acids, may potentiate the expression of Ia antigens by macrophages in the presence of lymphokine (57).

Studies In Vivo

Adjuvant Arthritis

The release of lysosomal enzymes from synovial cells and invading PMNs engaged in phagocytosis of immune complexes helps initiate and perpetuate inflammation and joint tissue injury in patients with RA (59). The reduction by PGE of endocytosis-induced enzyme release in vitro suggested that PGE might suppress inflammation in vivo. Prostaglandin E_1 and PGE_2 prevent progression of adjuvant-induced arthritis and cartilage destruction in rats (60,61). Cyclic AMP treatment also directly suppresses inflammation in several animal models. Prostaglandin$_{2a}$, F$_{2\alpha}$ which does not increase the cellular levels of cAMP in vitro, does not influence adjuvant arthritis. Furthermore, when doses of theophylline (which maintains cellular cAMP) and PGE$_1$, which singly do not affect adjuvant arthritis, were used together, inflammation and cartilage damage were prevented (62). Although these studies suggest that PGE suppresses adjuvant disease by increasing cAMP levels, the precise mechanisms whereby PGE protects these animals remains unknown. The fact that PGE prevents pannus formation in the animal model (61) suggests an effect on the immune response itself. Since depletion of suppressor T cells exacerbates adjuvant disease (63), PGE may enhance or substitute for T-suppressor activity. In addition, glass-adherent cells from mouse spleen suppress responses to mitogen of nonadherent cells (64). The effect is mimicked by dibutyryl cAMP and PGE$_1$ and blocked by indomethacin, which suggests that mitogen-activated suppressor cells regulate T-cell responses via the production of PGE and subsequent increases in cAMP.

Murine Lupus

The F$_1$ hybrid (NZB/W), which results from the mating of New Zealand Black (NZB) with New Zealand White (NZW) mice, spontaneously develops a disease remarkably similar to SLE in humans, which is characterized by the appearance of antibodies to nuclear antigens and the subsequent development of immune complex-mediated glomerulonephritis. The immune defect in these animals may be characterized as an imbalance in which B-cell activity (humoral antibody responses) is excessive and T-cell activity (cell-mediated immunity) is suppressed. Because of the evidence suggesting that PGE can enhance T-cell activity and suppress B-cell function, it was considered that PGE might prove useful in the treatment of NZB/W mice (murine lupus). When animals were treated with pharmacological doses of PGE$_1$, they were protected against the development of anemia, nephritis, and death. Treatment prevented the glomerular deposition of immunoglobulins and complement (monitored by immunofluorescence), and the development of the proliferative glomerulonephritis characteristic of untreated NZB/W mice (65,66). Both male and female mice benefitted from PGE$_1$ therapy. The protective effect of PGE$_1$ in the treatment of NZB/W mice has been confirmed in several laboratories (67-70).

It was subsequently shown (71) that PGE$_1$ treatment of female NZB/W mice with established nephritis (beginning at 23-27 weeks of age) prevents the progression of renal disease and prolongs survival significantly. Review of the kidney histology in these studies indicates that PGE$_1$ treatment stabilizes the histopathological changes; i.e., there was neither progression nor regression of the renal lesion during the 6-month treatment period. Small doses (4.0 μg SC twice daily) of the stable derivative 15-MPGE$_1$ can also retard progression of murine lupus when treatment is begun after disease is established (72).

The reasons for the beneficial effects of PGE$_1$ treatment of murine lupus are not known. T-Cell proportions decrease with age in NZB/W mice, and there appears to be a specific loss of suppressor T cells and decreased spleen cell responsiveness to T-cell mitogens. Prostaglandin$_1$ E$_1$ treatment maintains an appropriate balance of T- and B-cell concentrations and preserves spleen cell responses to several mitogens, which may be one of the mechanisms by which PGE$_1$ alters the course of murine lupus (73). Female NZB/W mice 3 months of age or older do not respond with a delayed hypersensitivity reaction to DNA injected intradermally and their lymphocytes do not produce migration inhibitory factor (MIF) when stimulated with DNA in vitro. Prostaglandin$_1$ E$_1$ treatment (200 µg twice daily for 2-12 weeks) induces these cell-mediated immune responses (74). Treated mice exhibit delayed hypersensitivity skin reactions to DNA, and spleen cell cultures from a majority of treated animals release MIF following exposure to DNA. These studies further indicate that PGE$_1$ treatment of NZB/W mice allows the expression of absent or suppressed cell-mediated responses. In addition, in a study (75) using the enzyme terminal deoxynucleotidyl transferase (Tdt; polymerizes DNA without template direction and is ordinarily restricted to primitive lymphoid cells) to identify pre-T cells, it was shown that PGE$_1$ treatment of NZB/W mice could reverse abnormalities in the differentiation of early lymphoid cells. In addition, short-term treatment (1-5 days) of NZB/W mice with PGE$_1$ increases thymocyte responsiveness to mitogens and alloantigens. Prostaglandin$_1$ appears to have little or no effect on the medullary fraction of mature thymocytes. Rather, the data suggest that PGE$_1$ increased functional maturity of immature cortical thymocytes (76).

It would be simplistic to consider that PGE$_1$ is replacement therapy (that was thought to be the mechanism for the dramatic effects of corticosteroids on the symptoms of rheumatoid arthritis when cortisone was first used 40 years ago). Nonetheless, peritoneal macrophages from NZB/W mice spontaneously produce less PGE than peritoneal macrophages from immunologically normal mice. Reduced PGE synthesis is seen as early as 2 months and becomes more profound as disease progresses (77).

However, PGE$_1$ exerts its striking protective effect despite the fact that treatment does not alter the final level of circulating antibodies to native DNA. It is of interest that PGE$_1$ treatment *delays* the development of significant levels of antiDNA antibodies from the usual 18-24 weeks to 35-44 weeks of age. The delay in treated mice coincides with a delayed increase in spleen B-cell numbers (73) and may indicate the direct elimination or inhibition of a specific clone of B cells. Indeed, PGE$_1$ treatment of mice appears to reduce lymphopoiesis (78). That PGE$_1$ treatment can have *selective* effects on immune responses is suggested by the fascinating observations of Izui and colleagues (68): An important antigen-antibody system in NZB/W mice includes the major envelope glycoprotein, gp70, of endogenous retroviruses and the corresponding antibody. Large amounts of both are deposited with complement in diseased glomeruli, and circulate as immune complexes. NZB/W mice treated with PGE$_1$ have far lower levels than untreated controls of circulating gp70 immune complexes (68). MRL/1 mice responded similarly, but BXSB mice (a strain in which males are more susceptible to disease) had high levels of circulating gp70 immune complexes and did not benefit from PGE$_1$ treatment. It appeared most likely that PGE$_1$ treatment did not change antigen formation or quantity. Rather, treatment seemed to selectively inhibit the humoral response to xenotropic viral gp70. In MRL/1 mice, PGE$_1$ suppresses immunoglobulin G$_1$ (IgG$_1$) antibody and does not affect IgG$_2$ production. Since IgG$_2$ is the major subclass of antiDNA antibodies in these animals, this may be why antiDNA antibody levels are not reduced by PGE$_1$ treatment.

In light of these observations in animals, it is of interest that the continuous intravenous infusion of PGE$_1$ improved renal function in patients with chronic glomerulonephritis (79) and with rapidly progressive glomerulonephritis (80). In addition, PGE$_1$ infusion suppressed dermal vasculitis in patients who had not responded to more traditional therapy (81).

Hypersensitivity and Foreign Body-Type Granulomatous Inflammation

The effect of systemically administered prostaglandins has been examined on the development of hypersensitivity and foreign body-type granulomas in mice (82). Foreign body-type granulomas were induced in mice by the embolization of Sephadex beads, whereas the hypersensitivity or immune granuloma was generated by the embolization of *Schistosoma mansoni* eggs. The hypersensitivity granuloma is a well-established model of cell-mediated immune reactions, whose development and modulation involve helper/effector and suppressor T-lymphocyte subsets (83). By employing these models and allowing granulomas to develop in a synchronous phase, the immunoregulating role of several arachidonate metabolites could be examined on the initiation, maintenance, and resolution of chronic lesions. The granuloma size around embolized schistosome eggs increases linearly over a 16-day study period. In 15-methyl-PGE_1-treated animals, hypersensitivity granulomas are dramatically suppressed, reaching a mean area by day 16 postchallenge of only 30% that of the control. In contrast, immune granuloma development in PGF_2-treated animals is augmented at days 4 and 8 postchallenge by 60 and 39%, respectively. The most striking evidence that the two prostaglandins manipulate an immune component of the hypersensitivity lesion stems from studies examining the development of foreign body-type granuloma in the treated mice. Neither 15-methyl-PGE_1 nor PGF_2 affected the proliferative response of the granuloma to the less immunogenic polysaccharide bead, Sephadex. The fact that the hypersensitivity-type granuloma lesion was suppressed, whereas the nonspecific foreign body granuloma was not is most likely related to a difference in lymphocyte involvement. The hypersensitivity lesion is a response to a natural granuloma-inducing nidus that results in highly active T cells, whereas the response to the foreign body granuloma lacks specific T-lymphocyte sensitization. In the hypersensitivity granuloma, as in all cell-mediated immune responses, lymphocytes are necessary (84). Thus, PGE-induced alterations in lymphocyte numbers and function were studied. As the normal hypersensitivity lung lesions developed over the 16-day study period, total spleen cells increased. In contrast, splenic lymphocytes did not increase in 15-methyl-PGE_1-treated animals. In control animals, the percentage of splenic T lymphocytes remained constant over the 16-day study period, wherreas B lymphocytes increased modestly. In those animals treated with PGF_2, a general decrease in total T lymphocytes was found, but the B-cell percentage increased. Treatment with PGE_1 decreased B lymphocytes dramatically and increased total T lymphocytes. These observations are similar to those made in NZB/W mice treated with PGE (73). In an effort to examine the means whereby eicosanoids modulate the development of the granuloma, a series of lymphocyte sensitization/transfer experiments were performed. Experiments were designed to determine whether PGE treatment affected granuloma development via the induction or elicitation arm of the immune system: Spleen cells from donor mice sensitized by schistosome egg challenge were adoptively transferred to naive mice, pulmonary granulomas induced, and the animals treated with $15MPGE_1$. The adoptively transferred, sensitized lymphocytes did enhance the normal granulomatous response, whereas the response in the $15MPGE_1$-treated animals was suppressed. Prostaglandin treatment was also shown to influence the induction of immunoreactive lymphocytes: In this study, spleen cells recovered from mice that received schistosome eggs and PGE treatment were transferred to normal mice and examined for their ability to alter the normal development of the granuloma. As previously observed, spleen cells from the untreated sensitized donor gave an enhanced inflammatory response, whereas spleen cells from 15MPGE$_1$-treated donors significantly suppressed the ability to adoptively transfer this delayed-type hypersensitivity response.

The in vivo kinetics of Ia antigen expression by granulomatous macrophages isolated from synchronous pulmonary lesions in treated and untreated animals were studied. The percentage of granuloma macrophages isolated from control mice expressing Ia antigen increased significantly during the 16-day study period. Animals receiving exogenous PGF$_{2\alpha}$ demonstrated an increase in the percentage of granuloma macrophages expressing Ia antigen when examined during the early development of the granuloma. The percentage of Ia antigen-positive granuloma macrophages were shown to increase by 46% at day 4. In contrast, the expression of Ia antigen by granuloma macrophages isolated from 15MPGE$_1$-treated animals was suppressed by approximately 70%. This paralleled the cellular infiltrate observed as the synchronous lesions developed in animals on various treatment protocols. The suppression of Ia antigen-bearing granuloma macrophages by exogenous 15MPGE$_1$ was found to be dose dependent, with as little as 15 μg/kg resulting in the suppression of Ia antigen. Since PGE acts therapeutically in rats with established adjuvant arthritis and in NZB/W mice with established nephritis, it was of interest to assess the effect of 15 MPGE$_1$ on *preformed* hypersensitivity lesions. Pulmonary granulomas were allowed to develop in mice for 8 days before eicosanoid therapy was initiated. This protocol allowed for the vigorous development of the immune response before treatment. Treatment with 15 MPGE$_1$ resulted in an involution of the normal response. In addition, the percentage of Ia antigen-positive granuloma macrophages isolated from these animals was significantly suppressed, reaching a mean of only 30% of the control value at day 16. Treatment with PGF$_{2\alpha}$ did not result in a significant therapeutic effect. These observations demonstrate that certain eicosanoids can arrest ongoing cell-mediated immune reactions.

DIETARY MANIPULATION OF ENDOGENOUS PROSTAGLANDINS

Arachidonic acid is the major fatty acid substrate for cyclooxygenase and lipoxygenase in cells from individuals on standard Western diets. An approach to the modulation of the generation and activities of eicosanoids is to provide substrates alternative to arachidonate for oxidative metabolism. Modification of the tissue fatty acid composition has in fact been shown to affect the synthesis of eicosanoids derived from arachidonic acid as well as to lead to the generation of compounds derived from fatty acids other than arachidonic acid (85). An example of this kind of manipulation is that of essential fatty acid deficiency in which deprivation of linoleic acid leads to a deficiency of arachidonic acid and the impairment of prostaglandin synthesis. Essential fatty acid deficiency causes many pathological changes, but it also reduces the severity of inflammatory reactions in experimental animals (86). It has also been shown that fasting has a salutary effect on the symptoms of patients with RA (87), and that dietary energy restriction in mice extends life and enhances immune responsiveness which is associated with decreased PGE$_2$ synthesis (117). Female mice exhibited more basal synthesis of PGE$_2$ per milligram of protein than male mice. Since fasting or the induction of essential fatty acid deficiency are not likely to be popular therapies, it might be more prudent to modify or supplement rather than delete lipid intake.

ANIMAL STUDIES

Early epidemiological studies demonstrated that Greenland Eskimos ingesting a diet in which the lipids are largely derived from marine sources rich in n-3 fatty acids incorporate large quantities of n-3 fatty acids in their tissues. The ability of dietary lipids to alter the formation of prostaglandins suggested that the modification of dietary lipids might have beneficial effects on inflammatory and autoimmune diseases. The concept was supported by observations of a striking beneficial effect by dietary marine lipids, given as menhaden fish oil, on autoimmune glomerulonephritis in NZB/W F_1 hybrid mice (88) and MRL/1pr mice (89), which are models for lupus nephritis. It was also demonstrated (90) that both pure eicosapentaenoic acid (EPA) and docosahexaenoic acid (DHA) are capable of protecting NZB/W mice from the development of nephritis to the same extent as whole fish oil preparations. However, dietary marine lipids do not suppress all experimental autoimmune processes nor all inflammatory reactions in general. This was shown in studies (91) of the induction of inflammatory arthritis by immunization of rats with type II collagen. The incidence of arthritis was approximately 50% in control rats, whereas in animals receiving dietary marine lipids, the incidence of disease was 85%. Despite the increased incidence, the severity and course of the arthritis was similar in dietary and control groups. In a mouse model of type II collagen-induced arthritis, fish oil did suppress the incidence of arthritis in female mice (92). Under certain conditions, dietary marine lipids also alter antibody formation (93). Fish oil-fed rats immunized with egg albumin produced four- to eight-fold greater titers of both IgE and IgG anti-egg albumin antibodies than beef tallow-fed control animals. This led to an enhanced Arthus reaction to egg albumin in fish oil-fed animals compared to the beef tallow-fed controls. It also has been reported (94) that casein-induced amyloidosis in mice is alleviated by marine lipid diets.

The mechanisms for the modification of immune and inflammatory reactions by dietary marine lipids are not completely understood. It was recognized from early work that these lipids impaired the synthesis of thromboxane A_2 by human platelets. These results indicate that incorporation of n-3 fatty acids into tissue impairs the utilization of arachidonate by cyclooxygenase and this inhibitory effect of marine lipids has been demonstrated in several tissues in experimental systems. It has also been shown that marine lipid diets reduce the formation of leukotrienes in inflammatory exudates and by stimulated leukocytes. It appears that EPA is a good substrate for lipoxygenases. Sulfadopeptide leukotriene generation in an immune complex reaction in rat peritoneal cavities was not significantly altered by fish oil feeding, but the sulfadopeptide leukotrienes derived from arachidonate were reduced and replaced in part by sulfadopeptide leukotrienes derived from EPA. Substitution of the less active LTB_5 for LTB_4 would be expected to have an anti-inflammatory effect.

Certain plant seed oils are enriched in γ-linolenic acid (γLA), which can be converted to dihomo-γ-linolenic acid (D-γ-LA) and then to monoenoic eicosanoids such as PGE_1 and thromboxane A_1 (TxA_1). The 5 desaturase enzyme which converts D-γ-LA to arachidonic acid (AA) is far less active in man than in rodents (95). Thus, the potential for D-γ-LA to be converted to PGE_1 (rather than PGE_2) is even greater in humans than animals. Although the biological activities of corresponding members of the monoenoic and dienoic series are in many cases qualitatively similar, they differ markedly in others. For example, PGE_1 inhibits and PGE_2 does not influence the aggregation of human platelets in vitro, and TxA_1 is less active than TxA_2 in eliciting vasoconstriction and platelet aggregation. Further, PGE_1 is more potent than PGE_2 in its ability to increase cellular cAMP (96), an action, which as noted, limits leukocyte effector function in humans and inflammation and tissue injury in animal models. Differences in the biological effects of fatty acid precursors for these PGEs have also been noted in vivo and in vitro. Arachidonic acid, precursor for PGE_2, induces platelet aggregation, whereas D-γ-LA, precursor for PGE_1, inhibits platelet aggregation in humans (97). The administration of plant seed oil containing 9% γ-LA suppresses adjuvant arthritis in rats (98) and γ-LA enrichment of the diet reduces inflammation in a unique animal model—the rat subcutaneous air pouch—that serves as a synovial cavity substitute (99).

The synovial pannus found in the joints of patients with rheumatoid arthritis is an inflammatory and invasive aggregation of connective tissue, small blood vessels, hyperplastic synovial cells, lymphocytes, plasma cells, and macrophages (100). It is much like a nonmetastatic tumor, and is likely responsible in large part for the irreversible destruction of joints seen in many rheumatoid arthritis patients. That pannus is an aggressive tissue is borne out by the cartilage and bone damage it appears to cause in rheumatoid arthritis patients and by the observations that the rheumatoid synovium can invade primary cultures of autologous tendon slices and can grow upon, invade, and destroy several layers of sterile rat gut in vitro. The cause of rheumatoid arthritis is unknown and the reasons why cells invade the synovium and synovial cells proliferate in rheumatoid arthritis patients have not been defined. Experimental evidence does indicate that products exported by monocytes, macrophages, lymphocytes, and platelets help regulate synovial cell proliferation (101).

Synovial fibroblasts from rheumatoid arthritis patients have some characteristics similar to cells which have been exposed to tumor-promoting agents. Combined epidemiological and experimental evidence supports the importance of fatty acids in tumor growth, although the precise relationships are not clear. Thus, fatty acids and eicosanoids have varying effects in vitro and in animals studies depending on the doses used and the tumor type studied. The accumulated experimental evidence indicates that fatty acids and eicosanoids can regulate tumor growth (102). Addition of D-γ-LA to human synovial cells in culture reduces PGE_2, increases PGE_1, and restrains interleukin 1-stimulated cell growth (103). The antiproliferative effect of D-γ-LA is in large part prevented by the addition to cells of indomethacin. However, fatty acids themselves, exclusive of their eicosanoid metabolites, are able to influence cell function (104). Thus, some of the effects of these precursor fatty acids on cell function and immune/inflammatory responses probably are caused directly by modifications in the membrane lipid composition rather than changes in eicosanoid production. For example, D-γ-LA suppresses the interleukin 2 production of human peripheral blood mononuclear cells in vitro (105), suppresses the proliferation of interleukin 2-dependent T lymphocytes, and reduces the expression of activation markers on T lymphocytes (106) directly, in a manner which is independent of conversion to prostaglandins. The observations indicate that fatty acids can modulate immune responses by acting directly on T cells, and suggest that alteration of cellular fatty acids may be a worthwhile approach to the control of inflammation.

STUDIES IN HUMANS

Studies in human volunteers ingesting a fish oil supplement demonstrated a reduction in the release of arachidonic acid from peripheral blood neutrophils (107). Leukotriene B_4 synthesis by stimulated neutrophils was reduced by nearly 60% and adherence of neutrophils to endothelial cell monolayers in tissue culture was markedly inhibited in individuals taking dietary supplements (approximately 5 g/day n-3 fatty acids; Eskimos ingest 5-10 g/day of n-3 fatty acids throughout their lifetime). All of these effects would be expected to contribute to an anti-inflammatory action by marine lipids. Three separate placebo-controlled studies in which patients with RA were treated with fish oil supplements indicate that the marine lipid has modest but significant anti-inflammatory effects (107-109). In addition, the synthesis of 5-lipoxygenase products, including LTB_4, is reduced by peripheral blood leukocytes harvested from these patients and stimulated in vitro (109-110). In another study (111), the production by peripheral blood monocytes of a lipid mediator of inflammation, platelet-activating factor, was reduced significantly in patients treated with fish oil supplements. A study done in England, however, failed to show a beneficial effect from fish oil supplements in patients with RA (112). In the most detailed clinical trial (109), a daily supplement of 2.7 g EPA and 1.8 g of DHA (15 capsules daily) was given to 21 patients with RA; 19 patients began the study with identical-appearing placebos. The background diet of the patients was unchanged. The therapeutic regimens were switched at the end of 14 weeks, after a 4-week washout period. At the end of the study, those patients who took the lipid supplement showed an improvement in mean time to onset of fatigue by 156 min, and the number of tender joints decreased by 3.5. Although the responses were modest, the beneficial effects of the fish oil supplementation were seen even after the 4-week washout period. Thus, the design of the study probably masks some of the beneficial effects of fish oil therapy, since patients given placebo after the fish oil would have had the effects of the fish oil treatment during the placebo period. In addition, the decrease in the number of tender joints correlated with neutrophil LTB_4 production; that is, the reduction in LTB_4 generation by neutrophils was greatest in patients who had the best clinical responses. The authors conclude that fish oil supplements are well tolerated and influence inflammation and disease activity in patients with RA, and they suggest that increasing the daily dosage might improve disease activity even more. Such studies are being undertaken now. Thus, although the results of these studies are not dramatic, they do generate some encouragement.

As noted, fish oil supplements do result in a dramatic alleviation of autoimmune glomerulonephritis in inbred strains of mice. Because of the experimental findings, a trial of dietary marine lipids was carried out in patients with mild SLE, and reported in preliminary form (113). In the 1-year study, no significant protective effects of dietary marine lipid supplements were observed compared to patients receiving placebo. A possible explanation for the differences in the response of murine lupus and human lupus to supplements of fish oil is that the quantity of marine lipids ingested during the clinical trials was insufficient. It is possible that marine lipid preparations containing higher quantities of the n-3 fatty acids might be more effective.

As mentioned, plant seed oils enriched in γ-LA have been shown to suppress inflammation and joint tissue injury in animal models. Some experience is available from human studies also. A placebo-controlled study from Denmark (114) indicated that 20 patients given a γ-LA supplement (360 mg/day), in the form of primrose seed oil, for 12 weeks received no benefit from such therapy. It is of interest that although only three patients improved clinically, all but two of the remaining patients were able to complete the study without resorting to other monosteroidal anti-inflammatory drugs (NSAIDs). Thus, although the study was considered to be "negative," the results suggested that the γ-LA supplement might substitute for NSAID treatment. In a double-blind placebo-controlled study done in Glasgow, Scotland (115), 16 patients with RA received 540 mg/day of γ-LA as primrose seed oil and 15 patients received 450 mg/day γ-LA and 240 mg/day of eicosapentaenoic acid. Patients took four capsules three times daily for 1 year. Patients were kept on their usual dose of NSAIDs and their physicians were allowed to alter the dose according to clinical responses. Patients did not exhibit changes in objective measures of their disease activity, but over 90% of patients in the treatment groups felt subjective improvement in their condition at 12 months, at which time 50% of treated patients had either stopped or reduced substantially the NSAID dose. In a preliminary study (116) designed to investigate the effect of a γ-LA supplement on leukocyte function, PGE_2 and LTB_4 production by stimulated leukocytes was reduced markedly, and six of seven RA patients appeared to respond favorably over a 12-week period to treatment with 1.1 g/day of γ-LA in the form of borage seed oil (nine capsules daily); the study was open and not placebo controlled. Unlike the other studies done with smaller doses of γ-LA, RA patients given borage seed oil did exhibit reductoins in the duration of painful morning stiffness and the number of tender, swollen joints. It is possible that the lack of placebo control is responsible for these results; the larger dose of γ-LA used in the study may help explain the apparent favorable responses.

Clinical trials done to date indicate that the oils can be given without adverse effects. However, experience teaches that the longer a given therapy is utilized, the greater the incidence of adverse effects. Certain potential pitfalls must be understood. Although Greenland Eskimos have a low incidence of acute myocardial infarction, they have a relatively high incidence of death due to cerebral hemorrhage. Whether or not this is due to the altered eicosanoid profile in their cells is not clear. It is clear that Eskimos are probably not protected from coronary artery disease simply because of their high intake of EPA and DHA. Greenland Eskimos also have low concentrations in their cells of arachidonic acid, which do not increase appreciably when they eat a traditional Western diet, and which causes EPA proportions in their cells to drop substantially. Other unknown factors, perhaps including impaired delta-5-desaturase activity, surely play a role in protecting the Eskimo population from coronary artery disease. Because ingestion of large amounts of n-3 fatty acids can prolong the bleeding time, there has been concern about spontaneous or excessive bleeding during surgery or as a result of trauma in people taking these supplements. Bleeding has not been observed during clinical trials with fish oil supplements so far, and the increase in bleeding time is similar to that produced by the ingestion of therapeutic doses of aspirin.

Supplementation of diet with long-chain polyunsaturated fatty acids increases the likelihood of lipid peroxidation with its associated toxic effects on cells. It is not known whether an increased requirement for an antioxidant (such as vitamins E and C) accompanies an increased ingestion of long-chain n-3 and n-6 unsaturated fatty acids. Further, because these novel fatty acids can reduce inflammatory and immune responses, the question arises as to whether these supplements can supress the immune system below its normal level of competence. Susceptibility to infection has not been observed as yet, but this must be considered a potential adverse effect.

As noted, there are theoretical reasons for suggesting that the alteration of dietary essential fatty acids may produce anti-inflammatory effects similar to the NSAIDs now in use. In fact, further benefits might derive from suppression of leukotriene production, an effect not seen with most NSAIDs. In addition, fewer gastric side effects might be expected, since other less inflammatory prostaglandins, especially those of the E series, might be available for the protection of gastric mucosa cells. It is possible that larger doses of the oils than used so far may be more beneficial, and it is certain that it will be necessary to treat patients in a controlled manner for a much longer time. It must never be forgotten that RA is a disease characterized by remissions and relapses and that establishment of long-term, multicenter, placebo-controlled studies of large numbers of patients is the only way to determine whether or not any form of therapy is useful to RA patients. Careful clinical studies based on thoughtful scientific findings must be developed in order to separate sense from nonsense in the field of dietary therapy.

REFERENCES

1. Vane JR (1976). Prostaglandins as mediators of inflammation. In: Advances in Prostaglandin and Thromboxane Research. B. Samuelsson and R. Paoletti eds. Raven Press, New York, p 791.
2. Kunkel SL, Chensue SW (1983). Prostaglandins and the regulation of immune responses. Adv Inflamm Res 7:93.
3. Dale HH (1929). Some chemical factors in the control of the circulation. Lancet 1:1285.
4. Ferreira SH (1972). Prostaglandins, aspirin like drugs and analgesia. Nature New Biol 240:200.
5. Zurier RB (1982). Prostaglandins, immune responses and murine lupus. Arthritis Rheum 25:804.
6. Hedqvist P (1970). Studies on the effect of prostaglandins E_1 and E_2 on the sympathetic neuromuscular transmission in some animal tissues. Acta Physiol Scand 345(Suppl 79):1.
7. Robert A, Nezamis JE, Lancaster C, Hanchar AJ (1979). Cytoprotection by prostaglandins in rats. Prevention of gastric necrosis produced by alcohol, HCl, NaOH, hypertonic NaCl, and thermal injury. Gastroenterology 77:433.
8. Kloeze J (1967). Influence of prostaglandins on platelet adhesiveness and platelet aggregation. In: Prostaglandins, Proceedings of the II Nobel Symposium, 1966, S. Bergstrom and B. Samuelsson, eds. Interscience, London, p 271.
9. Foreman JC, Hallett MD, Mongard JL (1977). The relationship between histamine secretion and ^{45}calcium uptake by mast cells. J Physiol 271:193.
10. Lichtenstein LM, DiBarnardo R (1971). The immediate allergic response: In vitro action of cyclic AMP and other drugs on the two stages of histamine release. J Immunol 107:1131.
11. Marone G, Thomas LL, Lichtenstein LM (1980). The role of agonists that activate adenylate cyclase in the control of cAMP metabolism and enzyme release by human polymorphonuclear leucocytes. J Immunol 125:2277.
12. Rivkin I, Rosenblatt J, Becker EL (1975). The role of cyclic AMP in the chemotactic responsiveness and spontaneous motility of rabbit peritoneal neutrophils. *J Immunol* 115:1126.
13. Zurier RB, Weissman G, Hoffstein S, Kammerman S, Tai HH (1974). Mechanisms of lysosomal enzyme release from human leucocytes. J Clin Invest 53:297.

14. Lehmeyer JE, Johnston RB Jr (1978). Effect of antiinflammatory drugs and agents that elevate intracellular cyclic AMP on the release of toxic oxygen metabolites by phagocytes: Studies in a model of tissue-bound IgG. Clin Immunol Immunopathol 9:482.
15. Goodwin JS, Kaszubowski PA, Williams RC (1979). Cyclic adenosine monophosphate response to prostaglandin E_2 on subpopulations of human lymphocytes. J Exp Med 150: 1260.
16. Goto T, Herberman RB, Maluish A, Strong DM (1983). Cyclic AMP as a mediator of prostaglandin E-induced suppression of human natural killer cell activity. J Immunol 130:1350.
17. Katz P, Zaytoun AM, Fauci AJ (1982). Mechanisms of cell mediated cytotoxicity. I. Modulation of natural killer cell activity by cyclic nucleotides. J Immunol 129:287.
18. Ham EA, Soderman DD, Zanetti ME, Dougherty HW, McCaulcy E, Kuehl FA (1983). Inhibition by prostaglandins of leukotriene B_4 release from activated neutrophils. Proc Natl Acad Sci USA 80:4349.
19. Samuelsson B (1983). Leukotrienes: Mediators of immediate hypersensitivity reactions and inflammation. Science 220:568.
20. Bryant RE, Sutcliffe MC (1974). The effect of 3'5'-adenosine monophosphate on granulocyte adhesion. J Clin Invest 54:1241.
21. Boxer LA, Allen JM, Schmidt M, Yoder M, Baehner RL (1980). Inhibition of polymorphonuclear leukocyte adherence by prostacyclin. J Lab Clin Med 95:672.
22. Serhan CN, Radin A, Smolen JE, Weissman G (1982). Leukotriene B_4 is a complete secretagogue in human neutrophils: A kinetic analysis. Biochem Biophys Res Commun 107: 1006.
23. Cotran RS, Majno G (1964). A light and electron microscopic analysis of vascular injury. Ann NY Acad Sci 116:750.
24. Fantone JC, Kunkel SL, Ward PA, Zurier RB (1980). Suppression by prostaglandin E_1 of vascular permeability induced by vasoactive mediators. J Immunol 125:2591.
25. DiRosa M, Groud JP, Willoughby DA (1971). Studies of the mediators of the acute inflammatory response induced in rats in different sites by carrageenin and turpentine. J Pathol 104:15.
26. Bonta IL, Parnham MJ (1975). Time dependent stimulatory and inhibitory effects of prostaglandin E_1 on exudative and tissue components of granulomatous inflammation in rats. B J Pharmacol 65:465.
27. Zurier RB, Hoffstein S, Weissman G (1973). Suppression of acute and chronic inflammation in adrenalectomized rats by pharmacologic amounts of prostaglandins. Arthritis Rheum 16:606.
28. Robak J, Trakka EK, Daniel Z (1980). The influence of three prostaglandin biosynthesis stimulators on carrageenin induced edema of rat paw. Biochem Pharm 29:1863.
29. Fantone JC, Kunkel SL, Weingarten B (1982). Inhibition of carrageenin-induced rat footpad edema by systemic treatment with prostaglandins of the E series. Biochem Pharmacol 31:3126.
30. Kunkel SL, Thrall RS, McCormick JR, Ward PA, Zurier RB (1979). Suppression of immune complex vasculitis in rats by prostaglandins. J Clin Invest 64:1525.
31. Kunkel SL, Zanetti M, Sapin C (1982). Suppression of nephrotoxic serum nephritis in rats by prostaglandin E_1. Am J Pathol 108:240.
32. Kravis T, Zvaifler N (1974). Alteration of rabbit PCA reaction by drugs known to influence intracellular cyclic AMP. J Immunol 113:244.
33. Camussi G, Bussolino F, Tetta C, Caligariscappio F, Coda R, Macchiorlatti E, Alberton M, Roffinello C, Segoloni G (1983). Effect of prostacyclin (PGI_2) on immune-complex-induced neutropenia. Immunology 48:625.
34. Camussi G, Tetta C, Bussolino F (1983). Inhibitory effect of prostacyclin (PGI_2) on neutropenia induced by intravenous injection of platelet-activating-factor (PAF) in the rabbit. Prostaglandins 25:343.

35. Hirose T, Aoki E, Domae M, Masayoshi I, Ikeda T, Tanaka K (1983). The effect of prostacyclin infusion on increased pulmonary vascular permeability following microembolization in dogs. Prostaglandins Leukotrienes Med 11:51.
36. Johnson A, Malik AB (1982). Pulmonary edema after glass bead microembolization: Protective effect of granulocytopenia. J Appl Physiol Respir Environ Exer Physiol 52: 155.
37. Fletcher JR, Ramwell PW (1980). The effects of prostacyclin (PGI_2) on endotoxin shock and endotoxin-induced platelet aggregation in dogs. Circ Shock 7:299.
38. Campo A, Kim Y, Azar SH, Vernier RL, Michael AF (1983). Prevention of the generalized Schwartzman reaction in pregnant rats by prostacyclin infusion. Lab Invest 48:705.
39. Henney CS, Bourne HR, Lichtenstein LM (1971). The role of cyclic AMP in the specific cytolytic activity of lymphocytes. J Immunol 108:1526.
40. Gordon D, Bray MA, Morley J (1976). Control of lymphokine secretion by prostaglandins Nature 262:401.
41. Bray MA, Gordon D, Morley J (1978). Prostaglandins as regulators in cellular immunity. Prostaglandin Med 1:183.
42. Rappaport RS, Dodge GR (1982). Prostaglandin E inhibits the production of human interleukin 2. J Exp Med 155:943.
43. Baker PE, Fahey JV, Munck A (1982). Prostaglandin inhibition of T cell proliferation is mediated at two levels. Cell Immunol 61:52.
44. Kunkel SL, Chensue SW, Phan SH (1986). Prostaglandins as endogenous mediators of interleukin 1 production. J Immunol 136:186.
45. Knudsen PJ, Dinarello CA, Strom TB (1986). Prostaglandins posttranscriptionally inhibit monocyte expression of interleukin 1 activity by increasing intracellular cyclic adenosine monophosphate. J Immunol 137:3189.
46. Goodwin JS, Webb DR (1980). Regulation of immune responses by prostaglandins. Clin Immunol Immunopathol 15:106.
47. Rozengurt E (1986). Early signals in the mitogenic response. Science 234:161.
48. Wang T, Sheppard JR, Foker JE (1978). Rose and fall of cyclic AMP required for onset of lymphocyte DNA synthesis. Science 201:155.
49. Rozengurt E, Legg A, Strang G, Courtenay-Luck N (1981). Cyclic AMP: A mitogenic signal for Swiss 3T3 cells. Proc Natl Acad Sci USA 78:4392.
50. Yoneda T, Mundy GR (1979). Monocytes regulate osteoclast activating factoir production by releasing prostaglandins. J Exp Med 150:338.
51. Stobo JD, Kennedy MS, Goldyne ME (1979). Prostaglandin E modulation of the mitogenic response of human T cells. J Clin Invest 64:1188.
52. Zurier RB, Dore-Duffy P, Viola MV (1977). Adherence of human peripheral blood lymphocytes to measles infected cells. Enhancement by prostaglandin E_1. N Engl J Med 296: 1443.
53. Dore-Duffy P, Berube M-L, Siok C, Zurier RB (1984). Oral administration of prostaglandin E_2 to humans: Effects on peripheral blood leucocyte function. J Lab Clin Med 104:283.
54. Thompson PA, Jelinek DF, Lipsky PE (1984). Regulation of human B cell proliferation by prostaglandin E_2. J Immunol 133:2446.
55. Jelinek DF, Thompson PA, Lipsky PE (1985). Regulation of human B cell activation by prostaglandin E_2. Suppression of the generation of immunoglobulin secreting cells. J Clin Invest 75:1339.
56. Snyder DS, Beller DI, Unanue ER (1982). Prostaglandins modulate macrophage Ia expression. Nature 299:163.
57. Kunkel SL, Chensue SW, Plewa M, Higashi G (1984). Macrophage function in the Schistosoma mansoni egg-induced pulmonary granuloma. Role of arachidonic acid metabolites in macrophage Ia antigen expression. Am J Pathol 114:240.

58. Steeg PS, Johnson HM, Oppenheim J (1982). Regulation of murine macrophage Ia antigen expression by an immune interferon-like lymphokine: Inhibitory effect of endotoxin. J Immunol 129:2402.
59. Weissman G (1972). Lysosomal mechanisms of tissue injury in arthritis. N Engl J Med 286:141.
60. Zurier RB, Quagliata F (1971). Effects of prostaglandin E_1 on adjuvant arthritis. Nature 234:304.
61. Zurier RB, Ballas M (1973). Prostaglandin E_1 suppression of adjuvant arthritis: Histopathology. Arthritis Rheum 16:251.
62. Bonta IL, Parnham MJ, van Vliete L (1978). Combination of theophylline and prostaglandin E_1 as inhibitors of the adjuvant induced arthritis syndrome of rats. Ann Rheum Dis 37:212.
63. Kayashima K, Koga T, Onoue K (1976). Role of T lymphocytes in adjuvant arthritis. I. Evidence for the regulatory function of thymus derived cells in induction of the disease. J Immunol 117:1878.
64. Webb DR, Jamieson AT (1976). Control of mitogen induced transformation. Characterization of a splenic suppressor cell and its mode of action. Cell Immunol 24:45.
65. Zurier RB, Damjanov I, Sayadoff DM, Rothfield NR (1977). Prostaglandin E_1 treatment of NZB/NZW mice. II. Prevention of glomerulonephritis. Arthritis Rheum 20:1449.
66. Zurier RB, Sayadoff DM, Torrey SB, Rothfield NR (1977). Prostaglandin E_1 treatment of NZB/NZW mice. I. Prolonged survival of female mice. Arthritis Rheum 20:723.
67. Hurd ER, Johnston JM, Okita JR, MacDonald PC, Ziff M, Gilliam JN (1981). Prevention of glomerulonephritis and prolonged survival in New Zealand Black/New Zealand White F_1 hybrid mice fed an essential fatty acid deficient diet. J Clin Invest 67:476.
68. Izui S, Kelley VE, McConahey A, Dixon FJ (1981). Selective suppression of retroviral gp70-anti-gp70 immune complex formation by prostaglandin E_1 in murine systemic lupus erythematosus. J Exp Med 152:1645.
69. Karmali RA, Hanrahan R, Volkman A, Smith N (1981). Regulation of autoimmunity and development of antibodies to DNA in NZB/W F_1 mice. Prog. Lipid Res. 20:655.
70. Kelley VE, Winkelstein A, Izui S (1979). Effect of prostaglandin E on immune complex nephritis in NZB/W mice. Lab Invest 41:531.
71. Zurier RB, Damjanov I, Miller PL, Biewer BF (1979). Prostaglandin E_1 treatment prevents progression of nephritis in murine lupus erythematosus. J Clin Lab Immunol 2:95.
72. Zurier RB, Gionfriddo M, Miller P (1980). Treatment of NZB/W ("lupus") mice with 15S-15 methyl PGE_1. Prostaglandins Med 4:381.
73. Krakauer KA, Torrey SB, Zurier RB (1978). Prostaglandin E_1 treatment of NZB/W mice. III. Preservation of spleen cell concentrations and mitogen-induced proliferative responses. Clin Immunol Immunopathol 11:256.
74. Adelman N, Ksiazek J, Cohen S, Yoshida T, Zurier RB (1980). Prostaglandin E_1 treatment of NZB/W F_1 hybrids: Induction of in vitro and in vivo cell mediated immune responses to DNA. Clin Immunol Immunopathol 17:353.
75. Whittum J, Goldschneider I, Greiner D, Zurier RB (1985). Developmental abnormalities of terminal deoxynucleotidyl transferase positive bone marrow cells and thymocytes in New Zealand Mice: Effects of prostaglandin E_1. J Immunol 135:272.
76. Whittum-Hudson J, Ballow M, Zurier RB (1989). Effect of PGE_1 treatment on in vitro thymocyte function of normal and autoimmune mice. Immunopharmacol (in press).
77. Dore-Duffy P, Guha A, Rothman BL, Zurier RB (1989). Synthesis of prostaglandin E by peritoneal macrophages from NZB/W mice. Life Sci (in press).
78. Winkelstein A, Kelley VE (1980). The effects of PGE_1 on lymphocytes in NZB/W mice. Clin Immunol Immunopathol 17:212.
79. Niwa T, Maeda K, Nasotuka Y (1982). Improvement of renal function with PGE_1 infusion in patients with chronic renal disease. Lancet 1:687.

80. Niwa T, Maeda K, Asada H, Yamamoto M, Yamada K (1983). Beneficial effects of PGE_1 in rapidly progressive glomerulonephritis. N Engl J Med 308:969.
81. Roberts WN, Hauptman HW, Ruddy S (1989). Reversal of the vasospastic component of lupus vasculopathy by prostaglandin E_1 infusion (abstr). Arthritis Rheum 32:574.
82. Chensue SW, Kunkel SL, Ward PA, Higashi G (1983). Exogenously administered prostaglandins modulate pulmonary granulomas induced by Schistosoma mansoni eggs. Am J Pathol 111:78.
83. Chensue SW, Wellhausen SR, Boros DL (1981). Modulation of granulomatous hypersensitivity. Participation of Ly1+ and Ly2+ T lymphocytes in the suppression of granuloma formation and lymphokine in the suppression of granuloma formation production in *Schistosoma mansoni* infected mice. J Immunol 127:363.
84. Chensue SW, Kunkel SL (1983). Arachidonic acid metabolism and macrophage activation. Clin Lab Med 3:677.
85. Robinson DR (1987). Lipid mediators of inflammation. Clin Rheum Dis NA 13:385.
86. Good RA (1981). Nutrition and immunity. J Clin Immunol 1:3.
87. Hafstrom I, Ringertz B, Gyllenhammar H, Palmblod J, Harms-Ringdahl M (1988). Effects of fasting on disease activity, neutrophil function, fatty acid composition, and leukotriene biosynthesis in patients with rheumatoid arthritis. Arthritis Rheum 31:585.
88. Prickett JD, Robinson DR, Steinberg AD (1983). Effects of dietary enrichment with eicosapentaenoic acid upon autoimmune nephritis in female $NZBxNZW/F_1$ mice. Arthritis Rheum 26:133.
89. Kelley VE, Ferretti A, Izui S, Strom TB (1985). A fish oil diet rich in eicosapentaenoic acid reduces cyclooxygenase metabolites and suppresses lupus in MRL-1pr mice. J Immunol 134:1914.
90. Robinson DR, Tateno S, Patel B (1987). The effects of dietary marine lipids on autoimmune disease. In: Polyunsaturated Fatty Acids and Eicosanoids, W.E.M. Lands, ed. American Oil Chemists' Society, Champaign, Illinois.
91. Prickett JD, Trentham DE, Robinson DR (1984). Dietary fish oil augments the induction of arthritis in rats immunized with type II collagen. J Immunol 132:725.
92. Leslie CA, Gonnerman WA, Ullman MD, Cathcart E (1985). Dietary fish oil modulates macrophage fatty acids and decreases arthritis susceptibility in mice. J Exp Med 162:1336.
93. Prickett JD, Robinson DR, Bloch KJ (1982). Enhanced production of IgE and IgG antibodies associated with a diet enriched in eicosanpentaenoic acid. Immunology 46:819.
94. Cathcart ES, Leslie CA, Meydani SN, Hayes KC (1987). A fish oil diet retards experimental amyloidosis, modulates lymphocyte function, and decreases macrophage arachidonate metabolism in mice. J Immunol 139:1850.
95. Stone KJ, Willis AL, Hart M, Kirtland SJ, Kernoff PBA, McNichols GP (1979). The metabolism of dihomo- -linolenic acid in man. Lipids 14:174.
96. Newcombe DS, Ciosek CP, Ishikawa Y, Fahey JV (1975). Human synoviocytes: Activation and desensitization by prostaglandins and L-epinephrine. Proc Natl Acad Sci USA 72:3124.
97. Willis AL, Comai K, Kuhn DC, Paulsrud J (1974). Dihomo-gamma-linolenate suppresses platelet aggregation when administered in vitro or in vivo. Prostaglandins 8:509.
98. Kunkel SL, Ogawa H, Conran PB, Ward PA, Zurier RB (1981). Suppression of chronic inflammation by evening primrose oil. Prog. Lipid Res 20:885.
99. Tate G, Mandell BF, Schumacher HR, Zurier RB (1986). Suppression of experimental urate crystal (UC) inflammation by prostaglandin E_1 (PGE_1) and dietary manipulation. Arthritis Rheum 29:147 (abstract).
100. Harris ED, Jr (1976). Recent insights into the pathogenesis of the proliferative lesion in rheumatoid arthritis. Arthritis Rheum 19:68.
101. Krane SM, Goldring SR, Dayer J-M (1982). Interactions among lymphocytes, monocytes and synovial cells in the rheumatoid synovium. In: Lymphokines. E. Pick and M. Landy, eds. Academic Press, New York, p 75.

102. Goodwin JS, Ceuppens J (1983). Regulation of the immune response by prostaglandins. J Clin Immunol 3:295.
103. Baker DG, Tate G, Laposata M, Zurier RB (1986). Suppression of human synovial cell proliferation by dihomogamma linolenic acid. Clin Res 34:615A.
104. Meade CJ, Mertin J (1978). Fatty acids and immunity. Adv Lipid Res 16:127.
105. Santoli D, Zurier RB (1989). Prostaglandin E (PGE) precursor fatty acids inhibit human IL-2 production by a PGE-independent mechanism. J Immunol 143:1303.
106. Santoli D, Phillips PD, Colt TL, Zurier RB (1990). Suppression of interleukin-2 dependent human T cell growth by E series prostaglandins (PGE) and their precursor fatty acids: Evidence for a PGE-independent mechanism of inhibition by the fatty acids. J Clin Invest 85:424.
107. Lee TH, Hoover RL, Williams JD (1985). Effect of dietary enrichment with eicosapentaenoic and docosahexaenoic acids on in vitro neutrophil and monocyte leukotriene generation and neutrophil function. N Engl J Med 312:1217.
108. Kremer JM, Biganoette J, Michalek AV (1983). Effects of manipulation of dietary fatty acids on clinical manifestations of rheumatoid arthritis. Lancet 1:184.
109. Kremer JM, Jubiz W, Michalek A, Rynes RI, Bartholomew LE, Biganoette RD, Timchalk M, Beeler D, Lininger L (1987). Fish oil fatty acid supplementation in active rheumatoid arthritis. Ann Int Med 106:497.
110. Kremer JM, Jubiz W (1988). The effect of different doses of fish oil fatty acid ingestion on neutrophil LTB_4 and LTB_5 generation from stimulated neutrophils in normals. Arthritis Rheum 30:S57.
111. Sperling RI, Weinblatt M, Robin J-L, Ravalese J, Hoover RL, House F, Coblyn JS, Fraser PA, Spur BW, Robinson DR, Lewis RA, Austen KF (1987). Effects of dietary supplementation with marine fish oil on leukocyte lipid mediator generation and function in rheumatoid arthritis. Arthritis Rheum. 30:988.
112. Darlington LG, Ramsey NW (1987). Olive oil for rheumatoid patients? Br J Dermatol 26:129.
113. Moore GF, Yarboro C, Sebring NG, Steinberg AD, Robinson DR (1987). Eicosapentaenoic acid in the treatment of SLE. Arthritis Rheum 30:S33.
114. Hansen TM, Lerche A, Kassis V, Lorenzen I, Sondergard J (1983). Treatment of rheumatoid arthritis with PGE_1 precursors cis-linoleic acid and gamma linolenic acid. Scand J Rheumatol 12:85.
115. Belch JJF, Ansell D, Madhok R, O'Dowd A, Sturrock RD (1988). Effects of altering dietary essential fatty acids on requirements for nonsteroidal antiinflammatory drugs in patients with rheumatoid arthritis: A double blind placebo controlled study. Ann Rheum Dis 47:96.
116. Pullman-Mooar S, Laposata M, Lem D, Holman RT, Leventhal LJ, DeMarco D, Zurier RB (1990). Alteration of the cellular fatty acid profile and the production of eicosanoids in human monocytes by gamma linolenic acid. Arthritis Rheum 33:1526.
117. Meydani SN, Lipman R, Blumberg TB, Taylor A (1990). Dietary energy restriction decreases ex vivo spleen prostaglandin E_2 synthesis in Emory mice J Nutr 120:112.

14
Vitamin E and the Immune Response

Simin Nikbin Meydani and Jeffrey B. Blumberg
USDA Human Nutrition Research Center on Aging, Tufts University, Boston, Massachusetts

INTRODUCTION

In the early 1920s, tocopherol (vitamin E), as its Greek name implies, was discovered when it was noticed that rats failed to reproduce when fed a rancid lard diet unless whole wheat was added to the preparation. Subsequently, it was found that the wheat germ oil contained all of the "vitamin" properties of the wheat, and vitamin E was isolated in 1936. Vitamin E is now accepted as the generic term for a group of tocol and tocotrienol derivatives possessing some degree of vitamin activity. The most active compound is α-tocopherol. Although many theories have been proposed to explain the activity of vitamin E, the most widely accepted explanation for its function is that it acts in concert with a number of enzymes, such as gluthathione peroxidase, superoxide dismutase, and catalase, to defend the cell against the damaging effects of oxygen radicals. In this fashion, vitamin E is thought to aid the body in maintaining its normal defenses against disease and environmental insults. Vitamin E deficiency is associated with damage to many cells, particularly muscle, nerve, and red blood cells. It is important to recognize that the qualitative and quantitative effects of vitamin E are dependent upon its interrelationships with selenium, sulfur amino acids, polyunsaturated fatty acids, and the status of other antioxidant defense systems.

There now exists substantial evidence in animals that vitamin E protects against the toxicity of environmental pollutants, reduces the formation of certain carcinogens, decreases thrombosis, and enhances the immune response. However, the degree to which these observations extrapolate directly to clinically relevant therapeutic applications is not well established. Nonetheless, it is of great interest to note that in experimental models almost every aspect of the immune system, including resistance to infection, specific antibody responses, splenic plaque-forming cells, in vitro mitogenic responses of lymphocytes, reticuloendothelial system clearance, and phagocytic index, have been shown to be altered by vitamin E deficiency and enhanced by increases in tocopherol intake.

THE ROLE OF VITAMIN E IN IMMUNE FUNCTION: ANIMAL STUDIES

Laboratory Animal Studies

Studies in different species of experimental animals using deficient as well as higher than recommended levels of vitamin E indicate that tocopherol is involved in the maintenance of the immune function. Segagni (1955) reported that vitamin E-supplemented rabbits produced antibodies earlier to typhoid vaccine, *Staphylococcus*, and O-streptolysin than those fed control diets, although no difference in peak antibody level was found between the two groups. Similar results in rabbits were later reported by Solano (1957) using *Vibrio cholerae*, *Salmonella typhi*, and heterologous erythrocyte vaccines. Tengerdy et al. (1973) showed that vitamin E-deficient mice had lower plaque-forming cells (PFC) and hemagglutination (HA) titer in response to sheep red blood cell (SRBC) injection than mice fed a sufficient amount of vitamin E. Supplementation with additional amounts of vitamin E further increased both PFC and HA. The adverse effect of vitamin E deficiency on humoral immunity was restored to normal by vitamin E supplementation but not by the synthetic antioxidant N,N-diphenyl-p-phenylenediamine (DPPD). Later, Tengerdy et al. (1978) reported that vitamin E supplementation (150-300 mg/kg) of chickens fed a commercial stock diet (43 mg/kg of vitamin E) increased survival against *Escherichia coli* infection. The increased protection correlated with elevated HA titer and a faster clearance of *E. coli* from the blood. Similar results were obtained when chickens were immunized with SRBCs. In mice, vitamin E supplementation (120-360 mg/kg) significantly increased percent survival against infection with *Diplococcus pneumoniae* type I (Heinzerling et al. 1974). Tengerdy et al. (1984) demonstrated that the immunostimulatory effect of vitamin E is due in part to its inhibition of prostaglandin (PG) synthesis in bursa and spleen. We have also observed that PGE_2 synthesis is affected by vitamin E in the mouse (Meydani et al., 1986a). Further support for a PG-mediated effect of vitamin E was obtained by a demonstration that aspirin, a cyclooxygenase inhibitor, also decreased mortality from *E. coli* infection in chickens.

Corwin and Shloss (1980a,b) showed that vitamin E acts directly as a mitogen for murine lymphoid cells and will also enhance lymphocyte proliferation induced by other mitogens such as lipopolysaccharide (LPS), concanavalin A (Con A), and phytohemagglutinin (PHA). They further explored the mechanism of the mitogenic effect of vitamin E by comparing its effect with that of other antioxidants (Corwin and Shloss, 1980b). In vitro, tocopherol quinone (oxidized tocopherol) was as effective in enhancing lymphocyte proliferation as tocopherol. Torolox C (an analog of tocopherol without the isoprene side chain) and butylated hydroxytoluene were ineffective, whereas DPPD proved stimulatory. Thus, it appears that the mitogenic effect of tocopherol cannot be explained solely by its antioxidant function. However, these experiments did not support a PG-mediated effect of tocopherol, as the addition of indomethacin had no effect on lymphocyte proliferation and the in vitro addition of tocopherol did not decrease PGE_2 synthesis. Moriguchi et al. (1990) have recently reported that high levels of vitamin E induce a macrophage-activating factor-like material in rats.

Bendich et al. (1986) demonstrated that while 15 mg/kg diet of vitamin E was adequate to prevent myopathy in SHR rats, optimal lymphocyte proliferation to PHA and Con A was only obtained at much higher levels of vitamin E (50-200 mg/kg). In mice, dietary vitamin E was shown to enhance helper T-cell activity (Tanka et al., 1978). These studies indicate that the dietary tocopherol requirement for maintenance of optimal immune responsiveness in rodents and chickens may be higher than the levels recommended for normal growth and reproduction.

Lafuze et al. (1983) injected rabbits with N-formylmethionyl leucyl phenylalanine, a chemoattractant which causes neutropenia, and found that animals treated with vitamin E had less neutropenia as well as less severe decreases in the mean blood pressure and respiratory rate than controls. They noted that neutrophils from the vitamin E-treated rabbits adhered less to the endothelium. The vitamin E-treated rabbits also had higher 6-keto-$PGF_{1\alpha}$ (PGI_2) level than nontreated rabbits, which might contribute to the observed effect.

Eskew et al. (1985) examined the effect of vitamin E or selenium deficiency in rats on lymphocyte proliferation and antibody-dependent chicken red blood cell (CRBC) lysis and found that a deficiency of either nutrient depressed lymphocyte proliferation with a combined deficiency having the most suppressive effect. The double deficiency also decreased cell viability during the culture period. It was suggested that the nutrient deficiencies increased CRBC lysis via an increased formation of oxygen intermediates. Eskew et al. (1986) also looked at the combined effect of vitamin E deficiency and ozone exposure on different cell-mediated immune responses and found that while vitamin E deficiency or ozone exposure alone did not have a significant effect on splenic antibody-dependent cell-mediated cytotoxicity (ADCC), a combined treatment significantly depressed spleen ADCC. No such interaction was observed on the mitogenic responses of splenocytes. Therefore, it appears that the vitamin E requirement for optimal immune function might be even higher under conditions in which lipid peroxidation and oxidative stress are increased.

Other Animal Species

The immunostimulatory effect of vitamin E has also been demonstrated in other species (Tengerdy, 1990). Pigs supplemented with vitamin E showed enhanced blastogenic proliferation of peripheral lymphocytes to PHA (Larsen and Tollersrud, 1981) but not antibody response to sheep red blood cells (Bonnette et al., 1990). Vitamin E deficiency in dogs decreased the blastogenic response to Con A attributable to a serum factor that could be washed from the cell surface of depressed lymphocytes.

Reddy et al. (1986) studied the effect of weekly oral supplementation of dl-α-tocopheryl acetate (1400-2800 mg) or intramuscular (IM) injections of dl-α-tocopherol (1400 mg) on lymphocyte proliferation to PHA in calves. The injected dose of tocopherol significantly enhanced the mitogenic response to PHA, although the oral route was ineffective. It is not clear whether the stimulatory effect of the intramuscular injection was due to resulting higher cellular tocopherol levels as no tocopherol measurements were reported. In vitro, added dl-α-tocopherol (5-500 μg/L/10^5 cells) did not enhance the mitogenic response to PHA. This lack of an in vitro effect of tocopherol might be due to the mitogen used or to inadequate incorporation of tocopherol into the cells. In the same study, serum from tocopherol-supplemented calves inhibited infectious bovine rhinotracheitis viral replication more effectively in tissue culture than serum from unsupplemented calves. These findings indicate that vitamin E supplementation might be beneficial in increasing the resistance to some cattle diseases.

In a follow-up study, Reddy et al. (1987a) looked at the effect of oral supplementation of calves from birth to 24 weeks of age with different levels of vitamin E (0-500 IU/day of either dl-α-tocopherol before weaning or dl-α-tocopheryl acetate after weaning) on the mitogenic response of lymphocytes to T- and B-cell mitogens, as well as on antibody development to anti-bovine herpes virus type 1 vaccine. Even though the vitamin E-supplemented groups had slightly higher antibody titer, a significant effect was observed only at 125 IU/day of vitamin E, and there was no difference in general health or mortality between different groups. The effect of vitamin E on lymphocyte proliferation to T- and B-cell mitogens was not dose dependent or consistent, although an overall stimulatory effect of vitamin E was observed when the means were averaged over the entire period of the study. This effect of vitamin E was associated with an overall decrease in the serum cortisone level. Reddy et al. (1987b) have concluded that supplementation (with 125 IU/day) is a cost-effective way to enhance immunological performance and decrease stress. They also suggest that the dietary requirement of vitamin E for dairy calves similarly be increased to 125 IU/day.

Afzal et al. (1984) found in rams that dl-α-tocopheryl acetate used as an adjuvant to *Brucella ovis* vaccine decreased overall infectivity against an experimentally induced infection compared to *Brucella ovis*-Freund's incomplete adjuvant preparation. This protective effect of vitamin E was not directly related to an increase in antibody titer but rather appeared to be mediated by effects on cellular and local immunity. It is of interest that injection of vitamin E without the vaccine also decreased infectivity albeit less than the *Brucella ovis*-vitamin E adjuvant; a vitamin E injection was more effective than an oral supplement (Tengerdy, 1983).

Aging Animal Models

One of the biological changes associated with aging is increased free radical formation with subsequent damage to cellular processes. Numerous studies have expounded on the free radical theory of aging and the role of antioxidants, including vitamin E, on the life expectancy of rodents (Blumberg and Meydani, 1986). Oxygen metabolites, especially H_2O_2, produced by activated macrophages depress lymphocyte proliferation. Free radical formation associated with aging may be an underlying factor in the depressed immune response observed in aged rodents. Tocopherol decreases H_2O_2 formation in polymorphonuclear cells. These issues have been further discussed in a recent review (Meydani et al., 1990a).

It has been suggested by Harman (1982) that vitamin E and other antioxidants may increase longevity by influencing the immune system and reducing age-related diseases. An immunological basis for many age-associated diseases such as amyloidosis, atherosclerosis, and cancer has been proposed by Walford et al. (1981). Vitamin E supplementation has been shown to be protective against some of these diseases in animals. For example, Ip (1985) showed that vitamin E deficiency increases 7,12-dimethylbenz[a]anthracene (DMBA)-induced mammary adenocarcinomas and decreases the effectiveness of selenium supplementation in reducing DMBA-induced carcinogenesis. Horvath and Ip (1983) showed that vitamin E supplementation decreased lipid peroxidation and potentiated the prophylactic action of selenium against mammary carcinogenesis. Ip (1982) has also shown that vitamin E deficiency increases the risk of the development of mammary tumors, especially in rats fed diets high in polyunsaturated fatty acids. The protective effect of vitamin E appears to be due to its antioxidant effect rather than its effect on enzymes involved in DMBA detoxification. Meydani et al. (1986b) found that while 40% of old mice fed 50 mg/kg vitamin E had kidney amyloidosis, a common age-related pathological feature, none of the mice fed 500 mg/kg vitamin E had evidence of amyloid deposits. An increase in the average life span of short-lived autoimmune-prone NZB/NZW mice receiving vitamin E supplements was reported by Harman (1980).

These observations prompted us to evaluate the effect of vitamin E supplementation on the cell-mediated immune response of aged mice (Meydani et al., 1986a). We found that 500 ppm dietary vitamin E supplementation of 24-month-old C57BL/6j mice for 6 weeks significantly increased splenocyte proliferation to Con A and LPS but not to PHA relative to control animals fed 30 ppm of the vitamin. In addition, vitamin E supplementation significantly increased delayed cutaneous hypersensitivity (DCH) to 2,4-dinitro-7-fluorobenzene. This immunostimulatory effect of vitamin E was associated with an increased production of interleukin 2 (IL-2) and a decreased production of PGE_2 (Table 1). No stimulatory effect of vitamin E was noted on natural killer cell (NK)-mediated cytotoxicity; however, when the mice were immunized with SRBCs (a condition associated with increased oxidative stress) prior to assessment, the supplemented mice had a greater NK-mediated cytoxicity (Meydani et al., 1988).

We have recently extended these experiments (unpublished data) by comparing the effect of an in vitro addition of tocopherol (4 μg/ml) on the mitogen-induced proliferative response to splenocytes from young and old mice fed corn oil or fish oil diets. While tocopherol alone was not mitogenic, it significantly enhanced the mitogenic response of PHA and Con A (Table 2). Vitamin E caused a greater increase in young mice than in old mice on both diets. This effect might be due to a greater utilization and/or incorporation of tocopherol in the cells from young mice. Furthermore, a higher percentage increase in mitogen-induced proliferation was observed in mice fed corn oil than in those fed fish oil. This difference could be partially due to

Table 1 Effects of Vitamin E on Immune Responsiveness of 24-Month-Old Mice

Parameters	Control	Dietary vitamin E[a]	
		30 ppm	500 ppm
Serum α-tocopherol	236 ± 39 μg/dl	71	194[b]
Delayed hypersensitivity	59.9 ± 13.8%	36[b]	75
T-cell lymphocyte proliferation	119,611 ± 35,491 cpm	5[b]	38
B-cell lymphocyte proliferation	25,074 ± 5,149 cpm	24[b]	85
Ex vivo splenic PGE_2 synthesis	2.60 ± 0.08 μg/g	123[b]	89
Interleukin 2	27 ± 4 unit/ml	44[b]	85

[a]All values expressed as percent of 3-month-old control group (fed 30 ppm vitamin E).
[b]Significantly different from control and other experimental group, P ≤0.05.
Source: Data adopted from Meydani et al., 1986a.

Table 2 Percent Increase in Mitogen-Induced Splenocyte Proliferation by In Vitro Addition of α-Tocopherol (4 μg/ml)

Age	Diet	Percent increase in response	
		PHA	Con A
Young	Corn oil	131	416
Old	Corn oil	94	191
Young	Fish oil	83	244
Old	Fish oil	0	10

Mice were fed semisynthetic diets containing 10% by weight of corn oil or 8.8% fish oil + 1.2% corn oil. Cells were incubated with tocopherol 4 hr prior to the addition of mitogens and cultured for 72 hr. Percentages are calculated using counts per minute from cultures in the presence of α-tocopherol relative to those in the absence of α-tocopherol from the same animal.

a higher tocopherol requirement associated with fish oil consumption (Meydani et al., 1987a). These studies indicate that vitamin E supplementation improves the impaired immune response of aged mice. Further studies are required to determine the optimal level as well as the effect of long-term supplementation with vitamin E on the immune response of aged rodents.

THE ROLE OF VITAMIN E IN IMMUNE FUNCTION: CELLS IN CULTURE

The main body of research on the role of vitamin E in immune function has focused on the effect of vitamin E supplementation either in vitro or in vivo on different aspects of humoral and cell-mediated immunity such as antibody production, lymphocyte proliferation, phagocytosis, and bacterial killing and resistance. However, more recent studies have addressed the effect of vitamin E on immune cell-mediated injury to other cells as well as to their own membrane components.

Vitamin E appears to play a protective role against the oxidation of the macrophage membrane. Coquette et al. (1986) demonstrated that rat peritoneal macrophages contain 298 ± 18 ng vitamin E/mg protein. The tocopherol content of these cells decreased by 40% when they were exposed to oxygen-generating agents. Sepe and Clark (1986) reported that vitamin E protected against membrane damage caused by the oxidative products of neutrophils in a liposome model cell system.

Yamada et al. (1981) have noted that immune-triggered neutrophils adhere to and damage endothelial cells. Boogaert et al. (1984) found that human umbilical vein endothelial cells pretreated with α-tocopherol were protected against the cytotoxic effect of complement-activated neutrophils. The cytotoxic effect of neutrophils, presumably due to reactive oxygen radicals produced during their activation, is enhanced in the presence of platelets. Vitamin E not only protected endothelial cells from the damage caused by neutrophils, it also abolished the exaggerating effect of platelets. This action of vitamin E appears to be due to an increased production of PGI_2 by endothelial cells. When endothelial cells are exposed to oxidative stress (Boogaerts et al. 1984; Triau et al. 1988), they synthesize more PGI_2, perhaps as a defensive/

protective response against injury. Meydani et al. (1987b) have shown that vitamin E supplementation in mice increases lung PGI_2 synthesis.

Leb et al. (1985) demonstrated that preincubation of human mononuclear phagocytes with α-tocopherol decreased PMA-induced cytotoxicity. Furthermore, target erythrocytes incubated with α-tocopherol were also more resistant to PMA-induced monocyte cytotoxicity. This effect of tocopherol appears to be due to a reduction of H_2O_2 formation. However, α-tocopherol was not effective in reducing monocyte ADCC, presumably because nonoxidative injury is more important in ADCC.

Vitamin E provides protection against transplantation of virus-transformed Balb/3T3 (K3T3) tumor cells. This protective action requires an increase in Fc- and C_3 b-receptor-mediated phagocytosis and the expression of Ia antigen (Gebremichael et al., 1984). Yogeeswaran and Mbawuike (1986) and Mbawuike et al. (1988) have hypothesized that vitamin E modulates the expression and function of some of these important membrane molecules such as the glycolipids. Yogeeswaran and Stein (1980) noted that cell surface glycoconjugates are important components of the tumorogenic and metastatic potential of tumor cells. Therefore, they examined the effect of vitamin E in vitro on cell surface glycosphingolipids (GSL) and found a dose-dependent decrease in GSL biosynthesis and cellular expression. These changes observed in GSL might underlie the increased antigenicity (as measured by increased humoral antibody production) reported in mice for vitamin E-treated K3T3 cells (Mbawuike, 1984). It has also been reported that pretreatment of K3T3 cells with vitamin E increases their binding to tumor-specific antisera (Mbawuike et al., 1988). Kurek and Corwin (1982) reported that vitamin E-supplemented mice were protected against transplantation of K3T3 tumor cells, presumably due to stimulation of their immune response by the vitamin.

Similar effects of vitamin E on the metabolism and cell surface expression of glycoconjugates have been demonstrated in $HepG_2$ cells (Yogeeswaran et al., 1987). Furthermore, Iwama et al. (1985) showed that vitamin E deficiency causes alteration of glycosaminoglycans in rat aorta. Yogeeswaran and Reddy (1988) reported that vitamin E increased glycoconjugate biosynthesis in association with increased IL-2-dependent cell growth in an IL-2-dependent cell line. Since glycolipids are important in cell differentiation, cell growth, and cell-cell interaction and glycan groups serve as antigenic determinants, these findings may have important implications for understanding the mechanism of the immunostimulatory effect of vitamin E.

THE ROLE OF VITAMIN E IN IMMUNE FUNCTION: HUMAN STUDIES

Clinical Trials

Studies of the effects of vitamin E on the immune response in humans are limited. An early report by Baehner et al. (1977a) showed that in vivo supplementation with vitamin E could depress the bactericidal activity of leukocytes without affecting other blood chemistry and hematological parameters. They hypothesized that directed movement and phagocytosis by polymorphonuclear leukocytes (PMNs) are attenuated by the auto-oxidative damage to the cell membrane by endogenously derived H_2O_2, and that administration of vitamin E may prevent this damage via scavenging of reduced oxygen radicals. They administered 1600 IU daily for 7 days to three volunteers and found their isolated PMNs were hyperphagocytic (measured by uptake of LPS-coated paraffin oil particles) but killed *Staphylococcus aureus* 502A less effectively than controls, suggesting that less H_2O_2 was available to damage PMNs or kill bacteria. H_2O_2-Dependent stimulation of the hexose monophosphate shunt, H_2O_2 release from phagocytizing PMNs, and fluoresceinated Con A cap formation promoted by H_2O_2 damage to microtubules were all diminished, but the release of superoxide from phagocytizing PMNs was not reduced in the vitamin E group. It is difficult to assess the dichotomy between the depressant effect on PMN killing in vitro and the reduced PMN autotoxicity leading to improved phagocytosis. Boxer et al. (1979a) suggest these results indicate that the stable reduction product of oxygen, H_2O_2, may be responsible for modulating PMN motile functions.

Prasad (1980) studied the effect of a daily, 3-week treatment of 300 mg dl-α-tocopherol acetate on delayed hypersensitivity in five young boys (13-18 years) and on the bactericidal activity of peripheral leukocytes and cell-mediated immunity in 13 men (25-30 years). The vitamin E supplementation decreased leukocyte bactericidal activity, the release of acid phosphatase activity, and PHA-stimulated lymphocyte proliferation but did not alter the delayed hypersensitivity of the skin to an intradermal injection of PHA. The results of this trial reveal a discrepancy between the in vivo and in vitro results of cell-mediated immunity parameters. Interestingly, two subjects showed clinical improvement in their symptoms of asthmatic attacks and nasal allergy, respectively.

Vitamin E deficiency has been suggested to contribute to alterations in neonatal PMN function through peroxidative damage to the cell's membrane (Oski, 1980). Newborn infants, especially premature babies, have a low status of vitamin E and neonatal PMNs have been shown to be deficient in phagocytosis, bactericidal activity, and chemotaxis (Miller, 1979). These defects may play a role in determining the high susceptibility to infections of the newborn infant by impairment of host defenses. Chirico et al. (1983) administered 120 mg/kg dl-α-tocopherol (divided into single doses of 20 mg/kg intramuscularly on days 2, 3, 4, 7, 10 and 13 after birth) to 10 of 20 healthy premature infants and assessed neutrophil phagocytosis at 2, 5, 14, and 30 days of age. In the treated and untreated infants no differences were found in PMN function before treatment with vitamin E, although phagocytosis, bactericial activity, and chemotaxis were lower than in 30 adult controls. At 5 days of age, the untreated infants maintained a low index and frequency of phagocytosis, whereas these parameters were significantly increased in the group receiving vitamin E. However, at 14 and 30 days, phagocytosis was normal in both groups of infants with no differences being noted in bactericidal activity, NBT reduction, random movement, chemotaxis, or metabolic activity. Thus, vitamin E appeared to accelerate the normalization of phagocytic function during the first week of life in the newborn.

Zimlanski et al. (1986) supplemented 20 institutionalized elderly women (63-93 years) with 100 mg dl-α-tocopherol acetate twice daily and assessed serum proteins and immunoglobulin concentrations after 4 and 12 months. Vitamin E increased total serum protein with the principal effect on α_2- and β_2-globulin fractions occurring at 4 months. No significant effects were noted on the levels of immunologlobulins and complement C3, although another group administered vitamin C (400 mg daily) with vitamin E displayed significant increases in IgG and complement C3 levels.

Harman and Miller (1986) supplemented 103 elderly patients from a chronic care facility with 200 or 400 mg daily α-tocopherol acetate, but did not see any beneficial effect on antibody development against influenza virus vaccine. Unfortunately, data on the health status, medication use, antibody levels, and other relevant parameters were not reported. Payette et al. (1990) have reported a negative correlation between dietary intake of vitamins D and E and interleukin 2 production in vitro in free-living elderly individuals. However, the majority of their subjects had no detectable level of IL-2, which raises questions about the health status of the subjects. Furthermore, direct supplementation would be needed to assess the relevance of this type of observation. We conducted a 30-day placebo-controlled, double-blind vitamin E supplementation (800 IU/day) trial of healthy elderly subjects in which in vivo and in vitro indices of immune response were evaluated in each subject before and after supplementation (Meydani et al., 1990b). The analysis of the data indicated that vitamin E supplementation improved the delayed hypersensitivity skin response as well as the mitogenic response of lymphocytes to Con A and IL-2 production, which correlated with the decrease in prostaglandin E_2 production and plasma lipid peroxides.

Epidemiological Studies

The use of vitamin E supplements in high doses by healthy individuals, although deemed inappropriate by most nutrition professionals, is widely promoted and, along with vitamin C supplements, represents the most popular nutrient supplement (Hartz and Blumberg, 1986; Willett et al., 1981). Goodwin and Garry (1983) studied a population of healthy older adults (65-94 years) consuming megadoses of vitamin supplements and did not see any correlation between vitamin E intake and DCH, mitogen stimulation, serum antibodies, or circulating immune complexes. Persons taking megadoses of vitamin E ($>5 \times$ RDA) had lower absolute circulating lymphocyte counts than the rest of the population. However, the study was complicated by the fact that several vitamin supplements at megadose levels were used by each subject and the interaction between different nutrients present confounded the variables. The same complications may have been operating in the study by Payette et al. (1990). It has been suggested that some megadose nutrients may act as nonspecific adjuvants, the effects of which diminish with time.

Chavance et al. (1984, 1985, 1989) conducted community-based surveys on the relationship between nutritional and immunological status in 100 healthy subjects over 60 years of age. They reported that plasma vitamin E levels were positively correlated with positive DCH responses to diphtheria toxoid, *Candida*, and *Trichophyton*. In men only, positive correlations were also observed between vitamin E levels and the number of positive DCH responses. Subjects with tocopherol levels greater than 135 mg/L were found to have higher helper-inducer/cytotoxic-suppressor ratios. Blood vitamin E concentrations were also negatively correlated with the number of infectious disease epidsodes in the preceding years.

Immunological Role of Vitamin E in Disease States

Evidence has been accumulating that oxidant damage to tissues underlies the pathology of several human diseases, including many associated with altered immune function, e.g., amyloidosis, rheumatoid arthritis, and cancer. Vitamin E deficiency in premature infants is now recognized as a key factor in hemolytic anemia, rotrolental fibroplasia syndrome, and bronchopulmonary dysplasia. The precise role played by free radicals and H_2O_2 in such disorders or immune injury to the kidney and lung is not resolved, although they are formed and they interact with PG, leukotrienes, interleukins, and other modulators of immune function. Vitamin E may be beneficial to host defense mechanisms by preventing the infection-induced increase in tissue PG production from arachidonic acid (Likoff et al., 1978; Tengerdy et al., 1978; Meydani et al., 1986b).

Vitamin E could affect PG production by interfering with its synthesis. Prostaglandin production requires an active oxygen species and lipid peroxides (such as the PG intermediate PGG_2) can stimulate synthesis by providing an oxygen species to enhance the activity of the rate-limiting enzyme, cyclooxygenase. Swartz et al. (1985) administered 800 IU vitamin E or placebo daily to 30 healthy adults for 8 weeks and observed a dramatic decline in plasma 6-keto-$PGF_{1\alpha}$, the principal stable degradation product of prostacyclin, in the treatment group. Vitamin E may reduce prostacyclin production through its antioxidant activity via diminishing the levels of peroxide needed for activation of arachidonic acid. A similar inverse relationship between serum vitamin E and other PGs, e.g., PGE_2 and $PGF_{2\alpha}$, has been noted in animal studies (Hope et al., 1975; Machlin, 1978; Meydani et al., 1986, 1991). However, Lauritsen et al. (1987) found oral supplements of 1920 IU α-tocopherol daily for 2 weeks in eight patients with active ulcerative colitis did not affect the disease-induced elevations of PGE_2 or leukotriene B_4 in the lumen. Goetzl (1980) reported that vitamin E bidirectionally modulates the activity of the lipoxygenase pathway of human neutrophils in vitro. He further noted that normal plasma concentrations of vitamin E enhanced the lipoxygenation of arachidonic acid, whereas higher concentrations exerted a suppressive effect consistent with α-tocopherol's role as a hydroperoxide scavenger. While these data mostly support the influence of vitamin E on the arachidonic acid cascade, less evidence is available to explain the involvement of superoxide in neutrophil chemotaxis, the modulating action of platelet-activating factor and tumor necrosis factor on oxidant production by phagocytes, and oxidant involvement in T-lymphocyte activation (Halliwell, 1987).

Mowat and Baun (1971), Hill et al. (1974), and others have demonstrated abnormal PMN function in diabetes, including defective phagocytic uptake and chemotactic responses. Kitahara et al. (1980) found that monocytes from diabetic patients produced higher chemoluminescence peaks and generated more superoxide anion upon phagocytic challenge than did controls. Hill et al. (1983) administered 25 IU α-tocopherol/kg/day orally for 2-3 weeks to seven diabetic patients with consistently depressed monocyte chemotactic responses. The vitamin E treatment doubled monocyte random motility and chemotactic responsiveness toward zymosan-activated serum to levels comparable to normal controls, suggesting this defective function may partially be a result of auto-oxidative membrane damage.

Spielberg et al. (1979) described an infant boy with congenital glutathione synthetase deficiency who had episodic profound neutropenia accompanying infections. Boxer et al. (1979b) treated this patient with 400 IU (approximately 30 IU/kg) α-tocopherol acetate as an oral, single daily dose for 3 months. Prior to the treatment, the abnormal leukocytes exposed to phagocytic challenge released more H_2O_2, fixed less opsonized zymosan particles, killed bacteria less effectively, and demonstrated impaired microtubule assembly. These functional abnormalities disappeared after the administration of vitamin E and no neutropenia occurred during subsequent infections. The patient was continued on the vitamin E therapy and was noted to have no further episodes of bacterial infections for 18 months (compared to six episodes the year prior to treatment). The investigators suggested this evidence supports the idea that in glutathione-deficient leukocytes vitamin E protects against nonspecific oxidant damage to membranes and nonmembranous structures (e.g., microtubules) by hastening the destruction of excess peroxide during phagocytosis. This suggestion was supported by Oliver (1980) who further studied the cytoskeletal defects associated with glutathione synthetase deficiency in this patient and found normal microtubule assembly during the resting phase but damage to the structure from excessive peroxide production during stimulated phagocytic activity. Vitamin E protected against cytoskeletal damage incurred during phagocytosis but did not normalize other cellular functions dependent upon glutathione.

Free radical damage is thought to be involved in the initiation and promotion of many cancers. The increased incidence of cancer among older adults has been postulated to be in part, due to the increasing level of free radical reactions with age and the diminishing ability of the immune system to eliminate the altered cells. Although controlled human studies on vitamin E and cancer are very limited, epidemiological data suggest that higher intakes of vitamin E (and other dietary antioxidants) may decrease the risk for certain cancers, particularly cancers of the breast, colon, lung, and stomach (Salonen et al., 1985; Stahelin et al., 1984; Wald et al., 1984; Kok et al., 1987; Lopez et al., 1985; Menkes et al., 1986). Knekt et al. (1988) assessed blood vitamin E levels and subsequent cancer incidence in a longitudinal study of 21,172 men in Finland. Vitamin E was measured from stored blood samples of 453 subjects who developed cancer during the 6- to 10-year study period and 841 matched controls. Adjusted relative risks in the two highest quintiles of blood vitamin E concentrations compared to all other quintiles were 0.7 for all cancers and 0.6 for cancers unrelated to smoking.

CONCLUSIONS

There is now substantial evidence indicating that the tocopherol status influences the immune response. Tocopherol deficiency in rodents and mammals compromises immune function. Supplementation with higher than recommended dietary levels of tocopherol stimulate both humoral and cell-mediated immunity resulting in enhanced in vivo antibody production, delayed hypersensitivity skin test, and resistance to some bacterial and viral-induced infections in animal models. This evidence has led to questions about the adequacy of the current recommended dietary guidelines for vitamin E, especially under conditions in which oxidative stress is increased. It is not surprising that the immune system might require a different level of tocopherol for its optimal function than other organ systems. White blood cells are particularly rich in polyunsaturated-containing phospholipids prone to oxidative destruction. The mounting of an immune response requires membrane-bound receptor-mediated communication between cells as well as between protein and lipid mediators which can be directly or indirectly affected by tocopherol status. However, although several possibilities have been proposed, the exact nature of the tocopherol effect has not been determined. Tocopherol could effect the immune system through its antioxidant function either by decreasing reactive oxygen metabolites such as H_2O_2 and/ or by altering the formation of arachidonic acid metabolites such as PG, both of which have been shown to suppress immune responsiveness. However, the immunostimulatory effect of tocopherol cannot be fully explained by its antioxidant function, as other antioxidants do not produce similar actions. Interestingly, cyclooxygenase inhibitors such as aspirin and indomethacin have been shown to enhance several parameters of cell-mediated immunity and vitamin E has been shown to decrease PG production in immune cells (Likoff et al., 1978; Meydani et al., 1986a). On the other hand, Corwin and Shloss (1980b) were not able to demonstrate a PG-mediated mechanism for the vitamin E effects they observed. The work by Yogeeswaran and Reddy (1988) of vitamin E-induced changes in cell surface glycoconjugates suggests another possible mechanism of action for vitamin E; i.e., changes in membrane receptor molecules involved in the immune response.

The mechanisms of the vitamin E effect on immune responsiveness need to be further explored and their relative contributions to the immunostimulatory action of vitamin E determined. More research effort must be focused on the effect of vitamin E on the immune response of humans. While a substantial amount of work has been completed in animal models, very few human trials have been conducted and most of them suffer from inadequate sample size and lack of appropriate controls. Data are especially lacking in elderly subjects and in individuals exposed to environmental conditions involving oxidative stress.

REFERENCES

Afzal M, Tengerdy RP, Ellis RP, Kimberling CV, Morris CJ (1984). Protection of rams against epidimymitis by a *Brucella ovis*-vitamin E adjuvant vaccine. Vet Immunol Immunopathol 7:293-304.

Baehner RL, Boxer LA, Allen JM, Davis J (1977). Autooxidation as a basis for altered function by polymorphonuclear leuckocytes. Blood 50:327-335.

Bendich A, Gabriel E, Machlin LJ (1983). Effect of dietary level of vitamin E on the immune system of the spontaneously hypertensive (SHR) and mormotensive Wistar Kyoto (WKY) rats. J Nutr 113:1920-1926.

Bendich A, Gabriel E, Machlin LJ (1986). Dietary vitamin E requirement for optimum immune response in the rat. J Nutr 116:675-681.

Blumberg J, Meydani SN (1986). Role of dietary antioxidants in aging. In: Bristol-Myers Nutrition Symposia: Nutrition and Aging. Vol. 5. H. Munro and M. Hutchinson, eds. Academic Press, New York, pp 85-97.

Bonnette ED, Korngay ET, Lindemann MD, Notter DR (1990). Influence of two supplemental vitamin E levels and weaning age on performance, humoral antibody production, and serum cortisol levels of pigs. J An Sci 68:1346-1353.

Boogaerts MA, Van de Broeck J, Deckmyn H, Roellant C, Vermylen J, Verwilghen RL (1984). Protective effect of vitamin E on immune triggered granulocyte mediated endothelial injury. Thromb Haemost 51:89-92.

Boxer LA, Harris RE, Baehner RL (1979a). Regulation of membrane peroxidation in health and disease. Pediatrics 64:S713-S718.

Boxer LA, Oliver JM, Spielberg SP, Allen JM, Schulman JD (1979b). Protection of granulocytes by vitamin E in glutathione synthetase deficiency. N Engl J Med 301:901-905.

Chavance M, Brubacher G, Herbeth B, Vernhes G, Mikstacki T, Dete F, Fournier C, Janot C (1984). Immunological and nutritional status among the elderly, In: Lymphoid Cell Functions in Aging. A. L. de Wick, ed. Eurage, Paris, pp 231-237.

Chavance M, Brubacher G, Herberth B, Vernhes G, Mistacki T, Dete F, Fournier C, Janot C (1985). Immunological and nutritional status among the elderly. In: Nutrition, Immunity, and Illness in the Elderly. R. K. Chandra ed. Pergamon Press, New York, pp137-142.

Chavance M, Herbeth B, Fournier C, Janot C, Vernhes G (1989). Vitamin status, immunity, and infections in an elderly population. Eur J Clin 43(12):827.

Chirico G, Marconi M, Colombo A, Chiara A, Rondini G, Ugazio AG (1983). Deficiency of neutrophil phagocytosis in premature infants: Effect of vitamin E supplementation. Acta Paediatr Scand 72:521-524.

Coquette A, Vray B, Vanderpas J (1986). Role of vitamin E in the protection of the resident macrophage membrane against oxidative damage. Arch Int Physiol Biochem 94:529-534.

Corwin LM, Shloss J (1980a). Influence of vitamin E on the mitogenic response of murine lymphoid cells. J Nutr 110:916-923.

Corwin LM, Shloss J (1980b). Role of antioxidants on the stimulation of the mitogenic response. J Nutr 110:2397-2505.

Eskew ML, Scholz RW, Reddy CC, Todhunter DA, Zarkower A (1985). Effects of vitamin E and selenium deficiencies on rat immune function. Immunology 54:173-180.

Eskew ML, Scheuchenzuker WJ, Scholtz RW, Reddy CC, Zarkower A (1986). The effects of ozon inhalation on the immunological response of selenium and vitamin E-deprived rats. Environ Res 40:274-284.

Gebremichael A, Levy EM, Corwin LM (1984). Adherent cell requirement for the effect of vitamin E on in vitro antibody synthesis. J Nutr 114:1297-1305.

Goetzel EJ (1980). Vitamin E modulates lipoxygenation of arachidonic acid in leukocytes. Nature 288:183-187.

Goodwin JS, Garry TJ (1983). Relationship between megadose vitamin supplementation and immunological function in a healthy elderly population. Clin Exp Immunol 51:647-653.

Halliwell B (1987). Oxidants and human disease: Some new concepts. FASEB J. 1:358-364.

Harman D (1980). Free radical theory of aging: Beneficial effect of antioxidants on the lifespan of male NZB mice; role of free radical reactions in the deterioration of the immune system with age and in the pathogenesis of systemic lupus erythematosus. Age 3:64-73.

Harman D (1982). The free-radical theory of aging. In: Free Radicals in Biology Vol 5. W. A. Pryor, ed. Academic Press, New York, pp 255-273.

Harman D, Miller RW (1986). Effect of vitamin E on the immune response to influenza virus vaccine and incidence of infectious disease in man. Age 9:21-23.

Hartz S, Blumberg J (1986). Use of vitamin and mineral supplements by the elderly. Clin Nutr 5:130-136.

Heinzerling RH, Tengerdy RP, Wick LL, Lueker DC (1974). Vitamin E protects mice against Diploccocus pneumonia type I infection. Infect Immun 10:1292-1295.

Hill HR, Sauls HS, Dettloff JL, Quie PG (1974). Impaired leukotactic responsiveness in patients with juvenile diabetes mellitus, Clin Immunol Immunopathol 2:395-403.

Hill HR, Augustine NH, Rallison ML, Santos JI (1983). Defective monocyte chemotactic responses in diabetes mellitus. J Clin Immunol 3:70-77.

Hope WC, Dalton C, Machlin LJ, Filipski RJ, Vane FM (1975). Influence of dietary vitamin E on prostaglandin synthesis in rat blood. Prostaglandins 10:557-561.

Horwarth PM, Ip C (1983). Synergestic effect of vitamin E and selenuim in the chemoprevention of mammary carcinogenesis in rats. Cancer Res 43:5335-5341.

Ip C (1982). Dietary vitamin E intake and mammary carcinogenesis in rats. Carcinogenesis 3:1453-1456.

Ip C (1985). Attention of the anticarcinogenic action of selenium by vitamin E deficiency. Cancer (letters) 25:325-331.

Iwama M, Honda A, Ohoshiaki Y, Sakai T, Mori Y (1985). Alterations in glycosaminoglycans of the aorta of vitamin E-deficient rats. Atherosclerosis 55:115-123.

Kelleher J, Losowsky MS (1978). Vitamin E in the elderly. In: Tocopherol, Oxygen and Biomembranes. C. DeDuve, O. Hayaishi, eds. Elsevier/North-Holland, Biomedical Press, Amsterdam, pp 311-327.

Kitahara M, Eyre HJ, Lynch RE, Rallison ML, Hill HR (1980). Metabolic activity of diabetic monocytes. Diabetes 29:251-256.

Kok FJ, Van Duijn C, Hofman A, Vermeeren R, de Bruijn AM, Valkenburg HA (1987). Micronutrients and the risk of lung cancer. N Engl J Med 316:1416.

Knekt P, Aromaa A, Maatela J, Aaran R, Nikkari T, Hakama M, Hakulinen T, Peto R, Saxen E, Teppo L (1988). Serum vitamin E and risk of cancer among Finnish men during a ten-year follow-up. Am J Epidemiol 127:28-41.

Kurek MP, Corwin LM (1982). Vitamin E Protection against tumor formation by transplanted murine sarcoma cells. Nutr Cancer 4:128-139.

Lafuze JE, Weisman SJ, Alpert LA, Baehner RL (1984). Vitamin E attenuates the effects of FMLP on rabbit circulating granulocytes. Pediatr Res 18:536-540.

Larsen HJ, Tollersrud S (1981). Effect of dietary vitamin E and selenium on the phytohaemagglutinin response of pig lymphocytes. Am J Vet Sci 31:301-305.

Lauritsen K, Laursen LS, Bukhave K, Rask-Madsen J (1987). Does vitamin E supplementation modulate in vivo arachidonate metabolism in human inflammation? Pharmacol Toxicol 61:246-249.

Leb L, Beatson P, Fortier N, Newburg PE, Snyder LM (1985). Modulation of mononuclear phagocyte cytotoxicity by alpha-tocopherol (vitamin E). J Leuk Biol 37:449-459.

Lehman J, McGill M (1982). Biomedical and ultrastructural alterations in platelets, reticulocytes, and lymphocytes from rats fed vitamin E-deficient diets. J Lipid Res 23:299-306.

Leichter J, Angel JF, Lee M (1978). Nutritional status of a select groups of free-living elderly people in Vancouver. Can Med Assoc J 118:40-43.

Likoff RO, Mathias MM, Neckles CP (1978). Vitamin E enhancement of immunity mediated by the prostaglandins. Fed Proc 37:829.

Lopez-S A, Le Gardeur BY, Johnson WD (1985). Vitamins and lung cancer. Am J Clin Nutr 41:854.

Machlin L (1978). Vitamin E and prostaglandins. In: Tocopherol, Oxygen, and Biomembranes. C. de Dure and O. Hayaishi, eds. Elsevier/North-Holland Biomedical Press, Amsterdam, pp 208-215.

Mbawuike IN (1984). Mechanisms of Vitamin E Protection Against Transplanted Murine Sarcoma Cells. Ph. D. Dessertation, Boston University, Boston, Massachusetts.

Mbawuike IN, Corwin LM, Yogeeswaran G (1988). Vitamin E induced alterations in antigenicity, and sialoglycoconjugates of Kirsten Murine Sarcoma Virus-transformed Balb/3T3 cells. BBA (in press).

Menkes MS, Comstock GW, Vuilleumier JP, Helsing KJ, Rider AA, Brookmezer R (1986). Serum beta-carotene, vitamins A and E, selenium, and the risk of lung cancer. N Engl J Med 315:1250-1254.

Meydani M, Macauley J, Blumberg JB (1986). Influence of dietary vitamin E, selenium and age on regional distribution of α-tocopherol in the rat brain. Lipids 21:786-791.

Meydani SN, Meydani M, Verdon CP, Shapiro AC, Blumberg JB, Hayes KC (1986a). Vitamin E supplementation suppresses prostglandin E_2 synthesis and ehnances the immune response in aged mice. Mech Ageing Dev 34:191-201.

Meydani SN, Cathcart ES, Hopkins RE, Meydani M, Hayes KC, Blumberg JB (1986b). Antioxidants in experimental amyloidosis of young and old mice. In: Fourth International Symposium of Amyloidosis. Glenner GG, Asserman EP, Benditt E, Calkins E, Cohen AS, and Zucker-Franklin D, eds. Plenum Press, New York, pp 683-692.

Meydani SN, Shapiro AC, Meydani M, McCauley J, Blumberg JB (1987a). Effect of age and dietary fat (fish oil, corn oil, and coconut oil) on tocopherol status of C57BL/6Nia mice. Lipids 22:345-350.

Meydani SN, Shapiro AC, Meydani M, Blumberg JB (1987b). Effect of fat type and tocopherol supplementation on tocopherol status and eicosanoid synthesis in lung. Producings of the American Oil and Chemical Society on Polyunsaturated Fatty Acids and Eicosanoids. WEM Lands, ed. AOCS Champaign, Illinois, pp 438-441.

Meydani SN, Yogeeswaran G, Liu S, Baskar S, Meydani M (1988). Fatty oil and tocopherol induced changes in natural killer cell mediated cytotoxicity and PGE_2 synthesis in young and old mice. J Nutr 118:1245-1252.

Meydani M, Meydani SN, Shapiro AC, Macauley JB, Blumberg JB (1991). Influence of dietary fat, vitamin E, ethoxyquin and indomethacin on the synthesis of prostaglandin E_2 in brain regions in the mouse. J Nutr 121:438.

Meydani SN, Meydani M, Blumberg JB (1990a). Antioxidants and the aging immune response. Adv Exp Biol Med 262:57-67.

Meydani SN, Barkland MP, Liu S, Meydani M, Miller RA, Cannon JG, Marrow FO, Rocklin R, Blumberg JB (1990b). Vitamin E supplementation enhances cell-mediated immunity in healthy elderly subjects. Am J Clin Nutr 52:557.

Miller ME (1979). Phagocytic function in the neonate: Selected aspects. Pediatrics 64:5709-5712.

Mowat AG, Baum J (1971). Chemotaxis of polymorphonuclear leukocytes from patients with diabetes mellitus. N Engl J Med 284:621-627.

Oliver J (1980). Reduced glutathione in specific cellular processes. Ann Intern Med 93:337-340.

Oski FA (1980). Anemia in infancy: iron deficiency and vitamin E deficiency. Pediatr Rev 1:247-253.

Payette H, Rola-Plesszczynski M, Ghadirian P (1990). Nutrition factors in relation to cellular and regulatory immune variables in a free-living elderly population. Am J Clin Nutr 52:927-932.

Prasad JS (1980). Effect of vitamin E supplementation on leukocyte function. Am J Clin Nutr 33:606-608.

Reddy PG, Morrill JL, Minocha HC, Morrill MB, Dayton AD, Frey RA (1986). Effect of supplemental vitamin E on the immune system of calves. J Dairy Sci 69:164-171.

Reddy PG, Morrill JL, Frey RA (1987a). Vitamin E requirements of dairy calves. J Dairy Sci 70:123-128.

Reddy PG, Morrill JL, Minocha HC, Stevenson JS (1987b). Vitamin E is immunostimulatory in calves. J Dairy Sci 70:993-999.

Salonen JT, Salonen R, Lappetelainen R, Maenpaa PH, Alfthan G, Puska P. (1985). Risk of cancer in relation to serum concentrations of selenium and vitamin A and E: Matched case-control analysis of prospective data. Br Med J (Clin Res) 290(6466):417-420.

Segagni E (1955). Vitamin E effect on Vaccination. Minerva Pediatr 7:985-987.

Sepe S, Clark RA (1985). Oxidant membrane injury by the neutrophili myeloperoxidase system. II: Injury by stimulated neutrophils and protection by lipid-soluble antioxidants. J Immunol 134:1896-1901.

Solano G (1957). Effects of vitamins on antibody production in rabbits to Vibrio choleral. Int Z Vitamin Forsch 27:373-375.

Spielberg SP, Boxer LA, Oliver JM, Schulman JD (1979). Oxidative damage to neutrophils in glutathione synthetase deficiency. Br J Haematol 42:215-223.

Stahelin HB, Rosel F, Buess E, Brubacher G (1984). Cancer, vitamins and plasma lipids: Prospective Basel study. JNCI 73:1463-1468.

Swartz SL, Willett WC, Hennekens CH (1985). A randomized trial of the effect of vitamin E on plasma prostacyclin (6-keto-$PGF_{1\alpha}$) levels in healthy adults. Prostaglandins Leukotr Med 18:105-111.

Tanka J, Fuyiwara H, Torisu M (1979). Vitamin E and immune response: Enhancement of helper T cell activity by dietary supplementation of vitamin E in mice. Immunology 38:727-734.

Tengerdy RP, Heinzerling RH, Brown GL, Mathias MM (1973). Enhancement of the humoral immune response by vitamin E. Intern Arch Allergy 44:221-232.

Tengerdy RP, Heinzerling RH, Mathias MM (1978). Effect of vitamin E on disease resistance and immune responses. In: Tocopherol, Oxygen, and Biomembranes, C. de Duve and O. Hayaishi, eds. Elsevier/North-Holland Biomedical Press, Amsterdam, pp 191-200.

Tengerdy RP, Meyer DL, Lauverman LH, Lueker DC, Nockels CF (1983). Vitamin E enhances humoral antibody response to Clostridium perfringens, type D in sheep. Br Vet J 139: 147-151.

Tengerdy RP, Mathias MM, Nockels CF (1984). Effect of vitamin E on immunity and disease resistance. In: Vitamins, Nutrition and Cancer. A. Prasad, ed. Krager, Basel, pp 123-133.

Tengerdy RP. Immunity and disease resistance in farm animals fed Vitamin E supplement. Adv Exp Med Biol 262:103.

Triau JE, Meydani SN, Schaefer EJ (1988). Oxidized low density lipoproteins stimulate prostacyclin production by adult human vascular endothelial cells. Arteriosclerosis 8:810-818.

Wald NJ, Boreham J, Hayward JL, Bulbrook RD (1984). Plasma retinol, beta-carotene and vitamin E levels in relation to the future risk of breast cancer. Br J Cancer 49:321-324.

Willett W, Sampson L, Bain C, Rosner B, Hennekens C, Witschie J, Speizer F (1981). Vitamin supplement use among registered nurses. Am J Clin Nutr 34:1121-1125.

Willett WC, Polk BF, Underwood B, Stampfer MJ, Pressel S, Rosner B, Taylor JO, Scheider K, Hames CG (1984). Relation to serum vitamins A and E and carotenoids to the risk of cancer, N Engl J Med 310:430-434.

Yamada O, Moldow CF, Sachs T, Craddock PR, Boogaerts MA, Jacob HS (1981). Deleterious effects of endotoxin on cultured endothelial cells. Inflammation 5:115-119.

Yogeeswaran G, Mbawuike IN (1986). Altered metabolism and cell surface expression of glycosphingolipids caused by vitamin E in cultured murine (K 3T3) reticulum sarcoma cells. Lipids 21:643-647.

Yogeeswaran G, Reddy GS (1988). Correlation of increased glycosylation and stimulation of growth by alpha-D-tocopherol (αT) in CTL cell lines. FASEB J 2:A638.

Yogeeswaran G, Stein BS (1980). Glycosphingolipids of metastatic variant RNA virus-transformed non producer Balb/3T3 cell lines: Altered metabolism and cell surface exposure. J Natl Cancer Inst 65:967-976.

Yogeeswaran G, Triau JE, Koul O (1987). Modulation of glycosylation by α-d-tocopherol delivered to hepatoma cell line via human lipoproteins versus bovine serum. Fed Proc 46:2201.

Ziemlanski S, Wartanowicz M, Klos A, Raczka A, Klos M (1986). The effects of ascorbic acid and alpha-tocopherol supplementation on serum proteins and immunoglobulin concentrations in the elderly. Nutr Int 2:1-5.

15
Copper and Immunity

Tim R. Kramer
Beltsville Human Nutrition Research Center, U.S. Department of Agriculture, Beltsville, Maryland

W. Thomas Johnson
Grand Forks Human Nutrition Research Center, U.S. Department of Agriculture, Grand Forks, North Dakota

INTRODUCTION

Findings indicating an impaired host defense system in copper deficiency come from studies in humans and animals. Children with the Menkes syndrome, a rare congenital disease resulting in copper deficiency, frequently die from pneumonia (1). Copper deficiency in humans is accompanied by bacterial infections, diarrhea, and bronchopneumonia (2-5). Bactericidal activity by neutrophils is decreased in copper-deficient cattle, ewes, and lambs (6,7). Jones and Suttle (8) and Newberne et al. (9) used small laboratory animals to study in more detail the findings of impaired host defense against infectious organisms in copper deficiency. Using the rat model, Newberne et al. (9) suggested that increased susceptibility to *Salmonella typhimurium* in copper deficiency was caused by decreased macrophage activity. Reduced numbers of splenic antibody-producing cells have been found in copper-deficient mice (10,11). Lukasewycz and coworkers demonstrated that, in mice, copper deficiency reduced the proliferation of mitogen-stimulated B lymphocytes (11,12); reduced the number of splenic T lymphocytes (12), and responsiveness to T-lymphocyte mitogens (11,12); reduced responsiveness and stimulator activity of splenic T lymphocytes in the one-way mixed lymphocyte reaction (13); and impaired cell-mediated immunity to leukemia cells (14). A relationship to reduced interleukin 2 production has been suggested (15). Based on the above findings, we have pursued the effects of copper deficiency on the cell-mediated immune system in a rat model.

COPPER-DEFICIENT RAT MODEL

Using a low-copper basal diet similar to that used for mice by Lukasewycz and coworkers (10-15), a series of experiments were completed using weanling inbred Lewis rats. The findings of these experiments as described subsequently show an orderly progression of biological changes associated with copper deficiency (16); the influences of reduced food intake, sex, and iron on these changes; and the influences of plastic-adherent cells, erythrocytes, and latex particles on in vitro proliferation of concanavalin A (Con A)-stimulated splenic T lymphocytes in copper deficiency.

For these experiments, weanling Lewis rats were purchased from a commercial source and handled as previously described (17). Purified copper-deficient (0.6 μg Cu/g diet) and copper-adequate (5.6 μg Cu/g diet) diets contained 21.3% casein protein, 5% safflower oil, adequate (50 μg/g diet) and excess (300 μg/g diet) iron, and other nutrients as listed (17,18). Hematological and biochemical analyses were completed (17,18). Collection of lymphoid cells and analysis for mitogen-induced proliferation of T lymphocytes were also done (17). Data were analyzed by either Student's t-test or by analysis of variance (ANOVA).

PROGRESSION OF CHANGES IN COPPER DEFICIENCY

Anemia, depressed serum or plasma ceruloplasmin activity, depressed serum or plasma copper and iron, depressed liver copper, elevated liver iron, depressed cytochrome

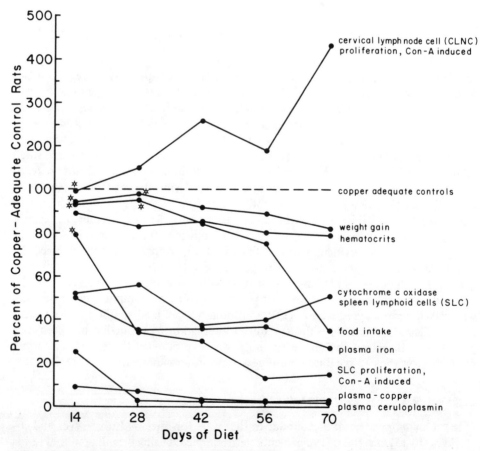

Figure 1 Progression of biological changes during copper deficiency (17). Values marked with a star are not significantly different from controls.

Copper and Immunity

c oxidase activity, and copper/zinc superoxide dismutase in lymphoid cells have been commonly found in young male copper-deficient rats (17,19-25). In our studies of young male Lewis strain rats, indicators of copper deficiency were a combination of dietary, anthropometrical, hematological, biochemical, and immunological variables. Significant differences between copper-deficient and copper-adequate rats were first displayed by hematological and biochemical indices, followed by immunological functions and last by dietary intake and growth (Fig. 1). Upon completion of 14 days of dietary regimen, rats fed low copper showed reduced hematocrits, plasma copper and iron, plasma ceruloplasmin activity, and cytochrome c oxidase activity of spleen lymphoid cells collected on a density gradient (Ficoll-Hypaque). With low copper-fed rats, changes in the proliferation of spleen lymphoid and cervical lymph node

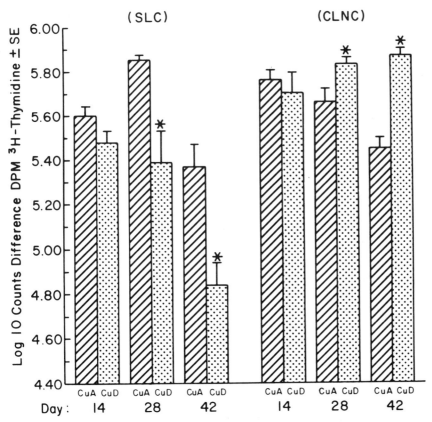

Figure 2 Progression of proliferation changes during copper deficiency of spleen lymphoid cells (SLCs) and cervical lymph node cells (CLNCs) stimulated with concanavalin A (17). Male Lewis rats were fed ad libitum either copper-adequate (CuA, 5.6 μg Cu/g diet) or copper-deficient (CuD, 0.6 μg Cu/g diet) diets. Counts difference DPM of SLCs and CLNCs showing highest [^{3}H]thymidine incorporation following stimulation with optimal dose of concanavalin A for peak proliferation. Counts difference was determined by subtracting the value of unstimulated cells from the value of concanavalin A-stimulated cells. Values between CuA and CuD groups within a cell type and time period were determined by Student's t-test. Standard error of the mean for each treatment group is indicated. Asterisk (*) indicates a difference between CuA and CuD responses ($p < 0.05$) at given times.

cells stimulated by Con A were not found until day 28 of dietary regimen. Reduction in food intake and growth were not found in rats fed low copper until dietary regimen day 42.

Proliferation of spleen lymphoid and cervical lymph node cells stimulated by Con A was influenced by low dietary copper (Fig. 2). Upon completion of dietary regimen day 28, proliferation of spleen lymphoid cells stimulated with multiple doses of Con A for peak proliferation was significantly lower in cells from copper-deficient rats than in cells from copper-adequate rats. In contrast to spleen lymphoid cells, proliferation of cervical lymph node cells stimulated with multiple doses of Con A was significantly higher in cells from copper-deficient rats than in cells from copper-adequate rats. Causes for these contrasting responses by spleen lymphoid and cervical lymph node cells stimulated by Con A from copper-deficient rats are unclear and need further investigation. However, the changes in proliferation of lymphoid cells following stimulation by Con A suggest that the ability of these cells to react to specific antigens may be altered by copper deficiency.

EFFECT OF FOOD INTAKE ON BIOLOGICAL CHANGES IN COPPER DEFICIENCY

Because young male Lewis rats fed a diet low in copper for 42 days consumed less food than copper-adequate control rats, an experiment was performed to determine the influence of reduced food intake on biological changes in copper deficiency. The suppressed weight gain of young male Lewis rats fed a diet low in copper for 42 days was found to be caused by reduced food intake alone (Fig. 3). Age- and weight-matched rats fed restricted amounts of copper-adequate diet, equivalent to the amount consumed by rats fed the copper-deficient diet, showed no greater weight gain than the copper-deficient rats. Both the food-restricted and copper-deficient rats consumed less food and gained less weight than copper-adequate rats. In contrast, the impaired hematological, biochemical, and immunological functions in copper-deficient rats were caused by low dietary copper and not reduced food intake. Copper-deficient, but not food-restricted rats, showed depressed hematocrits, serum copper and iron, serum ceruloplasmin activity, and proliferation of spleen lymphoid cells stimulated by Con A. Therefore, suppressed proliferation of spleen lymphoid cells stimulated by Con A was not related to reduced protein-energy intake, but to copper deficiency per se.

INFLUENCE OF RAT GENDER ON EXPRESSION OF COPPER DEFICIENCY

Anemia in rats (26) and suppressed immunity in mice (14) were less severe in copper-deficient females than males. We, therefore, performed experiments to determine the influence of the gender of the rat on the hematological, biochemical, and immunological changes observed in copper deficiency. The sex of young Lewis rats influenced the biological changes observed in copper deficiency (27) in a manner that anemia was present in copper-deficient male rats but not female rats (Fig. 4). Copper-deficient male rats showed severe depression of hematocrits and hemoglobin, whereas female copper-deficient rats showed only modest declines. In contrast, serum copper, iron, and ceruloplasmin activity were severely depressed in both male and female

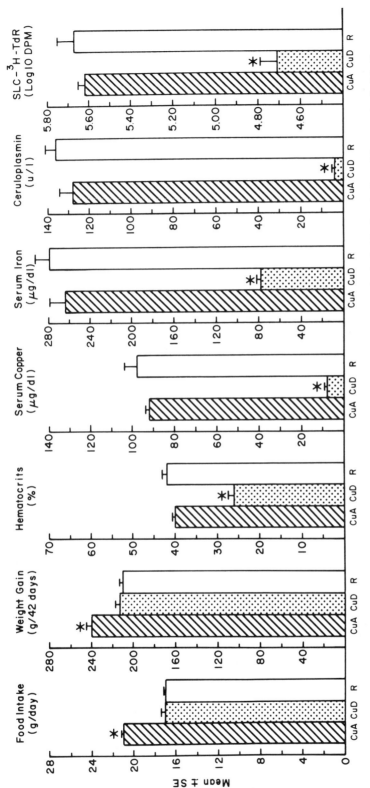

Figure 3 Influence of restricted food intake over a 42-day period on weight gain, hematological, biochemical, and immunological indices in copper-deficient male Lewis rats (17). Data were analyzed by using a one-way ANOVA. The restricted (R) food intake group received the copper-adequate diet (CuA, 5.6 μg Cu/g diet), but were limited to the amount consumed by the copper-deficient (CuD, 0.6 μg Cu/g diet) group. Standard error of the mean for each treatment group is indicated. Asterisk (*) indicates a difference ($p < 0.05$) between that treatment group and the other two.

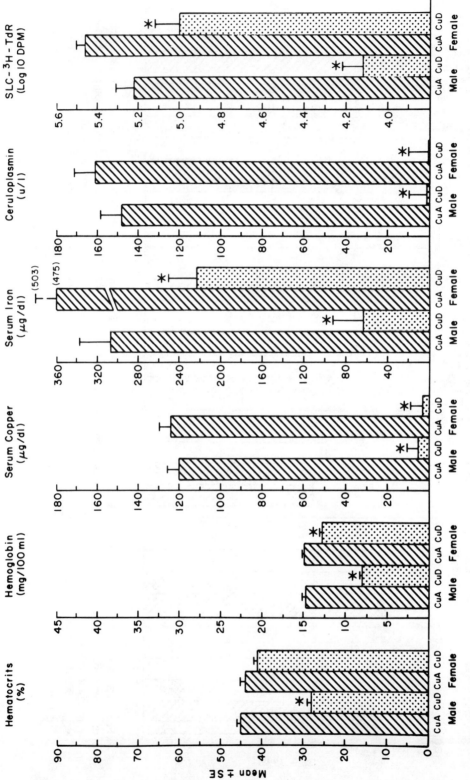

Figure 4 Influence of the sex on the animal on hematological, biochemical, and immunological responses in Lewis rats after 42 days on a copper-adequate (CuA, 5.6 μg Cu/g diet) or copper-deficient (CuD, 0.6 μg Cu/g diet) diet (27). Standard error of the mean for each treatment group is indicated. Asterisk (*) indicates a difference ($p < 0.05$) between that treatment group and the other within a given sex group. Data were analyzed using a two-way ANOVA.

Copper and Immunity

copper-deficient rats. In comparison to copper-adequate rats of the same sex, copper-deficient male and female rats showed decreased proliferation of spleen lymphoid cells stimulated by Con A. Interestingly, the decrease was greater in cells from copper-deficient male rats than in cells from copper-deficient female rats. Thus, cellular immunity is not compromised to the same extent by copper deficiency in female as it is in male rats. One reason for this difference may be better iron utilization in female copper-deficient rats. To explore the mechanism of suppressed proliferation of T lymphocytes in copper deficiency, we investigated the possible influence of iron on this phenomenon.

INTERACTION BETWEEN IRON AND COPPER

Anemia and reduced serum iron are characteristics of copper deficiency in the rat. High dietary iron did not correct these conditions in male Lewis rats fed diets low in copper (Fig. 5). Copper-deficient male rats fed adequate (50 μg Fe/g diet) and excess (300 μg Fe/g diet) iron had lower hematocrits and serum iron than did copper-adequate rats fed adequate and excess iron. Serum copper, iron, and ceruloplasmin activity and cytochrome c oxidase activity of spleen lymphoid cells were reduced in copper-deficient rats fed adequate and excess iron. Excess dietary iron also did not correct the suppressed proliferation of spleen lymphoid cells stimulated by Con A from copper-deficient rats.

Since a direct approach of feeding excess iron did not clarify the role of iron in suppressed proliferation of T lymphocytes in copper deficiency, an indirect approach was attempted. Three groups (10 rats/group) of weanling male Lewis rats were fed either copper-adequate or copper-deficient diets, containing adequate or deficient iron, for 5 weeks. A fourth group was fed a diet deficient in copper and iron for 3 weeks, followed by 2 weeks of diet adequate in copper but deficient in iron.

Rats fed adequate iron and low copper showed reduced hematocrits, hemoglobin, and serum iron (Fig. 6). Severe reductions in hematocrits, hemoglobin, and serum iron were exhibited by rats fed low copper and low iron for 3 weeks, followed by 2 weeks of adequate copper. Serum copper and ceruloplasmin activity were reduced in rats fed low-copper, adequate, and deficient iron diets. Rats fed low-iron, adequate-copper diets during weeks 4 and 5 of dietary regimen showed increased serum copper and ceruloplasmin activity.

As in earlier experiments, copper-deficient rats fed adequate iron showed suppressed proliferation of spleen lymphoid cells stimulated by Con A. However, increased proliferation with stimulation by Con A was found with spleen lymphoid cells from low-iron copper-deficient and copper-replenished rats (see Fig. 6). The finding of increased proliferation of T lymphocytes from dually copper- and iron-deficient rats prevents a clarification of the role of altered iron metabolism on suppressed proliferation of T lymphocytes in copper deficiency. This experiment did yield the interesting finding of increased T-lymphocyte proliferation in rats fed low-iron diets, which could be interpreted as indicating a negative modulatory role for iron on splenic T lymphocytes. These studies also indicate a potential interaction between iron and copper in the control of T-lymphocyte proliferative responses.

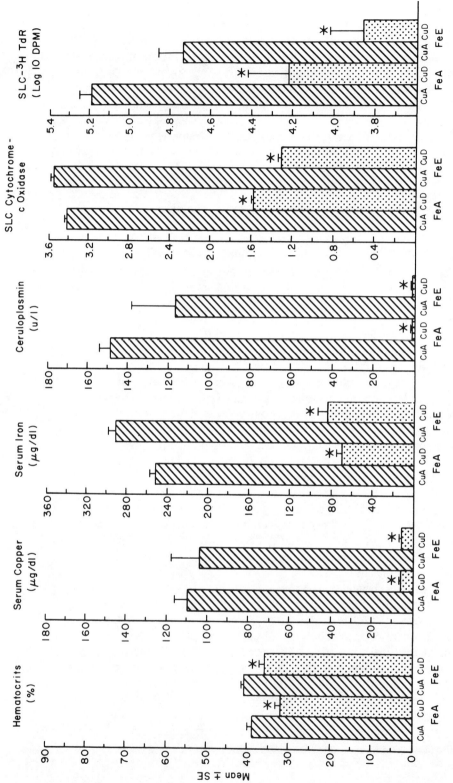

Figure 5 Influence of dietary iron on hematological, biochemical, and immunological responses in male Lewis rats after 42 days on copper-adequate (CuA, 5.6 μg Cu/g diet) and copper-deficient (cuD, 0.6 μg Cu/g diet) diets within iron-adequate (FeA, 50 μg Fe/g diet) or iron-excess (FeE, 300 μg Fe/g diet). Cytochrome c oxidase activity equals nmoles reduced cytochrome c oxidized/10^6 cells/min. Standard error of the mean for each treatment group is indicated. Asterisk (*) indicates a difference ($p < 0.05$) between copper groups within each iron group. Data were analyzed using a two-way ANOVA.

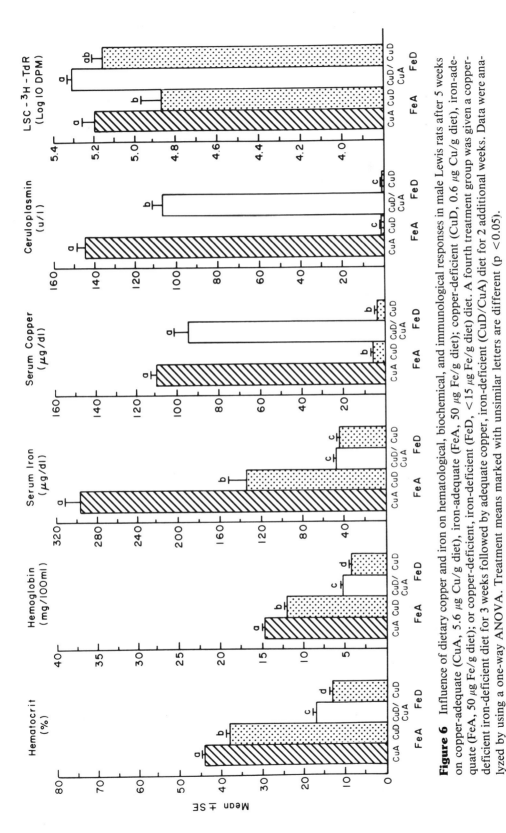

Figure 6 Influence of dietary copper and iron on hematological, biochemical, and immunological responses in male Lewis rats after 5 weeks on copper-adequate (CuA, 5.6 μg Cu/g diet), iron-adequate (FeA, 50 μg Fe/g diet); copper-deficient (CuD, 0.6 μg Cu/g diet), iron-adequate (FeA, 50 μg Fe/g diet); or copper-deficient, iron-deficient (FeD, <15 μg Fe/g diet) diet. A fourth treatment group was given a copper-deficient iron-deficient diet for 3 weeks followed by adequate copper, iron-deficient (CuD/CuA) diet for 2 additional weeks. Data were analyzed by using a one-way ANOVA. Treatment means marked with unsimilar letters are different (p <0.05).

ROLE OF MACROPHAGES IN ALTERED IMMUNE RESPONSE IN COPPER DEFICIENCY

The influence of splenic macrophages on proliferation, stimulated by Con A, of spleen lymphoid cells collected by density gradient (Ficoll-Hypague) from copper-deficient rats was questioned. As in earlier experiments, the proliferation of spleen lymphoid cells stimulated by Con A was lower for cells from copper-deficient than copper-adequate rats (Fig. 7A). Suppressed proliferation, stimulated by Con A, of spleen lymphoid cells from copper-deficient rats was not, however, alleviated following removal of phagocytic plastic-adherent cells (Fig. 7B) from the spleen lymphoid cell suspension (17). Furthermore, proliferation, stimulated by Con A, was equivalent for spleen lymphoid cells (SLCs) from copper-deficient rats and nonadherent spleen lymphoid cells (NASLCs; minimal number of macrophages) from both copper-deficient and copper-adequate rats. Thus, we infer that depressed proliferative responses in copper deficiency were associated with impaired enhancer function (possible interleukin 1 production) by plastic-adherent spleen lymphoid cells (macrophages) on T lymphocytes.

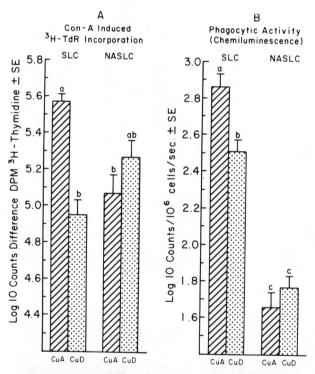

Figure 7 Proliferation of concanavalin A-stimulated (A), and phagocytic activity (B), of density gradient collected spleen lymphoid cells (SLCs) and plastic-nonadherent spleen lymphoid cells (NASLCs) of copper-adequate (CuA, 5.6 µg Cu/g diet) and copper-deficient (CuD, 0.6 µg Cu/g diet) male Lewis rats (17). Data were analyzed using a two-way ANOVA. Treatment means with different letters are different ($p < 0.05$).

Copper and Immunity

INFLUENCES OF ERYTHROCYTES AND LATEX PARTICLES ON T-LYMPHOCYTE PROLIFERATION IN COPPER DEFICIENCY

Ebert (28) reported that small numbers of sheep red blood cells added in vitro augmented the proliferation of T lymphocytes stimulated by phytohemagglutinin. We performed experiments to determine whether suppressed proliferation of splenic T lymphocytes in copper deficiency could be corrected by the presence of intact erythrocytes. The experimental model involved weanling male Lewis rats fed ad libitum copper-adequate and copper-deficient diets for 6 weeks.

Suppressed proliferation, stimulated by Con A, of spleen lymphoid cells from copper-deficient rats was alleviated by the in vitro presence of intact erythrocytes or latex particles (Figs. 8 and 10). Reduced proliferation, stimulated by Con A, of splenic T lymphocytes from copper-deficient rats was alleviated when resident splenic erythrocytes were present in the in vitro culture (Fig. 8). Suppressed proliferation, stimulated by Con A, of splenic T lymphocytes from copper-deficient rats was evident following removal of splenic erythrocytes from the spleen cell suspension by density

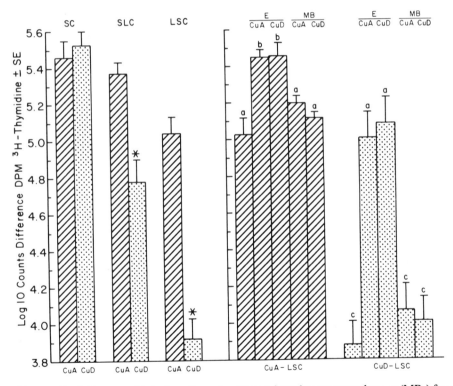

Figure 8 Influence of intact erythrocytes (Es) and erythrocyte membranes (MBs) from copper-adequate (CuA) and copper-deficient (CuD) rats on proliferation of concanavalin A-stimulated spleen lymphoid cells from CuA and CuD rats. SCs represents spleen lymphoid cells with resident splenic erythrocytes. Splenic erythrocytes were removed from SLCs (spleen lymphoid cells) and LSCs (lysed spleen cells) by density gradient centrifugation or lysis with NH_4Cl, respectively. Asterisk (*) indicates difference ($p < 0.05$) by Student's t-test. Treatment means marked with different letters are different ($p < 0.05$) by two-way ANOVA.

gradient (Ficoll-Hypaque) collection (SLCs) or by lysis of erythrocytes with 0.87 NH$_4$Cl (LSCs).

In vitro addition of intact peripheral blood erythrocytes (E, 10^6 cells) from copper-deficient and copper-adequate rats to NH$_4$Cl-treated LSCs from copper-adequate and copper-deficient rats caused enhanced proliferation of splenic T lymphocytes stimulated by Con A (Fig. 8). The degree of enhanced proliferation was more for LSCs from copper-deficient rats than for cells from copper-adequate rats; hence, a compensatory effect was found. Enhanced proliferation, stimulated by Con A and treated in vitro with erythrocytes, of LSCs from copper-deficient rats was equivalent to proliferation of LSCs, without the presence of intact erythrocytes, from copper-adequate rats. Suppressed proliferation, stimulated by Con A, of LSCs from copper-deficient rats was not alleviated by the addition of either erythrocyte membranes (Fig. 8) or lysate (Fig. 9).

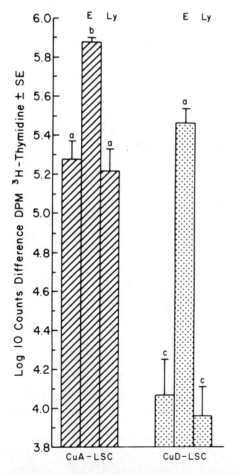

Figure 9 Influence of intact erythrocytes (Es) and erythrocyte lysate (Ly) from CuA male Lewis rats on proliferation of concanavalin A-stimulated lysed spleen cells (LSCs, erythrocyte lysed with NH$_4$Cl) from CuA and CuD rats. Treatment means marked with different letters are different (p<0.05) by two-way ANOVA.

Copper and Immunity

Enhanced proliferation, stimulated by Con A, of spleen lymphoid cells from copper-deficient rats was also observed when latex particles were added in vitro to the lymphoid cell cultures (Fig. 10). The mechanism has not been defined for enhanced proliferation of spleen lymphoid cells stimulated by Con A following in vitro exposure to intact erythrocytes or latex particles. These data appear to reflect an increase in suppressor cell activity, which Webb and Brooks (29) have described as a natural macrophage like suppressor cell which inhibits response to Con A in the absence of erythrocytes in culture. We have found that copper-deficient rats required four times as many latex particles compared to copper adequate rats to produce a maximal response (30).

In summary, copper deficiency in the rat caused suppressed splenic and enhanced cervical lymph node T-lymphocyte proliferation. Those changes were observed after hematological and biochemical changes but before impaired growth. Suppressed splenic T-lymphocyte proliferation in copper deficiency was not caused by decreased

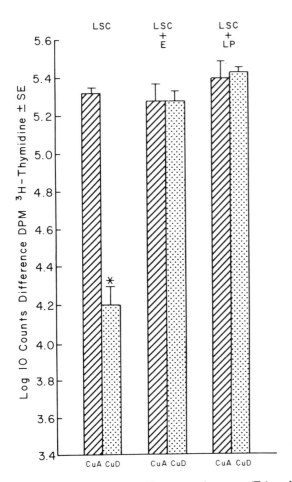

Figure 10 Influence of intact erythrocytes (Es) and latex particles (LPs) on proliferation of concanavalin A-stimulated lysed spleen cells (LSCs, erythrocytes lysed with NH_4Cl) from CuA and CuD rats. Values between CuA and CuD groups within a cell-treatment combination were determined by Student's t-test. Asterisk (*) indicates a difference between CuA and CuD responses ($p < 0.05$) of LSCs.

food intake, and was not corrected by high iron intake. Although splenic T-lymphocyte proliferation was decreased in copper-deficient male and female rats, it was decreased more markedly in copper-deficient male rats. Suppressed splenic T-lymphocyte proliferation in copper deficiency was influenced by the presence of plastic-adherent lymphoid cells (macrophages). Suppressed in vitro proliferation of splenic T lymphocytes in copper deficiency was alleviated when intact erythrocytes or latex particles were added to the lymphoid cell culture, but not when either erythrocyte membranes or lysate were added. It is not known if splenic macrophages are required for the enhanced proliferation of splenic T-lymphocytes upon the addition of intact erythrocytes or latex particles. Studies are needed to determine the role of splenic macrophages and their interaction with T lymphocytes on suppressed splenic T-lymphocyte proliferation in copper deficiency.

CONCLUSIONS

Thus, studies on the effect of copper deficiency in the rat suggest that copper has a specific regulatory role in the development and expression of immune reactions which is both qualitatively and quantitatively separate from other general effects on numerous biological processes. Specificity is suggested by the fact that the immune function of the spleen but not the cervical lymph node lymphocyte is affected (17) and the restriction of anemia and the most profound immune effects to the male rat. Further, we have determined that the effects on the immune function were not directly related to anemia and that iron deficiency appears not to be the principal cause of immune dysfunction (27). As suggested above, however, the sex difference may be related to better iron utilization in the female rat, although the basis of this phenomenon remains to be explored and probably is complex, since sex hormones could also influence immune response. Recently, Bala et al. (31) confirmed our observations on decreased mitogenesis in the copper-deficient rat. Interestingly, these investigators found an increase in the relative percentage of macrophages in the copper-deficient group which seems consistent with our hypothesis that the naturally occurring macrophagelike suppressor cell is increased during copper deficiency (30). In addition, in this study, a decrease of $CD4^+$ T cells was noted as a very early event occurring even before anemia was produced, whereas a decrease in $CD8^+$ T cells was found only in the context of reduced thymus, enlarged spleen, and reduced hematocrit. However, there was no simple relationship between lymphocyte profile and immune response, since T-cell ratios were normal in the copper-deficient females, whereas responsiveness to mitogen in vitro was depressed. The finding of increased interleukin 2 receptor- and transferrin receptor-bearing lymphocytes in copper deficiency may suggest a possible basis for the apparent sequestration of less reactive immune cells to the spleen. While the critical mechanism of copper interaction in immunity will require further study, the present evidence suggests that such investigations will elucidate key regulatory events in the normal immune response.

REFERENCES

1. Pedroni E, Bianchi E, Ugazio AG, Burgio GR. Immunodeficiency and steely hair. Lancet 1:1303-1304, 1975.
2. Graham GG, Cordano A. Copper depletion and deficiency in the malnourished infant. Johns Hopkins Med J 124:139-150, 1969.

3. al-Rashid RA, Spangler J. Neonatal copper deficiency. N Engl J Med 285:841-843, 1971.
4. Karpel JT, Peden VH. Copper deficiency in long-term parenteral nutrition. J Pediatr 80:32-86, 1972.
5. Yuen P, Lin HJ, Hutchison JH. Copper deficiency in a low birthweight infant. Arch, Dis Child, 54:553-555, 1979.
6. Boyne R, Arthur JR. Effects of selenium and copper deficiency on neutrophile function in cattle. J Comp Pathol 91:271-276, 1981.
7. Jones DG, Suttle NF. Some effects of copper deficiency on leucocyte function in sheep and cattle. Res Vet Sci 31:151-156, 1981.
8. Jones DG, Suttle NF. The effect of copper deficiency on the resistance of mice to infection with *Pasteurella haemolytica*. J Comp Pathol 93:143-149, 1983.
9. Newberne PM, Hunt CE, Young VR. The role of diet and the reticuloendothelial system in the response of rats to *Salmonella typhimurium* infection. Br J Exp Pathol 49:448-457, 1968.
10. Prohaska JR, Lukasewycz OA. Copper deficiency suppresses the immune response of mice. Science 213:559-561, 1981.
11. Lukasewycz OA, Prohaska JR. Lymphocytes from copper-deficient mice exhibit decreased mitogen reactivity. Nutr Res 3:335-341, 1983.
12. Lukasewycz OA, Prohaska JR, Meyer SG, Schmidtke JR, Marder SM, Marder P. Alterations in lymphocyte subpopulations in copper deficient mice. Infect Immun 48:644-647, 1985.
13. Lukasewycz OA, Kolquist KL, Prohaska JR. Splenocytes from copper-deficient mice are low responders and weak stimulators in mixed lymphocyte reactions. Nutr Res 7:43-52, 1987.
14. Lukasewycz OA, Prohaska JR. Immunization against transplantable leukemia impaired in copper-deficient mice. J Natl Cancer Inst 69:489-493, 1982.
15. Lukasewycz OA, Prohaska JR. Immune response in copper deficiency. NY Acad Sci 587:147, 1990.
16. Vyas D, Chandra RK. Thymic factor activity, lymphocyte stimulation response and antibody producing cells in copper deficiency. Nutr Res 3:343-349, 1983.
17. Davis MA, Johnson WT, Briske-Anderson M, Kramer TR. Lymphoid cell functions during copper deficiency. Nutr Res 7:211-222, 1987.
18. Johnson WT, Kramer TR. The effect of copper deficiency on erythrocyte membrane proteins. J Nutr 117:1085-1090, 1987.
19. Dempsey H, Cartwright GD, Wintrobe MM. Studies on copper metabolism, XXV. Relationship between serum and liver copper. Proc Soc Exp Biol Med 98:520-523, 1958.
20. Mills CF, Murray G. The preparation of a semi-synthetic diet low in copper for copper-deficiency studies with the rat. J Sci Food Agric 11:547-552, 1960.
21. Owen CA Jr, Hazelrig JB. Copper deficiency and copper toxicity in the rat. Am J Physiol 215:334-338, 1968.
22. Alfaro B, Heaton FW. Relationships between copper, zinc and iron in the plasma, soft tissues and skeleton of the rat during Cu deficiency. Br J Nutr 29:73-85, 1973.
23. Boyne R. Changes in leucocyte cytochrome oxidase activity associated with deficiency of copper in laboratory and farm animals. Res Vet Sci 24:134-138, 1978.
24. Prohaska JR. Changes in tissue growth, concentrations of copper, iron, cytochrome oxidase and superoxide dismutase subsequent to dietary or genetic copper deficiency in mice. J Nutr 113:2148-2158, 1983.
25. Prohaska Jr. Changes in Cu, Zu-superoxide dismutase, cytochrome C oxidase, glutathione peroxidase and glutathione transferase activities in copper-deficient mice and rats. J Nutr 121:355, 1991.
26. Fields M, Lewis C, Scholfield DJ, Powell AS, Rose AJ, Reiser S, Smith JC. Female rats are protected against the fructose induced mortality of copper deficiency. Proc Soc Exp Biol Med 183:145-149, 1986.

27. Kramer TR, Johnson WT, Briske-Anderson M. The influence of iron and the sex of rats on hematological, biochemical and immunological changes during copper-deficiency. J Nutr 118:214-221, 1988.
28. Ebert EC. Sheep red blood cells enhance T-lymphocyte proliferation. Clin Immunol Immunopathol 37:203-212, 1985.
29. Webb PJ, Brooks CG. Macrophage-like suppressor cells in rats. I. Inhibition of natural macrophage-like suppressor cells by red blood cells. Cell Immunol 52:370, 1980.
30. Kramer TR, Johnson WT, Briske-Anderson M. Erythrocytes and latex particles enhance blastogenesis of concanavalin-A stimulated spleen lymphoid cells from copper deficient rats. Nutr Res 10:303, 1990.
31. Bala S, Failla ML, Lunney JK. Alterations in splenic lymphoid cell subsets and activation antigens in copper-deficient rats. J Nutr 121:745, 1991.

16

Modulation of Differentiation Antigen Expression and Function of Immune Cells Following Short and Prolonged Alcohol Intake During Murine Retroviral Infection

Ronald R. Watson, Maria C. Lopez, Olalekan E. Odeleye, and Hamid Darban

University of Arizona College of Medicine, Tucson, Arizona

INTRODUCTION

Chronic alcohol intake affects a variety of immune functions (1). This modification in immunological function suggests that these alterations might be used as markers to identify severe alcohol abusers. The immune alterations caused by the direct effects of ethanol, its biochemical metabolites, or associated condiments may be an etiological factor in the increased incidence of diseases, including oral, esophageal, and hepatic cancers and immunodepressive diseases observed in alcohol abusers. Some of these effects may be related to other elements in the diet or their interactions (1-4). Much of the work relating to cellular immune functional change has been done in patients with alcoholic hepatitis and liver dysfunction (5,6). Therefore, conclusions from these studies may only be potentially indicative of changes which may occur in people with chronic consumption of alcohol. Patients with alcoholic liver disease are known to have reduced skin test reactivity to common antigens (7,8) and poor sensitization to dinitrochlorobenzene (7-10). However, upon clinical recovery from alcoholic hepatitis, positive skin test responses increase (8). However, whether reduced sensitization in alcoholism occurs as the result of undernutrition, the toxic effects of ethanol, or severe liver injury, this immune deficiency may have some diagnostic value (when combined with other types of biological measures), and furthermore may be relevant to disease resistance (5). Since improvement in hepatic function usually parallels nutritional recovery, the relative contribution of such factors to reduction in delayed hypersensitivity is difficult to measure. However, chronic alcoholics, even prior to the development of liver cirrhosis, while showing little detectable impairment of delayed hypersensitivity, do exhibit reduced E-rosette formation (11). We have been interested in the possibility that alcohol-induced immunosuppression may be a risk factor in the development of tumors (12) because of observations in vitro suggesting discrete immunoregulatory effects (13,14).

A strong indication that a high intake of alcohol in the absence of liver damage could cause a rapid change in the cellular immune function is suggested by the studies of Sorrel and Leevy (15). They showed that lymphocyte mitogenesis was increased upon addition of ethanol or acetaldehyde to cell cultures in vitro. Interestingly, mononuclear cells from alcoholics with inactive cirrhosis did not show increased mitogenesis when ethanol was added in vitro. These observations have since been confirmed using leukocyte migration tests (16). These data may indicate loss of responsiveness with continued exposure in vivo.

Human studies conducted in our laboratories on the effects of dietary ethanol have shown that the relative proportion of T-helper cells may be significantly increased in long-term alcohol consumption, particularly in the setting of liver damage (Table 1) (17). This is supportive of earlier in vitro data suggesting decreased E-rosette formation by lymphocytes in the presence of ethanol metabolites (11) and recent data (14) indicating the discrete effects of alcohols in vitro on human lymphocyte subpopulations. Our studies had also shown that B- and T-cell mitogenesis was not similarly affected to any significant degree in ongoing alcoholism (17). Studies of mild/moderate alcohol use over a long period of use are much needed to carefully define the effects of alcohol on cellular immune functions in animal models and humans. This could be potentially very important in diseases of long latency where immunodeficiency may play a key role in disease etiology. In particular, we wondered whether alcohol consumption might affect acquired immunodeficiency of retroviral origin. At least one group of AIDS patients, i.e., drug abusers, are likely to have been alcohol abusers at some time. If drugs of abuse, including alcohol, compromise the immune system, their use may be a predisposing factor in progression of HIV disease (18,19). We, therefore, have developed a defined murine model (20-22). We now report the effect of various levels of ethanol intake with and without retroviral infection on some immune cells and functions in C57Bl/6 mice.

Table 1 T-Lymphocyte Subsets Isolated from Blood of Alcohol Consumers

Group	T-helper lymphocytes (CD4$^+$)	T-suppressor lymphocytes (CD8$^+$)	T-helper/ T-suppressor
Lifelong abstainers (10)	40 ± 3.8	27 ± 2.7	1.7 ± 0.3
Previous alcohol abusers (10)	47 ± 2.0	28 ± 1.9	1.9 ± 0.2
Current alcohol abusers (10)	44 ± 3.8	25 ± 2.6	2.2 ± 0.5
Patients with alcoholic liver disease or pancreatitis (9)	60 ± 3.6[a]	16 ± 3.1[a]	5.9 ± 1.6[a]

Male subjects were classified in four groups. The number of subjects in each group is shown in parentheses.
Values are mean ± SE.
[a]Significantly different from life-long abstainers group ($p < 0.05$).
Source: Modified from Ref. 17.

THE MURINE MODEL

Mice of susceptible strains develop an acquired immunodeficiency syndrome (AIDS), termed murine-AIDS (MAIDS), following infection with LP-BM5 murine leukemia virus (MuLV) (23-32). The virus preparation that causes MAIDS includes a mixture of replication-competent ecotropic and mink cell focus-inducing murine leukemia virus and a defective virus (31). Mice infected with LP-BM5 MuLV presented lymphadenopathy and immune dysfunction characterized by polyclonal B-cell activation with hypergammaglobulinemia, impaired antigen-specific responses of B cells, failure of B cells to respond to normal T cells, and impaired responses to T and B cell mitogens (23).

Female C57B1/6 mice at 3-4 weeks of age, obtained from the Charles River Laboratories, were infected when they were 4-5 weeks old. Infection of adult C57/BL6 mice with LP-BM5 leads to the rapid induction of clinical symptomatology with virtually no latent phase (21-28).

Groups of mice were fed the Lieber-DeCarli diet (20) containing 0, 4, 5, or 6% (v/v) ethanol and made isocaloric by the addition of dextrin maltose. Mice fed the 6% ethanolic diet became severely dehydrated and died before the evaluation point at 7 weeks and the data obtained were not reported. We have reported vitamin E deficiency as a possible complication of this diet (33). One-half of the mice in each group were infected intraperitoneally with LP-BM5 MuLV on the day of initiation of dietary ethanol supplementation.

Spleens were collected in RPMI-1640 medium from dissected mice and mononuclear cells were obtained by gently teasing with tweezers. Cell suspensions were washed with RPMI, and red blood cells were lysed by ammonium chloride. The remaining cell suspensions were washed once with cold RPMI and counted with eosin Y to prepare desired viable cell concentrations ($1-2 \times 10^6/0.1$ ml/tube) for lymphocyte and macrophage surface marker determinations and were quantified by indirect immunofluorescence using monoclonal antibodies specific for total T cells (rat IgG_{2b} antimouse Thy 1.2 antigen), T-helper cells (L3T4; rat IgG_{2b} antimouse CD4 antigen, GK1.5 clone) or T-suppressor cells (Lyt-2; rat IgG_{2a} antimouse CD8 antigen). Total macrophages and activated macrophages were measured with antimurine antigen (Ag) of Mac-1 and Mac-2 monoclonal antibodies. The numbers of cells expressing interleukin 2 receptors (IL-2R) were determined by using rat IgG_{2a} monoclonal antibodies (clone AMT-13). Mature T cells that express CD5 antigen were determined by indirect immunofluorescence using a rat antimouse monoclonal antibody (Lyt-1). Fluorescein isothiocyanate labeled goat antirat immunoglobulin was used as second antibody. B Cells that express surface IgG or IgM were recognized by an indirect assay using an affinity-purified rabbit antimouse antibody and a fluorescein conjugated goat antirabbit antibody, as described previously (30,31).

Effect of Chronic Ethanol Exposure on the Percentage of Splenic Lymphocytes

Our first study was designed to evaluate the effect on the immune system of chronic ethanol administration for 3 or 7 weeks. There were no differences in spleen weight among the groups that received ethanol for 3 or 7 weeks. Also, there were no differences in spleen weight between the control groups in both experiments. But the cell number was statistically significant higher ($p < 0.01$, data not shown) in the control

Table 2 Percentage of Lymphocytes and Macrophages in the Spleen of Mice Chronically Exposed to Dietary Ethanol for 3 Weeks

Dietary ethanol (%)	Total (Thy 1.2)	Helper (CD4$^+$)	Suppressor (CD8$^+$)	Activated lymphocytes (IL-2 R)	Macrophages	Stimulated macrophages	B Cells
0	46.0 ± 7.8	24.6 ± 3.6	14.5 ± 5.0	0.37 ± 0.5	3.4 ± 0.7	0.45 ± 0.4	15.4 ± 3.7
4	50.7 ± 10.4	26.7 ± 3.1	11.8 ± 1.9	0.37 ± 0.5	2.7 ± 1.7	0.24 ± 0.17	13.8 ± 3.2
5	44.6 ± 12.5	28.9 ± 2.7	9.7 ± 1.7	0.51 ± 0.41	3.8 ± 1.0	0.39 ± 0.2	15.1 ± 1.5

Mice fed a 6% Leiber-DeCarli diet lose weight and died by 7 weeks.
Values shown as mean ± SD.

group for 7 weeks exposure than in the control group for 3 weeks exposure. We could not find statistically significant differences in the percentages of T and B cells and macrophages (Table 2) in the spleens of mice that received ethanol for 3 weeks. Nevertheless, a tendency to a lower percentage of CD8$^+$ cells was observed, which became significant when the absolute number of CD8$^+$ cells were considered (Table 4). After 7 weeks of ethanol consumption, an increase in the percentage of Thy 1.2$^+$ and CD4$^+$ cells was observed in the spleen of those mice that received 5% ethanol (Table 3). When the absolute number of cells specifically stained was analyzed, we failed to see this increase (Table 5), perhaps due to the fact that the total number of cells in the spleen was decreased ($p < 0.01$) in this experimental group when compared to the control group (data not shown).

Table 3 Percentage of Lymphocytes in the Spleens of Mice Chronically Fed Ethanol for 7 Weeks

Dietary ethanol (%)	Total (Thy 1.2)	Helper (CD4$^+$)	Suppressor (CD8$^+$)	Activated lymphocytes (IL-2 R)	Macrophages	Stimulated macrophages	B Cells
0	32.6 ± 4.2	17.6 ± 4.5	6.3 ± 2.6	0.3 ± 0.2	3.0 ± 0.7	0.57 ± 0.38	14.1 ± 3.1
4	31.4 ± 2.2	18.9 ± 2.1	4.5 ± 2.4	0.8 ± 0.5	2.8 ± 0.4	0.76 ± 0.6	15.4 ± 4.9
5	45.7 ± 7.5[a]	24.0 ± 4.4[a]	7.6 ± 1.0	0.5 ± 0.3	3.6 ± 0.2	0.64 ± 0.5	22.2 ± 3.7

Mice fed a 6% Leiber-DeCarli diet lost weight and died by 7 weeks.
Values shown as mean ± SD.
[a]Significantly different from untreated group ($p < 0.05$).

Table 4 Effects of 3 Weeks of Ethanol Consumption in Mice on the Absolute Numbers of Splenic Lymphoid Subsets

Dietary ethanol (%)	Total (Thy 1.2)	Helper (CD4$^+$)	Suppressor (CD8$^+$)	Activated lymphocytes (IL-2 R)	Macrophages	Stimulated macrophages	B Cells
0	34.0 ± 9.0	18.0 ± 5.0	10.64 ± 3.8	1.0 ± 1.5	2.6 ± 0.7	0.3 ± 0.3	12.0 ± 4.0
4	44.0 ± 12.0	25.0 ± 9.0	10.32 ± 2.6	0.2 ± 0.2	6.2 ± 7.4	0.2 ± 0.1	13.0 ± 7.0
5	23.0 ± 8.0	15.0 ± 3.0	5.0 ± 1.6[a]	0.2 ± 0.2	5.5 ± 8.1	0.2 ± 0.1	7.8 ± 1.9

Mice fed a 6% Leiber-DeCarli diet lost weight and died by 7 weeks.
Values shown as mean × 10^6 cells/spleen ± SD.
[a]Significantly different from control group ($p < 0.05$).

Table 5 Effects on the Absolute Numbers of Splenic Lymphoid Subsets of 7 Weeks of Ethanol Consumption in Mice

Dietary ethanol (%)	Total (Thy 1.2)	Helper (CD4$^+$)	Suppressor (CD8$^+$)	Activated lymphocytes (IL-2 R)	Macrophages	Stimulated macrophages	B Cells
0	36.0 ± 8.0	19.0 ± 4.0	7.0 ± 3.1	0.3 ± 0.2	3.2 ± 0.8	0.6 ± 0.3	15.0 ± 4.0
4	33.0 ± 9.0	20.0 ± 5.0	4.2 ± 1.6	0.8 ± 0.5	3.0 ± 1.7	0.8 ± 0.5	17.0 ± 12.0
5	37.0 ± 6.0	19.0 ± 3.0	6.2 ± 0.8	0.4 ± 0.2	2.9 ± 0.3	0.5 ± 0.4	18.0 ± 4.0

Mice fed a 6% Leiber-DeCarli diet lost weight and died by 7 weeks.
Values shown as mean × 10^6 cells/spleen ± SD.

Combined Effects of Ethanol and Retroviral Infection on Lymphoid Cells

In our second study, we investigated the possible role of ethanol as a cofactor in the immunosuppression caused by murine leukemia virus. Mice were fed the Lieber-DeCarli diet supplemented with sucrose or 5% (v/v) ethanol for 5 days per week. They were fed Purina Rat Chow and water provided ad libitum for the remaining 2 days of the week. The feeding routine was repeated for 12 weeks, the duration of the experiment. One-half of the mice in each group were infected with LP-BM5 MuLV on the day of initiation of dietary ethanol supplementation.

We observed a significant increase in spleen weight and cell number in the virus-infected mice (data not shown). The effect was remarkable on spleen weight and interestingly ethanol administration slightly slowed down this effect.

Murine AIDS infection induced by LP-BM5 MuLV significantly reduced the percentage of total T cells (Thy 1.2) (p <0.01), whereas increased the percentage of IL-2R$^+$ lymphocytes, CD4$^+$, and CD8$^+$ cells (Table 6). However, dietary ethanol in the infected mice prevented the virus-induced increase in CD4$^+$ and CD8$^+$ cells compared to infected mice fed the control diet. Interestingly, the percentage of total T cells was much less than the sum of the percentage of CD4$^+$ plus CD8$^+$ in the virus-infected mice (see Table 6). This result suggests the presence of Thy 1.2$^-$ CD4$^+$ cells in these mice as has recently been described by Holmes et al.

Table 6 Percentage of Lymphocytes in the Spleen of Mice Fed a 5% Ethanol Diet and Infected with a Murine Retrovirus

Treatment group	T Cells			
	Total (Thy 1.2)	Helper (CD4$^+$)	Suppressor (CD8$^+$)	Activated (IL-2R$^+$)
None	42.2 ± 4.3	21.5 ± 3.4	16.2 ± 1.7	0.9 ± 1.7
Ethanol	32.8 ± 8.4[a]	21.8 ± 2.9	15.5 ± 1.2	2.3 ± 2.5
Retrovirus	25.5 ± 5.0[a]	30.5 ± 2.5[a]	31.5 ± 6.5[a]	12.0 ± 1.6[a]
Retrovirus with ethanol	29.5 ± 5.0[a]	21.5 ± 2.2[b]	20.6 ± 3.2[b]	9.8 ± 2.1[a]

Values shown as mean ± SD.
[a]Significantly different from untreated group (p <0.05).
[b]Retrovirus-infected, ethanol-fed significantly different from retrovirus-infected group fed control diet (p <0.05).

CONCLUSIONS

Our results indicate that low levels of dietary ethanol in long-term studies could only induce limited changes in the percentage of various lymphocyte subsets in the spleens of mice exposed to different levels of alcohol in the diet. At levels sustainable over weeks or months without causing death, chronic ethanol-containing diets did not modify dramatically the percentage or the absolute number of most splenic lymphocyte subsets in C57BL/6 mice. However, there were increases in the percentages of cells that specifically bear Thy 1.2 and CD4 antigens after 7 weeks. These results suggest that either the lymphoid cells adapted to the effects of chronic exposure or the level of ethanol and its metabolites were not sufficient to cause differential long-term changes in cell subtypes. Ethanol can cause nutritional deficiency even with the high levels of nutrients of the Lieber-Decarlo diet (33). Nevertheless, these results contrast with changes in the relative ratio of T subsets observed with higher levels of ethanol (7% V/V or 35% of daily caloric intake) (29) after 1 week of exposure. However, such high intake levels have been studied only after very brief exposures of 7 days because, as we mentioned above, when we used such high levels of ethanol in the diet, mice became dehydrated and died before 7 weeks. In vivo studies involving short-term ethanol use show that very high ethanol consumption and its attendant weight loss and dehydration cause changes in the relative numbers of splenic lymphocyte subsets (29,30). On the contrary, our present observations of limited changes in the relative numbers of various lymphocyte subsets due to chronic ethanol use are in agreement with a previous human study, reinforcing the theory that the immune system could partially adapt and, hence, bypass the effect of chronic low-level exposure to ethanol (17). However, chronic ethanol consumption in a setting of malnutrition, major weight loss, or organ dysfunction may be expected to induce more significant changes in immune function. Specifically ethanol-induced malnutrition may affect immunoregulation in HIV disease (34).

Retroviral infection as described here significantly changed splenic lymphocyte subsets, altering not only the normal relationship between T-cell subsets, but their functionality as has been described previously (21-27). Retroviral infection preferentially lowered the apparent percentage of total T cells while increasing in T-helper and T-suppressor cells, which yielded a greater combined percentage than total T cells. This result may suggest blocking of Thy 1.2 antigen or the appearance of an abnormal population, in agreement with the finding of the group of Morse, which has recently described a subset of Thy 1.2^- $CD4^+$ cells in LP-BM5 MuLV-infected mice (32). The chronic ethanol exposure regimens with regular withdrawal episodes used here only modified the percentage of splenic total T lymphocytes significantly, and did not exacerbate the changes induced by retroviral infection. However, since in recent studies (35,36) we have noted that retroviral infection may promote tumor development in chronic alcohol consumption and that β-carotene and canthaxanthin thin can partially offset this effect, it seems highly likely that there are significant immunosuppressing effects of alcohol that could promote further immune deregulation in AIDS.

ACKNOWLEDGMENTS

The support of a grant from the Alcohol Drug Abuse and Mental Health Administration, Bethesda, Maryland, (AA08037), and a fellowship-sustaining MCL from Conicet

(Consejo Nacional de Investigaciones Cientificas y Tecnicas, Argentina) is gratefully recognized. We also thank Dr. R. A. Yetter of the Veterans Administration Hospital, Baltimore, Maryland, for providing the viral inoculum.

REFERENCES

1. Watson RR. Ethanol, immunomodulation and cancer. Prog Food Nutri Sci 12:189-209, 1988.
2. Sanchis R. The role of liquid diet formulation in the post natal ethanol exposure of rats via mother's milk. J Nutr 119:82-88, 1989.
3. Mohs ME, Leonard TK, Watson RR. Interrelationships among alcohol abuse, obesity, and type II diabetes mellitus: Focus on native americans world review of nutrition and diabetes. 56:93-172, 1988.
4. Mohs ME, Watson RR. Change in the nutrient status and balance associated with alcohol abuse. Diagnosis of Alcohol Abuse. Boca Raton, FL. CRC Press, 125-146, 1989.
5. Watson RR. Alcohol and cellular immune response. In: Watson RR, ed. Nutrition, Disease Resistance and Immune Functions. Marcel Dekker, New York, pp 313-324, 1984.
6. Zetterman RK, Sorrell MF. Immunologic aspects of alcoholic liver disease. Gastroenterology 81:616-624, 1981.
7. Berenyi MR, Straus B, Cruz D. In vitro and in vivo studies of cellular immunity in alcoholic cirrhosis. Am J Dig Dis 19:199-205, 1974.
8. Snyder N, Bessoff J, Dwyer JM, Conn HO. Depressed delayed cutaneous hypersensitivity in alcoholic hepatitis. Am J Dig Dis 23:353-358, 1978.
9. Straus B, Berenyi MR, Huang JM, Straus E. Delayed hypersensitivity in alcoholic cirrhosis. Am J Dig Dis 16:509-516, 1971.
10. Scheinberg MA. Delayed hypersensitivity in alcoholic cirrhosis. Am J Dig Dis 17:760, 1972.
11. Lang JM, Rushcer H, Hasselmann JP, Grandjean P, Bigel P, Mayer S. Decreased autologous rosette-forming T lymphocytes in alcoholic cirrhosis: Absence of correlation with other T cell markers and with delayed cutaneous hypersensitivity. Int Arch Allergy Appl Immunol 61:337-343, 1980.
12. Mufti JI, Darban HR, Watson RR. Alcohol, cancer, and immunomodulation. Crit Rev Hem Oncol 9:243-261, 1989.
13. Mufti SI, Prabhala R, Moriguchi S, Sipes IG, Watson RR. Functional and numerical alterations induced by ethanol in the cellular immune system. Immunopharmacology 15:85-93, 1988.
14. Prabhala RH, Watson RR. Effects of various alcohols applied in vitro on human lymphocyte subtype and mitogenesis progress in clinical and biological research. Prog Clin Biol Res 325:155-163, 1990.
15. Sorrell MF, Leevy CM. Lymphocyte transformation and alcoholic liver injury. Gastroenterology 63:1020-1025, 1972.
16. Actis GC, Ponzetoo A, Rizzetto M, Verme G. Cell mediated immunity to acetaldehyde in alcoholic liver disease demonstrated by leukocyte migration test. Am J Dig Dis 23:883-886, 1978.
17. Watson RR, Jackson JC, Hartmann B, Sampliner R, Mobley D, Eskelson C. Cellular immune functions, endorphins, and alcohol consumption in males. Alcoholism; Clin Exp Res 9:248-254, 1985.
18. Pillai RM, Watson RR. In vitro immunotoxicology and immunopharmacology: studies on drugs of abuse. Toxicol Lett 53:269-283, 1990.
19. Watson RR. Immunomodulation by alcohol: A cofactor in development of AIDS after retrovirus infection. In: Cofactors in HIV-I Infection and AIDS. CRC Press, 1989, pp 47-54.

20. Lieber CS, DeCarli LM. The feeding of alcohol in liquid diets: Two decades of application and 1982 update. Alcohol Clin Exp Res 6:523-531, 1982.
21. Watson RR. Murine models for Acquired Immune Deficiency Syndrome. Life Sci 44: i-xiii, 1989.
22. Watson RR. A murine retrovirus model for studies of the role of cofactors and ethanol in AIDS development. NIDA Res Monogr 96:166-80, 199
23. Mosier DE, Yetter RA, Morse HC III. Retroviral induction of acute lymphoproliferative disease and profound immunosuppression in adult C57BL/6 mice. J Exp Med, 161: 766-784, 1985.
24. Klinken SP, Fredrickson TN, Hartley JW, Yetter RA, Morse HC III. Evaluation of B cell lineage lymphomas in mice with a retrovirus-induced immunodeficiency syndromes, MAIDS. J Immunol 140:1123-1131, 1988.
25. Buller RML, Yetter RA, Fredrickson TN, Morse HC III. Abrogation of resistance to severe mouse pox in C57BL/6 mice infected with LP-BM5 murine leukemia viruses. J Virol, 61:383-387, 1987.
26. Mosier DE. Animal models for retrovirus-induced immunodeficiency disease. Immunol Invest 15:233-261, 1986.
27. Mosier DE, Yetter RA, Morse HC III. Functional T-lymphocytes are required for a murine retrovirus-induced immunodeficiency disease (MAIDS). J Exp Med 165:1737-1742, 1987.
28. Cerny A, Hugin AW, Hardy RR, Hayakawa K, Zinkernagel RM, Makino M, Morse HC III. B Cells are required for induction of T cell abnormalities in a murine retrovirus-induced immunodeficiency model. J Exp Med 171:315-320, 1990.
29. Watson RR, Prabhala RH, Abril E, Smith TL. Changes in lymphocyte subsets and macrophage functions from high, short-term dietary ethanol in C57B1/6 mice. Life Sci 43:865-870, 1988.
30. Mufti SI, Prabhala R, Moriguchi S, Sipes IG, Watson RR. Functional and numerical alterations induced by ethanol in the cellular immune system. Immunopharmacology 15: 85-94, 1988.
31. Hartley JW, Fredrickson TN, Yetter RA, Makino M, Morse HC III. Retrovirus-induced murine acquired immunodeficiency syndrome: Natural history of infection and differing susceptibility of inbred mouse strains. J Virol 63:1223-1231, 1989.
32. Cerny A, Hugin AW, Holmes KL, Morse HC III. CD4+ T cells in murine acquired immunodeficiency syndrome: Evidence for an intrinsic defect in the proliferative response to soluble antigens. Eur J Immunol 20:1577-1581, 1990.
33. Eskelson CD, Odeleye OE, Watson RR, Earnest D, Chrapil MY. Is the Leiber-de Carlo liquid ethanol diet adequate in Vitamin E? Alcohol Alcoholism 25:444, 1990.
34. Mohs ME, Watson RR. Ethanol induced malnutrition a potential cause of immunosuppression during AIDS. Prog Clin Biol Res 325:433-444, 1990.
35. Muffi SI, Watson RR. Effect of ethanol consumption and retroviral infection on carcinogenesis and its possible inhibition by an immunostimulant, canthaxanthins: Definition of a murine model. Prog Clin Biol Res 325:283-304, 1990.
36. Watson RR, Nguyen TH. Suppression by morphine and ethanol of tumor cell cytotoxic activity released by macrophages from retrovirally infected mice upon in vitro stimulation by beta carotene. Prog Clin Biol Res 325:79-91, 1990.

17
The Effect of Experimental Zinc Deficiency on Development of the Immune System

Kimberly G. Vruwink, Carl L. Keen, and M. Eric Gershwin
University of California, Davis, California

Jean Pierre Mareschi
BSN Groupe, Paris, France

Lucille S. Hurley
*University of California, Davis, California, and
BSN Groupe, Paris, France*

INTRODUCTION

During the last decade, it has become well established that adequate perinatal zinc nutriture is essential for normal immune ontogeny. Much of this evidence has been derived by using the mouse and the rhesus monkey as model systems. Indeed, prenatal zinc deficiency has a marked effect on the immune system, resulting in hypoplastic lymphoid tissues, lower antibody responses, abnormal immunoglobulin profiles, and reduced cell-mediated immunity (1-5). These observations are of particular interest as marginal zinc deficiency has been reported in several human populations and may be correlated with human immune deficiency (4). In this chapter, we discuss (a) the effects of zinc deficiency on the immune system, with particular emphasis on the perinatal period; (b) potential mechanisms which may underlie these effects, and (c) evidence that zinc deficiency also occurs in humans and is responsible for some immune defects.

Much of the work presented and direction of this research has been inspired by the life and work of the late Lucille Shapson Hurley (97).

ZINC DEFICIENCY IN EXPERIMENTAL ANIMALS

General Development

It has been recognized for over 20 years that adequate dietary zinc is crucial for normal mammalian development. In 1966, Hurley and Swenerton, using the Sprague-Dawley rat as a model, demonstrated that severe maternal zinc deficiency during pregnancy results in litters with gross congenital malformations, including cleft lip and palate, brain and eye malformations, and numerous abnormalities of the heart, lung, and urogenital system (6). In addition to morphological abnormalities, biochemical and functional lesions in the young also occur as a result of maternal zinc deficiency (7). Zinc deficiency during suckling and early weaning periods also produces poor postnatal growth.

There does not appear to be an efficient homeostatic mechanism for mobilizing zinc from bone or soft tissue, which contains considerable amounts of zinc (8). Owing to the lack of mobilizable zinc, a constant dietary intake of zinc is needed in order to maintain normal plasma zinc concentrations. Plasma levels decrease by as much as 50% within 8 hr after institution of a zinc-deficient diet (9); thus, it is obvious that the effects of zinc deficiency in rats can occur very rapidly. In the pregnant rat, the rapid effect of dietary zinc deficiency on plasma zinc concentration also is reflected in a low concentration of zinc in uterine fluid, along with abnormal development of preimplantation embryos (7).

The biochemical mechanisms underlying abnormal development caused by zinc deficiency are not well understood, but alterations in nucleic acid synthesis, microtubule function, cell migration and growth, and increased cellular peroxidation rates have been proposed as contributing factors (7). Some of these aspects are discussed in Chapter 33 and other chapters.

Zinc Deficiency and Immune Function in Adult Animals

Experimental studies using adult animal models have linked inadequate zinc intake to abnormal immune function (Table 1). Involution of the thymus and small spleen weights are characteristic of zinc deficiency, and appear to be primarily due to an absence of white cells (10-12). Fewer total numbers of lymphocytes appear to be responsible for the lowered white count (11,12), and in fact the total number of neutrophils may be higher in zinc-deficient animals. T Lymphocytes and, therefore, cell-mediated immunity, are particularly susceptible to zinc deficiency, although other components of the immune system are also affected (10,12). It has been proposed that certain subsets of the T-cell population might be differentially affected—in particular, T-helper cells. In terms of percentages, Dowd et al. (12) reported no significant differences in T-helper versus T-suppressor/cytotoxic cells, using monoclonal antibodies specific for markers on each type of cell. Zinc-deficient calves with the genetic lethal trait A46 had lower numbers of B lymphocytes, and fluctuating ratios of T-helper/suppressor cells (13). Fernandes et al. (10) reported that zinc-deprived mice had fewer Thy 1.2^+ cells and high numbers of cells with Fc receptors. The percentages of autologous rosette-forming cells, which are a subset of immature T cells, increased over time as mice were fed a zinc-deficient diet (14).

Several in vitro techniques exist to measure lymphocyte function, including antibody production (as measured by plaque formation in response to an antigen)

Table 1 Zinc Deficiency and General Immune Defects[a]

Parameter	Effect	Species	References
I. Physiology			
A. Organ wt/g body wt			
thymus	↓	Mouse, rat	10,11,16
spleen	N	Rat	12,26
adrenal	↑	Mouse, rat	34-36
			10-14
B. Cell number			
splenocytes	N	Mouse, rat	
thymocytes	↓	Mouse, rat	
total WBC	N or ↓	Mouse, rat	
lymphocytes	↓	Mouse, rat	
T cells	↓	Mouse	
T_H cells	N	Rat	
Thy 1.2+ cells	↓	Mouse	
Fc receptor cells	↑	Mouse	
rosette-forming	↑	Mouse	
B cells	↓	A46 calves	
C. Hormones			
corticosteroids	↑	Mouse	34,35
thymic hormone	↓	Mouse, rat	11,32,33
II. Tests of Immune Function			
A. In vitro tests			
plaques	↓	Mouse, rat	10,15
	N	Rat	16
	↓	Guinea pig	17
mitogens			
T cell	↓ or N	Mouse, rat	16,19,12
B cell	↓ or N	Mouse, rat	18,19
PMN chemotaxis	↓	Human (AE)[b]	96
monocyte chemotaxis	↓	Human (AE)	96
NK cell activity	↓ or ↑	Mouse	10,26
B. In vivo challenges			
bacterial	↑	Mouse, rat	20,21
parasite	↑ or N	Mouse	22,24
skin antigens (DTH)	↓	Human (AE)	86
skin antigens (DTH)	↓	Guinea pig	17
III. Immune Products			
Interleukin 1	↑ or ↓	Mouse	27,29
Interleukin 2	↓ or N	Mouse, rat	12,29
Gamma globulin	↓	Guinea pig	17

[a]Compared to adequate zinc intake groups: ↓ = lower than; ↑ = higher than; N = no significant difference.
[b]AE = Acrodermatitis enteropathica.

using lymphocytes from spleen, thymus, or lymph nodes. Zinc-deprived mice showed fewer immunoglobulin G (IgG) (indirect) plaques, but also less IgM (direct) plaques, particularly when expressed per total spleen (10,15). When plaques were expressed per number of spleen white cells, the differences were not as significant, implying that the reduced function was due in part to the lower number of white cells found in the zinc-deficient spleen (16). A study by Verma et al. (17) also showed a lower plaque and hemagglutinating titer in zinc-deficient guinea pigs, even when expressed on a per cell basis. These animals also had altered serum protein profiles, with lower γ-globulin.

Mitogen responsiveness is another assay useful for measuring lymphocyte function, by quantitating the ability of T and B cells to proliferate under specific stimulation. Concanavalin A and phytohemagglutinin are two mitogens which activate T lymphocytes, and blast transformation in response to these mitogens is reduced in mice fed low zinc diets. Although T-cell proliferation is most affected by zinc deficiency in vitro (18), mitogen proliferation specific for B cells is also reduced (19).

In vivo tests of the immune system include challenging an animal to a pathogen to determine the ability of the immune system to respond. Animals that do not receive adequate zinc have an increased susceptibility to challenges from pathogens, including *Candida albicans* (20), *Francisella tularensis* (21), and *Trypanosoma cruzi* (22). Calves with a genetic zinc deficiency (lethal trait A46) do not have a normal secondary response to an antigen (13). In contrast, other more recent studies show that infections in zinc-deficient animals impair particular aspects of the immune system, but the zinc deficiency does not appear to affect the ability of an animal to respond to a vaccine (23), or alter the response of an animal to a parasite (24).

Fernandes (10) and Tapazoglou et al. (25) showed a low natural killer cell activity, whereas Chandra (26) found higher activity in zinc-deficient mice. Fernandes (10) also found depressed cytotoxic responses (which are mediated by T cells) to EL-4 tumor cells.

There are a number of physiologically active proteins produced by immune cells which are important for the total immune response, and several of these specific proteins have been studied in zinc-deficient adult animals. Dowd et al. (12) suggested that interleukin 2 (IL-2), a lymphokine involved in T-cell proliferation, and receptors associated with it, may require zinc as a cofactor. Flynn et al. (29) found lower levels of IL-1 and no change in IL-1, also in vitro, using cultures with zinc-depleted media. Winchurch et al. (27,28) found lower IL-2 levels in zinc-supplemented cultures, but higher levels of IL-1, and B-cell stimulation factor 1 from activated T cells. Zinc also induces interferon production in vitro (30), and tumor necrosis factor in a culture system (31).

The involution of the thymus is correlated with reduced thymic hormone (11). This putative hormone, released by the thymus and important for normal T-cell function and for normal immune development in the fetus, has a requirement for zinc (32,33), and is discussed in Chapter 33.

Weanling rats fed diets deficient in zinc had larger adrenal glands, higher levels of corticosteroids, and smaller thymuses than control rats (34-36). The adrenals increase in size during zinc deficiency, presumably as a response to stress. This results in an increased release of corticosteroids, which are known to inhibit the immune response; however, adrenalectomy does not prevent thymus involution in zinc-deficient animals (35).

Zinc Deficiency and Immune Function in Postnatal Development

Postnatal development of the immune system in rodents occurs primarily during the suckling period; in several studies (Table 2) by Beach et al. (37-39) lactating dams were fed a purified diet containing 2.5, 5.0, 9.0, or 100 μg zinc/g diet for the first 4 weeks postpartum. A fifth group of dams was included to control for maternal inanition, and were fed control diet in amounts equal to that consumed by zinc-deficient animals. Organ weights and immune function were measured in the offspring at the end of 4 weeks. Several organs were affected in the pups from females receiving diets severely, mildly, or marginally deficient in zinc, and the reduced body or organ weights could not be accounted for by lower food intake alone; zinc deficiency further significantly impaired the growth of the pups. The immune organs were altered to the greatest extent; the thymus was markedly involuted, and the spleen was much smaller than in controls. Organ weights are best expressed as a percent of total body weight, particularly when overall growth is decreased; however, even expressed relative to body weight, the immune organs were proportionately smaller in size than either control or restricted-fed organ weights (39). In the spleen of zinc-deficient mice, there were also lower numbers of T and B lymphocytes and of red cells as expressed per weight of the tissue or as expressed as total numbers (37).

Table 2 Effects of Zinc Deficiency During Perinatal Period[a]

Parameter	Effect	Species	References
I. Physiology			
Body weight and length	↓	Mouse	38-41
		Monkey	87
Organ wt/g body wt			
spleen, thymus	↓	Mouse	37-41
liver	slightly ↓	Mouse	38,39
heart, kidney	↑	Mouse	39
thymus histology	abnormal	Mouse	39
Spleen RBC/g spleen	↓	Mouse	37
Spleen WBC/g spleen	↓↓	Mouse	37
II. Tests of Immune Function			
Plaques			
direct, indirect	↓	Mouse	37,40,41
dextran (TCI)	↑	Mouse	40
Mitogens			
Con A, LPS, PWM, PHA	↓	Mouse	39
Con A, PWM, PHA	↓	Monkey	5
III. Immune Products			
Immunoglobulins			
IgA	↓↓	Mouse	37
IgM, IgG_{2a}	↓	Mouse	37
IgG_1	↑	Mouse	37
IgA, IgG	N	Monkey	5
IgM	↓	Monkey	5

[a]Compared to adequate zinc intake groups: ↓ = lower than; ↑ = higher than; N = no significant difference.

Consistent with alterations in the size of the immune organs, the immune function was changed as well in both the cell-mediated and humoral branches of the immune system. The spleen plaque response was lower in zinc-deprived animals than in controls. When the number of plaques was expressed per number of spleen cells, zinc deficiency still resulted in a significantly lower than normal response. Both T- and B-cell mitogen responses were lower in these mice at 4 weeks of age (37,39).

Quantifying immune proteins such as serum immunoglobulins is a direct method of measuring the effect of zinc deficiency in vivo. The immunoglobulin profiles of mice postnatally deprived of zinc from birth in the studies by Beach et al. (37) were abnormal, with alterations in various subclasses of immunoglobulin. Immunoglobulin A was the most affected, with no detectable levels even in marginally (9 μg Zn/g diet) zinc-deprived mice. Immunoglobulin M was low in the more severely (2.5 μg Zn/g) deprived animals, as was $IgG2_b$. In contrast, IgG1 levels in the low-zinc mice were significantly higher than control concentrations.

When postnatally deprived mice are given zinc-replete diets, the plaque response returns to normal, and thymus weights soon reach those of controls (40,41). Thus, it appears that postnatal zinc deprivation is reversible and does not result in persistent alterations of immune organs or immune function.

Deficiencies and Immune Function in Prenatal Development

Zinc

Zinc deficiency that occurs in utero in mice has effects on the immune system similar to those of early postnatal deprivation. A primary difference, however, is that some of the effects appear to be longer lasting and can be passed on to subsequent generations (Table 3).

The prenatal studies by Beach et al. (1-3) involved mice fed diets marginally deficient in zinc (5 μg Zn/g diet) during the last two-thirds of gestation, after which potential outcome was followed for the offspring. Restricted-intake controls (animals fed control diet in amounts equal to those consumed by zinc-deficient animals) were included to control for maternal inanition; potential lactational defects in dams caused by zinc depletion were controlled by cross-fostering pups to dams who had been fed control diet (100 μg Zn/g diet) throughout pregnancy. Once the pups were born, all dams were fed control diets ad libitum and all pups were weaned to the control diet.

The litters of zinc-deprived females were smaller and had higher mortality rates than those of controls. They also showed growth retardation and small spleens, thymuses, hearts, kidneys, livers, and lungs relative to body weight. After birth, when their mothers (and later themselves) received zinc-replete diets, catch-up growth occurred in all organs, but at different rates. By 1 week past parturition, relative (to body weight) weights of heart, liver, kidney, and brain were equal to or higher than those of controls. By week 4, the relative weights of lung and thymus were comparable to those of controls. Thymus white cell counts per milligram of tissue were lower at term, but also caught up quickly (1).

The spleen cell plaque response to antigens was diminished in pups from zinc-deficient dams in a manner similar to that seen in postnatally deprived mice (2,3). Immunoglobulin profiles were also altered, with decreased IgG2a, IgA, and IgM. Unlike postnatal deficiency, however, IgG1 levels were not increased in low-zinc pups

Table 3 Prenatal Zinc Deficiency and Immune Defects in Mice[a]

Parameter	Effect				References
I. Effects in Neonates					
A. Physiology					1
Body weight/length	↓ 25%[b]				
Organ wt/g body wt					
spleen, thymus	↓ 60%				
heart, kidney	↓ 30%, ↓ 50%				
liver	N				
lung, brain	↓ 40%, ↓ 20%				
Total spleen, thymus WBC	↓ 80%				
Spleen WBC/g spleen	N				
Thymus WBC/g thymus	↓ 30%				
B. Immune Function					
B-cell response	↓				42
II. Effects in Adult Mice (Persistant)					
A. Physiology	WK2[c]	WK4	WK6	WK10	
Body weight	N	↓	N	N	1
Organ weight					
spleen	↓	↓	↑	↑	
thymus	↓	↓	N	N	
heart, liver	↑	↑	N	N	
brain, kidney	N	N	N	N	
lung	↓	N	N	N	
Spleen, thymus WBC/g organ wt:		N			
B. Immune function	WK6	WK10	MO6		
Plaques-direct	↓ 60%	↓ 50%	↓ 40%		2
Immunoglobulins					
IgM	↓ 99%	↓ 99%	↓ 30%		2
IgG2a	↓ 40%	↓ 30%	N		3
IgA	↓ 50%	↓ 40%	N		3
IgG1, IgG2b	N	N	N		3

[a]Compared to adequate zinc intake groups: ↓ = lower than; ↑ = higher than; N = no significant difference.
[b]% = approximate change in zinc deficient mice compared to zinc adequate mice.
[c]WK = age in weeks, MO = age in months.

and did not differ from controls (2,3). A study by Keller and Fraker has shown that although a marginal zinc deficiency in utero does not impair the ability of B cells from the fetus to respond to an antigen, there are fewer B cells found in fetal liver (42).

The major contrast in the effects of postnatal and prenatal zinc deficiency is that prenatal zinc deprivation appears to have persistent effects in postnatal life even if offspring are fed a zinc-replete diet from birth. Alterations in immune function, particularly in low levels of IgM and spleen cell plaque responses, continued to be seen in these offspring throughout adulthood, at weeks 6 and 10, and even at 6 months of age. Furthermore, the effects on immunoglobulins and plaque responses were multigenerational and were still found in the third generation (2,3). Although the abnormalities diminished with time, both in the F1 adults as they became older, and also in subsequent generations, they remained significantly different from controls.

Haynes et al. reported that peripheral blood lymphocytes from rhesus monkey infants fed a marginally zinc-deficient diet (4 μg Zn/g diet) from conception through 12 months of postnatal life were characterized by low responses to phytohemagglutinin, concanavalin A, and pokeweed mitogen compared to lymphocytes of infants born to mothers fed diets containing 100 μg Zn/g diet. In addition, infants in the marginal zinc group had low serum IgM levels (see Table 2). Thus, with regard to the immune system, the response of a nonhuman primate model to zinc deficiency during early development is similar to that observed for rodent models (5).

POSSIBLE MECHANISMS FOR THE PERSISTENCE OF IMMUNE DEFECTS. What are potential causes for the persistent defects in the immune system resulting from prenatal zinc deficiency? The presence of the zinc ion in vitro appears to be necessary for normal immune function. Zinc itself can act as a weak mitogen (43), and enhances blastogenesis when added to media in culture systems in vitro (44); conversely, these responses are reduced in zinc-depleted media (19,45). Once lymphocytes have been stimulated, zinc becomes associated with, and may be required for, the new soluble proteins that are synthesized by the lymphocytes (46).

Both intra- and intercellular concentrations of zinc may have an effect on bacterial and viral activity and replication. It is well established that infection is associated with changes in zinc distribution; in particular, plasma zinc concentrations are lower and liver levels are higher as a result of acute-phase protein synthesis (47). It has been shown that macrophages are activated when zinc concentration is lowered (48). The zinc ion may be required for normal immunoglobulin structure and processing. For example, it is required for normal patching, capping, and secreting of immunoglobulin of B cells (49), and also promotes polymerization of IgM in vitro (50). However, the requirement for the presence of zinc ion would not explain the persistence of defects in adult immune function after gestational zinc depletion unless zinc metabolism had been altered in such a way that the zinc ion was not readily available to the cells or proteins.

There are several other possible explanations for the long-term effects found after prenatal zinc deficiency. First, the in utero defect could be caused by a lack of dietary zinc occurring during some critical period in development, resulting in permanent changes in chromatin. Several investigators have shown that zinc deficiency may compromise the structure and function of chromatin. For example, zinc has been shown to have a role in (a) nucleic acid synthesis (51), (b) maintaining the native structure of DNA and RNA (52,53), and (c) maintaining normal cell cycle kinetics (54). Zinc deficiency also leads to abnormal histone profiles and chromatin conformation (55) as discussed in this book. It also is becoming apparent that zinc is a component of many nonhistone proteins (56). Several nucleic acid-binding regulatory proteins contain metal-binding domains (57,58).

In addition, zinc is a structural component of many metalloenzymes, including those involved in gene replication, such as DNA and RNA polymerases and thymidine kinase, although the latter may be using zinc as a cofactor. Thus, zinc deficiency during a crucial period of development may depress the DNA synthesis or cell division required for normal organ development by acting through any of the above mechanisms (59). The immune system seems to be particularly vulnerable to changes which result in decreases in cell division. Furthermore, the persistence of the effects through several generations suggests that these defects have indeed occurred at the chromosomal level in a heritable way.

The persistence of the effects of zinc deficiency even after zinc repletion occurs also suggests that protein synthesis, or its regulation, may be altered, thus causing long-term changes in protein expression. These may include the immune proteins, such as antibodies and hormones. Studies in our laboratory seem to suggest that the regulation of another protein, metallothionein, may also be altered by prenatal zinc deficiency in a persistent fashion. Metallothionein is a low molecular weight protein which is characterized by about one-third cysteine amino acid residues. Metallothionein has been suggested to be a potential zinc storage pool (47). Gestational zinc deficiency altered the expression of metallothionein induction in adult animals, with a higher production in response to zinc injection, even after dietary zinc repletion (60). It is possible that metallothionein expression may be altered by changes in gene methylation, a heritable trait of genes (61). A similar change in immunoglobulin protein expression may also be occurring in these mice.

Giugliano and Millward (62) suggest that the effects of zinc deficiency may be due to reduced protein synthesis, perhaps from impaired insulin which requires zinc for its own synthesis and may also be due to an increased catabolic response resulting from higher levels of corticosterone. Steroids might also have a direct effect on the development of immune proteins, or they might play a role in the developing animal's zinc metabolism. For example, it is known that steroids can enhance the production of metallothionein (63). Thymic hormone is also required for normal lymphocytic development and may be persistently affected, but the persistence of the immune defects due to any of these effects would imply long-term changes of the hormonal milieu, for which there is little evidence.

A second possibility is that zinc deficiency during a critical period of development causes defects in immune organs that are not repairable, resulting in decreased immune function. Involution of the thymus, correlated with fewer thymocytes (lymphocytes), also occurs in the zinc-deficient fetal mouse (1,64). The number of cells may be reduced by zinc deficiency because lymphocytes are proliferating rapidly during development, and zinc-dependent enzymes required for this synthesis may become limiting. It has been speculated by Meftah and Prasad (65) that zinc deficiency might also cause a nucleotide phosphorylase deficiency, resulting in a buildup of nucleotides which is toxic to lymphocytes, and thus results in fewer thymocytes. Macrophages, in contrast, are present in high numbers in the thymus during zinc deficiency, and may be phagocytosing defective lymphocytes (11,64). Lymphocytes begin migrating and lodging in the thymus during midgestation in the mouse (the same period when Beach et al. (1–3) fed the mice zinc-deficient diets), and these lymphocytes increase exponentially in number until birth (66). Thymectomy during these critical periods of development resulted in a lower response to phytohemagglutinin and fewer plaques (direct and indirect) in thymectomized adult animals than in nonthymectomized mice. Some immune function does reappear over time, similar to results seen in the gestationally zinc-deficient mice (2). These similar results suggest that zinc deficiency during crucial periods may be causing a reduction in total number of T cells, or of certain T-cell subtypes. It would still be difficult to envision why decreasing T-cell pool size would cause immune defects to be passed on to subsequent generations unless the immune potential of the dam also alters in utero conditions which then affects the fetus. For example, involution of the thymus may result in persistently lower levels of thymic hormone production, which might have effects on fetal immune development.

A third possibility is that zinc deprivation during a critical developmental time period alters zinc metabolism which secondarily affects immune function, whereas dietary repletion of zinc does not repair the damage to the homeostasis of zinc. Again, the higher levels of metallothionein that were found in the gestationally zinc-deprived adult mice could provide a mechanism for alterations in zinc homeostasis. Since metallothionein function is closely tied to zinc metabolism, changes in the former may therefore alter the availability of zinc for immune proteins. This enhanced synthesis of metallothionein in the F1 mother may alter the zinc availability to the developing organs of her fetus, and therefore cause problems of zinc homeostasis to be passed on. Evidence for this hypothesis has not yet been recorded.

Other Nutrients and Ontogeny

There are many single-nutrient deficiencies which will impair immune function, including vitamins and minerals. The broader malnutrition of protein-calorie deprivation also has effects on the immune system. Similar to zinc deficiency, other nutrient deficiencies cause immune defects that appear to be reversible when the insult occurs in adult animals but are persistent when it occurs during development. There have not been many developmental studies that examine the persistence of the effects following nutritional repletion; however, zinc is not the only nutrient whose deficiency can result in persistence of immune defects. These will only be discussed briefly; for a longer discussion, please see other reviews (4,67,68).

PYRIDOXINE. Robson and Schwarz (69) fed rats a pyridoxine-deficient diet through gestation and then fed the offspring control diet for 3 months. Even after this time, the deficient progeny had lower mixed lymphocyte reactivity, and a lower graft-vs-host reaction than controls. When the rats were fed deficient diets through lactation, spleen cell number and plaque responses were also reduced.

LIPOTROPES. Lipotropes, including vitamin B_{12}, choline, methionine, and folic acid, also have long-term effects. Rats fed diets deficient in the above nutrients during gestation and lactation only had offspring smaller in size at 3 months of age, with smaller spleens and thymuses, and reduced cellularity of these organs despite dietary repletion. They also had higher mortality from *Salmonella typhimurium* challenges, fewer plaque and spleen mitogen responses, and lower antibodies than controls (70,71).

IRON. Other minerals have not been studied as thoroughly as has zinc for effects during ontogeny of immune function. Iron is one metal, however, that also has been used in prenatal immune studies. A prenatal and lactational iron deficiency in rats resulted in fewer plaques and lower serum levels of IgG and IgM than in controls despite repletion (72). Iron-deficient rats show a lower resistance to challenge by *Salmonella typhimurium* compared to controls (73).

COPPER. Copper deficiency during gestation or lactation has been studied, but appears to have no long-term effects on immune function, with no change in immune organ weights, IgG or IgM levels, or mitogen responses (74).

SELENIUM. Selenium deficiency is associated with a depression of humoral immune responsiveness, with lower eventual titers of antibody. Mice fed selenium-deficient diets during gestation and lactation had reduced growth and lower IgM and IgG responses to antigens in plaque assays than did mice fed these same diets only after weaning (75).

CALORIE RESTRICTION. Calorie restriction in pregnant rats also resulted in impaired cell-mediated immune responses in the offspring. There were reductions and alterations in ratios of T-helper, T-cytotoxic, and T-suppressor cells (76). Deprivation of energy during pregnancy also led to abnormal immunoglobulin synthesis which persisted into adulthood, and also through a second generation, similar to the effects of zinc deprivation (77). Protein deficiency during gestation followed by rehabilitation caused significantly smaller thymuses, lower IgG_{2a} and IgG_{2b} levels, and a reduced plaque and mitogen response (78). Protein-calorie malnutrition had similar effects, with smaller spleens and thymuses, lower plaques, and hemagglutinization. An intergenerational study (77) also showed that the plaque abnormalities persisted through the next generation of mice.

PROTEIN-ENERGY UNDERNUTRITION. Srivastava et al. (79) reported a lower content of poly A^+ RNA in the lymphoid organs of rat pups exposed to protein-energy undernutrition during their second week of life. However, despite the lower content of poly A^+ RNA, the translational efficiency of poly A^+ RNA was higher in the thymus and spleens from the undernourished pups. These results support the idea that undernutrition early in life can modulate the mechanism of mRNA, and hence protein synthesis in lymphoidal tissues.

It is possible that similar mechanisms could account for the persistent abnormalities resulting from various nutrient deficiencies. For example, the immune defects could be due to lower numbers of T lymphocytes caused by alterations in cell synthesis which have been affected by inadequate amounts of a number of essential nutrients. Still, each nutrient may be affecting immunity at various points in development, with each deficiency resulting in similar outcomes. If, however, zinc metabolism is persistently altered in gestational zinc deficiency, then other mechanisms must also be involved.

IMPLICATIONS FOR HUMANS

Epidemiology

Human zinc deficiency was first described in the 1960s by Prasad (80) in the Middle East. The patients' dietary intake of zinc was low, and phytates present in the food further reduced bioavailability of the zinc. Signs of deficiency included hypogonadism, sexual immaturity, and decreased growth. Marginal zinc intake has been reported even in developed countries (81). Several studies have indicated that the average zinc intake of some Americans is lower than recommended levels, particularly in women during periods of increased requirement such as pregnancy or lactation, and also in children from low-income families during infancy and periods of growth (82-85).

Zinc Linked to Immune Function in Humans

Zinc deprivation has been linked to signs of immune dysfunction and abnormalities in humans, similar to experimental animals. Effects in sickle cell anemia are discussed in Chapter 24. Patients with acrodermatitis enteropathica (a genetic disorder of zinc metabolism) provided a definitive link between zinc metabolism and immune function. Acrodermatitis enteropathica results in low serum zinc levels and is associated with defective cellular immune responses, both of which are improved with zinc supplementation (86). Children with this anomaly have thymic atrophy, abnormal serum immunoglobulin profiles, and impaired T-cell function, along with a higher than normal incidence of infectious disease (4,87). Another link between zinc and the immune system was observed in patients given total parenteral nutrition with formulas that did not contain adequate zinc. Abnormal cell-mediated immune responses occurred that were readily reversible with zinc supplementation (88,89).

Immune disorders found in conjunction with protein-energy malnutrition may be in part due to concurrent zinc deficiency, since zinc is one of many nutrients that is inadequate in the diets of such individuals. This was affirmed by clinical findings of low serum zinc levels in malnourished humans in developing countries. When supplemented with zinc alone, some of the immune deficiencies could be reversed (90, 91), resulting in accelerated thymus growth and an increased delayed hypersensitivity response (7).

A recent study evaluated zinc supplementation on immune parameters in marasmic children (92). The zinc-supplemented infants had higher levels of serum IgA, better response to skin tests, lower incidence of energy, and lower incidence of infections that did placebo-supplemented children. These results again indicate the critical role of zinc during development in human immune function, and also provide evidence that zinc deficiency accompanies protein-calorie malnutrition.

Children with the Down syndrome have low serum zinc and abnormal humoral and cell-mediated immune function. Compared to age-matched controls, affected children have low IgM levels, fewer lymphocytes and T cells, a reduced response to mitogens, and higher levels of IgA and IgG (93). Supplementation of zinc increased circulating T cells and thymic hormone and reduced recurrent infections (94).

Children with Hodgkin's disease had lower blood and hair zinc compared to age- and sex-matched control children (95). These patients also had abnormalities of cellular immunity, including a lower number of lymphocytes and proliferation and higher incidences of anergy to delayed-type hypersensitivity antigens. In fact, within Hodgkin's disease patients, the more unresponsive patients had lower serum zinc levels. Cause or effect is difficult to determine without further studies, but this provides another correlation between low serum zinc and immune dysfunction in humans.

FUTURE STUDIES

Since zinc deficiency during gestation causes a wide variety of abnormalities, it is likely that its role in development is not limited to a single mechanism. Similarly, the effects on the immune system are probably not caused by only one biochemical defect, but occur through several alterations. These issues are in chapter 33. Furthermore, an important and unresolved issue is whether there are "critical periods" during which a trace metal deficiency may be especially harmful to immune system development. Studies should be done to determine whether the altered immune function of animals subjected to dietary influences during critical periods can be reversed. The mechanisms responsible for these effects should also be investigated. Although the absence of zinc in utero results in modification of the immune response, does this affect an individual's response to pathogens? Furthermore, the question of whether other systems or proteins are significantly altered in a long-term fashion is of fundamental importance, with serious implications for human nutrition and development.

REFERENCES

1. Beach RS, Gershwin ME, Hurley LS (1982). Reversibility of developmental retardation following murine fetal zinc deprivation. J Nutr 112:1169.

2. Beach RS, Gershwin ME, Hurley LS (1982). Gestational zinc deprivation in mice: Persistence of immunodeficiency for three generations. Science 218:469.
3. Beach RS, Gershwin ME, Hurley LS (1983). Persistent immunological consequences of gestational zinc deprivation. Am J Clin Nutr 38:579.
4. Gershwin ME, Beach RS, Hurley LS (1985). Nutrition and Immunity. Academic Press, Orlando, Florida.
5. Haynes DC, Gershwin ME, Golub MS, Cheung ATW, Hurley LS, Hendrickx AG (1985). Studies of marginal zinc deprivation in rhesus monkeys. VI. Influence on the immunohematology of infants in the first year. Am J Clin Nutr 42:252.
6. Hurley LS (1981). Teratogenic aspects of manganese, zinc and copper nutrition. Physiol Rev 61:249.
7. Keen CL, Hurley LS (1989). Zinc and reproduction: Effects of deficiency on foetal and postnatal development. In: Zinc in Human Biology. C Mills ed. Springer-Verlag, London, pp 183-220.
8. Hurley LS, Swenerton H (1971). Lack of mobilization of bone and liver zinc under teratogenic conditions of zinc deficiency in rats. J Nutr 101:597.
9. Hurley LS, Gordon P, Keen CL, Merkhofer L (1982). Circadian variation in rat plasma zinc and rapid effect of dietary zinc deficiency. Proc Soc Exp Biol Med 170:48.
10. Fernandes G, Nair M, Onoe K, Tanaka T, Floyd R, Good RA (1979). Impairment of cell-mediated immunity functions by dietary zinc deficiency in mice. Proc Natl Acad Sci USA 76:457.
11. Mercalli ME, Seri S, Aquilio E, Cramarossa L, Del Gabbo V, Accinni L, Toniette G (1984). Zinc deficiency and thymus ultrastructure in rats. Nutr Res 4:665.
12. Dowd PS, Kelleher J, Guillou PJ (1986). T-Lymphocyte subsets and interleukin-2 production in zinc-deficient rats. Br J Nutr 55:59.
13. Perryman LE, Leach DR, Davis WC, Mickelsen WD, Heller SR, Ochs HD, Ellis JA, Brummerstedt E (1989). Lymphocyte alterations in zinc-deficient calves with lethal trait A46. Vet Immunol Immunopathol 21:239.
14. Nash L, Iwata T, Fernandes G, Good RA, Incefy GS (1979). Effect of zinc deficiency on autologous rosette-forming cells. Cell Immunol 48:238.
15. DePasquale-Jardieu P, Fraker PJ (1984). Interference in the development of a secondary immune response in mice by zinc deprivation: Persistence of effects. J Nutr 114:1762.
16. Carlomagno MA, McMurray DN (1983). Chronic zinc deficiency in rats: Its influence on some parameters of humoral and cell-mediated immunity. Nutr Res 3:69.
17. Verma PC, Gupta RP, Sadana JR, Gupta RKP (1988). Effect of experimental zinc deficiency and repletion on some immunological variables in guinea-pigs. Br J Nutr 59:149.
18. Zanzonica P, Fernandes G, Good RA (1981). The differential sensitivity of T-cell and B-cell mitogenesis to in vitro zinc deficiency. Cell Immunol 60:203.
19. Gross RL, Osdin N, Fong L, Newberne PM (1979). I. Depressed immunological function in zinc-deprived rats as measured by mitogen response of spleen, thymus, and peripheral blood. Am J Clin Nutr 32:1260.
20. Salvin SB, Rabin BS (1984). Resistance and susceptibility to infection in inbred murine strains. IV. Effects of dietary zinc. Cell Immunol. 87:546.
21. Pekarek RS, Hoagland AM, Powanda MC (1977). Humoral and cellular immune responses in zinc deficient rats. Nutr Rep Int 16:267.
22. Wirth JJ, Fraker PJ, Kierszenbaum F (1989). Zinc requirement for macrophage function: Effect of zinc deficiency on uptake and killing of a protozoan parasite. Immunology 68:114.
23. Coghlan LG, Carlomagno MA, McMurray DN (1988). Effect of protein and zinc deficiencies on vaccine efficacy in guinea pigs following pulmonary infection with Listeria. Med Microbiol Immunol 177:255.

24. El-Hag HMA, MacDonald DC, Fenwick P, Aggett PJ, Wakelin D (1989). Kinetics of nippostrongylus brasiliensis infection in the zinc-deficient rat. J Nutr 119:1506.
25. Tapazoglou E, Prasad AS, Hill G, Brewer GJ, Kaplan J (1985). Decreased natural killer cell activity in patients with zinc deficiency with sickle cell disease. J Lab Clin Med 105:19.
26. Chandra RK, Au B (1980). Single nutrient deficiency and cell-mediated immune responses. I. Zinc. Am J Clin Nutr 33:736.
27. Winchurch RA, Togo J, Adler WH (1987). Supplemental zinc (Zn2+) restores antibody formation in cultures of aged spleen cells. II. Effects on mediator production. Eur J Immunol 17:127.
28. Winchurch RA, Togo J, Adler WH (1988). Supplemental zinc restores antibody formation in cultures of aged spleen cells. III. Impairment of IL-2 mediated responses. Clin Immunol Immunopathol 49:215.
29. Flynn A, Loftus MA, Finke JH (1984). Production of interleukin-1 and interleukin-2 in allogeneic mixed lymphocyte cultures under copper, magnesium and zinc deficient conditions. Nutr Res 4:673.
30. Salas M, Kirchner H (1987). Induction of interferon-gamma in human leukocyte cultures stimulated by Zn^{+2}. Clin Immunol Immunopathol 45:139.
31. Scuderi P (1990). Differential effects of copper and zinc on human peripheral blood monocyte cytokine secretion. Cell Immunol 126:391.
32. Dardenne M, Pleau JM, Nabarra B, Lefrancier P, Derrien M, Choay J, Bach JF (1982). Contribution of zinc and other metals to the biological activity of the serum thymic factor. Proc Natl Acad Sci USA 79:5370.
33. Iwata T, Incefy GS, Tanaka T, Fernandes G, Menendez-Botet CJ, Pih K, Good RA (1979). Circulating thymic hormone levels in zinc deficiency. Cell Immunol 47:100.
34. DePasquale-Jardieu P, Fraker PJ (1979). The role of corticosterone in the loss in immune function in the zinc-deficient A/J mouse. J Nutr 109:1847.
35. DePasquale-Jardieu P, Fraker PJ (1980). Further characterization of the role of corticosterone in the loss of humoral immunity in zinc-deficient A/J mice as determined by adrenalectomy. J Immunol 124:2650.
36. Quarterman J, Humphries WR (1979). Effect of zinc deficiency and zinc supplementation on adrenals, plasma steroids and thymus in rats. Life Sci 24:177.
37. Beach RS, Gershwin ME, Makishima RK, Hurley LS (1980). Impaired immunologic ontogeny in postnatal zinc deprivation. J Nutr 110:805.
38. Beach RS, Gershwin ME, Hurley LS (1980). Growth and development in postnatally zinc-deprived mice. J Nutr 110:201.
39. Beach RS, Gershwin ME, Hurley LS (1979). Altered thymic structure and mitogen responsiveness in postnatally zinc-deprived mice. Dev Comp Immunol 3:725.
40. Zwickl CM, Fraker PJ (1980). Restoration of the antibody mediated response of zinc/caloric deficient neonatal mice. Immunol Commun 9:611.
41. Fraker PJ, Hildebrandt K, Luecke RW (1984). Alteration of antibody-mediated response of suckling mice to T-cell dependent and independent antigens by maternal marginal zinc deficiency: restoration of responsivity by nutritional repletion. J Nutr 114:170.
42. Keller PR, Fraker PJ (1986). Gestational zinc requirement of the A/J mouse: Effects of a marginal zinc deficiency on in utero B-cell development. Nutr Res 6:41.
43. Hart DA (1978). Effect of zinc chloride on hamster lymphoid cells: Mitogenicity and differential enhancement of lipopolysaccharide stimulation of lymphocytes. Infect Immun 19:457.
44. Malave I, Benaim IR (1984). Modulatory effect of zinc on the proliferative response of murine spleen cells to polyclonal T cell mitogens. Cell Immunol 89:322.
45. Flynn A (1984). Control of in vitro lymphocyte proliferation by copper, magnesium and zinc deficiency. J Nutr 114:2034.
46. Phillips JL (1981). Molecular distribution of cytoplasmic zinc in phytohemagglutinin-stimulated and unstimulated human lymphocytes. Biol Trace Element Res 3:225.

47. Cousins RJ (1985). Absorption, transport, and hepatic metabolism of copper and zinc: Special reference to metallothionein and ceruloplasmin. Physiol Rev 65:238.
48. Karl L, Chvapil M, Zukoski CF (1973). Effect of zinc on the viability and phagocytic capacity of peritoneal macrophages. Proc Soc Exp Biol Med 142:1123.
49. Maro B, Bornens M (1979). The effect of zinc chloride on the redistribution of surface immunoglobulins in rat B lymphocytes. FEBS Lett 97:116.
50. Eskeland T (1977). The effect of various metal ions and chelating agents on the formation of noncovalently and covalently linked IgM polymers. Scand J Immunol 6:87.
51. Swenerton H, Schrader R, Hurley LS (1969). Zinc-deficient embryos: Reduced thymidine incorporation. Science 166:1014.
52. Shin YA, Eicchorn GL (1968). Interactions of metal ions with polynucleotides and related compounds. XI. The reversible unwinding and rewinding of deoxyribonucleic acid by zinc (II) ions through temperature manipulation. Biochemistry 7:1026.
53. Anwander EHS, Probst MM, Rode BM (1987). Investigations of Zn (II) complexes with DNA/RNA bases by means of quantum chemical calculations. Inorgan Chimca Acta 137:203.
54. Falchuk KH, Fawcett DW, Vallee BL (1975). Role of zinc in cell division of Euglena gracilis. J Cell Sci 17:57.
55. Castro CE, Armstrong-Major J, Ramirez ME (1986). Diet-mediated alteration of chromatin structure. Fed Proc 45:2394.
56. Hanas JS, Hazuda DJ, Wu CW (1985). Xenopus transcription factor A promotes DNA reassociation. J Biol Chem 260:13316.
57. Berg JM (1986). Potential metal-binding domains in nucleic acid binding proteins. Science 232:485.
58. Berg JM (1986). More metal-binding fingers. Nature 319:264.
59. Eckhert CD, Hurley LS (1977). Reduced DNA synthesis in zinc deficiency: Regional differences in embryonic rats. J Nutr 107:855.
60. Vruwink KG, Hurley LS, Gershwin ME, Keen CL (1988). Gestational zinc deficiency amplifies the regulation of metallothionein induction in adult mice. Proc Soc Exp Biol Med 188:30.
61. Hamer DH (1986). Metallothionein. Ann Rev Biochem 55:913.
62. Giugliano R, Millward DJ (1987). The effects of severe zinc deficiency on protein turnover in muscle and thymus. Br J Nutr 57:139.
63. Karin M, Haslinger A, Holtgreve H, Richards RI, Krauter P, Westphal HM, Beato M (1984). Characterization of DNA sequences through which cadmium and glucocorticoid hormones induce human metallothionein-IIA gene. Nature 308:513.
64. Gossrau R, Merker HJ, Gunther T, Graf R, Vormann J (1987). Enzymatic and morphological response of the thymus to drugs in normal and zinc-deficient pregnant rats and their fetuses. Histochemistry 86:321.
65. Meftah S, Prasad AS (1989). Nucleotides in lymphocytes of human subjects with zinc deficiency. J Lab Clin Med 114:114.
66. Rothenberg E, Lugo JP (1985). Differentiation and cell division in the mammalian thymus. Dev Biol 112:1.
67. Gross RL, Newberne PM (1980). Role of nutrition in immunologic function. Physiol Rev 60:188.
68. Chandra RK (1986). Nutrition, immune response and outcome. Prog Food Nutr Sci 10:1.
69. Robson LC, Schwarz MR (1975). Vitamin B6 deficiency and the lymphoid system II. Effects of vitamin B6 deficiency in utero on the immunological competence of the offspring. Cell Immunol 16:145.
70. Newberne PM, Young VR (1973). Marginal vitamin B12 intake during gestation in the rat has longterm effects on the offspring. Nature 242:263.
71. Williams EAJ, Gebhardt BM, Morton B, Newberne PM (1979). Effects of early marginal methionine-choline deprivation on the development of the immune system in the rat. Am J Clin Nutr 32:1214.

72. Kochanowski BA, Sherman AR (1984). Phagocytosis and lysozyme activity in granulocytes from iron-deficient rat dams and pups. Nutr Res 4:511.
73. Baggs RB, Miller SA (1973). Nutritional iron deficiency as a determinant of host resistance in the rat. J Nutr 103:1554.
74. Prohaska JR, Lukasewycz OA (1989). Copper deficiency during perinatal development: Effects on the immune response of mice. J Nutr 119:922.
75. Mulhern SA, Taylor GL, Magruder LE, Vessey AR (1985). Deficient levels of dietary selenium suppress the antibody response in first and second generation mice. Nutr Res 5:201.
76. Filteau SM, Woodward B (1984). Relationship between serum zinc level and immunocompetence in protein-deficient and well-nourished weanling mice. Nutr Res 4:853.
77. Chandra RK (1975). Antibody formation in first and second generation offspring of nutritionally deprived rats. Science 190:289.
78. Olusi SO, McFarlane H (1976). Effects of early protein-calorie malnutrition on the immune response. Pediatr Res 10:707.
79. Srivastava US, Rakshit AK, Seebag M, Omoloko C, Thakur ML (1981). Metabolism of adenine nucleosides and nucleotides, nucleic acids and proteins in the thymus and spleen of neonatal progeny of dietary restricted rats. Nutr Rep Int 23:1035.
80. Prasad AS, Halsted JA, Nadimi M (1961). Syndrome of iron deficiency anemia, hepatosplenomegaly, hypogonadism, dwarfism and geophagia. Am J Med 31:532.
81. Sandstead HH (1973). Zinc nutrition in the United States. Am J Clin Nutr 25:1251.
82. Walravens PA, Hambidge KM, Koepfer DM (1989). Zinc supplementation in infants with a nutritional pattern of failure to thrive: A double-blind, controlled study. Pediatrics 83:532.
83. Cherry FF, Sandstead HH, Rojas P, Johnson LK, Batson HK, Wang XB (1989). Adolescent pregnancy: associations among body weight, zinc nutriture, and pregnancy outcome. Am J Clin Nutr 50:945.
84. Simmer K, Thompson RPH (1985). Maternal zinc and intrauterine growth retardation. Clin Sci 68:395.
85. Hinks LJ, Ogilvy-Stuart A, Hambidge KM, Walker V (1989). Maternal zinc and selenium status in pregnancies with a neural tube defect or elevated plasma alpha-fetoprotein. Br J Obstet Gyn 96:61.
86. Oleske JM, Westphal ML, Shore, S, Gorden D, Bogden JD, Nahmias A (1979). Correction with zinc therapy of depressed cellular immunity in acrodermatitis enteropathica. Am J Dis Child 133:915.
87. Hansen MA, Fernandes G, Good RA (1982). Nutrition and Immunity: The influence of diet on autoimmunity and the role of zinc in the immune response. Ann Rev Nutr 2:151.
88. Pekarek RS, Sandstead HH, Jacob RA, Barcome DF (1979). Abnormal cellular immune responses during acquired zinc deficiency. Am J Clin Nutr 32:1466.
89. Allen JI, Kay NE, McClain CJ (1981). Severe zinc deficiency in humans: Association with a reversible T-lymphocyte dysfunction. Ann Int Med 95:154.
90. Golden BE, Golden MHN (1979). Plasma zinc and the clinical features of malnutrition. Am J Clin Nutr 32:2490.
91. Golden MHN, Golden BE, Harland PSEG, Jackson AA (1978). Zinc and immunocompetence in protein-energy malnutrition. Lancet 1:1226.
92. Castillo-Duran C, Heresi G, Fisberg M, Uauy R (1987). Controlled trial of zinc supplementation during recovery from malnutrition: Effects on growth and immune function. Am J Clin Nutr 45:602.
93. Lockitch G, Singh VK, Puterman ML, Godolphin WJ, Sheps S, Tingle AJ, Wong F, Quigley G (1987). Age-related changes in humoral and cell-mediated immunity in Down syndrome children living at home. Pediatr Res 22:536.

94. Franceschi C, Chiricolo M, Licastro F, Zannotti M, Masi M, Mocchegiani E, Fabris N (1988). Oral zinc supplementation in Down's syndrome: restoration of thymic endocrine activity and of some immune defects. J Ment Def Res 32:169.
95. Cavdar AO, Babacan E, Gozdasoglu S, Erten J, Cin S, Arcasoy A, Ertem U (1987). Zinc and anergy in pediatric Hodgkin's disease in Turkey. Cancer 59:305.
96. Weston WL, Huff JC, Humbert JR, Hambidge KM, Neldner KH, Walravens PA (1977). Zinc correction of defective chemotaxis in acrodermatitis enteropathica. Arch Dermatol 113:422.
97. Keen CL (1989). Lucille Shapson Hurley, 1922-1988. J Nutr 119:1875.

Part III
Nutrient Modulation of Immune Response in Human Development and Disease

18
Malnutrition and the Thymus Gland

Gerald T. Keusch
New England Medical Center
Boston, Massachusetts

INTRODUCTION

The association between childhood malnutrition and thymic atrophy was clearly described almost 150 years ago (Simon, 1845), long before any role for the thymus gland (or indeed of the lymphocyte) in immunological responses was known (Miller, 1961). Beginning early in this century, many additional reports cemented the relationship between malnutrition due to food scarcity, or illness associated with cachexia, and thymic atrophy with depletion of thymic lymphocytes and disruption of the thymic architecture (Jolly and Levin, 1911; Jackson, 1925; Boyd, 1927, 1932). Once kwashiorkor, the most clinically severe form of protein-energy malnutrition, was recognized as a nutritional disease by Cicely Williams in 1933, it became possible to more fully document the postmortem pathology of the thymus gland lesions in the malnourished (Vint, 1937; Trowell et al., 1954; Watts, 1969; Mugerwa, 1971), and to investigate its functional consequences in the living (Smythe et al., 1971).

By the early 1960s, the importance of thymic involution had begun to be unraveled. With the recognition that lymphocytes were the key cellular instruments of cell-mediated immunity and that the thymus played a central role in cell-mediated immune responses (Miller, 1961) the stage was set to begin to consider malnutrition as an immunosuppressive disease mediated by thymic abnormalities with functional consequences similar to the effects of neonatal thymectomy or combined system disease. This concept was succinctly captured by Smythe et al. (1971) in their use of the term *nutritional thymectomy*. The purpose of this chapter is to describe the effects of malnutrition on the thymus gland, T lymphocytes, and cell-mediated immunity in humans. The discussion will focus on human malnutrition, since observations in animals may or may not be relevant to the human situation (Keusch et al., 1983).

THYMUS GLAND HISTOPATHOLOGY IN MALNUTRITION

The size of the thymus gland relative to body weight is greatest at birth, and although total thymus mass increases slightly during the first year of life, its size stabilizes even as the progressive process of physiological involution begins. Thymic involution is especially noticeable after puberty, with increasing fatty infiltration of the parenchyma, slight loss of organ weight but not volume due to replacement of gland tissue by fat, and depletion of thymic lymphoid cells (Steinmann, 1986). The autopsy data showing relative constancy of thymus size over the life span of humans are supported by imaging studies using penumomediastinography (Sone et al., 1980) or computed tomography (Moore et al., 1983). Constancy of thymus size in humans differs from reports in mice, in which the gland weight shrinks by over 90% during the life of the animal (Hirokawa, 1977). This example of species differences is another reason why the specific effects of malnutrition on the human immune system cannot be simply extrapolated from animal studies (Keusch et al., 1983).

A profound atrophy of the gland is superimposed on this normal process in the case of children suffering from protein-energy malnutrition (PEM) (Vint, 1937; Watts, 1969). Watts (1969), commenting on the thymus pathology in cases of severe kwashiorkor in which only remnants of the gland remained, made the analogy to an "autothymectomy." She evaluated 192 postmortem records of East African children less than 5 years of age. These children were autopsied at Mulago Hospital, Makerere University College Medical School, Kampala, Uganda, during the years 1966-1967, and in all cases evaluated both body and thymus weight were recorded. Children were classified into three groups as follows: (a) kwashiorkor, based on autopsy findings of edema, typical skin and hair changes of kwashiorkor, atrophy of the pancreas, and fatty infiltration of the liver (32 cases); (b) marasmus, based on gross wasting, absence of edema, and minimal or no hepatic fat (26 cases); (c) nonmalnourished (presumably normal) subjects, including acute infections, tumors, trauma, accidents (75 cases). The results were compared to reference data published by Boyd (1932), and to 23 East African neonates of mean age 5 days and 9 children, average age 3 years, who died suddenly. Gross thymus weight and the ratio of thymus weight in milligrams:body weight in kilograms were recorded (Table 1). Severe atrophy of the gland was present in all malnourished children. In addition, in those under 1 year of age, the gland was smaller and the thymus:body weight ratio was less in kwashiorkor patients as compared with marasmus patients.

Smythe et al. (1971), working in South Africa, clearly recognized that the effects of protein-energy malnutrition on the thymus gland could result in impairment of cell-mediated immunity, which in turn might explain the pattern of infection noted in such children; that is, "a tendency to gram-negative septicaemia, disseminated herpes-simplex infection, anergic or afebrile response to infection, and gangrene rather than suppuration." To explore this hypothesis, they examined postmortem tissues from 118 children, ages 4-47 months, who were divided into four groups based on cadaver weight as a percentage of the Boston standards of weight-for-age. Two groups were considered adequately nourished, one with a mean body weight-for-age of 102% of standard, and the second with no evidence of marasmus but a mean weight-for-age of 80% (range 70-90%). The latter group most probably consisted primarily of stunted children caused by prior malnutrition, who now had a relatively normal weight-for-height, although these data are not given in the publication. A third group

Table 1 Thymus Weight in Malnourished African Children

Subjects	No.	Age[a]	Weight[a] (kg)	Thymus weight[a] Reference (g)	Patients (g)	Thymus:body ratio (g/kg)
Neonates	23	5 days	3.0	10.9 (6.5-17.5)[b]	12.1	3.96
1 month to 12 months of age:						
Kwashiorkor	7	10 months	6.4	19.5 (5.5-29.9)	2.9	0.45
Marasmus	11	5 months	4.0		3.7	0.91
Adequate	20	6 months	6.3		8.7	1.37
13 months to 5 years of age:						
Kwashiorkor	25	21 months	8.5	28.0 (16.5-38.5)	2.7	0.32
Marasmus	15	21 months	7.4		2.7	0.36
Adequate	55	30 months	10.8		21.9	2.03
Sudden death	9	36 months	11.7		38.6	3.30

[a] = Mean Value.
[b] = (Range).
Source: Adapted from Watts, 1969.

was clinically marasmic, with a mean weight-for-age of 59%. The final group, classified as kwashiorkor, had a mean weight-for-age of 69%. The thymus gland weight in each patient was calculated as a percentage of the expected weight for cadaver length, using previously published reference standards (Stowens, 1966). These data are shown in Table 2. There was a progressive decrease in thymus weight as nutritional indices worsened in groups 1-4, along with decreases in the percentage of glands with normal histology, mean thickness of the thymic lobule, and the percentage with evidence of acute involution (based on small lobules, loss of corticomedullary differentiation, and diminished numbers of thymoctyes), with a concomitant increase in the percentage demonstrating chronic atrophy (defined as the presence of narrow withered lobules with indented edges, no corticomedullary differentiation, scanty thymocytes, and prominent fibrosis).

Similar histological findings were reported from South Africa by Schonland (1972), who suggested that there was a continuous spectrum of histological findings from normal glands to fibrosis and atrophy, depending on the duration and severity of the underlying malnutrition. Thus, thymic abnormalities would be expected to be more frequent and more profound in kwashiorkor patients compared to marasmic subjects, which is consistent with the findings reported by Watts (1969) and Mugerwa (1971) in East Africa and Smythe et al. (1971) from South Africa. Aref et al. (1982) autopsied 60 Egyptian children, ages 6-31 months, who died of gastroenteritis and/or pneumonia between 1976 and 1979. Twelve patients were classified as marasmic, 13 marasmic-kwashiorkor, 20 kwashiorkor, and 15 were considered to be nutritionally normal. Thymic weight was significantly lower in kwashiorkor ($p < 0.005$) compared to the two marasmic groups, which were significantly less than control ($p < 0.001$). The histology of the gland was more frequently indicative of severe and chronic atrophy as nutritional status deteriorated, as previously observed in East African and South African children.

Mugerwa (1971) described the histology in some detail. He reported that the loss of lymphocytes was primarily from the cortex, which resulted in a relative prominence

Table 2 Histological Characteristics of the Thymus Gland in Malnourished Children

	Nutritional status[a]			
	Normal	Prior pem[b]	Marasmus	Kwashiorkor
Mean body weight (%Std)	102 (27)[c]	82 (21)	59 (23)	69 (47)
Thymus weight (%Std)	96	69	37	30
Normal histology (% +)[d]	48	29	8	0
Acute involution (% +)	45	33	22	15
Lobule thickness (ξ)	1172	911	538	476
Chronic atrophy (% +)	7	38	70	85

[a]Based on cadaver body weight reported as a percentage of standard (age, sex matched). See text for criteria.
[b]Based on absence of clinical features of recent malnutrition but with a significantly decreased weight-for-age. These findings probably represent stunting due to prior malnutrition, and although the data are not given in the paper, it is likely this group would have had a more normal weight-for-height than weight-for-age.
[c](Number of Subjects).
[d](% +) = Percent with the finding.
Source: Adapted from Smythe et al., 1971.

of epithelial and reticular tissues, and that there was a blurring of the demarcation between cortex and medulla, with infiltration by fibroblasts in severely affected glands. In kwashiorkor subjects, Hassall's corpuscles, formed from the thymic epithelium, were reduced in number and poorly formed. Purtilo and Connor (1975) reviewed autopsy tissues sent to the Armed Forces Institute of Pathology in Washington, D.C., from Uganda, Brazil, the Philippines, Zaire, New Guinea, Panama, and the United States. In addition to noting the same characteristics described by Mugerwa, they also commented on frequently finding dilation of Hassall's corpuscles. Recent pathology studies by Linder (1987) in the United States and Jambon (1988) in Senegal confirm that Hassall's corpuscles are often cystic, dilated, and filled with amorphous debris in glands from subjects with severe PEM. Although the significance of structural changes in Hassall's corpuscles could not have been appreciated by Mugerwa in 1971, or even by Purtilo and Connor in 1975, it is now known that the thymic epithelial cells produce a number of thymic hormones affecting differentiation and maturation of thymic lymphocytes (Dardenne and Bach, 1981; Haynes et al., 1990).

A study of thymus pathology in malnourished children from Senegal (Jambon et al., 1988) used microscopic examination with an image analyzer to quantify the fibrous tissue invading the gland and employed this criterion, in addition to descriptions of architecture and density of lymphoid cells and Hassal's corpuscles, to classify the degree of involution in malnourished subjects. The terminology dramatically highlighted the findings: When the connective tissue comprised 50-75% of the gland, involution was considered severe, and when there was greater than 75% replacement of thymus by fibrous tissue, the involution was termed extreme. There was a progressive increase in the proportion of more profoundly affected glands as nutritional status deteriorated from marasmus, through marasmic-kwashiorkor, to fullblown kwashiorkor (Table 3).

In attempting to assess the immunological significance of the alterations in thymic structure in malnutrition, it is relevant to note the similarities of these changes in

Table 3 Thymus Gland Pathology in Senegalese Children with PEM

Diagnosis	No.	Thymus weight (% of reference)	Fibrosis (% positive)	Stage of involution		
				moderate	severe	extreme
Mild PEM	18	8.0 (68.5 ± 10)	21.9	15	3	0
Marasmus	15	1.7 (17.1 ± 2.4)	49.7	2	8	5
Marasmus-Kwashiorkor	11	3.0 (19.7 ± 4.7)	60.7	0	5	6
Kwashiorkor	14	1.4 (10.3 ± 1.6)	60.6	0	3	11

Source: Adapted from Jambon et al., 1988.

malnutrition to those occurring with aging and associated reduction in immunological function. With aging, there is gradual loss of lymphocyte density in the gland, macrophages appear prominent in the cortex and contain phagocytized fragments of pyknotic thymic lymphocytes (so-called starry sky macrophages), the medulla becomes smaller, and Hassall's corpuscles are frequently altered, with cystic changes. Nonetheless, the "involuted" gland continues to play a role in T-lymphocyte biology. First, it is known that adult thymectomy results in a T-lymphocyte deficiency, suggesting its presence is still needed for T-lymphocyte maturation (Bjorkholm et al., 1975). Second, thymocytes from "old" glands express the E-rosette receptor and are able to proliferate (Kendall, 1981). Third, the thymic epithelium from naturally involuted glands still makes thymic hormones (Steinmann, 1986).

The postmortem evidence of thymic wasting in malnourished children is also consistent with in vivo observations of the size of the thymic shadow on chest x-ray (Golden et al., 1977). Since the estimation of thymic size from a chest x-ray is not reliable, Golden et al., had films evaluated by two observers without knowledge of the clinical status of the patient, and several measures were used, including the ratio of thymus diameter to chest diameter, the size of the gland classified into small, medium, or large, and finally rank order. They observed that even after nutrional rehabilitation sufficient to correct anthropometric abnormalities, the thymus shadow was still small, but that a 4-week period of zinc supplementation thereafter resulted in rapid growth of the gland, easily visible by x-ray. Golden et al. concluded that PEM in Jamaican infants is accompanied by zinc deficiency and that this feature contributes to the observed thymic lesion and immunodeficiency and may need to be specifically treated. To evaluate this suggestion further, Jambon et al. (1988) measured zinc concentration in the gland by differential impulse polarography using thymus tissue frozen in liquid nitrogen and maintained at $-70\,°C$ until assayed. No significant difference in zinc content of the glands was found when patients were classified by clinical form of malnutrition or by deficit in weight-for-height. This suggests that diminished zinc content in the gland is not a necessary condition for thymic involution in PEM, at least in Senegal. However, serum zinc levels do not suggest a high prevalence of zinc deficiency in Senegal (Maire, 1982). Even so, the requirement for zinc in many of the metalloenzymes involved in nucleic acid synthesis, and the supportive role of zinc in protein synthesis, means that zinc supplementation could still play a role by affecting the rapidity of regeneration of the thymus gland once normal protein and energy intake is restored. The role of zinc in the biological activity of thymulin is discussed in Chapter 33.

PERIPHERAL LYMPHOID AGGREGATES

In a few publications, other peripheral lymphoid tissues have been studied histologically in malnourished subjects, including the spleen, tonsil, lymph node, and others (Smythe et al., 1971; Chandra, 1972; Work et al., 1973; Neumann et al., 1975; Purtilo and Connor, 1975; Aref et al., 1982). For example, Smythe et al. (1971) found a significant decrease in spleen weight in kwashiorkor cases, along with a decrease in mean lymphoid tissue area in the tonsil, appendix, and Peyer's patches in kwashiorkor as well as marasmus patients. Purtilo and Connor (1975) noted depletion of lymphocytes from the spleen, lymph nodes, and other lymphoid tissues (tonsils, appendix, Peyer's patches), with decreased germinal center activity. The most severe lymphoctye depletion occurred in kwashiorkor patients and in those with antemortem lymphopenia. Mugerwa (1971) also examined the abdominal lymph nodes in controls and kwashiorkor patients in Uganda. There was a reduction in the number and size of lymphoid follicles, with depletion of cells from the paracortical regions. Lymphoid follicles in the spleen and appendix were present, but were smaller in kwashiorkor compared to nonmalnourished subjects, and the cuff of small lymphocytes around the follicles seen in the controls was reduced or absent. Aref et al. (1982) saw the same atrophy of the tonsils, with depletion of subepithelial lymphocytes, and also observed a decrease in spleen weight, most marked in kwashiorkor patients and, to a lesser extent, in marasmic or marasmic-kwashiorkor patients. In addition, they noted a hypocellular bone marrow with increased fat, especially in marasmic subjects, a finding not confirmed by Purtilo and Connors (1975), who later found normocellular or hyperplastic marrows. Lymphocyte depletion was largely confined to the T-cell regions in these tissues, including the paracortical and periarteriolar lymphocytes (Smythe et al., 1971; Purtilo and Connor, 1975), especially in kwashiorkor cases (Aref et al., 1982). B-Cell regions were less affected, and although diminished in size as well, there was a relative preservation of the B-lymphocyte-rich germinal centers and primary follicles. Even so, there was a general correlation between abnormal thymic histology and reduced numbers of germinal centers (Smythe et al., 1971), most marked in kwashiorkor patients. Plasma cells were present in all tissues, regardless of nutritional status, with a trend toward fewer cells in the kwashiorkor patients, which however did not reach statistical significance. Chandra and Wadhwa (1989) have noted decreased production of secretory IgA and intraepithelial cells in PEM in association with increased bacterial binding to epithelial cells, which suggests that impaired mucosal immunity may contribute both to infection severity and to decreased immune function.

Since it is possible to clinically evaluate these lymphoid aggregates during life and to estimate tonsillar size, the loss of T lymphocytes from lymphoid aggregates noted in postmortem specimens could be indirectly assessed by visual inspection and rough quantitation of the size of the tonsils. Smythe et al. (1971) used the following grading system: grade 0 if just a trace of tonsils was seen, grade 1 if the tonsil was easily visible but did not extend beyond the faucial arch; grade 2 is the tissue was beyond the arch but not greater than midway between the arch and uvula; and grade 3 if the tonsil extended beyond this point. Three-quarters of the PEM children had grade 0 tonsils, and none had higher than grade 1 score. In contrast, control African children were uncommonly classified in grade 0 (only 13%), and nearly two-fifths were classified as grade 2 or above. This observation has been confirmed by others

(Chandra, 1972; Neumann et al., 1975; Work et al., 1973). While the size of these lymphoid tissues is markedly decreased in malnourished patients, they respond to appropriate nutritional rehabilitation by significantly increasing in size (Neumann et al., 1975).

CIRCULATING T LYMPHOCYTES IN MALNOURISHED CHILDREN

Malnourished children, unless severely ill or near death, are usually not leukopenic, nor specifically lymphopenic; total peripheral white blood cell counts are usually similar to better-nourished controls of the same age and sex (Keusch et al., 1983). For example, McMurray et al. (1981) studied a group of normal Columbian children and subjects with kwashiorkor, with maramus, or marasmus-kwashiorkor (Table 4) and found that total lymphocyte counts were within the normal range in all subjects. Although the mean count rose from admission to discharge after nutritional therapy, the extent of change was not significant. In contrast, when the proportion of T lymphocytes in circulation in peripheral blood has been estimated in malnourished children around the world (Chandra, 1974; Ferguson et al., 1974; Keusch et al., 1987), a consistent decrease in the percentage of sheep erythrocyte rosette-forming T cells has been found in kwashiorkor patients, often with normal values in those with marasmus. The low counts respond to nutritional rehabiliation by increasing to the normal range over weeks to a few months (Keusch et al., 1983).

If T lymphocytes are reduced in the circulation in children with kwashiorkor, and the lymphocyte number is relatively preserved, what are the non-T lymphocytes in the blood? It is quite clear that only a portion of these cells are B lymphocytes, and a number of studies have demonstrated normal numbers of B lymphocytes in malnourished hosts, consistent with the relative sparing of B-cell regions in peripheral lymphoid organs and the normal to elevated levels of serum immunoglobulins in these patients (Keusch et al, 1983). For example, Chandra (1977) reported that the percentage of B lymphocytes defined by the EAC rosette test was normal in malnourished children. Chandra (1977) later confirmed these findings, using a simple test to detect surface immunoglobulin (Ig) with fluorescein-tagged antihuman IgG, IgM, and IgA. By this assay, the percentage of Ig-positive B cells in a group of Indian children with PEM and edema was found to be equivalent to the percentage of B cells in a group of age-matched healthy Indian children. The remaining cells cannot be clas-

Table 4 Lymphocyte Counts in Colombian Children with PEM

Parameter	Normal	Marasmus	Marasmus-Kwashiorkor	Kwashiorkor
Number studied	25	11	11	21
Mean age (months)	44.2	33.7	35.4	44.2
(range)	(27-60)	(24-41)	(18-51)	(32-60)
Total lymphocytes on admission	4007 ± 329	5291 ± 793	4316 ± 772	3952 ± 58
Total lymphocytes on discharge		5952 ± 699	5533 ± 912	4422 ± 469

Source: Adapted from McMurray et al., 1981.

sified as either mature T or mature B cells by the methods used, and therefore have been termed "null" cells.

Chandra et al. (1982) have also characterized lymphocyte subpopulations by the use of monoclonal antibodies recognizing the CD3, CD4, and CD8 differentiation antigens (Table 5). They studied six children, aged 10-32 months, who had severe protein-energy malnutrition (weight-for-age and weight-for-height both less than 70% of the standard) due to reduced dietary intake of unstated etiology. Recent infection in these children was excluded by history, x-ray, and laboratory studies to detect acute-phase responses. Compared to 10 controls of the same age, there was a marked decrease in the percentage of cells reacting with the pan-T-cell antibody, T3 (CD3), in the malnourished subjects. This was the consequence of a profound decrease in T4 (CD4)-positive cells, and a less dramatic but still highly significant drop in T8 (CD8) cells. This resulted in a sharp reduction of the mean T4:T8 ratio to 0.87, a value comparable to that observed in a number of immunodeficiency states. Since the total lymphocyte count is not changed in the malnourished, these data also indicate a greater decrease in the number of mature marker-positive T lymphocytes of the helper compared to the suppressor-cytotoxic phenotypes. Wade et al. (1988) have used the same monoclonal antibodies to define lymphocyte subpopulations in Senegalese children with malnutrition, with infection, or in uninfected nonmalnourished African controls. The mean values for $T3^+$, $T4^+$, and $T8^+$ cells, and the T4/T8 ratio were altered in the same direction in malnourished compared to control children as those reported by Chandra et al. (1982), with little change in the values in the infected children. However, because of wide variation in individual values, there were no significant differences among the means. Further recent studies by Woodward et al. (1991) suggest that altered ratios of $CD4^+$ T lymphocytes to $CD8^+$ T lymphocytes is not the basis of depressed T-cell immunity in PEM in the mouse, or that these changes may be observed only in peripheral blood which was not analyzed in this study. Additional examination of subpopulations of CD4 and CD8 will be needed to verify this conclusion, however, and the relationship to human PEM is unknown.

IMMATURE LYMPHOCYTES IN PEM

Chandra (1979) was able to purify the null cells from peripheral blood lymphocyte populations by first removing B cells on an anti-immunoglobulin column and then eliminating T cells from the B-lymphocyte-depleted population by allowing them to form E-rosettes which could be sedimented and removed. The remaining null cells comprised over 50% of the initial population of lymphocytes in the malnourished patients, compared to less than 10% in healthy, well-nourished controls. Samples containing such high proportions of null cells also were found to be high in enzyme activity for terminal deoxynucleotidyl-transferase (TdT), an enzyme present in immature thymic, bone marrow, and some circulating lymphocytes, probably representing a population of prothymocytes. The TdT activity was 10 times higher in malnourished cells compared to controls (11.34 ± 2.42 versus 1.08 ± 0.07 $U/10^8$ cells), and the correlation between the TdT activity and the number of non-T/non-B null cells was excellent ($r = 0.78$, $p < 0.01$), strongly suggesting that these cells were immature undifferentiated lymphocytes of the T-cell lineage.

Chandra also observed that null cells from malnourished subjects, free of macrophages which were removed by allowing them to ingest carbonyl iron and subject-

Table 5 Lymphocyte Subpopulations in Protein-Energy Malnutrition

	Cells Reactive With Monoclonal Antibodies (%)							
	T3+		T4+		T8+		T4:T8	
Subjects	Before[a]	After[a]	Before	After	Before	After	Before	After
Malnourished (n = 6)	26 ± 2.5	65 ± 2.7	15 ± 6.5	41 ± 1.2	18 ± 0.1	22 ± 0.8	0.87 ± .11	1.86 ± 0.07
Controls (n = 10)	67 ± 4.3		41 ± 3.7		25 ± 2.3		1.98 ± 0.21	

[a]Before and after nutritional rehabilitation.
Source: Adapted from Chandra et al., 1982.

ing them to a magnetic force, were functional cytotoxic lymphocytes in a cell-mediated cytotoxicity assay using ^{51}Cr-labeled DBA/2 fibroblasts as the target (Chandra, 1977). Although the nature of the cell mediating this effect is not clearly defined, these data demonstrate that natural cytotoxic cells are present among the null cells in malnourished subjects.

Another cytotoxic cell found in the circulation which requires no previous sensitization is the natural killer (NK) cell, which recognizes and lyses certain neoplastic cell targets, such as the K-562 human erythroid leukemia. NK activity is associated with large granular lymphocytes, and while its origin from T- or B-cell precursors is uncertain, the NK cell appears to be under some control by thymic factors, since NK cytotoxicity is high in athymic nude mice and can be enhanced in normal mice by thymectomy. Natural killer activity is also regulated in vivo and in vitro by interferon. It might be predicted that nutritional thymectomy would lead to high NK activity which could be augmented in vitro by incubation of peripheral blood mononuclear cells with interferon. However, a report from Nigeria (Salimonu et al., 1982) found significantly reduced NK cell activity among marasmic or kwashiorkor patients compared to controls. Furthermore, and in contrast to normal cells, not only was there no effect of incubation of cells from malnourished subjects with interferon, there was even a highly significant decrease in NK activity when kwashiorkor cells were incubated with interferon. Although the mechanisms are not clear, these findings point to defects in thymic influences on cytotoxic cell populations in malnourished patients. This subject is discussed further in chapter 22.

In addition, some reports suggest that protein restricted diets may enhance NK cell activity (Norris et al., 1990). However, complexity in these issues has been shown by Petro et al. (1991), who found that while a lower dietary protein level promoted increased NK activity and IL-3 production in the mouse, specific cytotoxic T-lymphocyte development was slowed.

THYMIC HORMONES IN MALNOURISHED SUBJECTS

Few data have been reported on thymic hormones in malnutrition. Human studies were reported by Chandra in 1979. He assayed serum levels of thymulin (facteur thymique serique) by means of the biological assay of Bach and Dardenne, which measures the ability of the serum being tested to convert thy-1-negative azathioprine resistant rosette-forming splenocytes harvested from recently thymectomized mice into azathioprine sensitive thy-1$^+$ cells. In practice, the highest dilution of serum that restores azathioprine sensitivity is considered to the be titer of thymulin. Nine Indian infants with protein-energy malnutrition were studied, ages 9-30 months, of whom only two were edematous. Mean values ($\log_2$ reciprocal titer) for thymulin activity were 6.9 in controls and 4.7 in patients. In contrast, and using a similar assay, Maire et al. (1982) did not find alterations in thymulin activity among Senegalese children with protein-energy malnutrition who were also infected at the time of study.

Until more recently, then, the score stood at 1 to 1 and it was unclear whether or not thymic hormone levels were affected by PEM. A more recent study (Wade et al., 1988) may explain the discrepancy. Serum thymulinlike activity, measured in Senegalese children by the assay of Dardenne and Bach, was not significantly different among malnourished, infected, and control subjects. However, when thymulin was absorbed with an antithymulin monoclonal antibody, a significant residual "thymulinlike activity" was present in all subjects and attributed to "allogeneic factor," a thymulinlike activity produced during antigen-induced T-cell activation. By subtracting this value from the total thymulinlike activity "specific-thymulin activity" could be calculated, which was markedly depressed in the malnourished and infected groups compared to the African controls in Senegal. These control values were also significantly less than those of age-matched well-nourished Senegalese controls living in France, suggesting that mild malnutrition is also associated with reduced serum levels of thymulin. The authors also noted that these levels had little relation to peripheral T-lymphocyte subpopulations and that decreased circulating thymic hormone levels are not necessarily associated with lymphocyte phenotypic alterations.

Thus, the level of hormone in the thymic microenvironment itself is more likely to correlate with thymocyte induction and maturation. The amount of thymulin in the thymus gland has been directly determined by an immunohistochemical method (Jambon et al., 1988). Thymulin present in the cytoplasm of producing cells was recognized by a rabbit antibody raised to a synthetic thymulin. The antibody was then extensively adsorbed with acetone powders of human organs to eliminate nonspecific binding, especially to keratin. Fluorescein-tagged goat antibody to rabbit IgG was used to stain the tissues. Fluorescence episcopic microscopy was employed for semiquantitation of the number of thymulin-positive epithelial cells and Hassall's corpuscles and to determine the intensity of labeling. These parameters were combined into a qualitative index score (Table 6). Four groups of children dying with varying degrees of malnutrition were studied; mildly malnourished children served as the comparison group. Approximately 80% in each group had infections at the time of death, including bronchopneumonia, acute diarrhea, malaria, recent measles, and others. Regardless of clinical classification of malnutrition, however, all glands studied had markedly decreased thymulin index scores in comparison to the mild PEM control group, and in over 25% there was absolutely no thymulin staining detected. There was a close correlation between thymus weight and thymulin content. The authors considered the possibility that the time between death and autopsy might affect the ability to detect thymulin in situ. However, the glands were all obtained within a few hours of death (mean elapsed time 3 hr 29 min ± 35 min), and did not correlate with the content of hormone detected. Jambon et al. (1988) conclude that thymic

Table 6 Nutritional Status and Thymulin Content of Thymus Glands

Nutritional status	No.	Weight for height (% standard)	Weight for age (% standard)	Thymulin (index)
Mild malnutrition	18	81 ± 2.0	78 ± 4.6	51.6 ± 4.2
Marasmus	15	61 ± 1.6	52 ± 2.4	15.8 ± 2.8
Marasmus-Kwashiorkor	14	61 ± 1.3	55 ± 2.5	12.5 ± 3.8
Kwashiorkor	11	74 ± 1.7	74 ± 2.4	21.7 ± 6.5

Source: Adapted from Jambon et al., 1988.

involution in PEM is associated with diminished thymulin content, and that this is a direct cause of deficient cell-mediated immunity in severely malnourished patients. Recent studies by Kuvibidila et al. (1990) in an animal model have shown that iron deficiency (which is often profound in severe malnutrition) does not affect thymic endocrine function or T-cell subset ratio, although a decrease in immunocompetent lymphocytes was observed, suggesting that there are discrete events which regulate or deregulate thymic activity during the process of malnutrition.

EFFECTS OF THYMIC FACTORS ON LYMPHOCYTES FROM MALNOURISHED SUBJECTS

If thymic hormone deficiency is responsible for defective maturation of the T-lymphocyte system, then provision of hormone should correct some or all of the defects. Three studies (Jackson and Zaman, 1980; Olusi et al., 1980; Keusch et al., 1987) have indeed shown that thymic factors added to human peripheral blood lymphocytes in vitro increase the percentage of cells forming E-rosettes. These publications preceded the Jambon study, were carried out in Asia, Africa, and Latin America, and all concluded that maturational events were induced in vitro by the hormones. Jackson and Zaman (1980) studied 10 marasmic and 6 kwashiorkor Bangladeshi children, ages 14 months to 6 years, all of whom were clinically infected. Following 2 hr of incubation with 1 μg/ml of purified thymopoietin obtained from calf thymus, the percentage of E-rosettes rose from 39 to 49 (mean percent increase was 46%). E-Rosettes were in the normal range (>50%) in four marasmic patients, and the effect of thymopoietin was minimal (mean increase of E-rosettes was only 6%). Similarly, the effect of the hormone in 11 age-matched controls (mean value of E-rosettes of 54% in the absence of thymopoietin) was nil, with a 2% decrement after the addition of the hormone.

The other two studies employed a partially purified thymic preparation, thymosin fraction 5, which is known to contain at least a dozen peptides. In the first of these, Olusi et al. (1980) studied 30 Nigerian children with a mean age of 2.6 years, and clinical kwashiorkor. Although E-rosettes were severely depressed (mean 26%, with none greater than 40%), a brief 10-min incubation with 5 μg of thymosin fraction 5 was sufficient to increase the E-rosettes in 80% (24/30) of subjects to a new mean value of 50%. Over half of these patients corrected the E-rosettes into the normal range (>50%), with a mean of 55% in these individuals. The third study (Keusch et al., 1987) evaluated 33 Guatemalan children with acute PEM, mean age 9 months,

31 of whom were edematous and had a weight for age less than 70% of standard. Peripheral blood mononuclear cells were incubated with 20 or 200 µg of thymosin fraction 5 for 1 hr. Whereas the mean value for E-rosettes was 43% in these infants, the data were scattered and in nearly one-third 50% or more of the cells formed E-rosettes. The effect of thymosin fraction 5 was inversely related to the initial values for E-rosettes, and was directly related to the dose of the thymosin added (Fig. 1). The authors concluded that PEM resulted in "a maturational arrest of T-lymphocytes at the thymic level," and that defects in cell-mediated immunity and the T lymphocytes could be "considered to be, in part, an endocrine abnormality" and subject to correction by thymic hormone replacement therapy.

Cruz et al. (1987) determined E-rosettes and thymosin fraction 5 responses in eight Guatemalan children, aged 14-38 months, and followed these responses during a 1-month period of optimal nutritional rehabilitation. The methods employed were identical to those of Keusch et al. (1987). Mean percent of E-rosettes steadily increased from $35.6 \pm 10\%$ to $43.3 \pm 19\%$ from admission to week 4, but this improvement was not statistically significant ($F = 0.2868$, $p = 0.76$). Addition of thymosin fraction 5, 20 µg, resulted in an increase of $8.0 \pm 4.7\%$ on admission, prior to nutritional rehabilitation, occurring almost exclusively in those with initially low values. A curious finding in this study was that an increase of similar magnitude was measured at 2 and 4 weeks of nutritional therapy, indicating that thymosin-responsive cells persisted in circulation in many of these children. The response in individual children was quite variable; although in some there were parallel changes in clinical, nutritional, and immunological parameters, in others no obvious relationship could be detected. By the end of the 1-month period of nutritional therapy, the value of E-rosettes in the presence of thymosin fraction 5 was similar to that observed in marginally malnourished subjects serving as controls for the studies. Cruz et al. (1987) suggest that thymosin fraction 5 is insufficient by itself to rapidly restore the level of mature T lymphocytes, and that perhaps there would be a more dramatic impact of adding the different thymic hormones together in vitro or giving them therapeutically in vivo. It is of interest and possibly of relevance to this idea that the same thymic epithelial cells, including the Hassall's corpuscles, produce the several thymic peptides that are responsible for maturation and differentiation of the T-lymphocyte system. (Dardenne and Bach, 1981).

CELL-MEDIATED IMMUNE FUNCTION IN MALNOURISHED SUBJECTS

There is little need to extensively document the defective cell-mediated immune responses in malnourished subjects, as this has been the subject of many studies and has been reviewed many times (e.g., Keusch et al., 1983). The most frequently reported in vivo measure of cell-mediated immunity is delayed-type skin hypersensitivity (DTH) responses to either recall or neoantigens. The early observations were made in subjects who should have had positive tuberculin responses, demonstrating defective tuberculin reactions even in those with documented tuberculosis or following BCG vaccination (Jayalakshmi and Gopalan, 1958; Harland, 1965; Harland and Brown, 1965). Subsequent studies have confirmed this many times, with the defect residing

Malnutrition and the Thymus Gland

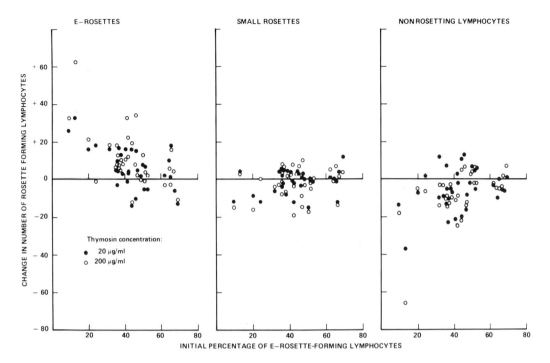

Figure 1 Change in number of E-rosettes due to in vitro incubation of peripheral blood mononuclear cells from Guatemalan children with acute protein-energy malnutrition with thymosin fraction 5 (TF-5). These data are plotted against the percentage of 5-rosetting lymphocytes in the sample without TF-5. The open circles represent data obtained with the high dose of TF-5 (200 μg/ml) and the closed circles are data with the low dose of TF-5 (20 μg/ml). E-Rosettes were defined as lymphocytes with three or more sheep erythrocytes attached; lymphocytes with one to two sheep erythrocytes were classified as small rosettes. Macrophages were clearly identified by feeding the cells latex particles; cells with ingested latex were excluded from the counts. The mean number of E-rosettes increased from 86.7 ± 5.1 in the control incubation, to 93.2 ± 4.2 in the presence of low dose TF-5, and to 98.2 ± 4.4 in the presence of high dose TF-5 (chi square [2 df] = 18.94, $p < 0.01$).

in the efferent limb of the DTH response (Edelman et al., 1973; Koster et al., 1981). The study by Koster et al. (1981) is particularly informative. Fifty severely malnourished Bangladeshi infants were randomized into four study groups and sensitized with 2 mg of dinitrochlorobenzene (DNCB) on day 2, 8, 15, or 22 of hospitalization. Nutritional rehabilitation began on admission, and all were given a bolus of vitamin A and daily oral multivitamins. Iron supplementation was started in week 2. The DNCB challenge was then performed 10 days after sensitization and again 2 and 4 weeks later. The results show that the later the initial sensitization was performed after beginning nutritional therapy, the greater the percent responding to challenge. Whereas only 29% of those sensitized on day 2 responded to challenge 1, and only 50% responded to challenge 2, 75% of those sensitized on days 8-22 responded to challenge 1 and 100% to challenge 2. Of particular interest, when the early sensitization group was subdivided by the total serum protein level, four of six with protein

>5.5 g/dl (mean 6.4 ± 0.22) responded, whereas none of eight with levels under 5.5 g/dl were positive.

The most common in vitro abnormality of cell-mediated immunity detected in patients with protein-energy malnutrition is a reduced proliferative response to mitogens or specific antigens (Keusch et al., 1983). Usually measured as the stimulation index, the incorporation of [^{3}H]thymidine in patients compared to controls in the presence of a mitogen such as phytohemagglutinin, the defect is more profound and more frequently observed in those with kwashiorkor compared to marasmus. This is presumably the consequence of the diminished number of mature, mitogen-responsive cells in circulation, although the predominance of suppressor over helper T lymphocytes may play a significant role. In some studies, humoral suppressor factors also have been postulated, but to date they have not been conclusively shown (Heyworth et al., 1975; Beatty and Dowdle, 1978). Based on data from mixing experiments with normal and kwashiorkor cells and serum, Beatty and Dowdle (1979) subsequently suggested that it was more likely that a factor needed for the proliferative response was missing from kwashiorkor serum rather than there being a specific inhibitor. This putative factor could be a specific nutrient, such as zinc or iron, or possibly a cytokine needed for activation of the immune response, or possibly transferrin, which is often depleted during acute-phase reactions and is required for cell proliferation.

The subject of cytokine production in malnourished subjects is becoming of interest, as methods have been developed to better assay these biologically active molecules. Reports have appeared suggesting that peripheral blood monocytes produce less IL-1 when activated by opsonized zymosan, *S. epidermidis*, or lipopolysaccharide endotoxin (Keenan et al., 1982; Kauffman, 1986). Bhaskaram and Sivakumar (1986) have also suggested that cells from malnourished patients may produce inhibitors of the lymphocyte-activating factor (LAF) response to IL-1. We may expect that data will become available to address these questions about cytokines and inhibitors in subjects with protein-energy malnutrition in the near future.

CONCLUSIONS

Available human data demonstrate that protein-energy malnutrition causes major changes in thymus gland structure, with marked decreases in the number of cortical lymphocytes, fatty infiltration, fibrosis, and diminution and alteration of Hassall's corpuscles. In addition, T-lymphocyte regions of peripheral lymphoid tissues including spleen, lymph node, tonsil, Peyer's patches, and appendix are depleted of lymphocytes. As a consequence, the number of mature circulating T lymphocytes is decreased, and all functions performed by these cells (e.g., proliferative responses to antigens or mitogens in vitro or delayed-type skin hypersensitivity responses in vivo) are significantly impaired. Although the mechanisms involved are not clear at the present time, thymic peptide hormone content in the gland, and probably in the serum as well, is decreased in protein-energy malnutrition, with a loss of maturation induction functions of the thymic microenvironment. The loss of mature peripheral blood lymphocytes is more evident in the CD4-positive cell subpopulation compared to the CD8-positive cell, with a significant reduction in the CD4:CD8 ratio. Incubation of peripheral blood lymphocytes with thymic hormone preparations such as thymopoietin or thymosin fraction 5 results in a significant increase in mature T lymphocytes detected by the E-rosette test. Immunosuppression in protein-energy malnutrition thus appears to be due to a loss of T-helper cells (CD4$^+$), a relative increase in T-suppressor cells (CD8$^+$), a probable decrease in the production of cytokines activating the immune response, and possibly due to suppressor humoral factors as well. The regulatory processes are not certain, and the role of specific nutrients such as zinc is not fully understood.

REFERENCES

Beatty DW, Dowdle EB (1978). The effects of kwashiorkor serum on lymphocyte transformation in vitro. Clin Exp Immunol 32:134-143.

Beatty DW, Dowdle EB (1979). Deficiency in kwashiorkor serum of factors required for optimal lymphocyte transformation in vitro. Clin Exp Immunol 35:433-442.

Bhaskaram P, Sivakumar B (1986). Interleukin-1 in malnutrition. Arch Dis Child 61:182-185.

Bjorkholm M, Holm G, Johansson B, Mellstedt H (1975). T-Lyphocyte deficiency following adult thymectomy in man. Scand J Haematol 14:210-215.

Boyd E (1927). Growth of the thymus. Am J Dis Child 33:867-879.

Boyd E (1932). The weight of the thymus gland in health and disease. Am J Dis Child 33:1162-1214.

Chandra RK (1972). Immunocompetence in undernutrition. J Pediatr 81:1194-1200.

Chandra RK (1974). Rosette-forming T lymphocytes and cell-mediated immunity in malnutrition. Br Med J 3:608-609.

Chandra RK (1977). Lymphocyte subpopulations in human malnutrition: Cytotoxic and suppressor cells. Pediatrics 59:423-427.

Chandra RK (1979). T and B Lymphocyte subpopulations and leukocyte terminal deoxynucleotidyl transferase in energy-protein undernutrition. Acta Paediatr Scand 68:841-845.

Chandra RK (1979). Serum thymic hormone activity in protein-energy malnutrition. Clin Exp Immunol 38:228-230.

Chandra RK, Gupta S, Singh H (1982). Inducer and suppressor T cell subsets in protein-energy malnutrition: Analysis by monoclonal antibodies. Nutr Res 2:21-26.

Chandra RK, Wadhura M (1989). Nutritional modulation of intestinal mucosal immunity Immunol Invest 18:119.

Cruz JR, Chew F, Fernandez R, Torun B, Goldstein AL, Keusch GT (1987). Effects of nutritional recuperation on E-rosetting lymphocytes and in vitro response to thymosin in malnourished children. J Pediatr Gastroenterol Nutr 6:387-391.

Dardenne M, Bach JF (1981). Thymic hormones. In: The Thymus Gland. Kendall MD, ed. Academic Press, London, pp 113-131.

Edelman R, Suskind R, Olson RE, Sirisinha S (1973). Mechanisms of defective delayed cutaneous hypersensitivity in children with protein-calorie malnutrition. Lancet 1:506-508.

Ferguson AC, Lawlor GJ Jr, Neumanmn CG, Oh W, Stiehm ER (1974). Decreased rosette-forming lymphocytes in malnutrition and intrauterine growth retardation. J Pediatr 85:717-724.

Golden MN, Jackson AA, Golden BE (1977). Effect of zinc on thymus of recently malnourished children. Lancet 2:1057-1059.

Haynes, BF, Denning SM, Le PT, Singer KH (1990). Human intrathymic T cell differentiation Semin Immunol 2:67.

Harland PS (1965). Tuberculin reactions in malnourished children. Lancet 2:719-721.

Harland PS, Brown RE (1965). Tuberculin sensitivity following BCG vaccination in undernourished children. East Afr Med J 42:233-238.

Heyworth B, Moore DL, Brown J (1975). Depression of lymphocyte response to phytohemagglutinin in the presence of plasma from children with acute protein energy malnutrition. Clin Exp Immunol 22:72-77.

Hirokawa K (1977). The thymus and aging. In: Immunology and Aging. Makinodan, T, Yunis E, eds. Plenum, New York, pp 51-72.

Jackson CA (1925). The Effects of Inanition and Malnutrition upon Growth and Structure. McGraw-Hill, Philadelphia.

Jackson TM, Zaman SN (1980). The in vitro effect of the thymic factor thymopoietin on a subpopulation of lymphocytes from severely malnourished children. Clin Exp Immunol 39:717-721.

Jambon B, Ziegler O, Maire B, Hutin MF, Parent G, Fall M, Burnel D, Duheille J (1988). Thymulin (facteur thymique serique) and zinc contents of the thymus glands of malnourished children. Am J Clin Nutr 48:335-342.

Jayalakshmi VT, Gopalan C (1958). Nutrition and tuberculosis. I. An epidemiologic study. Indian J Med Res 46:87-92.

Jolly J, Levin S (1911). Sur les modifications histologiques du thymus a la suite de jeune. CR Soc Biol 71:374-377.

Kauffman CA, Jones PG, Kluger MJ (1986). Fever and malnutrition: Endogenous pyrogen/interleukin-1 in malnourished patients. Am J Clin Nutr 44:449-452.

Keenan RA, Moldawer LL, Lyand RD, Kawamura I, Blackburn GL, Bistrian BR (1982). An altered response by peripheral leukocytes to synthesize or release leukocyte endogenous mediator in critically ill, protein malnourished patients. J Lab Clin Med 100:844-857.

Kendall MD (1981). Age and seasonal changes in the thymus. In: The Thymas Gland, Kendall MD, ed. Academic Press, Orlando, Florida, pp 21-35.

Keusch GT, Wilson CS, Waksal SD (1983). Nutrition, host defenses, and the lymphoid system. In: Advances in Host Defense Mechanisms. Vol 2. Gallin, JI, Fauci AS, eds. Raven Press, New York, pp 275-359.

Keusch GT, Cruz JR, Torun B, Urrutia JJ, Smith H Jr, Goldstein A (1987). Immature circulating lymphocytes in severely malnourished Guatemalan children. J Pediatr Gastroenterol Nutr 6:265-270.

Koster F, Gaffar A, Jackson TM (1981). Recovery of cellular immune competence during treatment of protein-calorie malnutrition. Am J Clin Nutr 34:887-891.

Kuvibidila S, Dardenne M, Savino W, Lepault F (1990). Influence of iron deficiency anemia on selected thymus functions in mice: Thymulin biological activity, T cell-subsets and thymocyte proliferation Am J Clin Nutr 51:228.

Linder J (1987). The thymus gland in secondary immunodeficiency. Arch Pathol Lab Med 111:1118-1122.

Maire B, Wade S, Bleiberg F, Dardenne M, Parent G, LeFrancois P, Carles C (1982). Absence of variation in facteur thymique serique activity in moderately and severely malnourished Senegalese children. Am J Clin Nutr 36:1129-1133.

McMurray DN, Watson RR, Reyes MA (1981). Effect of renutrition on humoral and cell-mediated immunity in severely malnourished children. Am J Clin Nutr 34: 2117-2126.

Miller JFAP (1961). Immunological function of the thymus. Lancet 2:748-749.

Moore AV, Korobkin M, Olanow W, Heaston DK, Ram PC, Dunnick NR, Silverman PM (1983). Age-related changes in the thymus gland. CT—pathologic correlation. AJR 141: 291.

Mugerwa JW (1971). The lymphoreticular system in kwashiorkor. J Pathol 105:105-109.

Neumann CG, Lawler GJ, Stiehm ER (1975). Immunologic responses in malnourished children. Am J Clin Nutr 28:89-104.

Norris JB, Meadows GG, Massey LK, Starky JR, Sylvester M, Lui SY (1990). Tyroxine-restricted and phenylalanine-restricted formula diet augments immune competence in healthy humans. Am J Clin Nutr 51:188-196.

Olusi SO, Thurman GB, Goldstein AL (1980). Effect of thymosin on T-lymphocyte rosette formation in children with kwashiorkor. Clin Immunol Immunopathol 15:687-691.

Petro TM, Schwacts KM, Schmid MJ (1991). Natural and immune anti-tumor interleukin production and lymphocyte cytotoxicity during the course of dietary protein deficiency or excess Nutr Res LL:6790.

Purtilo DT, Connor DH (1975). Fetal infections in protein-calorie malnourished children with thymolymphatic atrophy. Arch Dis Child 50:149-152.

Schonland M (1972). Depression of immunity in protein-calorie malnutrition: A post-mortem study. Environ Child Health 18:217-214.

Simon J (1845). Physiological Essay on the Thymus Gland. Renshaw, London.

Sone S, Higashirhara T, Morimoto S (1980). Normal anatomy of the thymus and anterior mediastinum by pneumonediastinography. AJR 134:81-89.

Smythe PM, Schonland M, Brereton-Stiles GG, Coovadia HM, Grace HJ, Loening WEK, Mafoyne A, Parent MA, Vos GH (1971). Thymolymphatic deficiency and depression of cell-mediated immunity in protein-calorie malnutrition. Lancet 2:939-943.

Stowens D (1966). Pediatric Pathology. Williams & Wilkins, Baltimore, Maryland.

Trowell HC, Davis JNP, Dean RFA (1954). Kwashiorkor. Edward Arnold, London.

Vint FW (1937). Post-mortem findings in natives in Kenya. East Afr Med J 13:332-340.

Wade S, Parent G, Bleiberg-Daniel F, Maire B, Fall M, Scheider D, Le Moullac B, Dardenne M (1988). Thymulin (Zn-FTS) activity in protein-energy malnutrition: New evidence for interaction between malnutrition and infection on thymic function. Am J Clin Nutr 47: 305-311.

Watts T (1969). Thymus weights in malnourished children. J Trop Pediatr 15:155-158.

Williams CD (1933). A nutritional disease of childhood associated with a maize diet. Arch Dis Child 8:423-433.

Work TE, Tfekwunigwe A, Jelliffe D, Jelliffe P (1973). Tropical problems in nutrition. Ann Intern Med 79:701-711.

Woodward BD, Miller RG (1991). Depression of thymus dependent immunity in wasting protein energy malnutrition does not depend on an altered ratio of helper ($CD4^+$) to suppressor ($CD8^+$) T cells or on a disproportionately large atrophy of the T cell relative to the B-cell pool. Am J Clin Nutr 53:1329.

19
Maturation of the Immune System in Breast-Fed and Bottle-Fed Infants

Susan Stephens
*Celltech, Ltd., Slough,
Berkshire, England*

INTRODUCTION

Many of the topics covered in this book concern problems associated with recognized nutritional deficiencies and their effects on the immune system. Most milk formulas available for feeding infants in the Western world are now considered to be complete with regard to all the conventional nutrional requirements of newborn infants. However, there are still many discrepancies between proprietary milk formulas based on cow milk (or soy protein) and fresh human milk. These differences can be divided into three main areas. First, cow milk proteins are foreign to the human infant, and proteins such as casein are known to be highly antigenic in the infant gut. Second (see Chap. 21), human milk contains a number of protective elements such as viable cells, immunoglobulins, lactoferrin, lactoperoxidase, and lysozyme. Although many of these are present in cow milk, few survive the heat treatment used in the preparation of milk formulas. Finally, a number of cytokines have been identified in human milk which are capable of affecting the growth and differentiation of cells in vitro, including epidermal growth factor and several lymphokines. There are good reasons to believe that while human milk and cow milk formulas are both considered nutritionally adequate, these three aspects of difference between them will modify the development of immunity in breast-fed and bottle-fed infants. In this chapter, the evidence suggesting that milk can modulate immune responses in infants will be reviewed: the data indicate that breast-feeding indeed has important effects on immunological development.

COMPONENTS OF HUMAN MILK AND COW MILK FORMULAS THAT MAY AFFECT IMMUNOLOGICAL DEVELOPMENT

Antigenicity of Cow Milk

During the first few weeks of life, the infant gut is more permeable to macromolecules than the adult gut and this results in increased uptake of food antigens (Eastham and

Walker, 1979). When infants are bottle-fed from birth, this means increased absorption of cow milk proteins. The immunogenicity of these proteins has been highlighted by the development of intolerance to cow milk in a small number of infants. Four major proteins may be involved; casein, α-lactalbumin, β-lactoglobulin, and bovine serum albumin (Goldman, 1977). However, even in infants with no obvious signs of allergy to cow milk, high concentrations of immunoglobulin G (IgG) antibodies to cow milk proteins are found in the serum (Kletter et al., 1971; Fällstrom et al., 1984). Phagocytosis of the resulting immune complexes causes release of lysosomal enzymes, which will then further increase gut permeability, not only to homologous proteins, but also to unrelated molecules (Tolo et al., 1977; Udall et al., 1981). This increased uptake of antigens from the gut will, therefore, lead to a general increase in the stimulation of the infants immune system.

Protective Factors in Human Milk

Several studies on infection rates in breast-fed and bottle-fed infants have indicated lower morbidity and mortality in breast-fed infants (Cunningham, 1979). This is particularly marked for gastrointestinal infections but also applies to systemic and respiratory tract infections (Watkins et al., 1979). A number of specific and nonspecific antimicrobial agents have been identified in human milk, and these will be discussed in detail in Chapter 35. However, two components (immunoglobulins and cells) will be mentioned briefly here as they are particularly relevant to immunological development. Milk contains large quantities of antibodies, mostly of the secretory immunoglobulin A (sIgA) class (Hanson and Winberg, 1972), but more recently IgG_4 has also been shown to be produced in the mammary gland (Keller et al., 1988). The maternal gut is an important site of stimulation for these antibodies, and gut-derived lymphoid cells primed to environmental antigens relocate in the mammary gland, where they secrete antibodies to organisms most likely to be encountered by the infant (Goldblum et al., 1975). These antibodies exert their protective effect within the gut of the infant by preventing microbial adhesion at the mucosal surface. However, whereas protecting the infant from infection, they also serve to prevent antigens from entering through the gut, thereby reducing stimulation and the subsequent proliferation and differentiation of lymphoid tissue in the infant. The level of these antibodies appears to change rapidly after birth (Ogura, 1987). Of current interest is the potential transfer of immunity to human immunodeficiency virus (HIV). Antibodies to HIV envelope glycoproteins have been demonstrated in seropositive women (Belac et al., 1990). However, the risk of transmission of the virus to the infant via this route has led to the recommendation of screening high-risk mothers (Seltzer and Benjamin, 1990), and has also contributed to the decline in human milk banks.

Human milk also contains large numbers of viable macrophages and lymphocytes (Smith and Goldman, 1968) which are capable of secreting effector molecules such as immunoglobulins in vitro (Ahlstedt et al., 1975; Slade and Schwartz, 1989). Whether viable cells are transferred to the circulation of the infant is not known but this remains a possibility (Hughes et al., 1988). Transfer of tuberculin sensitivity from TB-positive mothers to breast-fed but not bottle-fed infants (Mohr, 1973; Schlesinger and Covelli, 1977) has been observed, and this could be due to transfer of viable cells or soluble factors from milk. Purified protein derivative (PPD)-induced chemotactic factors can be produced by milk cells in vitro (Keller et al., 1984). However, these workers were unable to confirm the findings of Sclesinger and Covelli (1977) and suggest transplacental transfer of immunity may be more important (Keller et al., 1987).

Factors in Human Milk that Can Modulate Cell Function In Vitro

Several other soluble factors capable of modulating immune responses in vitro have been found in human milk. Emodi and Just (1974) demonstrated that milk lymphocytes produced as much interferon as peripheral blood lymphocytes when stimulated with Newcastle disease virus, and production of alpha and gamma interferons has subsequently been confirmed by other workers (Lawton et al., 1979; Keller et al., 1981). Milk cells also secrete prostaglandins E and F (Lucas and Mitchell, 1980). In addition, human colostrum and milk contain large quantities of epidermal growth factor (Carpenter, 1980; Klagsbrun and Shing, 1984), which as well as stimulating the maturation of epithelial cells (Heird and Hansen, 1977) is capable of enhancing antigen-driven lymphocyte proliferation (Acres et al., 1985). Interleukin 5 (IL-5), if present in human milk, could have an important role in switching B cells to IgA synthesis in the infants gut (Harriman and Strober, 1987). Pittard and Bill (1979a) have described a factor (possibly IL-5) which stimulates cord blood lymphocytes to differentiate into IgA-secreting cells. Also, enhanced urinary secretion of IgA has been demonstrated in breast-fed infants (Prentice, 1987). Juto (1985) has shown enhancement of B-cell proliferation and differentiation by milk components which may include IL-1 or B-cell growth and differentiation factors (possibly IL-4, IL-5, and IL-6). Interleukin 1 production by breast milk cells may, however, be lower than that by peripheral blood cells (Subiza et al., 1988). More recently, Mushata et al. (1989) have shown chemokinetic activity in milk which cross-reacts with tumor necrosis factor alpha (TNF-α). This cytokine has been shown to upregulate secretory component (Kvale et al., 1988) and could, therefore, potentially increase the concentration of IgA and IgM at the gut mucosa. In contrast, Crago et al. (1981) have described a factor in colostrum (possibly secretory component) which can inhibit proliferation and immunoglobulin production by peripheral blood lymphocytes. Whether these cytokines have a role in vivo is not yet known, but the possibility that milk may be important in the development of the infant immune system has been suggested by several workers (Roberts and Freed, 1977; Pittard and Bill, 1979b; Cederqvist, 1981; Tlaskalova-Hogenova et al., 1983; Schanler et al., 1986).

DEVELOPMENT OF IMMUNE RESPONSES IN NEWBORN BREAST-FED AND BOTTLE-FED INFANTS

Serum Immunoglobulins and Antibodies

Newborn infants have serum IgG concentrations similar to those of adults, but IgM and IgA concentrations are very low (Berg, 1969). The large quantities of IgA in milk do not seem to be absorbed into the serum of the breast-fed infant to any great extent (Yengar and Selvaraj, 1972; Ogra et al., 1978; Yap et al., 1979). In a detailed study of 15 breast-fed and 15 bottle-fed infants, bled sequentially from birth to 9 months of age, we found no significant differences between the two feeding groups in the development of serum IgG, IgM, and IgA (Table 1), suggesting that there was neither early absorption of milk immunoglobulins nor enhanced immunoglobulin production by the breast-fed infants.

Both groups of infants also respond equally well to systemic vaccination with antigens such as tetanus toxoid, producing high levels of specific IgG (Zoppi et al., 1983; Stephens et al., 1984), although when infants were fed with milk formulas containing low protein concentrations, responses to vaccination were lower than in breast-fed infants and more short lived (Zoppi et al., 1983). Recently, however, Pabst and Spady (1990) have reported that when infants were vaccinated with a conjugate vaccine, CRM-197 diphtheria-toxin *Hemophilus influenzae* type B polyribose phosphate, at 2.0-2.5 months of age, antibody levels at 7 and 12 months were significantly higher in breast-fed compared to bottle-fed infants. Further, there was no relationship between preimmunization antibody titer and titer at 7 months, demonstrating that the maternal antibody level did not interfere with the induction of response.

Serum antibody responses to antigens encountered in the gut, however, were significantly different in the two feeding groups. Higher levels of serum IgG antibodies to cow milk proteins in bottle-fed infants have already been mentioned. In addition, we have investigated the development of serum antibodies to lipopolysaccharide antigens from commensal strains of *Escherichia coli*, and shown that as early as 6 days of age, serum IgM antibodies were significantly higher in the bottle-fed group than the breast-fed group; this difference was maintained beyond 9 months (Fig. 1). Breast-fed infants weaned early, rapidly achieved similar antibody levels to the bottle-fed infants. Serum IgA antibodies to *E. coli* were also higher in the bottle-fed group (Stephens et al., 1984). There are two reasons for the higher antibody levels to components of the normal gut flora in bottle-fed infants. First cow milk antigens can cause increased gut permeability in infants (Eastham and Walker, 1979). Second, epidermal growth factor in breast milk may enhance maturation of the gut epithelium and thereby reduce permeability to macromolecules; work in rabbits suggests that this is an important mechanism during the first few days of life (Udall et al., 1981).

The importance of the microbial flora of the gut in modulating immunological development is well known (Rusch, 1981; Berg, 1983). The balance of microorganisms in the flora may be different for breast-fed and bottle-fed infants, with a higher proportion of lactobacilli in breast-fed infants and more *E. coli* and other Enterobacteriacae in bottle-fed infants (Bullen and Willis, 1971; Borriello and Stephens, 1984). Many of the Enterobacteriacae in the gut will produce endotoxins which can have a profound effect on the cells of the immune system (Lagrange et al., 1975; Kiyono et al., 1980; Rethy, 1983). *Escherichia coli* can also secrete biologically active molecules (bacterial cytokines) which are similar to the lymphokines released by cells of the immune system (Yoshida et al., 1975). Increased gut permeability in bottle-fed infants will, therefore, generally augment stimulation of lymphoid tissues. The observation that *total* serum immunoglobulin concentrations are similar in the two feeding groups may indicate that the immune system of the breast-fed infant is stimulated by alternative mechanisms (discussed below).

Secretory Immunoglobulins and Antibodies

Infants have low levels of immunoglobulins in secretions during the first few weeks of life; in fact, until highly sensitive radioimmunoassay techniques were developed, secretory immunoglobulins were undetectable before 2 weeks of age (Selner et al., 1968). Application of more sensitive techniques has produced conflicting reports on

Table 1 Development of Serum and Salivary Immunoglobulins in Breast-fed and Bottle-fed Infants

		Concentration of immunoglobulin in								
		Serum (µg/ml)					Saliva (µg/mg protein)			
Age	Feeding group	6 days	6 weeks	3 months	6 months	9 months	6 days	6 weeks	3 months	6 months	9 months
IgG	Breast	7240	4780	2920	3090	4400	1.6	0.7	0.3	0.4	0.5
	Bottle	7260	4710	3520	2980	3990	1.6	1.6	0.6	0.4	0.3
IgM	Breast	138	282	427	427	676	0.1	0.5	0.4	0.9	0.8
	Bottle	138	309	427	468	562	0.02	1.6	1.9	1.4	1.2
	p =						0.014		0.015		
IgA	Breast	1.9	69.2	115	166	195	2.34	36.2	22.9	22.4	17.4
	Bottle	1.7	91.0	112	148	178	0.05	53.7	39.8	17.0	15.2
	p =						<0.001		0.07		

Results are expressed as geometric means of immunoglobulin concentrations in serum and saliva from 15 breast-fed and 15 bottle-fed infants. Samples were assayed in duplicate by radioimmunoassay (Stephens et al., 1984). Total protein concentrations for saliva samples were estimated by a protein dye-binding technique (Stephens, 1986). Differences between the feeding groups were assessed by a pooled t-test.

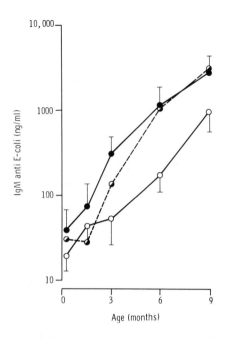

Figure 1 Serum IgM antibodies to *Escherichia coli* LPS antigens. Antibody concentrations were assessed by solid-phase RIA using a pool of "O" LPS antigens from six commensal strains of *E. coli*. Results are expressed as geometric means (±95% confidence intervals). ○——○ Breast fed exclusively for 4 months or more (n = 12); ◐——◐ Breast fed but fully weaned by 2 months (n = 3); ●——● Bottle fed from birth (n = 15). Differences between the groups were assessed by analysis of variance (p <0.001).

the development of IgA in the secretions of breast-fed and bottle-fed infants. Roberts and Freed (1977) reported significantly higher concentrations of IgA in the saliva and nasal secretions of breast-fed infants during the first week. Gross and Buckley (1980) suggested that this was due to contamination by milk IgA, and to overcome this problem they collected saliva samples at least 4 hr after feeding. However, in their study, although no significant differences were found between the groups overall, during the first week the concentration of IgA in the saliva of breast-fed infants was still three times higher than that of bottle-fed infants. Taylor and Toms (1984) also found higher concentrations of IgA in the nasal secretions from breast-fed infants at 1 week of age, and the highest levels did not correlate with the most recent feeding.

We have examined the development of immunoglobulin and specific antibody concentrations in saliva and nasal secretions from birth to 9 months (Stephens, 1986). In the breast-fed group, total IgM and IgA were significantly higher in both types of secretion at 6 days (see Table 1), and these levels did not correlate with the time since the last feed. The possibility of contamination of these samples with milk immunoglobulins remains, although some breast-fed infants still had high levels of IgA more than 4 hr after the last intake of milk. Binding of IgA to buccal epithelial cells may be responsible (Roberts et al., 1980) but increased local production, stimulated by the growth factors or lymphokines in milk, is a strong possibility, and a study of allotypic markers might identify the origin of the IgA detected. By 6 weeks of age, IgM and IgA concentrations had increased dramatically in all infants as a result of stimulation by environmental antigens and by colonization of the respiratory mucosae with microorganisms (Cebra et al., 1980). In saliva samples, concentrations of IgM were significantly higher in the bottle-fed group from 6 weeks to 9 months (see Table 1), although in nasal secretion samples IgM and IgA were similar in both groups (Stephens, 1986). These higher salivary immunoglobulin concentrations in bottle-fed infants could be due to stimulation of the salivary glands with cow milk proteins, resulting in a polyclonal expansion of local lymphoid tissue.

Specific antibodies in secretions to systemically administered antigens such as tetanus toxoid were low or undetectable ($<0.04\%$ of serum levels), indicating a very low level of transfer from serum. Specific antibodies to commensal strains of *E. coli* were also low, although IgA antibodies were detectable in the saliva of all infants by 6 weeks of age (Stephens, 1986). These antibodies were present in a significantly greater number of breast-fed than bottle-fed infants at 6 days, indicating either passive transfer by milk or increased local production. No differences were found between the groups beyond this age. The fact that antibodies to *E. coli* were present at such low concentrations in saliva and nasal secretions from these infants probably reflects the relatively low exposure rate of infants in European countries to these organisms. Mellander et al. (1985) found much higher levels in saliva from Pakistani infants, and a study comparing immunological development in breast- and bottle-fed infants in an area of high disease incidence such as Pakistan might well highlight further differences between the groups.

Lymphocyte Proliferative Responses In Vitro

The proliferation of peripheral blood lymphocytes in vitro has frequently been used as a measure of immunocompetence. Lymphocytes from cord blood and from newborn infants have a higher rate of spontaneous and mitogen-induced proliferation than cells from adults, an observation attributed to increased activation in vivo (Weber et al., 1973). The difficulties of obtaining large amounts of blood from newborn infants has meant that estimates of lymphocyte proliferation have frequently been made using single levels of each in vitro variable such as mitogen dose, cell concentration, and length of culture period. However, there are differences in the optimal conditions in vitro for infant and adult cells, and this can give misleading results when infant and adult responses are compared (Wara and Barrett, 1979). Similar problems arise when responses between breast- and bottle-fed infants are compared (Juto et al., 1982), and we were concerned that estimations using single point measurements might not reveal shifts in the dynamics of the responses. The development of microtechniques for the study of lymphocyte function (O'Brien et al., 1979) enabled us to investigate the development of lymphocyte responsiveness in more detail (Stephens et al., 1986). Peripheral blood mononuclear cells (PBMs) were isolated from heparinized venous blood, and spontaneous proliferation and proliferative responses to T- and B-cell mitogens, allogeneic lymphocytes, and antigen were measured. Cells were cultured in serum-free medium in Terasaki plates (20 μl) and proliferation was estimated by incorporation of [^{3}H]thymidine over a range of cell concentrations and periods of culture. The results indicated that while total numbers of white cells and percentages of lymphocytes were comparable for the two feeding groups, there were significant differences in the proliferative responses of the isolated PBM cells for all stimuli tested and these differences changed with age.

In newborn infants, spontaneous (background) proliferation and proliferative responses to stimuli affecting predominantly T cells (phytohaemagglutinin [PHA] and tetanus toxoid [TT] were significantly greater in the breast-fed group (shown for the peak day of culture in Fig. 2). This greater responsiveness occurred at all cell concentrations and on all days of culture, and therefore indicated an increase in the overall magnitude of the response rather than a shift in the dynamics. Responses to allogeneic lymphocytes (MLRs) were similar in total magnitude, but for breast-fed infants' maximal responses occurred earlier in the culture period. Since mitogens act preferentially on partially activated cells, this enhanced responsiveness in newborn breast-fed infants may well be due to an increased activation of T cells or their precursors in vivo, perhaps as a consequence of stimulation by the high levels of growth factors and lymphokines in colostrum and early milk. In support of this hypothesis, Pabst et al. (1989) have studied blastogenic responses in BCG-vaccinated infants and found a specific increase in responses of cells from breast-fed but not bottle-fed infants when they were vaccinated in the first month of life, but this difference was not apparent if they were vaccinated after this time. Although this increased proliferative response could theoretically reflect in vivo response to antigenic stimulation from microbial or viral sources, the finding that plasma lactoferrin, a known acute-phase protein, is not different between breast-fed and formula-fed infants up to 15 weeks of age makes this an unlikely explanation (Scott, 1989).

Responses to mitogens such as pokeweed mitogen (PWM) and *Staphylococcus aureus* strain Cowan (SAC) which affect B cells, showed no differences between the feeding groups at this age.

From 3 to 6 months of age, the lymphocyte response patterns reversed. All stim-

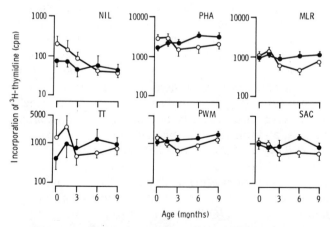

Figure 2 Proliferative responses of PBM cells to various stimuli in vitro. Cells were cultured in 20-μl hanging drop microcultures in serum-free medium only (NIL) and with the following stimuli: PHA 1 μg/ml; TT 2 ng/ml; Mitomycin-c-treated allogeneic lymphocytes (MLR) at 2 × 10^6 cells/ml; PWM 1 μg/ml; SAC 1/2000. Results are shown for the peak day of culture only and are expressed as geometric means ($\pm$95% confidence intervals) of [^{3}H]thymidine incorporated in 2 hr by cells from 15 breast-fed (○) and 15 bottle-fed (●) infants, cultured in duplicate at three cell concentrations. The significance of the interaction between feeding group and age (assessed by analysis of variance) is as follows: NIL, $p = 0.0013$; PHA, $p = 0.007$; SAC, $p = 0.014$; MLR, $p = 0.029$. Differences between groups (assessed by Bonferroni t-tests) PWM, 3, 6, and 9 months $p < 0.05$; TT 6 days, $p < 0.05$.

uli tested caused cells from bottle-fed infants to proliferate more vigorously than cells from breast-fed infants. This suggests that in these older infants, all types of cells were in a greater state of activation or maturation in vivo in the bottle-fed group. There are several reasons why responses in breast-fed infants might be lower at this time. First, there may be a decrease in the growth factors in mature human milk (Read et al., 1984). Second, factors in human milk such as secretory component may begin to have a supressive role on lymphocyte responses (Crago et al., 1981). A more likely explanation, however, is that the increased responses in the bottle-fed group are due to increased antigenic stimulation. This enhanced responsiveness corresponds with the period of increased serum antibody response to gut organisms in the bottle-fed infants.

Lymphocyte Function In Vitro

Immunoglobulin Production

Assessment of lymphocyte function in newborn infants using plaque assays has indicated that immunoglobulin production is deficient, and IgM is predominantly secreted by cord blood lymphocytes after PWM stimulation. Significant IgG production does not occur until 6 months (Andersson et al., 1981). To determine how the development of immunoglobulin secretion in vitro is affected by feeding group, PBM cells from breast-fed and bottle-fed infants were cultured in serum-free medium for 8 days and the immunoglobulins secreted into the supernatants were measured by radioimmunoassay. Figure 3 shows the spontaneous production of IgM and IgG by cells from infants aged between 3 and 9 months, the age when proliferation was higher in the bottle-fed group. At a concentration of 4×10^6 cells/ml, the supernatants contained an average of 100 ng/ml IgM, 800 ng/ml IgG, and 450 ng/ml IgA. There were no significant differences between the feeding groups, although IgM production was slightly higher in the bottle-fed group and IgG was slightly higher in the breast-fed group. Unfortunately, there was insufficient sample material to test immunoglobulin production by the cells from 6-day and 6-week-old infants, the age when lymphocyte proliferation was greatest in the breast-fed group.

Pokeweed mitogen enhanced IgM production in cultures from only three of nine breast-fed infants and one of seven bottle-fed infants. Production of IgG and IgA was not enhanced by PWM in either group. These results confirm that infant cells are rather unresponsive to this mitogen (Wu et al., 1976; Andersson et al., 1981). Tetanus toxoid, however, induced more than a twofold increase in total IgM production in 10 of 13 breast-fed and 4 of 8 bottle-fed infants tested (Fig. 4), although this higher proportion of responses in breast-fed infants was not significant. Tetanus toxoid, like PWM, did not stimulate an increase in total IgG or IgA production, nor were specific antibodies of any class detectable (<5 ng/ml), indicating that the IgM response to tetanus toxoid was polyclonal. When monocytes were depleted by plastic adherence, and B-cell growth and differentiation factors were added to the culture medium with tetanus toxoid, cells from two of five 9-month-old (bottle-fed) vaccinated infants secreted low levels of specific IgG (Stephens, 1984). Insufficient cells were available to separate T and B cells in order to obtain the optimal ratios of these cells necessary for in vitro antibody production, but the possibility of differences in immunoglobulin and specific antibody production in vitro between the feeding groups, particularly in the early neonatal period when proliferative responses are greater in breast-fed infants (Stephens et al., 1986; Pabst et al., 1989).

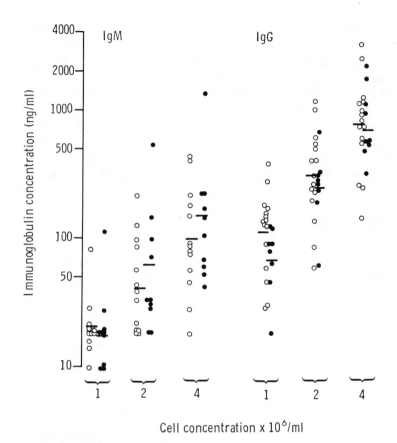

Figure 3 Spontaneous secretion of immunoglobulin in vitro by PBM cells from infants aged between 3 and 9 months. Cells were cultured in 20 μl hanging drop microcultures using serum-free medium and incubated for 8 days at 37°C with 5% CO_2 and 100% humidity. Supernatants from duplicate wells were pooled and concentrations of IgM and IgG were assessed by solid-phase RIA. ○ Breast fed; ● Bottle fed.

Gamma Interferon Production

Stimulation of the infant's immune system will cause release of various lymphokines such as interferons. Although secretion of alpha and beta interferons (IFN-α, IFN-β) by infant cells is comparable to that of adult cells (Bryson et al., 1980), production of gamma interferon (IFN-γ) has been reported as deficient until 6 months of age. Because IFN-γ is important in immune regulation as well as viral killing (Wallach et al., 1982), we have followed the development of IFN-γ production to determine the effect of breast- and bottle-feeding (Stephens et al., 1986). Pokeweed mitogen cells were cultured in 20-μl hanging drop cultures and stimulated with staphylococcal enterotoxin A (SEA), a potent inducer of IFN-γ. After 3 days, the quantity of IFN-γ in the supernatants was determined by immunoradiometric assay (Scott et al., 1985). With this stimulant, cells from all infants secreted large quantities of IFN-γ (>100 U/ml) as early as 6 days of age (Table 2), and in fact even cord blood lymphocytes produced as much IFN-γ as adult cells. There were no significant differences between breast-fed and bottle-fed infants, although bottle fed infants secreted slightly more IFN-γ, possibly due to the greater antigenic stimulation in vivo.

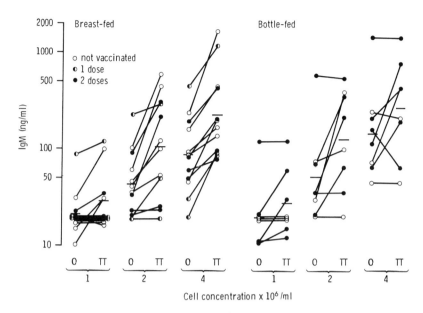

Figure 4 IgM production by PBM cells from breast fed and bottle fed infants in response to tetanus toxoid stimulation in vitro. Cultures were stimulated with immunopurified TT (2 ng/ml) and incubated as described for Figure 3.

Conclusions from the Study of Immune Responsiveness in Breast-Fed and Bottle-Fed Infants

Investigation of the effect of breast- and bottle-feeding on in vivo and in vitro immune responses has shown that breast-feeding has contrasting effects on the development of immunity. In the early neonatal period—up to 6 weeks of age—there is an enhancement of lymphocyte proliferative responses and an increase in the concentrations of IgM and IgA in the secretions of breast-fed infants. By 3 months of age, many immune responses are greater in the bottle-fed group, including higher serum antibody levels to cow milk proteins and to normal gut flora, higher salivary IgM, and greatly increased proliferative responses of PBM cells to all stimuli tested. It should be emphasized at this point that the two groups of infants in this study were comparable for all other factors which might be considered to affect immunological development, such as gestational age, birth weight, sex, standard of maternal care, and family history of allergy or other immunological disorders. Infection rates were also uniformly low in both feeding groups. It seems fair, therefore, to attribute the differences found between the groups to feeding method alone. The reasons why milk is likely to have contrasting effects on immunological development have been discussed in detail and are summarized now in Table 3. Growth factors and lymphokines in colostrum may have an important role in stimulating the development of the immune system in the newborn breast-fed infant at a time when the infant's immunological repertoire will be limited owing to immaturity and a lack of antigenic stimulation in utero. The unique system of passive protection of the infant by milk antibodies, however, will serve to "downregulate" specific immune responses by excluding potentially infectious organisms. In the bottle-fed infant, the immune system will receive its stimulus to proliferate and mature from direct antigenic stimulation, not

Table 2 IFN-γ Production In Vitro By Cells from Breast-fed and Bottle-fed Infants

	Cord blood	Age					
		6 days	6 weeks	3 months	6 months	9 months	Adult
	630						454
	(269,1472)						(191,1082)
Breast		239	327	387	208	272	
		(84,678)	(149,712)	(68,2177)	(109,395)	(73,1013)	
Bottle		357	316	493	325	520	
		(136,938)	(115,864)	(226,1073)	(181,582)	(243,1110)	

PBM cells were cultured for 3 days at 4×10^6 cells/ml with 250 ng/ml SEA, and the quantity of IFN-γ secreted into the supernatants was determined by immunoradiometric assay (Stephens, Duffy and Page, 1986). Results are expressed as geometric means in U/ml (with 95% confidence intervals) from between 7 and 12 samples per occasion, assayed in duplicate.

only from the relatively harmless cow milk proteins, but also from the microorganisms which colonize the infant within hours of birth. This may result in a similar final level of immunological maturity, but with a far greater risk to the infant. In addition, maturation factors in milk may affect the development of a primary response to particular vaccines, a fact which may be relevant to the future design of such products.

DEVELOPMENT OF ALLERGIC DISEASE IN BREAST-FED AND BOTTLE-FED INFANTS

Whereas the anti-infective role of breast-feeding is now well accepted, the role of breast milk in preventing the development of allergic disease is much more contraversial (Björksten, 1983). Many of the factors involved have been extensively reviewed (Businco and Cantani, 1984). Taylor et al. (1973) suggested that the development of allergic disease in infants was due to a transient IgA deficiency in early infancy, which could be reduced by breast-feeding (Soothill, 1976). Although some workers have found no differences between the incidence of allergic disease in breast-fed and bottle-fed infants (Fergusson et al., 1983; Gordon et al., 1982), diseases such as atopic eczema and asthma have generally been reported as being lower in breast-fed infants, particularly when the infants are selected for a family history of atopy (Chandra, 1978; Saarinen et al., 1979). IgE levels are also lower in breast-fed infants (Juto and Björkstein, 1979; Ostergaard, 1985).

It is now possible to resolve some of the apparent conflict if we accept that the development of allergic responses in infants is modified by human milk in the same way as other immune responses. The IgA antibodies in milk include antibodies with specificities for many different foods (McClelland and McDonald, 1976; Cruz, 1983; Fälth-Magnusson, 1989) and these will help to shield the breast-fed infant from the food antigens contained in a mixed diet. Conversely, although human milk will be generally less antigenic to the human infant than cow milk, many food antigens are transferred from the mother to the breast-fed infant in milk and have the potential to cause allergic reactions. These include cow milk proteins, egg proteins, theobromine from chocolate, and wheat and fruit antigens (Jakobsson and Lindberg, 1978). In fact, one exclusively breast-fed infant in our study (from a family with a history of atopy) developed severe eczema within 1 month of birth. This infant was found to

Table 3 Ways in Which Breast-Feeding May Modulate Immunological Development

	Upregulation		Downregulation	
Lymphokines				
IFN-γ		(Emodi and Just, 1974) (Lawton et al., 1979)	Suppressive factors secretory component	(Crago et al., 1981)
chemotactic factors		(Keller et al., 1981)		
IgA-stimulatory factor		(Keller et al., 1984)	Immunoglobulins antigen exclusion	(Soothill, 1976) (Hanson and Winberg, 1972)
Interleukin 1		(Pittard and Bill, 1979)		
B-cell growth factor		(Juto, 1985)		
B-cell differentiation factor			Dietary exclusion of foreign protein	(Kletter et al., 1971) (Eastham and Walker, 1979)
TNF-α		(Mushata et al., 1989)		
Epidermal growth factor Lymphocyte stimulation		(Carpenter, 1980) (Klagsbrun and Shing, 1984) (Acres et al., 1985)	Epidermal growth factor enhanced maturation of gut epithelium	(Heird and Hansen, 1977)
Prostaglandins E and F		(Lucas and Mitchell, 1980)		

be allergic to cow and soya milk, eggs, wheat, and citrus fruit and the eczema resolved when the mother avoided these foods (Sloper and Brostoff, 1985).

Finally, factors have now been identified in human milk from atopic mothers which can stimulate the secretion of IgE from PBM cells in vitro (Allardyce and Wilson, 1984). The possibility that these factors are active in vivo could be important for the potentially atopic infant. If so, then this may explain the conflicting reports on the incidence of allergy in infants from atopic families. When the infant comes from a family in which the father has a history of allergy, the risk to the infant of IgE-stimulating factors being transferred by breast-feeding will be much lower than if the mother has a history of allergic disease. Future studies on the role of breast-feeding in preventing allergy should, therefore, take into consideration which parent has a history of allergic disease.

CONCLUSIONS

The cow milk formulas currently available for feeding newborn infants are generally considered to be nutritionally adequate, but there are still multiple differences between these formulas and fresh human milk. Many of the differences involve components which are likely to have an effect on the infant's developing immune system. Lymphokines and epidermal growth factors in human milk can stimulate lymphoid cells in vitro, and in breast-fed infants they may be responsible for the increased secretory immunity and greater lymphocyte proliferative responses found during the first few weeks after birth. Specific antibodies in human milk (mainly sIgA) will provide passive protection for the infant, particularly against microorganisms encountered in the gut, but this protective effect will also reduce specific antigenic stimulation of the infant's own immune system. In addition to reducing exposure of the systemic immune system to gut organisms, breast-feeding also reduces the general antigenic load on the infant by the dietary exclusion of large quantities of cow milk protein. By 3 months of age, this increased exposure of bottle-fed infants to antigens results not only in higher levels of specific serum antibodies to gut organisms and cow milk proteins, but also significantly greater proliferative responses of lymphocytes in vitro, indicating a generally increased activation of lymphoid cells in vivo. In children from atopic families, it may also result in higher IgE levels and increased incidence of allergic disease.

There are thus contrasting effects of breast-feeding on the immune system of the infant: stimulation of general responsiveness by cytokines in milk and a reduction of specific responses by antigen exclusion. In bottle-fed infants, in whom antigenic stimulation forms the major stimulus for the immune system to proliferate and mature, a similar level of overall immunological maturity may be achieved, but not without added risks to the infant. In fact, in countries where the incidence of infectious diseases is high, this will constitute an extremely hazardous route of stimulation.

REFERENCES

Acres RB, Lamb JR, Feldman M. Effects of platelet-derived growth factor and epidermal growth factor on antigen-induced proliferation of human T-cell lines. *Immunology* 1985; 54:9-16.
Ahlstedt S, Carlsson B, Hanson LÅ, Goldblum RM. Antibody production by human colostral cells. I. Immunoglobulin class, specificity and quantity. Scand J Immunol 1975; 4: 535-539.

Allardyce RA, Wilson A. Breast milk supernatants from atopic donors stimulate cord blood IgE secretion in vitro. Clin Allergy 1984; 14;259-267.
Andersson U, Bird G, Britton S. A sequential study of human B lymphocyte function from birth to two years of age. Acta Paediatr Scand 1981; 70:837-842.
Bélac L, Bouquety JC, Georges AJ, Siopathis MR, Martin PMV. Antibodies to human immunodeficiency virus in the breast milk of healthy, seropositive women. Pediatrics 1990; 85:1022-1026.
Berg RD. Host immune response to antigens of the indigenous flora. In: Human Intestinal Microflora in Health and Disease. Hentges DJ (ed.). New York, Academic Press, 1983, pp 101-126.
Berg T. The immunoglobulin development during the first year of life. A longitudinal study. Acta Paediatr Scand 1969; 58:229-236.
Björksten B. Does breast feeding prevent the development of allergy? Immunol Today 1983; 4:215-217.
Borriello SP, Stephens S. The development of the infant gut flora; and the medical microbiology of infant botulism and necrotising enterocolitis. In: Microbes and Infections of the Gut. Goodwin CS (ed.). Blackwell Scientific, 1984, pp 1-26.
Bryson YJ, Winter HS, Gard SE, Fischer TJ, Stiehm ER. Deficiency of immune interferon production by leukocytes of normal newborns. Cell Immunol 1980;55:191-200.
Bullen CW, Willis AT. Resistance of the breast-fed infant to gastroenteritis. Br Med J 1971; 3:338-343.
Businco L, Cantani A. Prevention of atopy—current concepts and personal experience. Clin Rev Allergy 1984;2:107-123.
Carpenter G. Epidermal growth factor is a major growth-promoting agent in human milk. Science 1980;210:198-199.
Cebra JJ, Gearhart PJ, Halsey JF, Hurwitz JL, Shahin RD. Role of environmental antigens in the ontogeny of the secretory immune response. J Reticuloendothel Soc 1980;28:61s-71s.
Cederqvist LL. Breast-feeding influences the humoral immune response in the newborn. Am J Reproduc Immunol 1981;1:231-232.
Crago SS, Kulhavy R, Prince SJ, Mestecky J. Inhibition of the pokeweek mitogen-induced response of normal peripheral blood lymphocytes by humoral components of colostrum. Clin Exp Immunol 1981; 45:386-392.
Cruz JR. Specific immune response in human milk to oral immunization with food proteins. Ann NY Acad Sci 1983; 409:808-809.
Cunningham AS. Morbidity in breast-fed and artificially-fed infants. II. J Pediatr 1979; 95:685-698.
Eastham EJ, Walker WA. Adverse effects of milk formula ingestion on the gastrointestinal tract. An update. Gastroenterology 1979; 76:365-374.
Emödi G, Just M. Interferon production by lymphocytes in human milk. Scand J Immunol 1974; 3:157-160.
Fällstrom SP, Ahlstedt S, Carlsson B, Wettergren B, Hanson LÅ. Influence of breast-feeding on the development of cow's milk protein antibodies and the IgE level. Int Arch Allergy Appl Immunol 1984; 75:87-91.
Fälth-Magnusson K. Breast milk antibodies to foods in relation to maternal diet, maternal atopy and the development of atopic disease in the baby. Int Arch Allergy Appl Immunol 1989; 90:297-300.
Fergusson DM, Horwood LJ, Shannon FT. Asthma and infant diet. Arch Dis Child 1983; 58:48-51.
Goldblum RM, Ahlstedt S, Carlsson B, Hanson LÅ, Jodal U, Lidin-Janson G, Sohl-Akerlund A. Antibody forming cells in human colostrum after oral immunisation. Nature 1975; 257:797-799.
Goldman AS. Cow milk sensitivity: A review. Food and Immunology 1977; XIII Symposium Swedish Nutrition Foundation, pp 99-104.

Gordon RR, Ward AM, Noble DA, Allen R. Immunoglobulin E and the eczema-asthma syndrome in early childhood. Lancet 1982; 1:72-74.

Gross SJ, Buckley RH. IgA in saliva of breast-fed and bottle-fed infants. Lancet 1980; 2:543.

Hanson LA, Winberg J. Breast milk and defence against infection in the newborn. Arch Dis Child 1972; 47:845-848.

Harriman GR, Strober W. Interleukin 5, a mucosal lymphokine? J Immunol 1987; 139:3553-3555.

Heird WC, Hansen IH. Effect of colostrum on growth of intestinal mucosa. Pediatr Res 1977; 11:406.

Hughes A, Brock JH, Parrot DMV, Cockburn F. The interaction of infant formula with macrophages: effect on phagocytic activity, relationship to expression of Class II MHC antigen and survival of orally administered macrophages in the neonatal gut. Immunol 1988; 64:213-218.

Jakobsson I, Lindberg T. Cow's milk as a cause of infantile colic in breast-fed infants. Lancet 1978; 2:437-439.

Juto P. Human milk stimulates B cell function. Arch Dis Child 1985; 60:610-613.

Juto P, Björksten B. Lymphocyte activity and serum IgE in relation to feeding in infants. Lancet 1979; 2:102.

Juto P, Möller C, Engberg S, Bjorksten B. Influence of type of feeding on lymphocyte function and development of infantile allergy. Clin Allergy 1982; 12:409-416.

Keller MA, Gendreau-Reid L, Heiner DC, Rodriguez A, Short JA. IgG4 in human colostrum and human milk: continued local production or selective transport from serum. Acta Pediatr Scand 1988; 77:24-29.

Keller MA, Kidd RM, Bryson YJ, Turner JL, Carter J. Lymphokine production by human milk lymphocytes. Infect Immun 1981; 32:632-636.

Keller M, Kidd R, Reisinger D, Stewart D. PPD-induced monocyte chemotactic factor production by human milk cells. Acta Paediatr Scand 1984; 73:465-470.

Keller MA, Rodriguez AL, Alvarez S, Wheeler NC, Reisinger D. Transfer of tuberculin immunity from mother to infant. Pediatr Res 1987; 22:277-281.

Kiyono H, McGhee JR, Michalek SM. Lipopolysaccharide regulation of the immune response: Comparison of responses to LPS in germ-free, *Escherichia coli*-monoassociated and conventional mice. J Immunol 1980; 124:36-41.

Klagsbrun M, Shing Y. Growth-promoting factors in human and bovine milk. *In*: Growth and Maturation Factors. Vol. 2. New York, Wiley, 1984, pp 161-192.

Kletter B, Gery I, Freier S, Davies AM. Immune responses of normal infants to cow milk. II. Decreased immune reactions in initially breast-fed infants. Int Arch Allergy 1971; 40: 667-674.

Kvale D, Lovhaug D, Sollid LM, Brandtzaeg P. Tumor necrosis factor -α upregulates expression of secretory component, the epithelial receptor for polymeric Ig. J Immunol 1988; 140:3086-3089.

Lagrange PH, Mackaness GB, Miller TE, Pardon P. Effects of bacterial lipopolysaccharide on the immune induction and expression of cell mediated immunity. II. Stimulation of the efferent arc. J Immunol 1975; 114:447-451.

Lawton JWM, Shortridge KF, Wong RLC, Ng MH. Interferon synthesis by human colostral leucocytes. Arch Dis Child 1979; 54:127-130.

Lucas A, Mitchell MD. Prostaglandins in human milk. Arch Dis Child 1980; 55:950-952.

McClelland DBL, McDonald TT. Antibodies to dietary proteins in human colostrum. Lancet 1976; 2:1251-1252.

Mellander L, Carlsson B, Jalil F, Söderstrom T, Hanson LÅ. Secretory IgA antibody response against *Escherichia coli* antigens in infants in relation to exposure. J Pediatr 1985; 107: 430-433.

Mohr JA. The possible induction and/or acquisition of cellular hypersensitivity associated with ingestion of colostrum. J Pediatr 1973; 82:1062-1064.

Mushtaha AA, Schmalstieg FC, Hughes TK Jr, Rajaraman S, Rudloff HE, Goldman AS. Chemokinetic agents for monocytes in human milk: Possible role of tumour necrosis factor-α. Pediatr Res 1989; 25:629-633.

O'Brien J, Knight SC, Quick NA, Moore EH, Platt AS. A simple technique for harvesting lymphocytes cultured in Terasaki plates. J Immunol Methods 1979; 27:219-223.

Ogra SS, Weintraub DI, Ogra PL. Immunologic aspects of human colostrum and milk: Interaction with the intestinal immunity of the neonate. Adv Exp Med Biol 1978; 107:95-107.

Ogura H. Serum antibodies to Escherichia coli in breast-fed and bottle-fed infants. Acta Med Okayama 1987; 41:161.

Ostergaard PAA. Serum and saliva Ig-levels in infants of non-atopic mothers fed breast milk or cow's milk-based formulas. Acta Paediatr Scand 1985; 74:555-559.

Pabst HF, Spady DW. Effect of breast feeding on antibody response to conjugate vaccine. Lancet 1990; 336:269.

Pabst HF, Godel J, Croce M, Cho H, Spady DW. Effect of breast feeding on immune response to BCG vaccination. Lancet 1989; 1:295.

Pittard III WB, Bill K. Differentiation of cord blood lymphocytes into IgA-producing cells in response to breast milk stimulatory factor. Clin Immunol Immunopathol 1979a; 13:430-434.

Pittard III WB, Bill K. Immunoregulation by breast milk cells. Cell Immunol 1979b; 42:437-441.

Prentice A. Breast feeding increases concentrations of IgA in infants' urine. Arch Dis Child 1987; 62:792-795.

Read LC, Upton FM, Francis GL, Wallace JC, Dahlenberg GW, Ballard FJ. Changes in the growth-promoting activity of human milk during lactation. Pediatr Res 1984; 18:133-139.

Rethy L. Immunomodulant activity of endotoxins in man. Immunol Hung 1983; 23:15-53.

Roberts SA, Freed DLJ. Neonatal IgA secretion enhanced by breast feeding. Lancet 1977; 2:1131.

Roberts SA, Wincup G, Harries DA. Mucosal receptor for IgA in the breast-fed neonate. Early Hum Dev 1980; 4:161-166.

Rusch V. The 1st International workshop on regulation and modulation of immune activities and the 'Diehl triangle.' Microecol Ther 1981; 11:37-39.

Saarinen UM, Kajosaari M, Backman A, Siimes MA. Prolonged breast-feeding as prophylaxis for atopic disease. Lancet 1979; 2:163-166.

Schanler RJ, Goldblum RM, Garza C, Goldman AS. Enhanced fecal excretion of selected immune factors in very low birth weight infants fed fortified human milk. Pediatr Res 1986; 20:711-715.

Schlesinger JJ, Covelli HD. Evidence for transmission of lymphocyte responses to tuberculin by breast-feeding. Lancet 1977; 2:529-532.

Scott PH. Enzyme immunoassay of lactoferrin in newborn term infants: Reference values and influence of diet. Ann Clin Biochem 1989; 26:407.

Scott GM, Robinson JA, Secher DS, Ashburner CM, Abbott SR. Measurement of interferon from *in vitro* stimulated lymphocytes by bioassay and monoclonal antibody-based immunoassay. J Gen Virol 1985; 66:1621-1625.

Selner JC, Merrill DA, Claman HN. Salivary immunoglobulin and albumin: Development during the neonatal period. J Pediatr 1968; 72:685-689.

Seltzer V, Benjamin F. Breast feeding and the potential for human immunodeficiency virus transmission. Obstetrics and Gynecology 1990; 75:713-715.

Slade HB, Schwartz SA. Antigen-drive immunoglobulin production by human colostral lymphocytes. Pediatr Res 1989; 25:295-299.

Sloper KS, Brostoff J. Childhood eczema: A study of the effect of double-blind food challenges given to the mother of a breast-fed infant. Br Paediatr Asso 57th Ann Meet 1985, York, pp 111.

Smith CW, Goldman AS. The cells of human colostrum. I. *In-vitro* studies of morphology and function. Pediatr Res 1968; 2:103-109.

Soothill JF. Some intrinsic and extrinsic factors predisposing to allergy. Proc R Soc Med 1976; 69:439-442.

Stephens S. Influence of Human Milk on the Development of Immune Responses in Infants. PhD Thesis, Brunel University, Oxbridge, England, 1984.

Stephens S. Development of secretory immunity in breast-fed and bottle-fed infants. Arch Dis Child 1986; 61:263-269.

Stephens S, Brenner MK, Duffy SW, Lakhani PK, Kennedy CR, Farrant J. The effect of breast-feeding on proliferation by infant lymphocytes *in vitro*. Pediatr Res 1986; 20:227-231.

Stephens S, Duffy SW, Page C. A longitudinal study of interferon-γ production by peripheral blood mononuclear cells from breast-fed and bottle-fed infants. Clin Exp Immunol 1986; 65:396-400.

Stephens S, Kennedy CR, Lakhani PK, Brenner MK. *In-vivo* immune responses of breast-fed infants to tetanus toxoid antigen and to normal gut flora. Acta Pediatr Scand 1984; 73: 426-432.

Subiza JL, Rodriguez C, Figueredo A, Mateos P, Alvarez R, De La Concha EG. Impaired production and lack of secretion of interleukin 1 by human breast milk macrophages. Clin Exp Immunol 1988; 71:493-496.

Taylor B, Normal AP, Orgel HA, Stokes CR, Turner MW, Soothill JF. Transient IgA deficiency and pathogenesis of infantile atopy. Lancet 1973; 2:111-113.

Taylor CE, Toms GL. Immunoglobulin concentrations in nasopharyngeal secretions. Arch Dis Child 1984; 59:48-53.

Tlaskalová-Hogenová H, Šterzl J, Štěpánková R, Dlabac V, Větvička V, Rossmann P, Mandel L, Rejnek J. Development of immunological capacity under germfree and conventional conditions. Ann NY Acad Sci 1983; 409:96-113.

Tolo K, Brandtzaeg P, Jonsen J. Mucosal penetration of antigen in the presence or absence of serum-derived antibody. An *in vitro* study of rabbit oral and intestinal mucosa. Immunology 1977; 33:733-743.

Udall JN, Colony P, Fritze L, Pang K, Trier JS, Walker WA. Development of gastrointestinal mucosal barrier. II. The effect of natural versus artificial feeding on intestinal permeability to macromolecules. Pediatr Res 1981; 15:245-249.

Wallach D, Fellous M, Revel M. Preferential effect of gamma-interferon on the synthesis of HLA antigens and their mRNAs in human cells. Nature 1982; 299:833-836.

Wara DW, Barrett DJ. Cell-mediated immunity in the newborn: Clinical aspects. Pediatrics 1979; 64(suppl.):822-826.

Watkins CJ, Leeder SR, Corkhill RT. The relationship between breast and bottle feeding and respiratory illness in the first year of life. J Epidemiol Commun Health 1979; 33:180-182.

Weber TH, Santesson B, Skoog VT. The activation of fetal lymphocytes. Scand J Haematol 1973; 11:177-183.

Yap PL, Pryde A, Latham PJ, McLelland DBL. Serum IgA in the neonate. Molecular size, concentration and effect of breast-feeding. Acta Paediatr Scand 1979; 68:695-700.

Yengar L, Selvaraj RJ. Intestinal absorption of immunoglobulins by newborn infants. Arch Dis Child 1972; 47:411-414.

Yoshida T, Cohen S, Bigazzi PE, Kurasuji T, Amsden A. Inflamatory mediators in culture filtrates of *Escherichia coli*. Am J Pathol 1975; 81:389-400.

Zoppi G, Casparini R, Mantovanelli F, Gobio-Casali L, Astolfi R, Crovari P. Diet and antibody response to vaccination in healthy infants. Lancet 1983; 2:11-14.

20
Gliadin, Intestinal Hypersensitivity, and Food Protein-Sensitive Enteropathy

Riccardo Troncone
University of Naples, Naples, Italy

Karl Ziegler
Freie Universität Berlin, Berlin, Germany

Stephan Strobel
Institute of Child Health and Hospital for Sick Children, London, England

Anne Ferguson
University of Edinburgh and Western General Hospital, Edinburgh, Scotland

INTOLERANCE TO GLUTEN AND OTHER FOOD PROTEINS

Types of Wheat Intolerance

Any radical alteration in the diet is likely to influence gut physiology and gastrointestinal function as perceived by the subject. If the effects are disagreeable, there is, by definition, food intolerance (1). Some individuals have adverse clinical effects when they increase the cereal content of their diet—indeed an elimination diet which excludes wheat is said to cure the symptoms of some patients with the irritable bowel syndrome (2). Wheat gluten in a meal impairs the absorption of starch (3), and in a well-documented study of healthy and tuberculous volunteers, doses of 100-150 g gluten daily produced diarrhea and malabsorption, although jejunal biopsy histology remained normal (4). A syndrome of nonceliac gluten-sensitive diarrhea in patients with normal jejunal biopsy architecture (although some abnormalities of lymphoid cell counts) has also been described (5).

These conditions must be differentiated from the disorders in which wheat or gluten sensitivity is manifest as an enteropathy, with measurable changes in the histopathology of the jejunum after gluten has been withdrawn from the diet or re-introduced. Patients with celiac disease (permanent, life-long intolerance) and transient gluten-sensitive enteropathy (usually infants) exhibit an abnormal morphological response of the jejunal mucosa to what would in a healthy person be a harmless quantity of wheat or gluten in the diet. There is a great deal of evidence that in celiac disease, the enteropathy is likely to be immune mediated (6). Transient small intestinal mucosal damage with malabsorption occurs in infants who are intolerant of many foods. It is best documented as cow milk protein intolerance, but can also occur with soy, chicken, rice, fish, and egg (7,8). The importance of using objective criteria to establish any putative food intolerance has been recently discussed (30).

Food-Sensitive Enteropathy in Animals

Postweaning diarrhea with malabsorption is also an important clinical problem in veterinary practice. Many factors are likely to be involved, including viral and bacterial infections, and there is evidence that allergic reactions to foods contribute to diarrheal disease in young calves and pigs. Soya is an important postweaning food and both immunoglobulin E (IgE) (9) and precipitating, complement-fixing, serum IgG_1 antibodies (10) have been implicated in soya hypersensitivity. Soya challenge produced stunted villi, crypt hyperplasia, edema in the lamina propria, and lymphoid cell infiltrate (10,11), with similar crypt hyperplasia in the small intestine of preruminant calves fed with wheat gluten (11); these features suggested a role for delayed-type hypersensitivity (DTH) responses. Intermittent feeding of antigenic protein to young pigs creates conditions for the expression of DTH, and this is thought to be an important mechanism of postweaning diarrhea in this species (12,13).

Role of Immunopathology in Food-Sensitive Enteropathy

It seems likely that food protein-sensitive enteropathy has an immunological basis and our work, both in human celiac disease and on immunoregulation in mice, implicates induction of mucosal DTH as the underlying abnormality. The factor which leads to sensitization rather than tolerance could be an abnormality of T cells, antigen presentation, permeability of the epithelium, or an adjuvant effect of coincident infection. However, as we show below, in clinical as well as experimental work, it is likely that some other local factors are necessary in addition to sensitization to allow the full evolution of mucosal DTH as gluten-sensitive enteropathy.

INDUCTION AND MANIFESTATIONS OF INTESTINAL DELAYED-TYPE HYPERSENSITIVITY

Functions of GALT

The immune system of the gastrointestinal tract (GALT, gut-associated lymphoreticular tissue) generates protective responses to microorganisms and parasites and also creates a state of nonreactivity to many antigens, protecting the host from intestinal damage due to inappropriate immune responses. When the route of entry of antigen is through follicle-associated epithelium of Peyer's patches, there is suppression of systemic immunity, "oral tolerance" along with active intestinal immunization for harmless secretory IgA antibody. However, in some circumstances, enteric encounter with antigen induces a potentially immunopathogenic state; for example, IgE, IgG antibody, or T-cell-mediated immunity. When this type of immune response has been induced, ingress of antigen after a further feed may result in a local immune reaction with tissue damage—hypersensitivity.

Evaluation of Mucosal DTH

Currently, there are no standard methods for detecting the presence of antigen-specific T-effector cells in the mucosae. There is no evidence that cytotoxic T cells are involved in intestinal tissue damage even though their presence in the mucosae is well documented (14); secretion of lymphokines by activated T cells appears to be the mechanism of T-cell-mediated hypersensitivity in the gut (15,16), and more than a decade ago lymphokine-like activity was found to be present in organ culture fluid when celiac mucosal biopsies were cultured in the presence of gliadin (17). At the moment, the best available method for studying mucosal DTH is based on morphology. A distinct pattern of small intestinal mucosal damage has been observed in models such as allograft rejection, graft-versus-host reaction (GvHR), enteral challenge after immunization with protein antigen, and parasitic infections. The features described in some or all of these situations are hyperplasia of the crypts of Lieberkühn with or without shortening of the villi; an increase in the proportion of goblet cells; brush border enzyme deficiency; increased counts of intraepithelial lymphocytes (IELs) and mucosal mast cells; an increased mitotic index of IELs; and expression of class II antigens by crypt enterocytes (reviewed by Ferguson [18]). When these subtle changes are being studied, it is mandatory to use objective methods to examine biopsies.

Regulation of Mucosal Immunity

Immune responses to fed antigen are subject to several regulatory influences. Immunoregulatory T cells, dispersed in the mucosa as well as in the organized lymphoid tissues of the GALT, are critical to their induction and expression (19). Experiments with protein antigens have shown that there is also subtle alteration, "processing," of antigen as it crosses the gut epithelium, and such material is tolerogenic for cell-mediated immunity rather than immunogenic (20,21). The quantity of circulating antigen passing across a "leaky" epithelium may be important in the pattern of induction of immunity, although immunochemical properties of absorbed antigen are likely to be equally relevant. For example, the immature or diseased gut may yield antigenic moieties which are more immunogenic than normal instead of generating tolerogenic fragments. The above comments relate to systemic immunity. It is not yet known if mucosal DTH responses are activity suppressed or if there is simply an absence of any immunological effect in terms of induction or suppression.

Some years ago, we and others found that pretreatment of mice with cyclophosphamide and estrogen therapy reversed oral tolerance to ovalbumin (OVA) and at the same time induced local mucosal immune responses (as measured by a lymphocyte-migration technique, and by jejunal crypt hyperplasia and raised IEL count after antigen refeeding) (22,23). The mechanisms of immunomodulation differ in these two systems. Cyclophosphamide acts at the T-suppressor cell level, whereas estrogens activate the reticuloendothelial system and increase the antigen-presenting activity of macrophages.

In order to study these phenomena in other states of aberrant immunity, we examined immune responses to fed OVA in animals immunomodulated by means of a GvHR; by injection of the synthetic adjuvant N-acetyl-muramyl dipeptide (MDP); or in newborn animals which are immunologically inexperienced by virtue of age (24). All of these treatments prevented the induction of oral tolerance, as predicted from previous experience. In a parallel series of experiments, mice were orally immunized with a single dose of OVA, rested for 4 weeks, and then challenged with OVA in their drinking water. They were killed on day 10 and the presence or absence of intestinal DTH inferred from IEL counts and mucosal architecture measurements. Jejunal architecture was not altered by the antigen challenge, but MDP-treated and immature animals which had been sensitized to OVA and later reexposed to the same antigen had significantly higher intraepithelial lymphocyte counts than appropriate controls. Similar positive results were obtained by feeding OVA to neonatal mice (Fig. 1). Immaturity of immunoregulatory T-cell circuits is the most likely explanation for this finding, and the possible clinical implications are obvious.

MUCOSAL DTH IN A CLINICAL SETTING— GLUTEN CHALLENGE IN CELIAC DISEASE

Diagnostic Criteria for Celiac Disease

Clinically, it is only by manipulation of antigen encounter, usually of dietary protein antigens such as gluten or milk, and by repeat biopsies of the small intestinal mucosa, that a diagnosis of food protein-sensitive enteropathy is made. Strict diagnostic criteria for celiac disease demand a positive challenge test confirmed by biopsies (25). The histological and other features which change with dietary manipulation are very similar to those of experimental DTH, supporting the concept of T-cell-mediated tissue injury.

In order to fulfill the criteria laid down by the European Society for Paediatric Gastroenterology and Nutrition (ESPGAN) for celiac disease, at least three jejunal biopsies are therefore necessary—one taken at the time of diagnosis, one after a period on a gluten-free diet which should show complete restoration to normal, and one or more biopsies taken after reintroduction of gluten as a controlled gluten challenge to demonstrate the reappearance of the pathological features within 2 years. Usually, the histopathological changes associated with dietary manipulation are so striking that subjective comparison by an experienced pathologist is sufficient to confirm improvement or worsening of the pathology. It is, however, of interest to demonstrate objectively the consistent patterns of change in the jejunal mucosa, since this experience gained in human medicine is now being applied to the investigation of potentially similar food-sensitive enteropathies in domestic animals.

Jejunal Morphometry in Celiac Disease

The data summarized in Figures 1-5 have been obtained from routine diagnostic jejunal biopsies performed in the Gastro-Intestinal Unit of the University of Edinburgh (26). Patients with suspected or proven celiac disease have jejunal biopsy carried out by clinical investigation nurses on an outpatient basis. Biopsies are taken from the jejunum just distal to the ligament of Treitz using a Watson peroral biopsy capsule. The tissue obtained is divided into two. One part is examined with a dissecting microscope, then paraffin embedded, and processed for routine histopathology and counts of intraepithelial lymphocytes (IELs) (27). The other part is weighed, homogenized, and the disaccharidases lactase, sucrase, trehalase, and maltase are assayed as described by Dahlqvist (28). In prospective studies, we use a simple microdissection technique for measurements of villus and crypt sizes and crypt mitoses (29). However, insufficient material from treated and gluten-challenged celiacs had been processed by this method to present here and so the measurements were made on coded histological sections by using an eye-piece micrometer.

Food-Sensitive Enteropathy

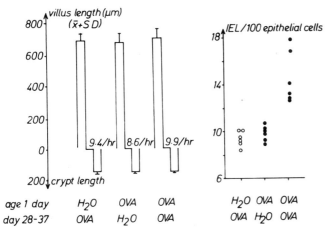

Figure 1 Gastrointestinal morphology and IEL infiltration after a neonatal OVA feed and challenge. *Left*: Morphology. There were no differences in villus or crypt lengths or crypt cell production rates in any of the treatment groups. *Right*: Intraepithelial lymphocytes. There is a significant rise in IEL count in the group of animals which have been fed on day 1 of life and challenged with OVA after 4 weeks ($p < 0.01$) (8.2–10.6/100 epithelial cells versus 12.4–18.2/100 epithelial cells). (From Ref. 24; used with permission.)

Gluten Withdrawal

In 11 patients with celiac disease, jejunal biopsy taken at the time of diagnosis (when the patients were ingesting normal, gluten-containing diets) are compared with biop-

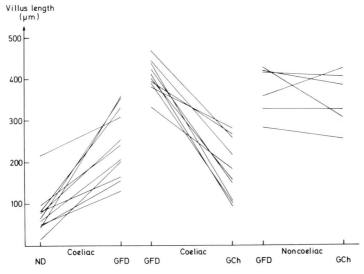

Figure 2 Effects of gluten-free and gluten-containing diets on lengths of jejunal villi. ND = normal diet (gluten containing); GFD = gluten-free diet (3-6 months); GCH = gluten challenge (approximately 20 g gluten daily for 3-6 months). (From Ref. 26; used with permission.)

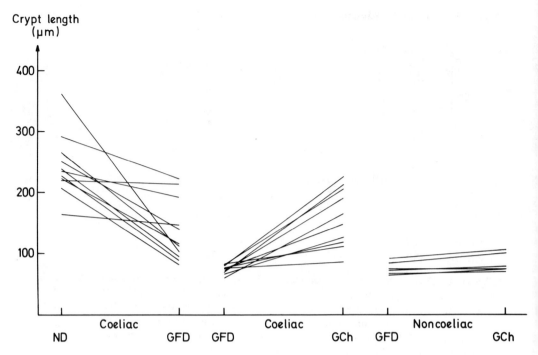

Figure 3 Effects of gluten-free and gluten-containing diets on lengths of jejunal crypts. ND = normal diet (gluten containing); GFD = gluten-free diet (3-6 months); GCH = gluten challenge (approximately 20 g gluten daily for 3-6 months). (From Ref. 26; used with permission.)

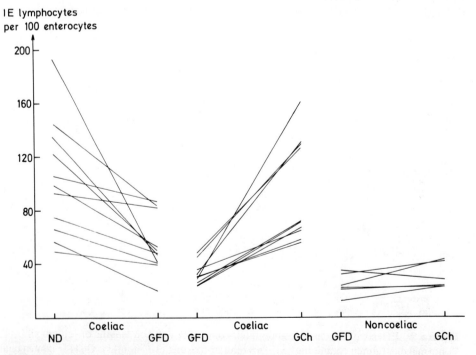

Figure 4 Effects of gluten-free and gluten-containing diets on IEL counts. ND = normal diet (gluten containing); GFD = gluten-free diet (3-6 months); GCH = gluten challenge (approximately 20 g gluten daily for 3-6 months). (From Ref. 26; used with permission.)

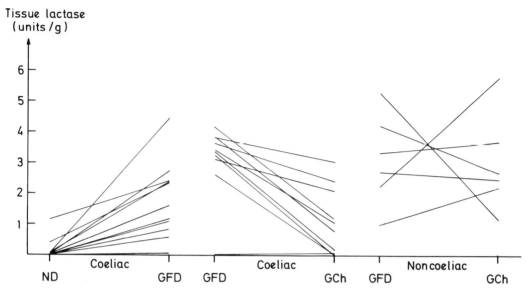

Figure 5 Effects of gluten-free and gluten-containing diets on jejunal lactase activity. ND = normal diet (gluten containing); GFD = gluten-free diet (3-6 months); GCH = gluten challenge (approximately 20 g gluten daily for 3-6 months). (From Ref. 26; used with permission.)

sies taken 3-6 months after prescription of a gluten-free diet. Patient compliance with diet is not always absolute but, as can be seen in Figures 2-6, and summarized in Figure 7, changes in virtually every case have occurred, comprising growth of villi, reduction in the length of crypts, reduction in IEL count, and increased activities of the brush border enzymes lactase and sucrase. Patients with untreated celiac disease had higher levels of serum antibodies to gliadin compared to treated patients, predominantly IgA and IgG in serum and IgA and IgM in jejunal aspirate and gut lavage fluid (31).

Gluten Challenge

The need for gluten challenge to confirm celiac disease in all patients is still debatable. However, even if an individual physician does not have a policy of carrying out gluten challenge in every likely celiac patient, there are certain groups of patients in whom such a procedure is mandatory (32). These include:

1. Patients in whom a gluten-free diet has been started without an initial diagnostic biopsy
2. Patients in whom the original biopsy is technically poor or in whom the histopathology is not classically that of celiac disease
3. Any patient in whom infection or immunodeficiency was present at the time of the original diagnosis of celiac disease
4. Patients with a strong personal or family history of atopic disease

Different techniques of gluten challenge have been used with similar results. We either continue to prescribe a gluten-free diet and add 20 g daily of gluten powder, or advise the patient to take a normal diet and after 1 or 2 months assess accurately the amount of gluten eaten by the patient—this should be between 15 and 20 g daily. If

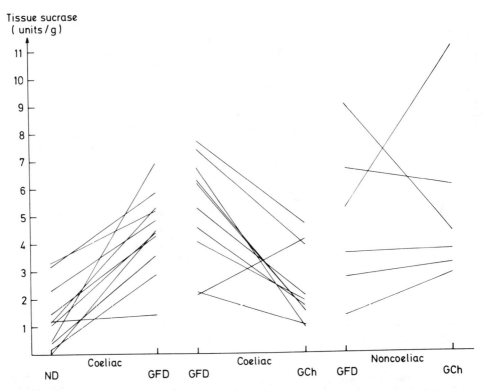

Figure 6 Effects of gluten-free and gluten-containing diets on jejunal sucrase activity. ND = normal diet (gluten containing); GFD = gluten-free diet (3-6 months); GCH = gluten challenge (approximately 20 g gluten daily for 3-6 months). (From Ref. 26; used with permission.)

gluten challenge is performed only in patients in whom a jejunal biopsy is normal at the time of gluten reintroduction, side effects are extremely rare and never serious. Figures 2-7 illustrate and summarize results of jejunal biopsy measurements in 16 patients who underwent gluten challenge, the biopsies being taken when a gluten-free diet was being ingested, and after 3-6 months of gluten reintroduction. Ten of the patients had sufficient clinical and pathological deterioration to establish the existence of gluten-sensitive enteropathy; i.e., to confirm celiac disease. In six patients, despite continuing ingestion of gluten for 2 years or longer, no clinical or biopsy deterioration occurred, and therefore they did not have celiac disease. The figures clearly illustrate the deterioration in all facets of morphology and biochemistry in the gluten-sensitive celiac patients, and the lack of significant alteration in these parameters in sequential biopsies taken several months apart from the nonceliac, presumed normal individuals.

DOSE-DEPENDENT GLUTEN-SENSITIVE ENTEROPATHY

Gluten-Sensitivity in Dermatitis Herpetiformis

Dermatitis herpetiformis (DH) is characterized by a symmetrical pruritic skin rash with subepidermal blisters and granular subepidermal deposits of IgA in remote,

Food-Sensitive Enteropathy

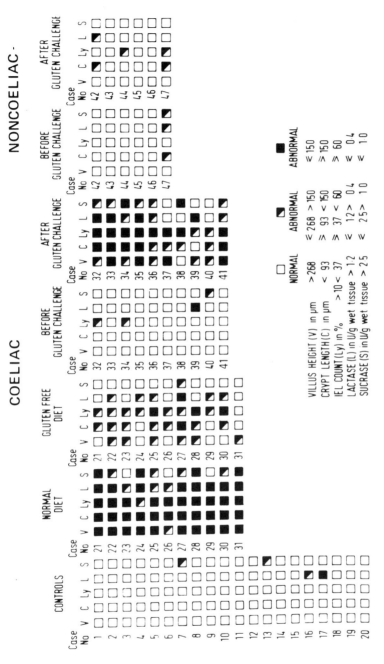

Figure 7 Diagrammatic representation of the results of gluten withdrawal and gluten challenge (data derived from Figs. 2-6). V = villus length; C = crypt length; Ly = IEL count; L,SGD = low activity of disaccharidases.

uninvolved skin. Most DH patients have abnormal small intestinal biopsy pathology, histologically indistinguishable from that of celiac disease and returning to normal after dietary exclusion of gluten. An interpretation of these observations is that most patients with DH also have celiac disease, but a minority are totally tolerant of gluten. Alternatively, there may be intestinal gluten sensitivity in all cases with a variable requirement of dietary gluten for its clinical expression (i.e., there is a latent enteropathy in the minority). A combination of objective tests of small intestinal architecture and function has been found to detect abnormalities in most DH patients, including some with histologically normal biopsy. However, some DH patients have no discernible abnormality (33).

Latent Gluten Sensitivity

Support for the existence of a degree of gluten sensitivity in all DH patients was provided by Weinstein in 1974 (32). He described "latent celiac disease" in two patients with DH who had a morphologically normal small intestinal mucosa when eating a normal diet. When they took a high-gluten diet for 22-30 weeks, jejunal biopsies became flat in both cases. However, there were unusual features in both of these patients. One man had Addison's disease in addition to DH and was receiving treatment with cortisone acetate and fluorohydrocortisone. The other patient was diabetic and taking tolbutamide. The normal diet of these subjects contained only 5-7 g gluten/day, and the "high-gluten" diet which unmasked latent celiac disease contained 20 g of gluten/day, an amount similar to that in the normal diet of most Europeans.

Further evidence of dose-related gluten-sensitive enteropathy emerged from an investigation of 15 subjects without overt small bowel disease in whom a normal diet was supplemented with 40 g gluten daily for 6 weeks (34). There were five normal volunteers, six normal first-degree relatives of celiac patients, and four patients with "altered immunity." Two of the celiac patient's relatives had unequivocal alterations in jejunal biopsies, with increased IEL counts, and xylose malabsorption, and both had diarrhea and lost weight when they took the extra gluten.

Studies of Gluten Loading in Volunteers and DH Patients

We have followed up these important reports of a state of latent celiac disease by studying volunteers and DH patients who had their diets supplemented with 20 g gluten powder daily for 2 weeks. Quantitative techniques were used to define the architecture, lymphocyte infiltrate, and brush border enzyme activities of jejunal biopsies before and after this gluten loading (35). There were 6 healthy controls and 11 patients with DH. Five DH patients also had celiac disease (cases 1-5). They had previously been shown to have an abnormal jejunal biopsy and had been prescribed a gluten-free diet for more than 5 years. None had required any drug for DH for at least 3 years. Six DH patients (cases 6-11) had normal jejunal biopsies while eating a normal diet, and all required drug therapy for control of skin symptoms.

After baseline jejunal biopsies had been taken, the volunteers and patients continued on their usual diet, to which was added 20 g of gluten powder (BDH Chemical Ltd., Poole, Dorset, England) daily for 2 weeks. Postgluten jejunal biopsies were collected on the fourteenth day. A 2-week, relatively low-dose regimen was selected for ethical reasons because we anticipated that gluten reintroduction or gluten loading would cause recrudescence of the skin lesions of DH.

Food-Sensitive Enteropathy

Biopsies were formalin fixed, paraffin embedded, and routine H&E stained sections prepared. These were examined and formally reported by a consultant pathologist. Intraepithelial lymphocyte (IEL) counts were performed on the H&E-stained sections (27); measurements of crypts, villi, and crypt mitosis were carried out on microdissected specimens (29); disaccharidases were assayed by the method of Dahlqvist (28).

Jejunal biopsies from five of the six volunteers were histologically normal pre- and postgluten loading, but in one subject the postgluten biopsy had short villi, long crypts, a striking increase in crypt mitoses, increased lamina propria lymphoid cell infiltrate, and reduced tissue disaccharidase activities. The IEL count rose from 24.4 pregluten to 35.1 postgluten.

In the DH patients on a gluten-free diet who had gluten challenge, morphometry and cell counts showed minor abnormalities in some prechallenge biopsies and all postchallenge biopsies were unequivocally abnormal, similar to the gluten challenge data for celiac patients described above. In five of the six DH patients with normal biopsies on a normal diet, there was no deterioration in the measurements of mucosal architecture after gluten loading, but in one case, villus length dropped from 531 to 308 μm and there were reductions in tissue disaccharidase activities after gluten loading.

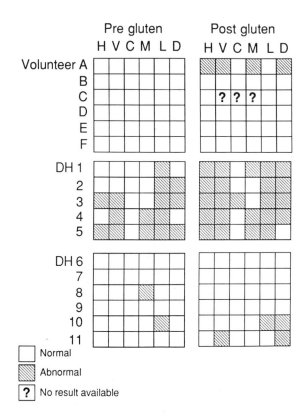

Figure 8 Diagrammatic representation of the results of biopsy assessments before and after the addition of 20 g gluten to the diet of volunteers and DH patients. H = histology; V = villus length; C = crypt length; M = count of crypt mitoses; L = IEL count; D = abnormally low activity of two or more disaccharidases.

The results obtained were examined in two ways. Statistical analysis of the results in the various clinical groups would be expected to show if there were any generalized toxic effect of gluten loading; none of the comparisons between pre- and post-gluten biopsies gave positive results. On the other hand, if individual measurements are considered as normal or abnormal, a distinct pattern emerges, as shown in Figure 8, with clearcut effects of gluten challenge in DH cases 1-5 and effects of gluten loading in volunteer A and in DH case 11. The results in case DH 10 are less convincing, there being only a reduction in disaccharidases after gluten loading, although this patient also had a high IEL count pregluten.

We have confirmed the existence of latent, dose-dependent gluten-sensitive enteropathy, and there can now be little doubt that doubling or trebling the amount of gluten in the diet can produce an enteropathy in some individuals. Further studies are needed, particularly in normal subjects and in relatives of celiac patients, to establish how often and why a change in the nature of the diet induces pathological features identical to those of celiac disease. On theoretical grounds it seems unlikely that doubling or trebling the quantity of an already-present antigen would induce a new, pathological immune state. More likely, there are local factors in the gut which segregate antigen from the small number of potentially reactive T cells, and that either lectinlike or some other properties of the dietary change allows the expression of mucosal DTH to gliadin. If this is correct, there should be evidence of altered immunity to gluten in individuals with latent celiac disease; for example, high titers of serum or secretory antigliadin antibodies. We have recently observed identical profiles of immunoglobulin concentrations and secretory antibodies of patients with DH and normal jejunal biopsies to gliadin compared with patients with untreated celiac disease, thus confirming that an inappropriate response to gliadin can indeed precede the appearance of histological abnormalities in the gut (36).

IMMUNOLOGICAL PROPERTIES OF GLIADIN FED TO MICE

Range of Immunological Effects of Feeding Antigen to Mice

When an antigen is first presented via the gut, the spectrum of effects on systemic immunity ranges from active sensitization to oral tolerance. Although as discussed above, host factors such as age (37), nutritional status (38), and immunoregulatory T-cell function (39) contribute to this variability, the dose and physicochemical nature of antigen are also relevant. Feeding antigen at the same time as cholera toxin (40,41) or an antigen which is a lectin, such as kidney bean lectin (42), primes rather than tolerizes humoral immunity; effects of these substances on systematic DTH have not been established.

The storage proteins of several cereals, including wheat gliadins, are complex antigens with some lectinlike properties and might, therefore, be predicted to sensitize rather than tolerize when fed even to healthy individuals. We have, therefore, investigated the immunological properties of gliadin when presented via the gut in mice (43). The experiments were undertaken to determine if feeding gliadin, either as a purified molecule or as a constituent of a standard gluten-containing diet, results in a state of specific immunological unresponsiveness.

Techniques Used for Experiments on Gliadin as a Tolerogen

Female mice from two colonies of BALB/c mice were used. These are referred to below as normal diet (ND) and gluten-free diet (GFD) mice. The ND mice were maintained on a standard rodent diet, which contains 2.8% gluten (CRM(X), Labsure Ltd., Poole, Dorset, England). A gluten-free colony was established in 1985; these animals were fed a gluten-free (GF) diet (Special Diets Service Ltd., Witham, Essex, England); only second- or later-generation mice were used for experiments. Gliadin for sensitization and challenge was fed either as pellets of standard gluten-containing diet or as commercial gliadin powder (BDH Chemical Ltd., Poole, Dorset, England) incorporated in agar pellets.

To study oral tolerance, a group of GFD mice received the gluten-containing diet for a week and thereafter were switched back onto the gluten-free diet; control mice continued on the gluten-free diet throughout. In a separate series of experiments, GFD mice received a single feed of gliadin powder (5, 25, and 125 mg). Mice were systematically immunized 7 days after the feed of gliadin in agar, or at the end of the week on gluten-containing diet, and 3 weeks later, humoral and cellular immune responses were assessed by ELISA and by skin testing.

Results of Experiments on Immunological Properties of Gliadin

When mice from the GFD diet colony were given a single feed of gliadin, there was a dose-dependent reduction in the cellular and humoral immune responses to subsequent parenteral immunization with gliadin in CFA (Fig. 9). Similarly, mice immunized at the end of the week on the gluten-containing diet showed marked suppression of both cellular and humoral immune responses after parenteral immunization with gliadin ($p < 0.001$) (Table 1).

Since 1 week on a normal, gluten-containing diet significantly reduced the capacity of GFD mice to mount a systemic immune response to gliadin, ordinary laboratory mice, ingesting a gluten-containing diet throughout life, may have similar immunological tolerance. To investigate this, the systemic immune responses after parenteral immunization of mice from the GFD and ND colonies were compared. Although ND mice, when immunized with gliadin, developed specific humoral and DTH responses, these were significantly less ($p < 0.001$) than the responses of mice reared on a gluten-free diet (Fig. 10).

The experiments presented above demonstrate that in respect to immunogenicity when systemically administered and tolerogenicity when fed, wheat gliadin is similar to many other protein antigens. The question of gliadin tolerogenicity was addressed by modifying the protocol which we have successfully used to document oral tolerance in mice to many different antigens, including ovalbumin, human serum albumin, β-lactoglobulin, cholera toxin, and gum arabic. However, since gliadin is poorly soluble in aqueous solutions, it was fed to mice as solid food or as gliadin powder incorporated in agar pellets. Mice reared on a gluten-free diet and fed 25 or 125 mg gliadin, showed a clear dose-dependent suppression of both cellular and humoral immune responses. Feeding mice a standard gluten-containing diet for 1 week (about 140 mg gluten daily) had similar effects. This latter experiment demonstrates that gliadin presented via the gut can induce oral tolerance even if still retained in the wheat

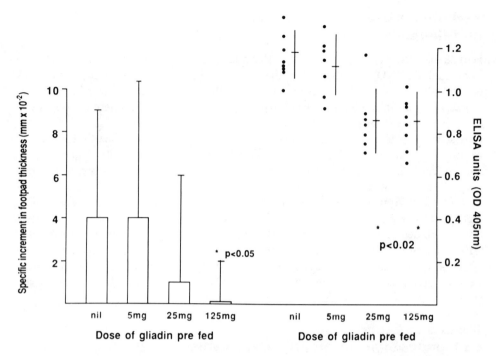

Figure 9 Tolerizing effect of a single feed of gliadin. *Left*: Systemic DTH responses 3 weeks after parenteral immunization. Results shown are mean specific increments in footpad thickness + 1 SD. *Right*: Serum IgG responses measured by ELISA 3 weeks after immunization. The responses in groups marked by asterisks are significantly different from those in mice not fed gliadin. (From Ref. 43; used with permission.)

grain, without having been previously alcohol extracted. Interestingly, we have also observed that sensitization in utero or shortly after birth also strongly affects responsiveness to gliadin (44), such that priming rather than tolerance is the outcome. It seems likely that this may be related to the size of the dose per minute in milk, or transplacental passage, but may also reflect timing, stage of development of the immune system, or other unidentified factors (20).

Table 1 Effect of Feeding Normal Gluten-Containing Diet (ND) on the Systemic Immune Responses to Gliadin of GFD Mice

	DTH (mm)		IgG antibody (OD405)	
	GFD throughout	1 week ND	GFD throughout	1 week ND
Adult mice	mean 0.27 (0.09)	0.08[a] (0.07)	1.208 (1.040-1.500)	0.693[a] (0.512-1.006)
Weanling mice	mean 0.15 (0.08)	0.06[b] (0.03)	0.930 (0.799-1.035)	0.738[b] (0.671-0.876)

Serum IgG antibody response was measured by ELISA 3 weeks after parenteral immunization and the results expressed as mean and range of individual OD405 readings. Systemic DTH response was also assessed 3 weeks after immunization, and the results shown are mean specific increment in footpad thickness (mm ± 1 SD).
[a]$p < 0.001$; [b]$p < 0.01$.
Source: From Ref. 43; used with permission.

Food-Sensitive Enteropathy

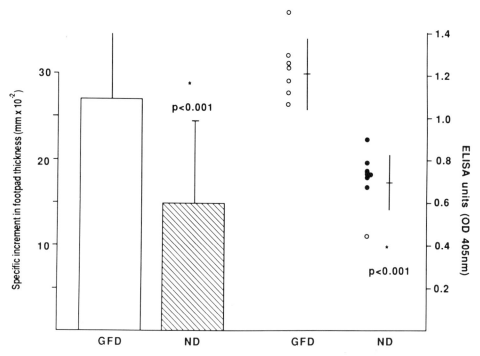

Figure 10 Systemic immune response to gliadin in mice reared on a gluten-containing diet. DTH (*left*) and antibody (*right*) responses 3 weeks after parenteral immunization with gliadin in mice from the gluten-free diet (GFD) and the normal diet (ND) colonies. DTH results are shown as mean specific increments in footpad thickness +1 SD. Antibody results are shown as individual OD405 readings in ELISA. Bars indicate mean +1 SD. (From Ref. 43; used with permission.)

Thus, despite its lectinlike physicochemical properties, gliadin behaves as an oral tolerogen in adults both if fed as purified molecule or as a constituent of a normal diet. These results have broad implications in addition to the demonstration that gliadin is indeed an oral tolerogen. Standard animal feeds, regardless of the manufacturer, usually contain gluten as a protein source. Our results show that in animals fed these diets, immune responses to parenterally administered gliadin are significantly suppressed. This finding has the practical implication that in vivo studies of immunogenicity and cross-reactivity of gliadins must be conducted in animals from gluten-free colonies.

ATTEMPTS TO INDUCE GLUTEN-SENSITIVE ENTEROPATHY

Rationale for These Experiments

Gluten intolerance in celiac disease is unequivocal. There is considerable evidence supporting an immunological basis for the gluten intolerance; i.e., supporting celiac disease as an important food-allergic state. However, it is still conceivable that the primary injury is toxic, and that all of the immunological phenomena which can be observed in celiac patients are the secondary result of injury to the small bowel epithelium by gluten. Nevertheless, the close resemblance between experimental T-cell-mediated immune damage to the small bowel and celiac disease does give further support to the immunological theory of gluten intolerance in this disease. It follows that by inducing local DTH to gluten in the gut, the pathological features of celiac disease should be reproduced.

Methods and Results of Attempts to Induce DTH to Gliadin in the Gut

In several different experiments, BALB/c mice from the colony reared on a gluten-free diet were immunized systemically with gliadin in CFA and challenged by feeding. We failed to produce any effect of the gluten-containing diet on intestinal mucosal architecture or IEL count. Similar negative results were obtained regardless of the method of parenteral immunization—subcutaneous, footpad, or intraperitoneally.

In another series of experiments we investigated whether, in addition to systemic immunity, other factors would be necessary in order to allow the expression of a specific mucosal cell-mediated response in the gut (45). In the first of such experiments, the effect of a concurrent graft-versus-host reaction (GvHR) was evaluated. BDF_1 mice were used—reared and maintained throughout on gluten-containing diet. They were given an intraperitoneal injection of gliadin in CFA and a boosting injection 3 weeks later. Control animals were immunized with ovalbumin an unrelated antigen not present in mouse diet. At the same time of the booster, a GvHR was induced in both groups of mice by the intraperitoneal injection of 1×10^8 C57BL6/J spleen cells. Mice were sacrificed 14 days later. Pieces of jejunum were obtained and processed as previously described. When compared to control mice, gliadin-immunized mice showed a striking increase both in crypt cell production rate (19.7 versus 7.0 metaphases/hr; $p < 0.01$), and in crypt depth (172 ± 10 versus $151 \pm 17\mu$; $p < 0.05$); a significantly higher count of IELs (17.3 ± 2.8 vs $13.8 \pm 2.2\%$; $p < 0.05$) were also noted in gliadin immunized mice in comparison to control animals.

In a second experiment, the mucosal immune status was modulated by the induction of intestinal anaphylaxis. BALB/c mice were used—maintained throughout on gluten-containing diet. They were given an intraperitoneal injection of gliadin in CFA and a boosting injection 3 weeks later; control animals were immunized with ovalbumin. At the same time of the booster, both groups of animals were infected by subcutaneous injection of 1000 larvae of *Nippostrongylus brasiliensis*; 10 days later, anaphylaxis was induced by the intravenous injection of *Nippostrongylus* antigens (400 worm equivalents). Twelve days after anaphylaxis induction, mice were sacrificed. Mice immunized with gliadin showed a striking increase in crypt cell production rate when compared to control mice immunized with ovalbumin (14.0 versus 6.9 metaphases/hr; $p < 0.05$). In this case, no significant differences were recorded in villus and crypt length and in IEL counts.

CONCLUSIONS

The results of clinical and pathological observations of patients undergoing gluten challenge and gluten loading and of our mouse experiments suggest that induction of a state of systemic DTH to gliadin is not sufficient for the full expression of intestinal cell-mediated immunity to gluten, with enteropathy. Additional factors also appear to be necessary, such as those occurring during graft-versus-host reaction or intestinal anaphylaxis. The mechanisms may be via enhanced antigen-presenting cell activity or increased mucosal permeability allowing gliadin present in the diet to come in contact with sensitized cells within the mucosa.

ACKNOWLEDGMENTS

We are indebted to Dr. W. T. H. Hekkens and to Dr. H. Weiser for providing us with purified gliadin.

Some of this work has been supported by grants from the Priory of Scotland of the Order of St. John, and from Fisons (UK) Pharmaceuticals.

REFERENCES

1. Food intolerance and food aversion. A joint report of the Royal College of Physicians and the British Nutrition Foundation. J R Coll Physicians Lond 1984;18:83-123.
2. Alun Jones V, McLaughlan P, Shorthouse M, Workman E, Hunter JO. Food intolerance. A major factor in the pathogenesis of irritable bowel syndrome. Lancet 1982;2:1115-1117.
3. Anderson IH, Levine AS, Levitt MD. Incomplete absorption of the carbohydrate in all-purpose wheat flour. N Engl J Med 1981; 304:891-892.
4. Levine RA, Briggs GW, Harding RS, Nolte LB. Prolonged gluten administration in normal subjects. N Engl J Med 1966;274:1109-1114.
5. Cooper BT, Holmes GKT, Ferguson R, Thompson RA, Allan RN, Cooke WT. Gluten-sensitive diarrhea without evidence of celiac disease. Gastroenterology 1980;79:801-806.
6. Howdle PD, Losowsky MS. The immunology of celiac disease. In: Wright R, Hodgson HJF, eds. Clinical Gastroenterology. Gastrointestinal and Liver Immunology. London, Bailliere Tindall, 1987;507-529.
7. Hutchins P, Walker-Smith JA. The gastrointestinal system. Clin Immunol Allergy 1982; 2:43-76.
8. Vitoria JC, Camarero C, Sojo A, Ruiz A, Rodriguez-Soriano J. Enteropathy related to fish, rice and chicken. Arch Dis Child 1982;57:44-48.
9. Kilshaw PJ, Sissons JW. Gastrointestinal allergy to soyabean protein in preruminant calves. Antibody production and digestive disturbances in calves fed heated soyabean flour. Res Vet Sci 1979;27:361-365.
10. Barratt MEJ, Strachan PJ, Porter P. Antibody mechanisms implicated in digestive disturbances following ingestion of soya protein in calves and piglets. Clin Exp Immunol 1978;31:305-312.
11. Kilshaw PJ, Slade H. Villus atrophy and crypt elongation in the small intestine of preruminant calves fed with heated soyabean flour or wheat gluten. Res Vet Sci 1982;33: 305-308.
12. Stokes CR, Newby TJ, Bourne FJ. The influence of oral immunization on local and systemic immune responses to heterologous antigens. Clin Exp Immunol 1983;52:399-406.
13. Roy JHB. Dietary sensitivities in the calf. In: Batt RM, Lawrence TLJ, eds. Function and Dysfunction of the Small Intestine. Liverpool, Liverpool University Press, 1984:95-132.
14. Ernst PB, Befus AD, Bienenstock J. Leukocytes in the intestinal epithelium: An unusual immunological compartment. Immunol Today 1985;6:50-55.
15. Elson CO, Reilly RW, Rosenberg IH. Small intestinal injury in the graft versus host reaction: An innocent bystander phenomenon. Gastroenterology 1977;72:886-889.
16. Mowat AMCI, Ferguson A. Hypersensitivity reactions in the small intestinal mucosa of the mouse. 6. Pathogenesis of the graft-versus-host reaction in the small intestinal mucosa. Transplantation 1981;32:238-243.

17. Ferguson A, MacDonald TT, McClure JP, Holden RJ. Cell-mediated immunity to gliadin within the small-intestinal mucosa in celiac disease. Lancet 1975;1:895-897.
18. Ferguson A. Models of immunologically driven small intestinal damage. In: Marsh MN, ed. Immunopathology of the Small Intestine. Chichester, England, John Wiley and Co. Ltd., 1987:225-252.
19. Mowat AMcI. The regulation of immune responses to dietary protein antigens. Immunol Today 1987;8:93-98.
20. Strobel S, Mowat AMcI, Drummond HE, Pickering MG, Ferguson A. Immunological responses to fed protein antigens in mice. II. Oral tolerance for CMI is due to activation of cyclophosphamide-sensitive cells by gut-processed antigen. Immunology 1983;49:451-456.
21. Bruce MG, Ferguson A. The influence of intestinal processing on the immunogenicity and molecular size of absorbed, circulating ovalbumin in mice. Immunology 1986;59:295-300.
22. Mowat AMcI, Ferguson A. Hypersensitivity in the small intestinal mucosa—V. Induction of cell mediated immunity to a dietary antigen. Clin Exp Immunol 1981;43:574-582.
23. Mowat AMcI, Parrott DMV. Immunological responses to fed protein antigens in mice. IV. Effects of stimulating the reticuloendothelial system on oral tolerance and intestinal immunity to ovalbumin. Immunology 1983;50:547-554.
24. Strobel S, Ferguson A. Modulation of intestinal and systemic immune responses to a fed protein antigen, in mice. Gut 1986;27:829-837.
25. Meeuwisse G. Diagnostic criteria in celiac disease. Acta Paediatr Scand 1970;59:461-64.
26. Ziegler K, Ferguson A. Celiac disease. In: Batt RM, Lawrence TLJ, eds. Function and Dysfunction of the Small Intestine. Liverpool University Press, 1984:149-166.
27. Ferguson A, Murray D. Quantitation of intraepithelial lymphocytes in human jejunum. Gut 1971;12:988-994.
28. Dahlqvist A. Method for assay of intestinal disaccharidases. Analyt Biochem 1964;7:18-25.
29. Ferguson A, Sutherland A, MacDonald TT, Allan F. Technique for microdissection and measurement in biopsies of human small intestine. J Clin Pathol 1977;30:1068-1073.
30. Ferguson A. Food sensitivity or self-deception? N Engl J Med 1990;323:476.
31. O'Mahony S, Arranz E, Barton JR, Ferguson A. Dissociation between systemic and mucosal humoral immune response in celiac disease. Gut, 1991;32:29.
32. Weinstein WM. Latent celiac sprue. Gastroenterology 1974;66:489-493.
33. Gawkrodger DJ, McDonald C, O'Mahony S, Ferguson A. Small intestinal function and dietary status in dermatitis herpetiformis. Gut 1991;32:377.
34. Doherty M, Barry RE. Gluten-induced mucosal changes in subjects without overt small-bowel disease. Lancet 1981;1:517-520.
35. Ferguson A, Blackwell JN, Barnetson RStC. Effects of additional dietary gluten on the small intestinal mucosa of volunteers and of patients with dermatitis herpetiformis. Scand J Gastroenterol 1987;22:543-49.
36. O'Mahony S, Vestry JP, Ferguson A. Similarities in intestinal humoral immunity in dermatitis herpetiformis without enteropathy and in coeliac disease. Lancet 1990;335:1487.
37. Strobel S, Ferguson A. Immune responses to fed protein antigens in mice. 3. Systemic tolerance or priming is related to age at which antigen is first encountered. Pediatr Res 1984;18:588-593.
38. Lamont AG, Gordon M, Ferguson A. Oral tolerance in protein deprived mice. 1. Profound antibody tolerance but impaired DTH tolerance after antigen feeding. Immunology 1987;61:333-37.
39. Strobel S, Mowat AMcI, Ferguson A. Prevention of oral tolerance induction to ovalbumin and enhanced antigen presentation during a graft-versus-host reaction in mice. Immunology 1985;56:57-64.

40. Elson CO, Ealding W. Cholera toxin feeding did not induce oral tolerance in mice and abrogated oral tolerance to unrelated protein antigen. J Immunol 1984;133:2892.
41. Lycke N, Holmgrem J. Strong adjuvant properties of cholera toxin on gut mucosal immune responses to orally presented antigens. Immunology 1986;59:301-308.
42. Grant G, Greer F, McKenzie N, Pusztai A. Nutritional response of mature rats to kidney bean (Phaseolus vulgaris) lectins. J Sci Food Agric 1985;36:409-414.
43. Troncone R, Ferguson A. Gliadin presented via the gut induces oral tolerance in mice. Clin Exp Immunol 1988;72:284-287.
44. Troncone R, Ferguson A. In mice, gluten in maternal diet primes systemic immune responses to gliadin in offspring. Immunology 1988;64:533-537.
45. Troncone R, Ferguson A. An animal model of gluten-induced enteropathy in mice. Gut 1991;32:871-875.

21
Macromolecular Antigen Absorption from the Gastrointestinal Tract in Humoral Immunodeficiency

Charlotte Cunningham-Rundles
The Mount Sinai School of Medicine, New York, New York

INTRODUCTION

In health, the mucous membranes of the mature gut are relatively impermeable to large dietary molecules owing to the intrinsic structure of this barrier and the mucosal immune system. The mucosal epithelium consists of several different types of cells—the border cells and goblet cells are the most common. The border cells with microvilli are the primary absorptive cells (1,2). The goblet cells contain and discharge a mucus, which probably constitutes a first defense against such harmful materials as parasites and micobial antigens (3). At the base of these cells is the basement membrane (1-3), which separates the epithelium from the subepithelium. Most available data support the view that the membranous epithelial cells (M cells) are important sites for limited absorption of protein antigens and for subsequent exposure of these antigens to the mucosal immune system (4). A second route of antigen absorption is via the columnar epithelial cells (5). Aside from these structural features which form the gastrointestinal barrier, the secretory immune system also fulfills a vital role against the excess absorption of antigens from the lumen of the intestinal tract. Secretory immunoglobulin A (IgA) in particular, which is produced in abundance by plasma cells lining the intestinal mucous surfaces, binds various dietary antigens (as well as microbial antigens), and thereby excludes them from being absorbed into the systemic compartment (6).

However, despite these barriers, a variety of antigenically intact molecules normally traverse the mature gut mucosa in small amounts by physiological transport mechanisms. Up to 0.01% of ingested dietary protein can be absorbed in the adult (6,7), and much more than this in infants (8). It has been shown in normal adults that at least part of the ingested dietary protein appears to maintain its original molecular weight, which suggests that enzymatic digestion of this fraction has not occurred

(7). However, the normal mechanisms can become greatly perturbed by many kinds of systemic or local pathological processes, and the increased intestinal absorption which results may be of critical importance in the pathogenesis and pathophysiology of various disease states. A leaky membrane might permit the absorption of numerous, essentially undigested substances, which could adversely effect more distant organs such as the skin, liver, kidneys, or joints. The systemic complications of atopy, cirrhosis, celiac disease, dermatitis herpetiformis, IgA nephropathy, chronic alcoholic liver disease, Crohn's disease, ileojejunal bypass, and Henoch-Schonlein purpura represent examples in which gastrointestinal hyperabsorption has been suspected (9-14).

We have been investigating a specific aspect of this phenomenon—the excess absorption of dietary proteins from the gastrointestinal tract which occurs in primary humoral immunodeficiency disease, particularly selective IgA deficiency and common varied immunodeficiency. In both of these diseases, secretory IgA is absent, or present in very low amounts. Our basic hypothesis is that the excessive systemic absorption of numerous antigens, which are normally confined to the lumen of the intestinal tract, is an integral part of primary humoral immunodeficiency disease and that the continual absorption of such antigens places unique strains upon both the remainder of the immune system and other organs. In these congenital immune disorders, varying perturbations of the systemic immune system can be detected which stem from the lack of mucosal IgA antibodies. Depending upon the completeness of the defect, and the range of compensations which can be called into play, varying immunological abnormalities can often be detected. In this chapter, a review of some of the perturbations we have found will be presented, and data from new analyses now ongoing will be described.

Work in Selective IgA Deficiency

Immune Complexes Containing Dietary Antigens

Immunoglobulin A deficiency is the commonest of the primary immune deficiency diseases, as it may affect as many as 1:400 individuals (15,54). In this disorder, both serum and secretory IgA are absent; as a result, the major immunoglobulin of the secretory mucosa is missing. Various compensations can be called into play (such as secretory IgM) (16), but if these compensations are inadequate, disease status may follow. An individual with IgA deficiency is, for example, more likely to develop allergies, sinopulmonary infections, or autoimmune disease (17-19). We have investigated the effect of absent IgA on the intestinal absorption of dietary antigens. In this work, we showed that bovine milk proteins (specifically identified in our work have been bovine gamma globulin and bovine casein) can be absorbed in large amounts from the diet in these patients, and that in the IgA-deficient subject, high titers of specific antibodies are raised and circulating immune complexes are formed which contain these milk antigens (20-21). For example, of 25 IgA-deficient patients with circulating immune complexes in the serum, 15 had sufficient milk antigen to be detected by a method as insensitive as agar diffusion.

In addition to patients who are totally deficient in IgA in both serum and secretions, there are other individuals who have a partial deficiency of IgA—some of these patients have a small amount of serum and/or salivary IgA. Since secretory IgA is a major means whereby dietary antigens are excluded from the blood, we investigated whether a correlation between the level of serum or salivary IgA could be made with the amount of IgG antibody in the serum directed to a specific milk antigen such as casein. This theme is developed by data shown in Figures 1-5. The IgA-deficient patients 1 and 2 (Fig. 1), who have no detectable serum or salivary IgA, have widely varying amounts of immune complex after milk ingestion. Similarly, patients with no serum IgA, but a small amount of salivary IgA (Fig. 2) or serum IgA but no salivary IgA (Fig. 3), or small amounts of both serum and salivary IgA (Fig. 5), or only slightly depressed amounts of serum or salivary IgA (Fig. 4) all have widely varying amounts of immune complex in their serum after milk ingestion. In studying these parameters for 20 IgA-deficient patients, we could not make any correlation between these data. In fact, there is no correlation between serum or salivary IgA and antigen absorption when studied this way (Table 1). The correlation which could be drawn, however, was the the *peak* of immune complex was strongly correlated with the titer of antimilk antibody ($p < 0.01$) (Fig. 6). From our data it was clear that some patients who have a slightly depressed serum IgA and a readily detectable salivary IgA can still have an apparently inadequate gastrointestinal barrier to exclude dietary antigens. Other IgA-deficient patients who lacked serum and secretory IgA had no obvious excess absorption in this test. Thus, it may be that individuals not normally considered to have significant IgA deficiency may have a physiologically relevant secretory IgA defect, and that other patients who have no serum IgA can have an apparently insignificant defect, presumably due to other local compensations (20-23).

Systemic Effects of Immune Complexes

The appearance of circulating immune complexes in the sera of IgA-deficient individuals after milk ingestion is not accompanied by any obvious clinical illness. Serum

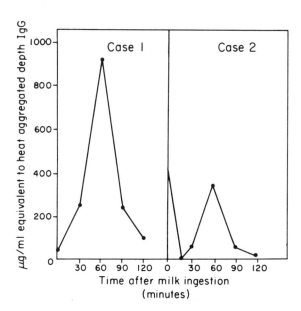

Figure 1 The level of circulating immune complex that was present in the sera of IgA-deficient patients after ingesting 100 ml of milk is shown. The time that each serum sample was obtained is given. The immunological parameters for each of the IgA-deficient patients included in these figures are given in Table 1. The level of immune complex is given in units (m) g/ml equivalent to heat-aggregated IgG. These patients had no detectable serum or salivary IgA.

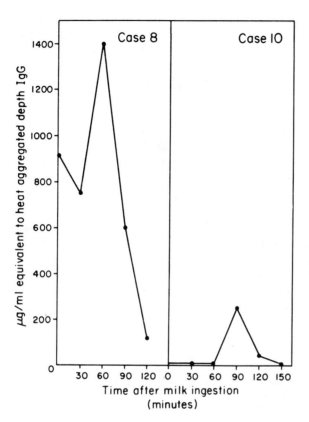

Figure 2 Same as for Figure 1. Patients 8 and 10 (Table 1) were tested. No serum IgA was found, but small amounts of salivary IgA were detected.

sickness does not develop (22) and individuals with IgA deficiency—most of whom are affected in this way—have no evidence of immune complex disease. This was (and is) a puzzling situation, and we attempted to determine if excess antigen absorption could be related to any clinical or laboratory parameter. We found that high levels of immune complexes and increased titers correlated with autoimmune disease the appearance of autoantibodies, neurologic disease, and arthritis (23).

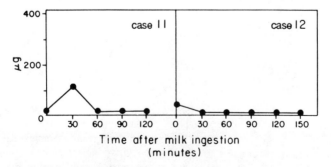

Figure 3 Same as for Figure 1. Patients 11 and 12 were tested. Variable amounts of serum were found, but no salivary IgA was detected for these patients.

Macromolecular Antigen from the GI Tract

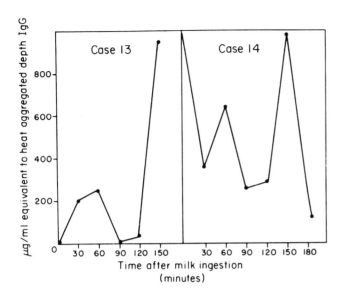

Figure 4 Same as for Figure 1. Patients 13 and 14 were tested. These patients had reduced amounts of serum and salivary IgA.

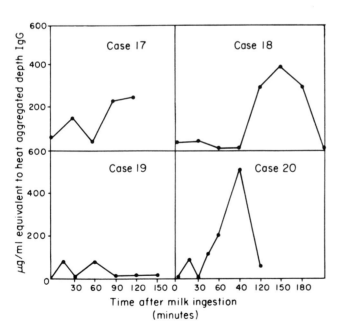

Figure 5 Same as for Figure 1. Patients 17-20, who had reduced but varying amounts of serum and salivary IgA, were tested.

Table 1 Laboratory Data on IgA-Deficient Patients

Patient number	Age	Sex	Serum immunoglobulins[a]			Salivary immunoglobulins[b]			Milk precipitins	Peak of immune complexes
			IgG	IgA	IgM	IgG	IgA	IgM		
Group 1										
1	19	F	1500	0	172	13	0	5	+	928
2	12	F	1096	0	187	0	0	5	0	320
3	52	F	1550	0	78	ND[c]	0	ND	0	480
4	20	M	1134	0	90	ND	0	ND	+	1280
5	13	F	1161	0	97	0.9	0	0	+	6400
6	11	M	664	0	103	1.5	0	0	+	6400
7	32	M	1489	0	33	ND	0	ND	0	1680
Group 2										
8	35	F	1685	0	153	1.7	2	0	+	1400
9	53	M	2300	0	220	<1	11	0	0	1700
10	52	F	1087	0	86	20	9	3	0	216
Group 3										
11	19	F	757	5	198	0	0	0	0	112
12	60	F	675	44	222	0	0	0	0	0
Group 4										
13	33	F	812	13	312	4	31	0	0	900
14	32	M	1420	10	105	ND	5	ND	+	1360
15	12	F	2940	19	165	18	6	0	0	6240
16	16	M	689	20	70	0	5	0	0	1360
17	35	F	910	31	165	ND	5	ND	0	230
18	35	M	775	32	55	ND	13	ND	0	400
19	32	M	747	48	132	<1	11	0	0	80
20	20	F	1220	76	80	40	5	5	0	528

[a]Normal range for serum immunoglobulins: IgG = 800-1800 mg/d, IgA = 90-450 mg/d, and IgM = 80-300 mg/d.
[b]Normal range for salivary immunoglobulins: IgG = 8.2 mg/d ± 1 SD 6.87; IgA = 4.9 mg/dL ± 1 SD 1.88; and IgM = 1.13 ± 1 SD 1.72.
[c]ND = not done.

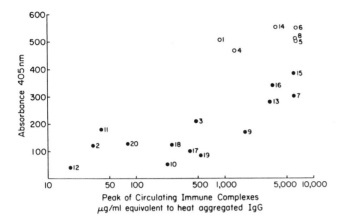

Figure 6 This illustration shows that the peak amount of immune complex that was detected in the serum of each patient of Table 1 (given on the abcissa on a log scale in µg/ml equivalent to heat-aggregated IgG) was related to the level of antibody to bovine milk proteins in these sera (shown on the ordinate, absorbance 405 nm). Sera that contained precipitating amounts of antibody to bovine milk proteins are shown with open circles (○).

The connection between chronic circulating immune complexes and these diseases is not understood. One way to explain the association would be to assume that since IgA-deficient individuals have more absorption of dietary antigens in general, the absorption of a diverse range of such antigens could promote the development of antibodies cross-reacting with internal tissues. The previous demonstration of serum antibodies in IgA deficiency to a bovine mucoprotein constituent of the fat globule membrane formed by the bovine mammary gland (24), and our demonstration of high levels of antichicken ovalbumin antibodies in IgA-deficient subjects (25), lend weight to this hypothesis. It is also possible that tissue damage by immune complexes could secondarily stimulate autoantibody production and provoke autoimmune disease. Among the group of patients having immune complexes and high titers of autoantibodies to bovine proteins, there were four individuals with neurological disease; this suggested that the chronic circulation of immune complexes could induce intermittent abnormalities of the cerebral vascular blood flow.

Anti-Idiotypes in IgA Deficiency Relating to Dietary Antigen

Since the IgA-deficient individual may have such a large amount of antigen entering the blood stream from the gastrointestinal tract, and most make a high level of antibodies to such antigens, we wondered if a corresponding autologous anti-idiotype was also being made. Specifically, we sought antibodies directed to the variable regions of anticasein antibodies, particularly those antibodies which would be blocked from binding to anticaseins by the addition of casein antigen itself. We did find such "site-directed" anti-idiotypes in the sera of the three IgA-deficient individuals in whom these were sought (26,27). Since the autologous anti-idiotypic antibodies we isolated could bind to anticasein antibodies in the place of certain casein antigens, it seemed likely that the large amount of immune complex in the blood could contain both dietary antigens and anti-idiotypic antibodies. While we have not searched for other anti-idiotypes (anti-antiovalbumin, for example) it seems most probable that numerous anti-idiotypes are present in the sera of such patients.

Since at least some anti-idiotypes made by the IgA-deficient individual are directed at the binding site of the primary antibody, it seems more likely that casein antigen and the anti-idiotype bind alternatively to the primary antibody, depending upon the serum concentration of the relative antigen at each point in time. After eating, a large amount of casein, for example, would be present, which would tend to displace the anti-idiotype. After a period of fasting, the amount of casein antigen in the blood might be lower, and the immune complex present would be more likely to contain idiotype and anti-idiotype. Figure 7 illustrates this alteration of antigen and idiotype in a schematic way.

The curious part of this phenomenon is the concomitant appearance of idiotype and anti-idiotype in the blood of an IgA-deficient individual at one time. If anti-idiotypes have a suppressive role in reducing idiotype (anticasein) production, why has this not apparently happened here? One explanation could be that the continued absorption of dietary casein continually stimulates the production of anticasein levels despite such controls as the anti-idiotypic antibodies can supply.

Absorption of a Dietary Peptide in IgA Deficiency

If antigenically intact molecules are absorbed into the circulation in IgA deficiency, it seems probable that dietary peptides could be also absorbed. We have investigated whether bovine β-casomorphin is absorbed in IgA deficiency.

Bovine β-casomorphin is an interesting peptide with μ-type opioid activity in opioid receptor-binding studies and isolated organ preparations. It was first isolated from bovine milk, infant milk formula, and enzymatic digests of bovine casein in 1979 (28-29). The peptide has been isolated and is known to correspond to residues 60-66 of β-casein. This peptide, like morphine, elicits naloxone-reversible analgesia after intracerebroventicular injection in rats. From the first reports of β-casomorphin in 1979, this unique peptide has stirred interest because it is a clear morphine-type agonist derived from a major dietary protein consumed in large quantities. But this intriguing possibility has been tempered by the objection that the peptide would have to be enzymatically and nondestructively cleaved from β-casein in the intestinal tract before any biological effect could be exerted (30-31). Furthermore, the β-casomorphin would have to be absorbed into the blood stream in sufficient amounts and survive

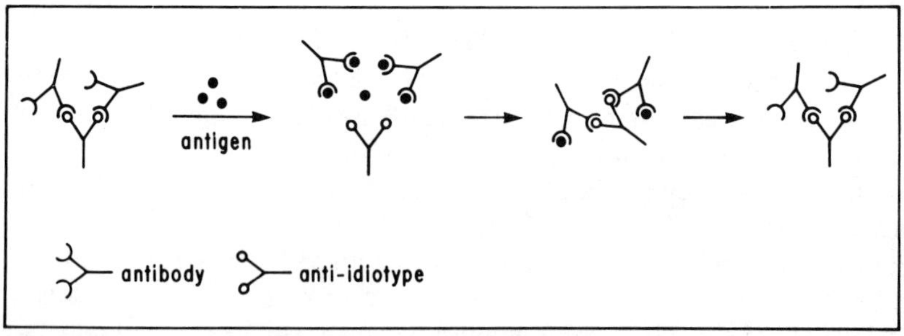

Figure 7 When fasting, the immune complexes of an IgA-deficient subject is predominantly composed of idiotype and anti-idiotype. As dietary antigen enters the blood stream, anti-idiotype is largely displaced by antigen, but as antigen concentrations are reduced, the immune complexes contain both idiotype and antigen. Eventually, as antigen disappears, the original balance of idiotype-anti-idiotype complex is restored.

serum enzymatic cleavage in order to exert a systemic effect. These objections are particularly pertinent since β-casomorphin is less potent pharmacologically than morphine, and more peptide on a molar basis would have to be available for an effect to be exerted (32). Recently, several reports have appeared which cast a new light on this question, and suggest that β-casomorphin could have biological effects, since it can be detected in various biological systems after the ingestion of β-casein (33,34).

Looking at this from another point of view, we have investigated whether antibodies to β-casomorphin are detectable in sera of IgA-deficient subjects. Using an enzyme-linked immunosorbent assay and pure β-casomorphin peptides, we have found that the sera of IgA-deficient patients have substantial amounts of both IgG and IgM antibodies to β-casomorphin. Comparing the amounts of antibodies to casein and β-casomorphin in IgA-deficient sera, we found that there is a strong statistical correlation between these antibody levels for IgA-deficient individuals ($p < 0.001$). This again reinforces the view that casein is the immunogen which supplies β-casomorphin, and that this peptide (either incorporated into large polypeptide fragment or present in peptide form) is absorbed into the blood where it has at least sufficient half-life to serve as an immunogen.

Other biologically active peptides have also been reported to exist in dietary sources. It seems possible that increased absorption of these peptides could occur in any situation of mucosal permeability.

Work in Hypogammaglobulinemia

Intestinal Hypermeability in Hypogammaglobulinemia

Hypogammaglobulinemia (or common variable immunodeficiency) is a fairly rare primary immunodeficiency in which serum levels of IgG, IgA, and IgM are all low; no antibodies are made (55).

Since patients with hypogammaglobulinemia also lack secretory IgA, one might expect that patients with this defect could have an equally excessive gastrointestinal permeability compared with the IgA-deficient patients. However, since hypogammaglobulinemic patients produce antibodies poorly or not at all, the ingested proteins would not elicit antibody production. Thus, these dietary antigens cannot engage in immune complex formation with endogenous immunoglobulin. For this reason, the absorbed antigens would not be eliminated via the mechanisms of immune complex clearance, and could potentially accumulate in the blood. In analyzing a series of such patients, it was shown that this prediction was true; very large amounts of bovine casein are found in the serum of hypogammaglobulinemic patients (Table 2) (36). The amount of foreign protein in these sera cannot be correlated with gastrointestinal disease nor to any specific immunological parameter. However, for still unknown reasons, the amounts of protein in the sera of hypogammaglobulinemic patients is closely associated with the presence of splenomegaly and/or lymphadenopathy (see Table 2). It seems possible that the continued absorption of external antigens could serve to stimulate the proliferation of lymphoid tissue (36).

Clearing of Antigen by Immunoglobulin Infusions

The fact that hypogammaglobulinemic individuals can absorb dietary antigen into the blood stream upon ingestion of specific dietary proteins can be demonstrated. To further investigate the presence and amounts of casein in sera of immunodeficient subjects, we have recently developed a monoclonal antibody to kappa casein, a molecule which in addition to binding calcium, has a role in stabilizing the micelle structure

Table 2 Bovine Antigens in Serum of Hypogammaglobulinemic Patients

Patient no.	Patient	ng casein/ml in serum	ng BGG/ml in serum	Spleen[a]	Immunoglobulin treatment
1	HK	1600	600	+ + +	IM
2	GM	1200	500	0	O
3	SSu	1080	250	+ +	IM
4	SF	980	700	+ +	IM
5	CL	1100	300	+ + +	IM
6	RR	970	ND	0	IM
7	JV	960	ND	0	IM
8	RD	960	ND	0	O
9	SK	1000	800	+ +	IM
10	TS	980	ND	0	IM
11	EW	1000	ND	0	IM
12	SSi	900	800	+ +	IM
14	EL	900	ND	0	IM
15	JK	600	ND	0	IM
16	SR	400	ND	+ +	IV
17	JO	400	ND	0	IV
18	TG	400	ND	+	IV
19	NB	290	ND	0	IV
20	OM	270	ND	+	IV

[a]Spleen + + + = enlarged by 6 cm or more (to umbilicus or below); + + = enlarged by 2-6 cm; + = just palpable; 0 = not palpable.

of milk. The antibody (IgG$_1$ kappa isotype) does not bind to other bovine milk products nor to human casein (56). In other studies, we have shown that when patients with hypogammaglobulinemia are infused with intravenous gamma globulin, a dietary antigen such as casein can be a major constituent of the immune complexes which appear immediately after infusion. As this occurs, there is a concomitant reduction in the amount of casein antigen in the blood. Figures 8 and 9 show results of this kind for two hypogammaglobulinemic patients (37). In these cases, the immune complexes formed could fix C3 and a significant drop in the level of serum C3 could be detected during the infusion of immunoglobulin (Table 3). This phenomenon occurs, however, despite the apparent absence of any infusion reaction.

If immune complex clearance is a mechanism whereby patients with hypogammaglobulinemia can eliminate foreign antigens from their blood stream, it might be possible that the infusion of intravenous immunoglobulin might result in an overall lowering of the amounts of these antigens in the blood. To study this, we have compared the amount of dietary casein and bovine gamma globulin in the sera of hypogammaglobulinemic patients treated with intramuscular immunoglobulin with the levels of these antigens (pretreatment) in sera of patients treated with intravenous immunoglobulin. We have concluded that substantially less of these antigens are found in the sera of the latter group. In Table 2, for example, the last five patients listed had been on intravenous gamma globulin and the other patients had been studied while receiving intramuscular immunoglobulin. Thus, five individuals treated with intravenous gamma globulin have much less casein or bovine gamma globulin antigen detectable in their sera (pretreatment) than do 18 other patients treated with intramuscular immunoglobulin replacement.

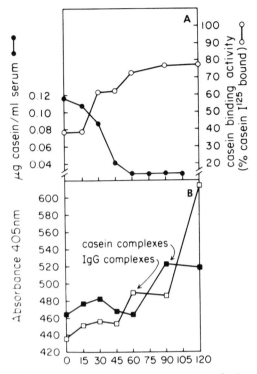

Figure 8 The serum of a hypogammaglobulinemic patient (who had ingested milk the previous day) was tested during the course of the intravenous infusion of immunoglobulin to determine if casein antigen (●—●) decreased as casein binding activity (0—0) increased (A). Similarly, we also determined if IgG immune complexes (□—□) and casein-containing immune complexes (■—■) increased during this period.

Alternative Mechanisms for Excess Absorption in Humoral Immunodeficiency

Why does this excessive absorption from the gastrointestinal tract occur? One clear reason is that secretory IgA is either absent or present in insufficient amounts in the intestinal tract. However, as discussed above, the quantitative amount of antigen in the blood cannot be correlated with either the amount of IgA in the blood or saliva in either IgA-deficient nor hypogammaglobulinemic patients. Furthermore, we have found that apparently similar patients with comparable immunological profiles and similar clinical status can have widely differing amounts of absorption of dietary antigens (22). For these reasons, we have proposed that there might be another mucosal lesion, possibly nonimmunological in nature.

To investigate this, we have studied the intestinal absorption of a molecular weight standardized preparation of polyethylene glycol (PEG) in patients with selective IgA deficiency and common varied immunodeficiency in collaboration with Dr. K.-E. Magnusson and Dr. B. Lindblad. This test was originally introduced as a probe for measuring intestinal permeability, since PEG is nonimmunogenic, nontoxic, not de-

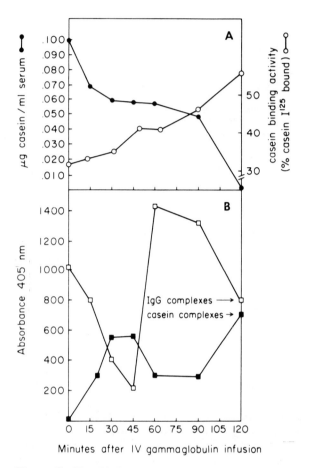

Figure 9 For this hypogammaglobulinemic patient, similar analyses were performed as in Figure 7. Again, the patient ingested milk prior to the intravenous immunoglobulin infusion. A and B show similar data collected as described in the legend for Figure 7.

graded by intestinal bacteria, not metabolized during or after passage through the investinal wall, and rapidly excreted in the urine (38). The different-sized molecular components of PEG cross the intestinal epithelium at different rates, allowing characterization of the differential passive permeability properties of the mucosa. Using the suggestions of Chadwick (39), Sundquist et al. (38) devised mathematical models for the absorption of PEG and methods for analyzing the data achieved have been published. This method has been used to examine the integrity of the gastrointestinal mucosa in patients with protozoal and bacterial infections, in Crohn's disease, in ileojejunal bypass, and in rheumatoid arthritis (32). Using different-sized PEGs (400- and 1000-Da mixtures), it has been possible to assess the general surface area of absorption of small molecules, and the possibility of increased passage of larger molecules, suggesting leakage or hyperabsorption in various diseases. Hyper-

Table 3 Complement Levels After Milk Ingestion and During Intravenous Immunoglobulin Infusion[a]

	Time	CH50	C1q	C3
Patient 1[b]	0	182	23	143
	15	175	23	152
	30	170	23	98
	45	163	22	109
	60	159	26	159
	90	162	24	146
	120	160	23	152
Patient 2	0	126	36	58
	15	125	31	58
	30	125	33	73
	45	117	28	13
	60	117	23	34
	90	111	35	43
	120	93	30	58

[a]Normal ranges for complement including 2 SD from the mean. CH50—50-110 U/ml, which includes 2 SD from the mean (80 U/ml); C1q—15.2-6.4 mg/dl, which includes 2 SD from the mean (20.8 mg/dl); C3—70-176 mg/dl, which includes 2 SD from the mean (123.0 mg/dl).
[b]Patients 1 and 2 are the same individuals tested as in Figs. 2 and 3.

absorption has been found to be characteristic of *Yersinia* infections, Crohn's disease, and surprisingly many patients with rheumatoid arthritis (untreated) and eczema (38-43).

Using the PEG absorption test, we have tested 18 hypogammaglobulinemic and 10 IgA-deficient patients. After ingestion of a standard amount of PEG of a mixture of molecular weight 400-1000, urine was collected for 6 hr; samples were frozen for analysis for determination of PEG content and molecular weight sizing was done by HPLC. The results are plotted as percent recovery in the urine, by molecular weight species, by means of a computer program. Our results show that the great majority of patients with hypogammaglobulinemia and IgA deficiency have distinct abnormalities of PEG absorption as compared to normal individuals. These abnormalities can be classified into one of three types:

Type 1: Reduced absorption of small and large molecular weight species
Type 2: Reduced absorption of small molecular weight species and increased absorption of large molecular weight PEG
Type 3: Normal absorption of low molecular weight but hyperabsorption of large molecular weight PEG
Type 4: Normal pattern

To summarize our results:

PEG Type	IgA Deficient	Hypogammaglobulinemia
Type 1	1	5
Type 2	3	2
Type 3	3	8
Type 4	3	3
TOTAL	10	18

Thus, 7 of 10 IgA-deficient and 15 of 18 hypogammaglobulinemic patients were found to have abnormal absorption patterns (Cunningham-Rundles, C. and K.-E. Magnusson, unpublished). These results indicate that nonimmunological lesions may be part of the abnormal absorption from the intestinal tract in these humoral immunodeficiency diseases. What structural lesions could be present? One possibility would be that structural changes due to chronic infections could explain these findings. Since secretory IgA is not present, bacterial colonies could flourish and produce local inflammation. Another interesting observation has been made which might also explain the hyperabsorption found. Giorgi et al. (44) have reported that the small

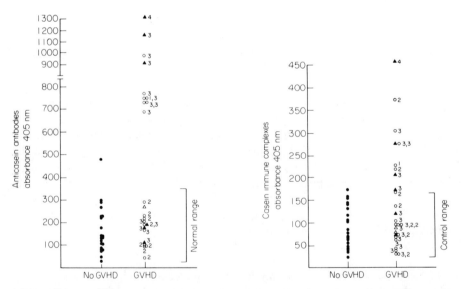

Figure 10 Antibody to bovine casein (absorbance 405 nm) was compared for 46 post transplantation sera drawn from 19 patients. Patients who did not develop GVHD are distinguished from those who did. The stage of GvH reaction for the latter patients is indicated for each sample (2-4). The range for normal controls is indicated. (○) Acute; (△), chronic; (▲) acute and chronic.

intestinal mucosa of children with IgA deficiency shows distinct pathological changes—some of these only recognizable at the ultrastructural level. Further work will need to be done to elucidate these questions.

Work in Bone Marrow Transplantation

The above sections describe data from patients with primary immune deficiency diseases which weaken the secretory immune barrier owing to a lack of IgA. However, in a variety of diseases, the secretory immune system becomes defective as a result of other processes. A good example of this state is presented by bone marrow transplant recipients. Here, the secretory immune system as well as systemic immunity are eliminated by a combination of chemotherapy and radiation. After transplantation, mucosal immunity is restored via donor cells, but this occurs slowly. In patients who develop graft-versus-host disease (GvHD), a clinical sequela of transplantation effecting up to 30% of recipients can occur (45). In such patients, secretory immunity is further impaired. The pathological changes affect the skin, gastrointestinal tract, liver lungs, and/or bone marrow (46) and mucosal immune defects have been documented (45-46). Part of this latter perturbation is due to a deficiency of secretory IgA (47), but the affected areas are also inflamed and ultimately may become scarred, resulting in permanent structural changes.

It is known that secretory IgA-producing plasma cells are restored more slowly posttransplantation in patients who develop GvHD (46-47). The immunological reasons for this failure are complex and involve both a greater depletion of IgA-producing cells in the lamina propria in patients with acute GvHD and a delay in the reconstitution of these cells by the donor's cells (46-47). An additional cause of the reduced

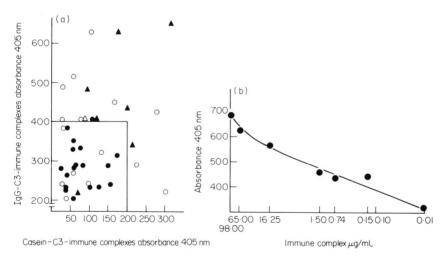

Figure 11 The amount of immune complex which contained bovine casein was analyzed by a C3 monoclonal ELISA for patients with and without GvHD. Control samples run in parallel were drawn from patients with other immune complex diseases. (○) Acute; (△) chronic; (▲) acute and chronic.

concentration of secretory IgA could be the presence of injured duct epithelium in exocrine glands such as the salivary glands and in the bile ducts (48). In addition, the nonspecific gastrointestinal epithelial damage which occurs as a common feature of GvH reactions could also permit excessive absorption of dietary antigens. As a result of each of these factors, systemic immunization with various dietary proteins could occur, and increased serum antibody titers to these substances could develop in the posttransplant period when the systemic immune system becomes engrafted. Further antigen absorption would then lead to the appearance in the sera of immune complexes containing antigens normally confined to the intestinal tract.

To address this question, we analyzed the sera of bone marrow transplanted recipients before and up to a year posttransplantation in order to determine whether evidence of excessive gastrointestinal permeability could be linked to GvHD. Specifically, we examined the possibility that increased antibody titers to bovine proteins or immune complexes containing these antigens could be related to the presence or stage of GvHD.

In these studies, we showed that post-bone marrow transplantation increased amounts of anticasein antibody (Fig. 10), and circulating immune complexes containing casein (Fig. 11) were found in the sera of patients who developed acute or chronic GvHD as compared to those patients who did not (49). That the presence of immune complexes is a hallmark of GvHD is shown by Figure 12. Here, the sera were tested for the presence of IgG immune complexes (Y axis) and for casein-containing complexes in experiments run at the same time in order to compare these two parameters. The boxed area of Figure 12a encloses those sera which had less of both IgG immune complex and casein-containing immune complex; it also encloses sera of all but one patient who did *not* have GvHD. (Figure 12b indicates a standard curve applicable to the IgG-G3 immune complex assays of Figure 12a.) Thus, with circulating immune complexes, especially immune complexes containing casein, GvHD is more likely to be present.

Although circulating immune complexes are known to be an important cause of tissue injury in numerous diseases (50), and immune complexes have been documented in blood and tissues in chronic GvHD (51-55), the connection between immune complexes and GvHD is not clear. Whether the demonstrated immune complexes could be involved in the further production of tissue injury in GvHD, or whether these complexes simply result from tissue damage, remains unsettled.

CONCLUSIONS

We have shown that patients who have defective secretory immunity due to a lack of secretory IgA have a particularly permeable gastrointestinal tract which allows the absorption of antigenically intact dietary macromolecules. While this situation resembles the physiological state of gastrointestinal hyperabsorption which normally exists in early infancy, individuals with primary immunodeficiency diseases have a defect in secretory immunity which persists throughout life. The systemic and immunological effects of the excess absorption of dietary antigens in these patients are diverse, have not been easily predictable, and probably are not yet entirely known.

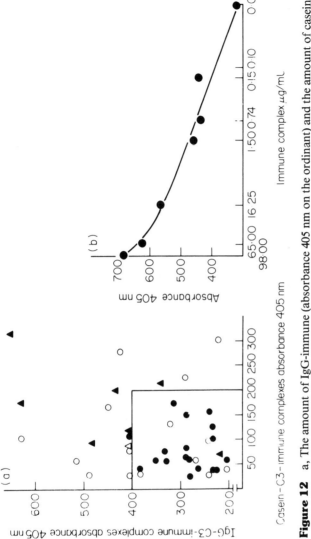

Figure 12 a, The amount of IgG-immune (absorbance 405 nm on the ordinant) and the amount of casein-containing immune complex (absorbance 405 nm on the asbcissa) were determined for sera of patients not having GvHD and for patients having GvHD. The boxed area is an arbitrary enclosure which groups together all but one of the patients who did not have GvHD. The symbols for this figure are the same as for Figures 9 and 10. b, For determining the amount of IgG immune complex which is present for the data of Figure 11, the standard curve for this experiment is given. Here, dilutions of heat-aggregated IgG were allowed to fix C3, and then were exposed to ELISA plates coated with anti-C3 antibody. The absorbance indicates the amount of immune complex which is present.

REFERENCES

1. Walker WA. Antigen absorption from the small intestine and gastro-intestinal disease. Pediatr Clin North Am 22:731-738, 1975.
2. Creamer B. Intestinal structure in relation to absorption. In: Biomembranes. Vol. 4A (Smith DH, ed.). New York, Plenum Press.
3. Glass JGB, Slomiany BL. Derangements of biosynthesis production and secretion of mucous in gastrointestinal injury and disease. In: Mucus in Health and Disease (Elstein M, Park DV, eds.). New York, Plenum Press, 1977.
4. Owen RL. Sequential uptake of horseradish peroxidase by lymphoid follicles of Peyer's patches in the normal unobstructed mouse intestine. Gastroenterology 72:440-451, 1977.
5. Specht W. Morphology of the intestinal wall. In: Intestinal Permeation (Kramer M. and Lauterbach F. eds.). Oxford, Experta Medica, New York, 1977.
6. Walker WA. Antigen uptake in the gut: Immunologic implications. Immunol Today, 2:30-34, 1981.
7. Husby S, Jensenins JC, Svehag SE. Passage of undergraded dietary antigen into the blood of healthy adults. Scand J Immunol 22:83-92, 1985.
8. Udall JN, Pang K, Fritze L. et al. Development of gastrointestinal mucosal barrier I. The effect of age in intestinal permiability to macromolecules. Pediatr Res 15:241-244, 1981.
9. Hall RP, Strober W, Katz SI, Lawley TJ. IgA containing circulating immune complexes in gluten sensitive enteropathy. Clin Exp Immunol 45:234-239, 1982.
10. Wands JR, LaMont JT, Mann E, Isselbacher K. Arthritis associated with intestinal bypass procedure for morbid obesity. Complement activation and character of circulating cryoproteins. N Eng J Med 294:121, 1976.
11. Triger DR, Alp MH, Wright R. Bacterial and dietary antigens in liver disease. Lancet 1: 60-62, 1972.
12. Gormly AA, Smith PS, Seymour AE, Clarkson AR, Woodroffe AJ. IgA glomerular deposits in experimental cirrhosis. Am J Pathol 104:50-54, 1981.
13. Cunningham-Rundles C. Failure of antigen exclusion. In: Food Allergy and Intolerance (Challacombs, Brostoff J, eds.). London, Balliere Tindall, pp 223-234, 1987.
14. Brandtzaeg P, Valnes K, Rognum TO, Bjerke K, Baklien K. The human gastrointestinal secretory immune system in health and diseases. Scand J Gastroenterol 114(suppl):17-38, 1985.
15. Hanson LA. Selective IgA deficiency. In: Primary and Secretory Immunodeficiency Disorders (Chandra RK, ed.). Edinburgh, Churchill Livingston, pp 62-84, 1983.
16. Brandtzaeg P, Fjellanger J, Giruldsen ST. Immunoglobulin M: Local synthesis and selective secretion in patients with selective IgA deficiency. Clin Exp Immunol 35:296-299, 1979.
17. Cassidy JT, Oldhan G, Plattsmill TAE. Functional assessment of a B cell, defect in patients with selective IgA deficiency. Clin Exp Immunol 35:296-299, 1979.
18. Ammann AJ, Hong R. Selective IgA deficiency: Presentation of 30 cases and review of the literature medicine. Medicine 50:223-229, 1971.
19. Ammann AJ, Hong R. Selective IgA deficiency and autoimmunity. Clin Exp Immunol 1:833-838, 1970.
20. Cunningham-Rundles C, Brandeis WE, Good RA, Day NK. Milk precipitins, circulating immune complexes and IgA deficiency. Proc Natl Acad Sci USA 75:3386-3389, 1978.
21. Cunningham-Rundles C, Brandeis WE, Good RA, Day NK. Bovine antigens and the formation of circulating immune complexes in selective IgA deficiency. J Clin Invest 64: 270-272, 1979.
22. Cunningham-Rundles C. Analysis of the secretory immune barrier in IgA deficiency, Ann Allergy 57:31-35, 1986.

23. Cunningham-Rundles C, Brandeis WE, Pudifin DJ, Day NK, Good RA. Autoimmunity in selective IgA deficiency: Relationship to anti-bovine protein antibodies, circulating immune complexes and clinical disease. Clin Exp Immunol 45:299-304. 1981.
24. Butler JE, Oskvig R. Cancer, autoimmunity and IgA deficiency, related by a common antigen-antibody system. Nature 249:830, 1974.
25. Pudifin DJ, Cunningham-Rundles C, Good RA. Circulating antibodies to chicken ovalbumin in IgA deficient subjects. Fed Proc 38:5263, 1979.
26. Cunningham-Rundles C. Naturally occurring autologous anti-idiotypic antibodies: Participation in immune complex information in selective IgA deficiency. J Exp Med 155: 771-719, 1985.
27. Cunningham-Rundles C, Cheung MKL. Cross-reactive idiotypes in immunoglobulin A-deficient sera. J Clin Invest 75:1722-1728, 1985.
28. Brantl V, Teschemacher H, Henschen A, Lottspeich F. Novel opioid peptides derived from casein (β-casomorphins). Isolation from bovine casein peptone. Hoppe-Seylers Z Phisiol Chem Bd 360:S1211-1216, 1979.
29. Henschen A, Lottspeich F, Brantl V, Teschemacher H. Novel opioid peptides derived from casein (b-casomorphins) II. Structure of active components from bovine casein peptone, Happe-Seylers Z Phisiol Chem Bd 360:1217, 1224, 1979.
30. Ziodrou C, Treaty RA, Klee WA. Opioid peptides derived from food protein in the exorphins. J Biol Chem 254:2446-2449, 1979.
31. Chang KJ, Cuatrecasas P, Weis ET, Chang JK. Analgesic activity of intracerebroventricular administration of morphiceptin and β-casomorphins. Correlation with the morphine (μ) receptor binding affinity. Life Sci 30:1547-1551, 1982.
32. Chang KJ, Su YS, Brent DA, Chang JK. Isolation of a specific m-opiate receptor peptide, morphiceptin, from an enzymatic digest of milk protein. J Biol Chem 260:9706-9712, 1985.
33. Svedberg J, DeHaas J, Leimenstoll G, Paul F, Teschemacher H. Demonstration of β-casomorphin immuno reactive materials in in vitro digest of bovine milk and in small intestine contents after bovine milk ingestion in adult humans. Peptides 6:825-830, 1985.
34. Hamel U, Keilwein G, and Teschemacher H. β-Casomorphin significance of proteinases originating from milk leucocytes and a comparison of the action of leucocyte, bacterial and natural milk proteinases on casein. J Dairy Res 52:101-112; 1985.
35. Grieve PA, Kitchen BJ. Proteolysis in milk: The significance of proteinases originating from milk leucocytes and a comparison of the action of leucocyte, bacterial and natural milk proteinases on casein. J Dairy Res 52:101-112, 1985.
36. Cunningham-Rundles C, Carr RI, Good RA. Dietary protein antigenemia in humoral immunodeficiency disease: Correlation with splenomegaly. Am J Med 76:181-185, 1984.
37. Cunningham-Rundles C, Carr RI. Dietary bovine antigens and immune complex formation after intravenous immunoglobulin in common varied immunodeficiency. J Clin Immunol 6:381-387, 1986.
38. Sundvist T, Mangusson KE, Sjodahl R, Stjernstrom I, Tagesson C. Passage of molecules through the wall of the gastrointestinal tract. II. Application of low molecular weight polyethylene glycol and a deterministic mathematical model for determining the intestinal permeability in man. Gut 21:208-214, 1980.
39. Chadwick VS, Phillips SF, Hofman AF. Measurements of intestinal permeability using low molecular weight polyethylene glycol (PEG 400) I. Chemical analysis and biological properties of PEG 400. Gastroenterology 73:241-246, 1977.
40. Magnusson KE, Sundqvist T, Sjodhal T, Tagesson C. Intestinal permiability studies and human disease. Monogr Allergy 17:250, 1981.
41. Magnusson KE, Sundqvist T, Sjodahl T, Tagesson C. Altered intestinal permeability to low-molecular weight polyethylene glycols (PEG 400) in patients with Crohn's disease. Acta Chir Scand 149:323-327, 1983.

42. Jacobson PG, Baher RWR, Lessaf MH, Ferret J, MacDonald DM. Intestinal permeability in patients with eczema and food allergy. Lancet 1:1285-1286, 1981.
43. Sundqvist T, Lindstrom F, Magnusson KE, Skoldstam L, Stjernstrom I, Tagesson C. Influence of fasting on intestinal permeability and disease activity in patients with rheumatoid arthritis. Scand J Rheumatol 11:33, 1982.
44. Giorgi PL, Catassi C, Sbarbat A, Bearzi I, Cinti S. Ultrastructural findings in the jejunal mucosa of children with IgA deficiency. J Pediatr Gastrointest Nutr 5:892-898, 1986.
45. O'Reilly RJ. Allogenic bone marrow transplantation: Current status and future directions. Blood 62:941, 1983.
46. Sullivan KM, Parkman R. The pathophysiology and treatment of graft-vs-host disease. Clin Hematol 12:775, 1983.
47. Beschorner WE, Yardley JH, Tutschka PJ, Santos GW. Deficiency of intestinal immunity with graft-vs-host disease in humans. J Infect Dis 114:38, 1981.
48. Izutsu KT, Sullivan KM, Schubert MM, Truelove EL, Shulman HM, Sale GE, Morton TH, Rice JC, Witherspoon RP, Storb R, Thomas ED. Disordered salivary immunoglobulin secretion and sodium transport in human chronic graft-vs-host disease. Transplantation 35:441, 1983.
49. Cunningham-Rundles C, O'Reilly R. Association of circulating immune complexes containing bovine proteins and graft-vs-host disease. Clin Exp Immunol 64:323-329, 1986.
50. Dixon FJ. Immune complex disease. J Invest Dermatol 59:413, 1973.
51. Cunningham-Rundles C, Brandeis WE, Safai B, O'Reilly RJ, Day NK, Good RA. Selective IgA deficiency and circulating immune complexes containing bovine proteins in a child with chronic graft-vs-host disease. Am J Med 67:883, 1979.
52. Tsoi M, Storb R, Jones E, Weiden PL, Shulman H, Witherspoon R, Atkinson K, Thomas ED. Disposition of IgM and complement at the dermoepidermal junction in acute and chronic graft-vs-host disease in man. J Immunol 120:1485-1491, 1980.
53. Manca F, Bacigalupo A, Van Lint MT, Trovatello G, Canterella S, Frassi F, Marmont A, Celada F. Circulating immune complexes in allogeneic marrow graft recipients. Transplantation 38:428, 1984.
54. Cunningham-Rundles C. Genetic aspects of immunoglobulin A deficiency. Adv Hum Genet 19:235, 1990.
55. Cunningham-Rundles C. Clinical and immunologic analysis of 103 patients with common variable immunodeficiency. J Clin Immunol 9:22, 1989.
56. Feng ZK, Cunningham-Rundles C. Production of a monoclonal antibody to bovine kappa casein. Hybridoma 8:223, 1989.

22
Natural Killer Activity in Protein-Calorie Malnutrition

Lekan Samusa Salimonu
University College Hospital, Ibadan, Nigeria

INTRODUCTION

A subpopulation of mononuclear cells from the circulating blood of normal human subjects have the ability to kill a wide spectrum of cultured tumor cells in vitro (Kiessling and Haller, 1978; Hersey, 1979) and virus-infected cells in vivo (Heberman et al., 1986; Trinchieri, 1989). Previously, some workers designated these cells as a subclass of T lymphocytes (West et al., 1977). It is now known that these cells, termed natural killer (NK) cells, are nonadherent (Kiessling et al., 1975), nonphagocytic lymphoid cells lacking the characteristic surface markers of mature lymphocytes (Kiessling et al., 1975). That NK cells are predominantly from the subpopulation of "null" cells have been confirmed by other workers (Kalden et al., 1977; Ozer et al., 1979) and other cell surface antigens such as CD16 (for type III) are used to define these cells (Lanier et al., 1986, Cassatella et al., 1989).

NK CELL ACTIVITY IN PROTEIN-CALORIE MALNUTRITION

As stated above, NK cells are known to be predominantly null cells because these cells do not usually express T-cell differentiation antigens (Ozer et al., 1979). Previous studies have consistently shown elevated blood levels of null cells in protein-calorie malnutrition (PCM), whereas the T lymphocytes were observed to be correspondingly diminished (Chandra, 1977, Salimonu et al., 1982c). It was to be expected that the NK cell activity in malnutrition would be higher than in healthy controls. The findings in the investigation of NK cell activities in 5 children having kwashiorkor, 14 having marasmus, and 16 healthy controls were contrary to such expectations (Salimonu et al., 1982a). The marasmic children as well as children having kwashiorkor had a high proportion of subjects with depressed NK cell activity. Six of the 14 marasmic children having kwashiorkor had very low NK cell activities (less than 2.5% specific lytic capacity). On the other hand, only 1 of the 16 control children had such low values (Salimonu et al., 1982a).

There is an abundance of evidence to show that natural killer cell activity may play an important role in tumor surveillance (Kiessling and Haller, 1978; Hersey, 1979). It is also known that NK cells may also play important role in graft-versus-host reactions. For instance, NK cells have been closely associated with the rejection of bone grafts (Kiessling et al., 1977). Natural killer cell activity has been implicated as the first line of defense against both bacteria and viruses (Herberman and Ortaldo, 1981). Depressed NK cell activity as reported in undernutrition (Salimonu et al., 1982a) would suggest a breakdown in the capacity of malnourished hosts to mount tumor surveillance and a reduced ability to reject transplanted tissues. Previous studies have, however, shown that, on the contrary, tumor or skin transplants are usually rejected more rapidly by protein- or amino acid-depleted experimental animals than in well-fed controls. For example, dietary amino acid deficiency has been found to increase resistance to transplantable tumors in mice (Theuer, 1971). Cooper et al. (1974) observed that skin transplants were rejected more rapidly in protein-deprived mice than in normal controls. Similarly, Fernandes et al. (1976) reported that NZB mice fed with a low-protein diet possessed greater capacity to produce graft-versus-host reactions and more vigorous cell-mediated "killer" cell immunity after immunization against DBA/2 mastocytoma cells than did NZB mice on normal protein diets. Recently, Norris et al. (1990) have shown that healthy human volunteers fed a phenylalanine- and tyrosine-restricted diet for 4 weeks showed enhanced natural killer cell activity compared to controls, which was correlated not only with increased NK cells, but also increased T cells, both $CD4^+$ and $CD8^+$, which may have related to recirculation into peripheral blood compartment. Blood protein status was unchanged.

It is possible, therefore, that despite the depressed NK cell activity other mechanisms are involved in tumor surveillance in protein-calorie malnutrition. For example, the enhanced rejection of transplantable tumors reported in protein- or amino acid-deficient animals may be due to a preferential suppression of antibody production in such animals (Jose and Good, 1971). It is possible that failure to produce tumor-specific "blocking" antibody is reflected in what appears to be hightened cell-mediated cytotoxicity against tumor antigens (Jose and Good, 1971, 1973). Since most investigations have suggested that anticancer immunity may depend upon $CD4^+$ T-cell response to tumor-specific antigens in association with class II major histocompatibility complex (MHC) molecules, leading to the production of interleukin 2 and interleukin 3 and the development of $CD8^+$ cytotoxic T lymphocytes (killing of cells expressing tumor-specific antigens in association with class I MHC determinants) as well as NK cells, Petro et al. (1991) have recently studied several cytotoxic functional changes during dietary protein deficiency or process. These rather complex studies in a mouse model indicate that while moderately low dietary protein levels had an enhancing effect on natural killing, higher levels of dietary protein were needed to produce an antitumor cytotoxic tumor response. In humans, Vaisman et al. (1990) found that acute short-term starvation was associated with reduced cellular cytotoxicity and was also depressed in patients with long-term anorexia nervosa. Further, cytotoxic function increased after refeeding.

INTERFERON LEVELS IN PCM

Interferon is known to play a major role in the induction of NK cells activities in both humans (Trinchieri and Santoli, 1978) and experimental animals (Zarling et al., 1979). Furthermore, most of the agents that have been observed to augment NK activity are known to be able to induce interferon production (Kirchner et al., 1977; Zarling et al., 1979). It is known that interferon is involved in the cytotoxic mechanism of NK cells (Peter et al., 1976; Bonnard et al., 1979) by acting as a boosting agent (Oehler et al., 1978) which triggers the development of pre-NK cells into mature NK cells (Burns et al., 1985).

Schlessinger et al. (1976) used Newcastle disease virus to induce interferon production in 9 severely marasmic infants and 31 well-nourished controls. They reported a significantly depressed interferon production in the marasmic infants. These findings were confirmed by Salimonu et al. (1982a), who observed no detectable levels of interferon in all but 3 (one marasmic and 2 normal sera) of the subjects studied (5 kwashiorkor, 14 marasmus, and 16 control). Interestingly, the three exceptional children had very high levels of circulating NK cell activity.

Chandra and Wadhwa (1989) have noted that impaired local and systemic immunity in protein-calorie malnutrition can result in decreased secretory IgA, fewer intraepithelial lymphocytes, and increased bacterial binding to epithelial cells and frequent gastrointestinal infection with decreased NK cell activity. These kinds of changes are also observed in certain vitamin A-deficient states often associated with malnutrition. Interestingly, Bowman et al. (1990) have noted that vitamin A deficiency in a rat model was associated with decreased NK activity and decreased interferon production. Although vitamin A status was not explored in our study, it is known that even mild vitamin A deficiency can be associated with increased mortality from respiratory and diarrheal infections (West et al., 1989).

Gammainterferon production is known to be regulated by a dynamic interaction between helper-, suppressor-, and interferon-producing cells (Luger et al., 1982). There is reduced thymic factor activity in protein-calorie malnutrition, which may impair the normal differentiation and maturation of the T-cell precursors (Chandra, 1979; Jackson and Zaman, 1980; Heresi and Chandra, 1980). For example, studies by Chandra (1983) have shown deficiency in the number and function of T-helper cells. This deficiency could be partly responsible for the depressed NK cell activity and the absence of detectable levels of interferon in the malnourished children. Thymic depletion in protein-calorie malnutrition is discussed further in a chapter in this book. Although Woodward et al. (1991) have suggested that altered T-cell immunity in an animal model of protein-calorie malnutrition is not associated with altered T-cell subsets or T/B cell ratio in spleen, lymph nodes, or recirculating pool, this study did not address lymphokine production. Furthermore, the effect of concomitant infection—a very real issue in malnourished human populations—was not a factor in this study.

EFFECT OF ADDING EXOGENOUS INTERFERON IN VITRO ON NK CELL ACTIVITY IN PCM

While normal well-nourished infants produced a significant increase in NK cell activity following treatment with exogenous interferon in vitro, this was not so in the

Table 1 Effect of Exogenous Interferon In Vitro on NK Level of Normal and Malnourished Infants

	Mean percentage specific lysis ± SE	
	Without interferon	Interferon added in vitro
Normal infants	11.20 ± 3.0	27.29 ± 6.0
Infants with kwashiorkor	8.85 ± 3.9	3.84 ± 1.7
Infants with marasmus	7.74 ± 2.1	8.93 ± 2.4

Note: P values calculated using Student's t = test: $p > 0.2$ = no effect of adding interferon on NK activity in marasmic PBLs compared to untreated, marasmic peripheral blood lymphocytes (PBLs). In contrast, $p < 0.02$ for a comparison between increased NK levels in normal, interferon-treated PBLs compared to similarly treated PBLs from marasmic children. $p > 0.05$ = no significant effect (slight suppression) of treating PBLs from kwashiorkor patients with interferon in vitro and comparing to the starting NK levels of PBLs from the same patients. In contrast, $p < 0.01$ for a comparison between the increased NK levels in normal, interferon-treated PBLs compared to the NK levels of interferon-treated PBLs from kwashiorkor donors. There were 16 children for normal controls, 5 and 14 for kwashiorkor and marasmus, respectively.
Source: Salimonu et al., 1982a; used with permission.

marasmic children nor in children with kwashiorkor (Table 1). Following the addition of exogenous interferon, enhancement of NK cell activity occurred in a greater proportion of normal children than in children having marasmus ($p < 0.025$) or kwashiorkor ($p < 0.01$) (Salimonu et al., 1982a). Interestingly, interferon addition was observed to suppress the NK cell activity in a large proportion (four out of five) of the children having kwashiorkor.

Apart from studies by Schlessinger et al. (1976) and Salimonu et al. (1982a), not much work has been done on interferon levels in PCM. Why interferon failed to function in the induction of NK cell activity of malnourished children is not clearly understood. It is possible that the NK cells of undernourished children have been accustomed to very low levels or that increased production during a prior period may have caused inhibition of response. Addition of large quantities of interferon in vitro, as employed by Salimonu et al. (1982a), may create a high dose tolerance by the NK cells. It is also possible, however, that addition of interferon did not activate the NK cells of malnourished children to lyse the target cells because the NK cell activity of these children never expressed mature activity owing to aborted development of the NK system. The NK system is known to be immature at birth and to develop during the first few months of life (Yabuhara et al., 1990). Alternatively, it may be that early demand on this population has led to paralysis of further response. The consequences of this could be highly significant, since NK activation has been implicated in host defense against primary infections (Wilson, 1986).

NK CELL ACTIVITY IN PCM AND SUSCEPTIBILITY TO INFECTION

Whether low NK cell activity in PCM has biological significance for susceptibility to infections is unknown. It can only be speculated from results of previous investigations (Wilson, 1986). It is well known that NK cell activity in mice could be boosted by innoculation of tumor cells and viruses as well as *C. parvum* and BCG (Herberman et al., 1977; Wolfe et al., 1977). Increased NK cell activity has also been reported in cases of experimental trypanosomiasis (Hatcher et al., 1981), in *Schistosoma mansoni* infections (Attallah et al., 1980), and upon challenge with *Histoplasma capsulatum* (Cozard and Lindsey, 1974). Many of these diverse stimulants appear to act indirectly by first inducing the production of interferon, which then activates NK cells (Djeu et al., 1980). Interestingly, neonatal cells have been shown to respond to interleukin 2, a gamma interferon inducer (Yabuhara et al., 1990).

Depressed NK cell activity in undernourished children even after interferon administration would predispose them to infections. There is circumstantial as well as biological evidence to indicate that nutritional deficiencies generally reduce the capacity of the host to resist the consequences of infections (Scrimshaw et al., 1968, Phillips and Wharton, 1968). Before now, several factors have been blamed for this lowered resistance. These include lowered antibody production (Scrimshaw et al., 1966) and reduced levels of immunoglobulins (Aref et al., 1970). Others include impaired tissue resistance, deranged phagocytic activity of polymorphonuclear neutrophils (Scrimshaw et al., 1959; Salimonu et al., 1982b), and depressed T-lymphocyte number and functions (Smythe et al., 1971; Keusch et al., 1977, Salimonu et al., 1982c).

As stated earlier, there is now evidence that (a) NK cell activity of circulating blood is normally enhanced following infections (Hatcher et al., 1981; Attalah et al., 1980) or addition of interferon (Herberman et al., 1980), (b) NK cell activity is depressed in undernutrition (Salimonu et al., 1982a), and the addition of interferon either has no effect or could cause enhanced depression of the activity (Salimonu et al., 1983); and (c) malnourished animals are highly susceptible to infections (Phillips and Wharton, 1968). It is, therefore, likely that apart from the other depressed immune states that reduce the resistance of malnourished animals to infection (Scrimshaw et al., 1968; Salimonu et al., 1982b,c), depressed NK cell activity would be another causative factor. Since the studies described here were undertaken in non-HIV-infected children, the AIDS virus was not a factor.

CORRECTION OF THE IMPAIRED NK CELL ACTIVITY AFTER NUTRITIONAL REPLETION

There is evidence that impaired immune mechanisms observed in PCM are usually corrected after management and nutritional recovery (Ferguson et al., 1974; Moore et al., 1977; Chandra, 1983). Natural killer cell activities were investigated in 8 children with kwashiorkor, 15 with marasmus, 17 children who had recovered from being marasmic, 10 children who had recovered from kwashiorkor, and 20 apparently healthy well-fed children. As in a previous study (Salimonu et al., 1982a), a high percentage of the malnourished children had very low NK cell activity. Only one of the 10 children who had recovered from kwashiorkor and 1 of the 17 recovered marasmic children had blood NK cell lytic activity that was less than 2.5%. In addition, one of the 20 control children had blood NK cell lytic activity of less than 2.5% (Salimonu et al., 1983).

As previously reported (Salimonu et al., 1982a), in vitro addition of exogenous interferon caused depression of the NK cell activity in a large population of (five out of eight) children having kwashiorkor. Slight enhancement of NK cell activity was observed in 10 out of the 15 marasmic children after exogenous interferon was added. The remaining five children showed no appreciable changes in the NK cell activity after interferon was added (Salimonu et al., 1983). After nutritional recovery, unlike the malnourished state, significant enhancement of NK cell activity was observed in both the children previously having marasmus or kwashiorkor and in well-fed children following in vitro addition of exogenous interferon (Table 2) (Salimonu et al., 1983).

The observation that depressed NK cell activity in PCM (Salimonu et al., 1982a) was corrected after nutritional repletion (Salimonu et al., 1983) may be explained by the considerable influence that PCM exerts on the growth and functions of body cells. Lymphoid organs such as bone marrow (Sood et al., 1965), the small intestine (Deo and Ramalingaswami, 1965), the thymus and other lymphoid aggregates (Hammar, 1921; Smythe et al., 1971; Olusi and McFarlane, 1976) are most affected. It is also known that if protein and calorie restrictions occur early in life, cell division and organ growth are severely affected (Winik, 1971). These cellular changes may be the direct result of the reduced availability of essential nutrients necessary for the synthesis of cellular components. Since NK cells are derived and dependent on bone marrow (Haller and Wigzell, 1977), such cellular changes would also affect the NK cells, as have been reported by Salimonu et al. (1983). In additiion to direct effects on thymus-derived T cells, protein-calorie malnutrition may indirectly affect NK cell maturation through negative effects on the thymus. Thymic hormones have been implicated in NK regulation through induction of receptors and lymphokine production (Serrate et al., 1987). Thus, thymus depletion may affect NK cell function.

We have also been interested in the role of plasma inhibitory factors in malnutrition. These substances appear to block the T-cell receptor (Salimonu, 1985; Salimonu and Akinyemi, 1986). We have speculated that such a substance might depress T-cell function or promote suppressor cell activation (Salimonu, 1986). It seems likely that such an inhibitory substance might affect NK cell function indirectly. The role of possible other inhibitors of NK cell activity, such as prostaglandins, in malnutrition is unknown at present, although these are of interest both because monocytes which are activated produce prostaglandins and because of the potential interaction between prostaglandins and thymic hormones (Homo-Delarche, 1990).

Thus, malnutrition has profound but not well-understood effects upon the NK system. Understanding of these effects is critical to a rational basis for future intervention.

Table 2 Effect of in Vitro addition of Exogenous Interferon on the NK Cell Activity of PBLs of Malnourished, Previously Malnourished but Recovered and Well-Fed Children

	% Specific lysis (Mean ± 1SD)	
	Without interferon	Interferon added in vitro
Well-fed children	12.83 ± 7.94	34.10 ± 6.35
Children having kwashiorkor	9.16 ± 6.91	3.51 ± 3.64
Children having marasmus	8.28 ± 6.24	12.54 ± 7.11
Children recovered from kwashiorkor	11.84 ± 10.18	31.21 ± 8.77
Children recovered from marasmus	12.70 ± 9.93	32.39 ± 8.90

Source: Salimonu et al., 1983; used with permission.

REFERENCES

Aref GH, Badr EL, Din MK, Hassan AI, Araby II. (1970). Immunoglobulins in kwashiorkor. J Trop Med Hyg 73:186-191.

Attallah AM, Lewis FA, Urritia-Shaw A, Folks T, Yeatman TJ (1980). Natural killer cell (NK) and antibody-dependent cell-mediated cytotoxicity (ADCC) components of Schistosoma mansoni infection. Int Arch Allergy Appl Immunol 63:351-354.

Bowman TA, Goonewardene M, Pasatiempo MG, Ross AC, Taylor CE (1990). Vitamin A deficiency decreases natural killer cell activity and interferon production in rats. J. Nutr. 120:1264.

Burns GF, Begley CG, Mackay IR, Triglia T, Werkmeister JA (1985). "Supernatural" killer cells. Immunol Today 6:370, 1985.

Cassatella MA, Anegon I, Curturi MC, Griskey P, Trinchieri G, Perussia B (1989). FcγR (CD$_{16}$) interaction with ligand induces Ca2^+ mobilization and phosphoinositide turnover in human natural killer cells. J Exp Med 169:549.

Chandra RK (1977). Lymphocyte subpopulations in human malnutrition cytotoxic and suppressor cells. Pediatrics 59:423-427.

Chandra RK (1979). Serum thymic hormone activity in protein energy malnutrition. Clin Exp Immunol 38:228-230.

Chandra RK (1983). Numerical and functional deficiency in T helper cells in protein energy malnutrition. Clin Exp Immunol 51:121-13.

Chandra RK, Wadhwa M (1989). Nutritional modulation of intestinal mucosal immunity. Immunol Invest 18(1-4):119.

Cooper WC, Good RA, Mariani T (1974). Effects of protein insufficiency on immune responses. Am J Clin Nutr 27:647-664.

Cozard GC, Lindsey TJ (1974). Effect of cyclophosphamide on Histoplasma capsulatum infections in mice. Infect Immun 9:261-265.

Deo MG, Ramalingaswami V (1965). Reaction of the small intestine to induced protein malnutrition in Rhesus monkeys. A study of cell population kinetics in the jejunum. Gastroenterology 49:150-157.

Djeu JY, Huang KY, Herberman RB (1980). Augmentation of mouse natural killer activity and induction of interferon by tumour cells in vivo. J Exp Med 151:781-789.

Ferguson AC, Lawlor GJ Jr, Neumann CG, Oh W, Stiehm ER (1974). Decreased rosette forming lymphocytes in malnutrition and intra-uterine growth retardation. J Pediatr 85:717-723.

Fernandes G, Yunis EJ, Good RA (1976). Influence of protein restriction on immune functions in NZB mice. J Immunol 116:782-790.

Haller O, Wigzell H (1977). Suppression of natural killer cell activity with radioactive strontium: Effector cells are marrow dependent. J Immunol 118:1503-1506.

Hammar JA (1921). The new views as to the morphology of the thymus gland and their bearing on the problem of the function of the thymus. Endocrinology 5:543-573, 731-760.

Hatcher FM, Kuhn RE, Cerrone MC, Burton RC (1981). Increased natural killer cell activity in experimental American trypanosomiasis. J Immunol 127:1126-1130.

Herberman RB, Ortaldo JR (1981). Natural killer cells: Their role in defense against disease. Science 214:24.

Herberman RB, Nunn ME, Holden HT (1977). Augmentation of natural cytotoxic reactivity of mouse lymphoid cells against syngeneic and allogeneic target cells. Int J Cancer 19:555-564.

Herberman RB, Ortaldo JR, Djeu JY, Holden HT, Jett J, Lang NP, Rubinstein M, Pestka S (1980). Role of interferon in regulation of cytotoxicity by natural killer cells and macrophages. Ann NY Acad Sci 350:63-71.

Herberman RB, Reynolds CW, Ortaldo J (1986). Mechanism of cytotoxicity by natural killer (NK) cells. Annu Rev Immunol 4:651.

Heresi G, Chandra RK (1980). Effects of severe calorie restriction on thymic factor activity and lymphocyte stimulation response in rats. J Nutr 110:1888-1893.

Hersey P (1979). Natural killer cells—A new cytotoxicity mechanism against tumors. Aust NZ J Clin Lab Invest 9:464-472.

Homo-Delarche F, Gagnerault MC, Bach JF, Dardenne M (1990). Thymic hormones and prostaglandins II. Synergistic effect on mouse spontaneous rosette forming cells. Prostaglandins 39:291, 1990.

Jackson TM, Zaman SN (1980). The in vitro effect of the thymic factor thymopoietin on a subpopulation of lymphocytes from severely malnourished children. Clin Exp Immunol 39:717-721.

Jose DG, Good RA (1971). Absence of enhancing antibody in cell mediated immunity to tumor heterografts in protein deficient rats. Nature 231:323-325.

Jose DG, Good RA (1973). Quantitative effects on nutritional protein and calorie deficiency upon immune responses to tumours in mice. Cancer Res 33:807-812.

Kalden JR, Peter HH, Roubin R, Cesarini JP (1977). Human peripheral Null lymphocytes. I. Isolation, immunological and functional characterization. Eur J Immunol 7:537-543.

Keusch GT, Urrutia JJ, Guerrero O, Casteneda G, Douglas SD (1977). Rosette forming lymphocytes in Guatemalan children with protein calorie malnutrition. In: Malnutrition and the Immune Response. Suskind RM (ed). Raven Press, New York, pp. 117-122.

Kiessling R, Klein E, Pross H, Wigzell H (1975). "Natural killer" cells in the mouse. II. Cytotoxic cells with specificity for mouse Moloney leukemia cells. Characterization of the killer cells. Eur J Immunol 5:117-121.

Kiessling R, Hochman PS, Haller O, Shearer GM, Wigzell H, Cudkowicz G (1977). Evidence for a similar or common mechanism for natural killer cell activity and resistance to haemopoietic grafts. Eur J Immunol 7:655-663.

Kiessling R, Haller O (1978). Natural killer cells in the mouse: An alternative immune surveillance mechanism? In: Contemporary Topics in Immunology. Vol. 8. Warner NL (ed). pp. 171-199.

Kirchner H, Hirt HM, Becker H, Munk K (1977). Production of an antiviral factor by murine spleen cells after treatment with corynebacterium parvum. Cell Immunol 31:172-176.

Lanier LL, Phillips JH, Hackett JR, Tutt JM, Kumar V (1986). Natural killer cells: Definition of a cell type rather than a function. J Immunol 137:2735.

Luger TA, Smolen JS, Chused TM, Steinberg AD, Oppenheim JJ (1982). Lymphocytes with either the helper ($T4^+$) or suppressor ($T8^+$) phenotype produce interleukin 2 in culture. J Clin Invest 70:470-473.

Moore DL, Heyworth B, Brown J (1977). Effect of autologous plasma on lymphocyte transformation in malaria and acute protein energy malnutrition. Immunology 33:777-785.

Oehler JR, Lindsay LR, Nunn ME, Holden HT, Herberman R (1978). Natural cell mediated cytotoxicity in rats. II. In vivo augmentation of NK cell activity. Int J Cancer 21:210-220.

Olusi SO, McFarlane H (1976). Effects of early protein calorie malnutrition on the immune response. Pediatr Res 10:707-712.

Ozer H, Strelkauskas AJ, Callery RT, Schlossman SF (1979). The function dissection of human peripheral null cells with respect to antibody-dependent cellular cytotoxicity and natural killing. Eur J Immunol 9:112-118.

Peter HH, Eife RR, Kalden JR (1976). Spontaneous cytotoxicity (SCNC) of normal human lymphocytes against a human melanoma cell line. A phenomenon due to a lymphotoxin-like mediator. J Immunol 116:342-348.

Petro TM, Schwartz KM, Schmir MJ (1991). Natural and immune anti-tumor interleukin production and lymphocyte cytotoxicity during the course of dietary protein deficiency or excess. Nutr Res 11:679.

Phillips I, Wharton B (1968). Acute bacterial infection in kwashiorkor and marasmus. Br Med J 1:407-409.

Salimonu LS, Ojo-Amaize E, Williams AIO, Johnson AOK, Cooke AR, Adekunle FA, Alm GV, Wigzell H (1982a). Depressed Natural killer cell activity in children with protein-calorie malnutrition. Clin Immunol Immunopathol 24:1-7.

Salimonu LS (1985). Soluble immune complexes, acute phase proteins and E rosette inhibitory substance in sera of malnourished children. Ann Trop Paediatr 5:137-141.

Salimonu LS (1986). Plasma inhibitory factos in malnutrition. In: Nutrition and Immunology. Chandra RK (ed). Liss. New York p 25.

Salimonu LS, Akinyemi A (1986). Lymphocyte number, E rosette substance and soluble immune complexes in protein calorie malnutrition, malaria, and measles. Nutr Inter 2:264-267.

Salimonu LS, Johnson AOK, Williams AIO, Adeleye, Iyabode G, Osunkoya BO (1982b). Phagocyte function in protein caloric malnutrition. Nutr Res 2:445-452.

Salimonu LS, Johnson AOK, Williams AIO, Adeleye, Iyabode G, Osunkoya BO (1982c). Lymphocyte subpopulations and antibody levels in immunized malnourished children. Br J Nutr 48:7-14.

Salimonu LS, Ojo-Amaize E, Johnson AOK, Laditan AAO, Akinwolere OAO, Wigzell H. 1983. Depressed Natural killer cell activity in children with protein-calorie malnutrition. II. Correction of the impaired activity after nutritional recovery. Cell Immunol 82:210-215.

Schlessinger L, Ohlbaum A, Grez L, Stechel A (1976). Decreased interferon production by leucocytes in marasmus. Am J Clin Nutr 29:758-761.

Scrimshaw NS, Taylor CE, Gordon JE (1959). Interaction of nutrition and infection. Am J Med Sci 237:367-403.

Scrimshaw NS, Taylor CE, Gordon JE (1968). Interactions of nutrition and infection. WHO Monogr Series 57:165-167.

Serrate SA, Schulof RS, Leonadaridis L, Goldstein AL, Sztein M (1987). Modulation of human natural killer cell cytotoxic activity, lymphokine production and interleukin 2 receptor expression by thymic hormones. J Immunol 139:2338.

Smythe PM, Schonland M, Brereton-Stiles GG, Coovadia HM, Grace HJ, Loening WEK, Mafoyane A, Parent MA, Vos GH (1971). Thymolymphatic deficiency and depression of cell mediated immunity in protein calorie malnutrition. Lancet 2:939-974.

Sood SK, Deo MG, Ramalingaswami V (1965). Anemia in experimental protein deficiency in the rhesus monkey with special reference to iron metabolism. Blood 26:421-432.

Theuer RC (1971). Effect of aminoacid restriction on the growth of female C57BL mice and their implanted BW 10232 adenocarcinomas. J Nutr 101:223-232.

Trinchieri G (1986). Biology of natural killer cells. Adv Immunol 47:187.

Trinchieri G, Santoli D (1978). Anti viral activity induced by culturing lymphocytes with tumour derived or virus transformed cells. Enhancement of human natural killer cell activity by interferon and antagonistic inhibition of susceptibility of target cells to lysis. J Exp Med 147:1314-1333.

West HW, Cannon GB, Kay D, Bonnard GD, Herberman RB (1977). Natural cytotoxic reactivity of human lymphocytes against a myeloid cell line: a Characterization of effector cells. J Immunol 118:355-361.

West KP, Howard JB, Sommer A (1989). Vitamin A and infection: Public health implications. Annu Rev Nutr 9:63.

Wilson LB (1986). Immunologic basis for increased susceptibility of the neonate to infection. J Pediatr 108:1.

Winik M (1971). Cellular growth during early malnutrition. Pediatrics 47:969-978.

Wolfe SA, Tracey DE, Henney CS (1977). BCG-induced murine effector cells. II. Characterization of natural killer cells in peritoneal exudates. J Immunol 119:1152-1158.

Woodward BD (1991). Depression of thymus-depend immunity in wasting protein-energy malnutritiion does not depend on an altered ratio of helper ($CD4^+$) to suppressor of the T-cell relative to the B-cell pool. Am J Clin Nutr 53:1329.

Vaisman N, Hohn T, Dayan V, Schattner A (1990). The effect of different nutritional states on cell-mediated cytotoxicity. Immunol Lett 24:37.

Yabuhara A, Kawai H, Komiyama A (1990). Development of natural killer cytotoxicity during childhood: Marked increases in number of natural killer cells with adequate cytotoxic abilities during infancy to early childhood. Pediatr Res 28:316.

Zarling JM, Eskra L, Borden EC, Horoszewicz J, Carter WA (1979). Activation of human natural killer cells cytotoxic for human leukaemia cells by purified interferon. J Immunol 123:63-70.

23
Modification of Lymphocyte Function by Fatty Acids—Biological and Clinical Implications

Pierre J. Guillou and John R. Monson
Imperial College of Science, Technology, and Medicine, London, England

Peter C. Sedman and Thomas G. Brennan
St. James University Hospital, Leeds, West Yorkshire, England

INTRODUCTION

It has been recognized for a number of years that modifications of the lipid composition of cell membranes can alter cell function in vitro (1,2). That such structural modifications might also influence leukocyte function has until recently stimulated only sporadic interest from immunologists (see also Chaps. 11 and 12). The development of techniques for studying molecular interactions at the lymphocyte cell surface represent convenient tools for studying the modulatory effects of lymphocyte membrane lipid composition. In parallel with these developments, the manufacture of lipid emulsions for administration to patients as part of the calorie source in intravenous feeding regimens has, perhaps fortuitously, provided an opportunity to study the effects of such changes in vivo in humans. Consideration of the effects of these lipid emulsions on immunological interactions both in vitro and in vivo may have important clinical implications in addition to the potential value they may have in elucidating the role played by lipids in cell membrane function. Such investigations may lead to novel therapeutic applications of lymphocyte membrane modification in patients suffering from malnutrition and malignant disease.

Our own interest in this area has evolved from efforts to administer total parenteral nutrition (TPN) to malnourished tumor-bearing patients in an attempt to augment the depressed antitumor lymphocytotoxicity observed in cancer patients. Because of the exciting prospects for adjuvant immunotherapy afforded by the recent explosion of interest in the use of biological response modifiers in such patients, nutritional support could be an important component of this approach. This chapter aims to describe the background and current status of research on the effects of fatty acids on leukocyte function in an attempt to intercalate some of the biological observations into certain clinical scenarios in sepsis and oncology. We have not addressed the role of plasma lipoproteins in the modulation of the immune response, since this has been reviewed elsewhere (3,4) and in other chapters in this volume (Chap. 11).

In the first instance, however, it may be of value to recall the observations which led to the widespread use of total parenteral nutrition.

Surgery, Cancer, Malnutrition, and the Background of Parenteral Nutritional Support

Malnutrition occurs commonly in the cancer patient, particularly when the tumor is relatively advanced or when the primary lesion originates in the gastrointestinal tract. Of a consecutive series of 72 preoperative patients awaiting surgery for gastrointestinal cancer, we found that almost 40% were suffering from malnutrition as defined by rather severe criteria, including either a greater than 15% loss of recall body weight, a serum albumin of less than 32 g L^{-1} and/or a serum transferrin of less than 2 g L^{-1} (5). This malnutrition may be a result either of alterations in metabolic expenditure or as a consequence of reduced intake (7). In tumor-bearing mice, malnutrition appears to affect albumin synthesis of the gene level (6). The theme of this whole volume attests to the fact that such a degree of malnutrition adversely influences both humoral and cellular aspects of the immune response (8,9). The malnourished patient undergoing surgery, which also has deleterious effects on many aspects of the immune response, is therefore subjected to a dual immunological insult. It was not perhaps unexpected that skin test anergy prior to surgery in such patients would correlate with the subsequent development of sepsis with all its attendant morbidity and mortality (10-12). Attempts to reverse this skin test anergy by means of nutritional supplementation was, therefore, an entirely logical extension of these observations. The clinical conditions of many of these patients, who were either unable or unwilling to eat normally, rendered the parenteral route of nutritional supplementation an attractive one. Using an intravenous nutritional regimen that employed glucose solutions as the sole nonprotein calorie source, Copeland and his colleagues claimed to be able to restore positive skin test reactivity to a panel of recall antigens in 50% of cancer patients (13). Similar results could be obtained by prolonged enteral feeding where possible (14). It was subsequently claimed that the outcome both in terms of the incidence of infection and response to tumor therapy was "better" in the responders than in the nonresponders (15). It is of interest that at the time of these studies few, if any, of the patients received lipid solutions as part of their calorie supply.

Since these early reports, numerous studies have examined the metabolic and clinical influences of TPN on the outcome of surgery. In a well-conducted trial of preoperative TPN in patients undergoing surgery for gastrointestinal cancer (16), the incidence of major septic complications and postoperative mortality were significantly lower in the TPN group than in the control (non-TPN) group. Moreover, this reduction in morbidity appeared to correlate with the restoration of immunological responsiveness as assessed by skin reactivity to recall skin test antigens, serum immunoglobulin levels, and serum levels of the C3A component of complement. Recent reviews (4,12,17) of all such studies have in general confirmed these conclusions, but it should be remembered that (a) the majority of reports have confirmed the description of their results to the preoperative period with little regard for the long-term (i.e., greater than 30 days) results of cancer treatment, and (b) few of these studies incorporated lipid emulsions into the TPN regimen.

Modifications of Lymphocyte Function by Fatty Acids

These two reservations should be borne in mind during the discussion which follows. However, at this point, it may be pertinent to describe the evolution of lipid emulsions as calorie sources in TPN regimens in order that the more recent reports questioning the use of TPN in cancer therapy may be viewed in perspective.

Lipid Emulsions in Total Parenteral Nutrition

The impetus for the provision of intravenous protein and energy substrates in the traumatized or septic patient is the maintenance or restoration of the lean body mass. The nitrogen-sparing effect of parenteral nutrition is now well established and amino acids are regarded as an essential part of any intravenous nutritional regimen. Furthermore, certain amino acids, specifically arginine, appear to enhance host anti tumor immunity and to promote survival (18,19), as discussed also elsewhere in this volume. However, an element of controversy has surrounded the nature of the optimal energy source which should accompany these amino acid solutions. The available alternatives are of course glucose, which has a number of clinical and metabolic disadvantages when used as the sole source of nonprotein calories, or the more recently developed lipid emulsions. Glucose and lipid solutions appear to have similar capacities for nitrogen sparing (20). However, in recent years, it has been recognized that ketone bodies are also a useful source of energy, and this has led a number of workers to support the administration of fat emulsions in TPN on the basis that fatty acids from the hydrolysis of triglycerides are the main source of ketones (21). Furthermore, and perhaps just as importantly in the light of subsequent observations, such solutions are an important source of essential fatty acids, particularly those which constitute major components of cell membranes such as linoleic acid and arachidonic acid (22). These, together with a number of other metabolic advantages (23), represent compelling reasons to incorporate lipid emulsions as at least part of the nonprotein calorie source during TPN. Currently, most workers employ regimens in which approximately 50% of the non-amino acid calories are supplied as glucose and 50% in the form of lipid emulsions, among which the most readily available has been Intralipid (Kabi-Vitrum, Stockholm), which is a mixture of soybean oil, egg phospholipid, and glycerol. The constituents of this solution are summarized in Table 1, from which it can be seen that the principal lipids are of the long-chain fatty acid type.

Subsequent to the emergence of lipid emulsions as a viable preparation for parenteral nutritional support, two very important issues have been raised in recent years.

Table 1

Constituents of Intralipid (20%)
1. Fatty acid source—soybean oil—200 g L^{-1}
2. Emulsifier—egg yolk phospholipid—12 g L^{-1}
3. To maintain isotonicity—glycerol—25 g L^{-1}

Fatty Acid Profile of Soybean Oil (%)

Linoleic acid (c18:2)	50	(– > arachidonic [c20:4] in vitro)
Linolenic acid (c:18:3)	8	(– > docosahexaenoic [c22:6] in vivo)
Oleic acid (c18:1)	26	
Palmitic acid (c16)	9	
Stearic acid (c18)	3	
Others	4	

The first concerns the suggestion that conventional lipid emulsions are immunosuppressive, an argument which continues to excite investigation. The second, and equally controversial, question surrounds the possibilities that when employed as an adjunct to cancer therapy, TPN may be deleterious to the medium and long-term outcome for tumor-bearing patients. In the light of recent observations concerning the role of antitumor cytotoxic cells in the immunosurveillance and treatment of malignant disease, it is conceivable that these two aspects of nutritional support may be interrelated.

Immunoregulatory Effects of Lipid Emulsions

A case report (24) on the occurrence of splenic lipidosis in a patient receiving TPN initially raised the possibility that reticuloendothelial and immunological responses might result from the administration of lipid emulsions. Other studies on the immunoregulatory effects of lipid emulsions were also prompted by a number of reports which suggested that essential fatty acids could influence some aspects of cell-mediated immunity. These investigations stemmed from the fact that the essential polyunsaturated fatty acids, linoleic acid (C18:2) and arachidonic acid (C20:4), are prostaglandin precursors that have a depressive effect on murine reticuloendothelial function when ingested (25). It was subsequently suggested that both the saturated and polyunsaturated fatty acids were capable of inhibiting the response of normal peripheral blood lymphocytes to stimulation with either specific (PPD) or nonspecific (PHA) mitogens in vitro in a dose-related manner (26). In these experiments, the polyunsaturated fatty acids appeared to suppress preferentially the proliferation of stimulated rather than unstimulated lymphocytes, an observation whose relevance may emerge later. Free fatty acids in culture medium are readily incorporated into cell membrane phospholipids (27). These substitutions in the cell membrane appear to modify the rate of patching and capping of H-2 surface antigens on murine lymphoma cell lines on exposure to fluorescinated alloantibodies. This has been interpreted as a reflection of the altered fluidity of the membrane consequent upon the modification of its fatty acid profile (28). These, and a number of other observations served as a springboard for the investigation of the effects of clinically administered lipid solutions on several aspects of the immune response.

A preliminary report from Dudrick's group claimed that the in vitro coculture of peripheral blood lymphocytes with relatively high concentrations of Intralipid not only did not inhibit lectin and varidase-induced lymphocyte transformation, but actually augmented it (29). Unfortunately, this report lacked adequate controls and the changes reported were minimal. Furthermore, the addition of linoleic acid to the cultures in equivalent concentrations to those known to be present in the lipid emulsion was found almost completely to inhibit lymphocyte transformation, an observation which was ignored in the discussion to the paper. Since this initial report, and because of its potential importance with regard to the recognizably high incidence of severe sepsis in malnourished patients undergoing TPN, a number of in vitro and in vivo studies have attempted to address this question from both experimental and clinical standpoints. Differences between the role of lipids in the formation of oxygen-reactive species and as intermediates in arachidonic acid metabolism appear to underly part of this issue (4). Review of this literature reveals a dichotomy in the evidence which can be summarized according to which type of leukocyte is under study.

Effects of Lipid Emulsions on Monocyte and Polymorphonuclear Cell Functions

In a study of the effects of a short (2-hr) infusion on Intralipid into healthy volunteers, the solution was found markedly to impair both the random migration of polymorphonuclear leukocytes and also that induced by a chemotactic stimulus (30). This phenomenon was also observed when the lipid emulsion was added in vitro. In the in vivo studies, the impaired chemotaxis appeared to correlated with the plasma levels of triglycerides in these subjects. These findings are compatible with previous in vitro observations that low concentrations of palmitic acid (C16.0) (which constitutes approximately 10% of the fatty acid composition of Intralipid) can selectively inhibit leukocyte chemotaxis (31). In order to investigate the basis of this depressed polymorphonuclear cell function in greater detail, Cleary and Pickering cultured human polymorphs for brief periods in the presence of varying concentrations of Intralipid equivalent to those obtained during in vivo administration (32). These workers reported that the phagocytic activity of polymorphs which had been preincubated with Intralipid was significantly impaired. Such cells expressed fewer Fc receptors and exhibited depressed oxidative metabolism. This contrasted with the results obtained when the respiratory studies were performed at the initiation of culture with the Intralipid present. These latter experiments revealed that hexose monophosphate shunt activity actually appeared to have been stimulated. Since neither of the other two constituents of Intralipid (egg phospholipid and glycerol) was found to have any effect on these parameters, it was concluded that the fatty acid components of the solution initially stimulated the oxidative burst of polymorphonuclear cells resulting in exhaustion of the metabolic pathways involved in respiration, phagocytosis, and Fc receptor availability. However, other considerations discussed below may render the postulated mechanism of Fc receptor distribution open to other interpretations.

Short-term infusions of Intralipid have also been reported to impair significantly monocyte chemotaxis and phagocytosis in seriously ill postoperative patients as well as healthy volunteers (33). Most authors have also commented upon the development of phagoliposomes in the leukocytes studied, and it has been suggested that these appearances are associated with the functional abnormalities. Both might be prevented by stimulation of the pathway for Intralipid catabolism via the tissue lipoprotein lipase system, but this has not yet been substantiated (34).

All these investigations seem compatible with the notion that lipid emulsions are at least in part responsible for the high incidence of septic complications seen in the malnourished immunocompromised recipient of lipid-based TPN. This hypothesis has received further support from an experimental murine study in which Intralipid was found seriously to impair bacterial clearance and result in highly significantly increased mortality from bacterial challenge (35). However, it should be noted that in these studies vast quantities of Intralipid were administered to the animals. These doses were quite unrealistic in clinical terms and resulted in the administration of quantities of fatty acids which can overwhelm the rodent reticuloendothelial system (36). Despite these constraints and the presentation of somewhat flimsy evidence to the contrary (37), the results of these investigations are almost entirely in favor of the opinion that the most commonly employed lipid emulsions do impair the phagocytic and chemotactic functions of polymorphonuclear leukocytes and monocytes.

Effects of Lipid Emulsions on Lymphocyte Function

In contrast to the effects of polymorph and monocyte function, the position with regard to the influence of lipid emulsions on lymphocyte function is much less clear. There is scant information on the effects of these lipid emulsions on B-lymphocyte function, response to B-cell growth factors, or capacity to produce antibody. Our own findings of lipid emulsions on natural killer, NK, and K-cell function will be described presently. The majority of in vivo studies of the changes occurring in lymphocytes in the presence of Intralipid have not revealed any deleterious effect of this solution on mitogen-induced T-lymphocyte transformation, although it may do so in vitro (29,34,38). Unfortunately, most reports have involved short (2- or 3-hr) infusions of Intralipid, this bears little relationship to its clinical use. However, with the exception of the later paper by Ota et al. (38), there were no reports on the influence of parenteral nutrition on lymphocyte subset distribution in malnourished patients. Equally, the only aspect of lymphocyte function which has been examined in this regard was that of transformation in response to standard mitogens in vitro. Despite the fact that such observations that existed had failed to demonstrate any consistent pattern of change of lymphocyte subset distribution or mitogenic responses, we wished to examine this for ourselves in the context of a prospective, randomized controlled clinical study. Our purpose in so doing stemmed from an interest in seeking means of augmenting endogenous immunological responses, particularly those with antitumor capacities, with a view to their potential clinical application in immunotherapeutic protocols.

Our study was designed as a 14-day prospective crossover trial in which half the patients were administered a lipid-based TPN regimen for the first 7 days followed immediately by 7 days of TPN using a wholly carbohydrate-based regimen. The remaining patients received the same regimens over the same time period but in the reverse order. The patients thus served as their own controls and were a heterogeneous group of patients suffering from sepsis or malignant disease in whom total parenteral nutrition was clinically indicated. The nutritional regimens were equicaloric and equinitrogenous and were prescribed on the basis of calculated metabolic energy expenditure for each individual patient daily. The immunological parameters which we examined included the distribution of T-lymphocyte subsets using a standard panel of monoclonal antibodies recognizing helper/inducer (CD4) and suppressor/cytotoxic (CD8) lymphocytes, and the production of the T-helper lymphokine interleukin 2 (IL-2) after 24 hr of lymphocyte stimulation with concanavalin A (Con A). Interleukin 2 was measured using a standard Gillis bioassay (39) based on the proliferation of the murine IL-2-dependent T-cell clone CTLL-2.

The findings of this study are reported in detail elsewhere (40), but in summary appeared to indicate that augmentation of all the immunological parameters occurred during the period of lipid-based TPN but not during the wholly carbohydrate-based TPN. Thus, the total numbers of circulating lymphocytes expressing CD3 appeared almost to double during the period of lipid-based TPN. This was largely attributable to a significant increase in the numbers of CD8-positive cells. No such changes were observed in the same patients during the periods of solely carbohydrate-based TPN. Simultaneously with these observations, we also found IL-2 production to be significantly elevated during TPN with the lipid-based regimen, there being no equivalent changes observed with the carbohydrate-based regimen (Fig. 1). At the time, it seemed a simple matter to attribute this increased IL-2 production to increased CD3-positive

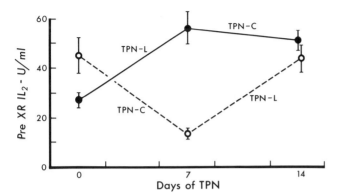

Figure 1 IL-2 content of supernatents from 24-hr cultures of Con A activated peripheral blood mononuclear cells in patients receiving total parenteral nutrition (means + s.e.). Solid lines refer to group 1 patients who received lipid-based TPN (TPN-L) for 7 days followed by 7 days of carbohydrate-based TPN (TPN-C). Dotted line refers to group 2 patients who received identical regimens but in the reverse order. Supernatant IL-2 content was significantly increased after 7 days TPN-L in both groups and tended to fall during TPN-C. (Used with the permission of the British Journal of Surgery.)

lymphocytes consequent upon the presence of the more "normal" metabolic environment afforded by the lipid-based regimen. As will unfold, subsequent studies have caused us to reexamine this interpretation, but we were encouraged by these findings to pursue a further study aimed at examining the influence of this lipid-based "immunorestorative" TPN regimen on lymphocyte-mediated antitumor cytotoxicity in cancer patients. There was no preexisting data on the effects of total parenteral nutrition on these more recently described aspects of the host response against tumors, and it seemed important to have such information for the reasons elaborated below.

Theoretical Rationale for Considering Nutritional Support During Immunotherapeutic Approaches to the Treatment of Malignant Disease

Like many others, we have been excited by the prospects for the exploitation of the stimulation of endogenous biological responses for tumor therapy (41). One such approach involves the ex vivo stimulation of vast numbers of autologous lymphocytes for several days with high-dose IL-2 during which time they become promiscuously cytotoxic toward tumor cells but not normal cells (42,43). The subsequent reinfusion of these lymphokine-activated killer (LAK) cells together with IL-2 has been followed by significant tumor regression in approximately 40% of over 200 patients so treated in at least two independent centers in the United States (44,45). We have been intrigued by the fact that this approach is almost universally successful in causing the regression of experimental animal tumors (46-48), whereas it fails to have demonstrable effects on the tumors in 60% of humans with advanced tumor burdens. Experimentally, the success or otherwise of adoptive cellular immunotherapy with LAK cells and IL-2 seems to be related to the cytolytic activity of the administered LAK cells (49). Accordingly, one possible explanation for the frequently observed clinical failure of adoptive cellular immunotherapy is that in these patients with advanced tumor burdens, autologous LAK cells are cytolytically inefficient, at least in comparison with those obtained from healthy individuals. Of course, in the experimental murine protocols, LAK cells are derived from the spleens of healthy syngeneic mice. Many aspects of the cellular immune response are impaired in tumor-bearing patients. This is particularly so in those patients suffering from advanced disease of gastrointestinal origin and who exhibit an impaired capacity for endogenous IL-2 production (50-51), so it came as little surprise to discover that the generation of LAK cells was also impaired in such patients (53). We, therefore, postulated that herein lay one possible explanation of the therapeutic failure of adoptive cellular immunotherapy with LAK cells in some patients. During this study, we were also able to confirm previous suggestions that basal NK cell activity in these patients was also impaired (54). This finding is important insofar as it is widely held that the precursor cell for much of the LAK cell activity seen after 3-4 days of lymphocyte culture in the presence of IL-2 is in fact the NK cell (55,56).

It is generally supposed that the immunodeficiencies described above in patients with advanced malignant disease are to a large extent attributable to malnutrition. We have recently confirmed this supposition with respect to LAK cell generation in patients with advanced gastrointestinal cancer, although even in nonmalnourished patients with localized disease impaired responses may also be observed, suggesting that other additional factors may be operative (4). The antitumor cytotoxicity of unfractionated peripheral blood mononuclear cells from these patients can be augmented by coculture in the presence of other biological response modifiers such as gamma interferon in addition to IL-2 (57). However, if, as traditional views would suggest, these impaired cytotoxic responses are the result of malnutrition, it would seem logical to attempt their correction by nutritional repletion.

A second reason for invoking the aid of nutritional support during immunotherapy for cancer results directly from the anorexia and malnutrition which frequently accompany the use of biological response modifiers in cancer therapy. For example, the administration of recombinant interferons together with cytotoxic agents in the treatment of advanced malignant melanoma caused anorexia and marked weight loss in over 80% of the patients in our experience (58,59). Similarly, LAK/IL-2 therapy is also associated with considerable toxicity and diminished nutritional intake. If these therapeutic modalities mediate some of their effects via the stimulation of cell-mediated antitumor cytotoxicity, then some of their benefit may be blunted by the influence of acute starvation in diminishing the cytotoxic efficacy of these leukocytes.

With these considerations in mind, it was then that we embarked on an investigation of the effects of our lipid-base "immunorestorative" TPN regimen on tumor-directed lymphocytotoxicity.

Effects of Lipid-Based TPN on Nonspecific Lymphocyte Responses and Tumor-Directed Lymphocytotoxicity in Patients with Gastrointestinal Cancer

The questions addressed by this second TPN study were twofold. First, could we reproduce the effects reported in our original study by administering 7 days of lipid-based TPN to a homogeneous group of gastrointestinal cancer patients? Second, were the augmented lymphocyte responses previously seen during lipid-based parenteral nutrition followed by identical trends in the generation of antitumor cytotoxic responses? To this end, 30 preoperative gastrointestinal cancer patients awaiting surgery gave informed consent to receive 7 days of total parenteral nutrition with the previously described lipid-based regimen. Lymphocyte function was quantified prior to initiating TPN and the assays repeated on completion of the 7-day period of TPN. For the purposes of this investigation, the assays of lymphocyte function which we selected consisted of measurement of lymphocyte transformation in response to a standard mitogen (Con A), IL-2 production in response to this mitogen, NK activity using the standard 4-hr ^{51}chromium-release assay against K562 cells, and last the generation of LAK cell activity following 3 days of lymphocyte culture in the presence of high-dose IL-2. Lymphokine-activated killer cell activity was also quantified using 4-hr ^{51}Cr release from the international reference target for LAK activity, DAUDI, as well as from a colorectal cancer cell line (COLO 320) wherever sufficient cells permitted. The patients were classified as either normally nourished or malnourished according to the criteria described previously. Following retrieval of the operative and pathological findings, the patients were subsequently categorized as suffering from localized or advanced disease according to whether or not the disease had spread to involve structures beyond the serosal layer. This was of importance because of our previous finding that it is patients with advanced disease who suffer the most marked perturbations of antitumor cytotoxicity.

The results of this study have been both surprising and disturbing (60). As with our first report, we were gratified to discover that this TPN regimen resulted in the augmentation of IL-2 levels in the supernatants of lectin-activated lymphocytes from these patients at the end of the 7-day feeding period, particularly in patients suffering from advanced disease. However, this appeared to be accompanied by diminished stimulation indices of the lectin-activated lymphocytes and was also in marked contrast to the effects of this regimen on NK activity. As can be seen from Figure 2, overall the spontaneous lysis of the NK target K562 by peripheral mononuclear cells from these patients was significantly impaired after 7 days of TPN. This was most marked with the lymphocytes from those patients with localized disease in whom, following a week of TPN, NK activity appeared to be reduced to levels approaching those normally observed in patients with advanced disease. Similarly, the killing of K562 by lymphocytes activated for 3 days in vitro with high concentrations of IL-2 was also significantly diminished following 7 days of TPN. When these same activated killer cells were used as effector cells against the DAUDI and COLO 320 cell lines, the same pattern was observed (Fig. 3). Again, suppressive effects of TPN on LAK activity appeared to be particularly prominent in those patients subsequently shown to have localized disease. In these patients, LAK cell generation is normally similar, if not slightly greater, than that seen in healthy individuals. Clearly, these findings give cause for concern on a number of counts.

First and most obviously, a major implication of this report is that this particular lipid-based TPN regimen should not be used to provide nutritional support for those patients being considered for treatment with biological response modifiers whose therapeutic effects are mediated via the generation of antitumor killer cells. This regimen is evidently deleterious to the generation of such effectors irrespective of the influence it may have on the phenotypic distribution of lymphocyte subsets and LAK precursors (38,40). A possible explanation for this phenomenon lies in the observation that modification of the killer cell membrane ratios of saturated to unsaturated fatty acids may be associated with changes in their lytic potential. In particular, moderate concentrations of oleic acid (C18:1) have been found to impair human NK function

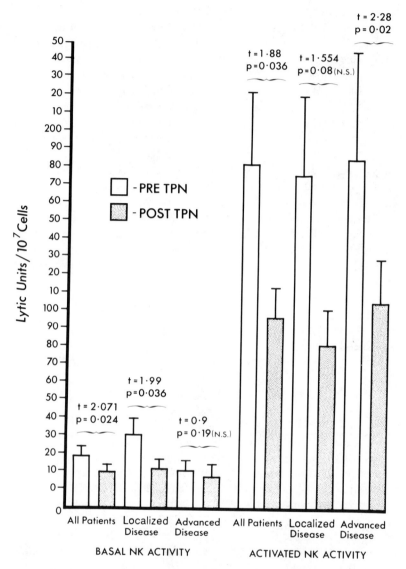

Figure 2 Basal and IL-2-activated cytotoxicity (+ s.e.) of peripheral blood mononuclear cells from preoperative patients suffering from gastrointestinal cancer before and after 7 days of total parenteral nutrition using a lipid-based TPN-regimen. (Used with the permission of Academic Press, London.)

in vitro (63). In addition, reduced fat intake in volunteers was found to increase NK cell activity (61,62). As will be alluded to further on, such modifications of the lipid profile of cell membranes result in diminution of the fluidity of the cell membrane. If NK cell membranes are rigidified by alteration of the lipid composition as described above, then the release of the natural killer cytotoxic factor thought to mediate NK activity is prevented even when effector-target cell binding is unimpeded (57,58). While prostaglandin production may be directly affected by dietary lipids, recent studies

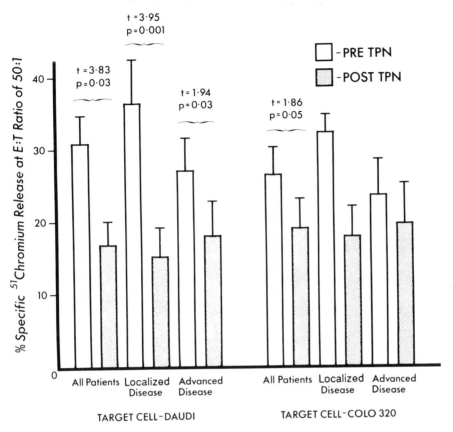

Figure 3 LAK activity (+ s.e.) of unfractionated peripheral blood mononuclear cells in patients suffering from gastrointestinal cancer before and after 7 days of preoperative intravenous nutrition with a lipid-based regimen. (Used with the permission of Academic Press Inc. London.)

by Meydani et al. (66) show that fish oil (n-3) ingestion, which decreases prostaglandin synthesis, is associated with marked suppression of cytokine production in vitro, so that effects on arachidonic acid metabolism are not an explanation of the results, which would in fact have predicted the reverse of the actual findings.

Second, these findings provide an additional perspective to recent publications challenging the contention that total parenteral nutrition in patients with malignant disease serves to improve responses to surgery and chemotherapy. As was stated earlier in this chapter, most of the published data relating to the supposed beneficial effects of TPN as an adjunct to surgery or chemotherapy for malignant disease concentrated on the immediate peritherapeutic period with no regard for the long-term outcome (16,67,68). More recently, several clinical studies have suggested that in fact the prognosis may be worse in parenterally fed patients for reasons unrelated simply to the presence of a central venous feeding catheter. In a study of TPN as an adjunct to the chemotherapy of metastatic colorectal cancer, the median survival time was significantly less in the intravenously fed group than in the control group (69). Whether or not lipid emulsions were included in this regimen is unclear. However, they certainly formed part of the protocol described by Shamberger and his colleagues in a well-designed controlled clinical trial of the use of TPN as an adjunct to surgery and chemotherapy in the treatment of sarcomas (70). The data from this study are most impressive with 71% of patients in the TPN group showing no evidence of disease at the conclusion of therapy compared with 86% in the control group. More importantly, however, the tumor recurrence rate in the TPN group was 80% at 1 year with a figure of 25% in the control group, the duration of remission in the TPN group being significantly less than in the nonfed group. Collective reviews of these and other reports on this subject have led a number of authors to question and indeed condemn the use of TPN in the cancer patient, their conclusion being that it is the TPN itself which is responsible for the attenuated prognosis in such patients (17,72,73).

Interestingly, some animal model studies have suggested that transfusion-related immunosuppression can be augmented with dietary manipulation based on increased lipid supplementation so that graft survival is improved (71). These studies constitute an exact counterpart to our studies in that a desired outcome—increased immunosuppression—is achieved by the same means, which in the cancer patient produces, or may produce, less resistance to tumor. Several clinical and experimental studies have suggested that the reason for this poorer prognosis is that TPN selectively nourishes the tumor at the expense of the host (74-76). Even cytokines thought to have antitumor potential, e.g., tumor necrosis factor, have sometimes been thought to enhance tumor growth (77). However, bearing in mind the putative physiological role of NK and LAK cells in the surveillance against micrometastasis deposits (78,79), it is tempting to speculate that the impaired maturation of these cytotoxic killer cells which we have observed following TPN may be an additional factor contributing to the rather worse prognosis seen in the parenterally fed patients.

The results of our recent investigation also raise questions concerning the interpretation of the data from our initial study on the effects of lipid-based TPN on lymphocyte function with specific reference to its influence on the production of IL-2. It will be recalled that in both the clinical studies (40,60) we have recorded augmented levels of IL-2 in the supernatants of Con A-activated peripheral blood lymphocytes following days of lipid-based TPN, an effect not seen with the carbohydrate-based regimen. It should be borne in mind that the CTLL-2 bioassay described by Gillis et al. (39) measures free unbound IL-2 which is present in the lymphocyte supernatant at the time of the assay. The free IL-2 content of a given supernatant must represent the residual balance between the IL-2 being elaborated and released by the activated T cells and that which is being bound by preexisting low-affinity receptors or newly generated high-affinity receptors on the surface of the activated T cells. Increased levels of IL-2 in the supernatant may, therefore, reflect not only increased production of IL-2, but also diminished binding of IL-2 to the high-affinity receptor. Accordingly, an alternative interpretation of the data shown in Figure 1 is that there is reduced binding of IL-2 to its receptor rather than increased production. This might have occurred as a consequence of some change occurring either in the expression or function of the IL-2 receptor during the lipid-based TPN. Such a hypothesis would also explain the reduced NK activity observed in vivo during the lipid-based TPN in our second study if it is assumed that IL-2 and other cytokines do play a physiological role in the maintenance of NK activity (80). The reduced capacity to stimulate LAK activity after lipid-based TPN compared with that prior to TPN might also be explained on the same basis.

Because of the known effects of different unsaturated fatty acids on leukocyte membranes in addition to the fact that lipid-emulsions adversely affect polymorph and monocyte function, it seems reasonable to suggest that the lipid emulsion is the component of the TPN regimen which is responsible for these modifications of lymphocyte function. Short-term fatty acid supplementation of volunteers has been shown to reduce cytokine production (81). The provision of at least some lipid is considered necessary to prevent essential fatty acid deficiency and provide nonprotein calories in most TPN regimens. We, therefore, felt that it was important to examine whether or not our hypothesis on the interference by lipid emulsions with IL-2 binding or IL-2 receptor function was tenable on the basis of in vitro studies using defined reagents. In addition, newer lipid formulations which reputedly provide the same number of calories but containing fewer long-chain fatty acids are now available for clinical use (82,83). We wished to investigate whether or not these newer formulations also possessed immunomodulatory properties.

Effects of Lipid Emulsions on Lymphocyte Responses in Vitro

That it was indeed the lipid component of the TPN which was responsible for these changes was established by a preliminary series of experiments in which the glucose, amino acid, and lipid sources were separately added at clinically obtained concentrations to healthy human lymphocyte cultures stimulated with Con A or IL-2. The effects of these components on lymphocyte proliferation and LAK cell induction were measured. Only the lipid emulsion (Intralipid) appeared to influence any of the parameters studied (Fig. 4). We have been unable to reproduce these effects by incorporating equivalent concentrations of either egg phospholipid or glycerol to those present in Intralipid into the cultures. We were thus left with the conclusion that it was the

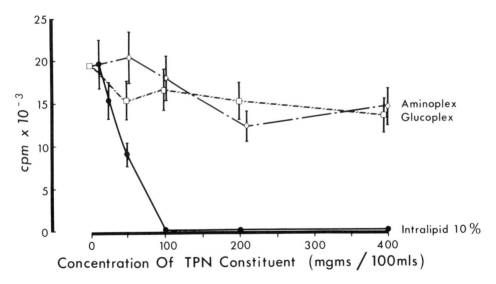

Figure 4 Effects of TPN constituents on generation of Con A blasts in vivo. Peripheral mononuclear cells from healthy donors were stimulated with Con A (20 μg/ml) in the presence of the amino acid source (Aminoplex 12, Geistlich, Chester), the glucose source (Glucoplea) and the lipid source (Intralipid, Kabivitrum, Stockholm). Cultures were harvested at 48 hr after pulsing with [^{3}H]thymidine overnight. Individual points represent mean + s.e. of five separate experiments. Only the Intralipid produces a significant suppression of the response at pharmacological concentrations (<100 mg/100 ml).

fatty acid component of the Intralipid which was exerting these effects. Recently, Kelley et al. (84) have reported that healthy volunteers fed increased alpha-linolenic acid (flax seed oil) showed suppressed lymphocyte response to mitogens and loss of delayed-type hypersensitivity response (skin test) after 56 days of the test diet.

We have, therefore, proceeded to examine these immunological effects in more detail in the presence of several commercially available lipid emulsions, including the standard Intralipid (KabiVitrum, Stockholm), a similar egg phospholipid/soybean emulsion, Lipofundin S (Braun, Melsungen, Germany), and a more recently developed emulsion in which only 50% of the calories are supplied as long-chain triglycerides, the remainder being present as medium-chain (C6-C10) triglycerides, MCT (Braun). In vitro, all three emulsions inhibited lymphocyte proliferation and LAK cell induction. However, as can be seen from Figure 5, these emulsions exert differential effects, the standard emulsions consistently producing greater levels of inhibition of the lymphocyte responses than the MCT. This does not appear to be due to toxicity, since the terminal cell recovery and viability is identical in the experimental cultures to those in the control cultures containing no lipid. Furthermore, the proliferation (as assessed by cell number and [^{3}H]thymidine uptake) of growth factor-independent lymphoblastoid cell lines such as K562, DAUDI and RAJI, is uninfluenced even by suprapharmacological concentrations of these emulsions, again tending to exclude a toxic effect. In contrast, the addition of the lipid emulsions to cultures of the IL-2-dependent murine T-cell line CTLL-2 produces dramatic effects. The proliferation of this clone is grossly impaired by the Intralipid and Lipofundin even at low con-

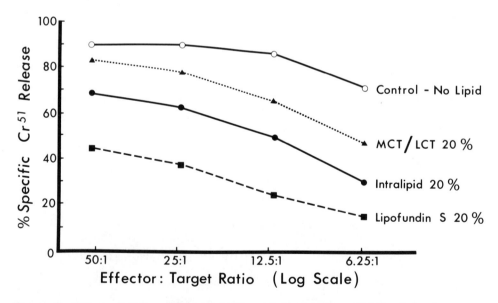

Figure 5 Effects of different lipid emulsions on the generation of LAK cells in vitro. Unfractionated peripheral blood mononuclear cells were incubated with 750 U/ml of recombinant IL-2 for 3 days then assayed in the 51Cr-release assay against Daudi as the tumor target. This is one representative of over 20 experiments in which the medium chain tryglyceride (MCT/LCT) solution consistently produces less inhibition of LAK activity than the standard soybean emulsions Intralipid and Lipofundin S.

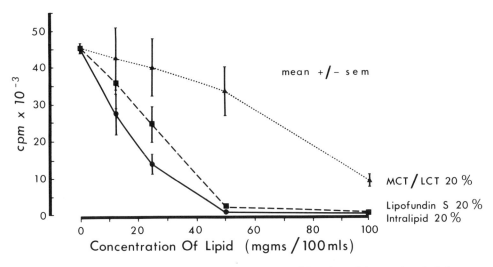

Figure 6 Effects of different lipid emulsions on the proliferation of the murine IL-2-dependent T-cell line CTLL-2 in the presence of a standard concentration of IL-2. Cultures were harvested at 36 hr after an overnight [^{3}H]thymidine pulse. Data points represent mean (+ s.e.) c.p.m. of duplicate wells from three separate experiments. All three lipid emulsions significantly diminish [^{3}H]thymidine uptake by CTLL-2 but the effect is much less marked with the MCT/LCT solutions than with the standard soybean emulsions.

centrations (Fig. 6). A similar trend can be seen with the MCT but is much less marked, a finding which has been consistently reproduced in our laboratory. Furthermore, exactly identical effects on human lymphocyte proliferation have been observed when these emulsions are added to cultures of resting lymphocytes incubated for 3 days in the presence of IL-2, the MCT again having significantly less suppressive influence than the soybean emulsions.

Because the lipid emulsions themselves impair the proliferation of the CTLL-2 cell line upon which the IL-2 bioassay is based, we have not yet been able to examine the effects of the lipid emulsions on IL-2 production in vitro to see if they parallel the in vivo findings. Clearly the carryover of the emulsion in the supernatant would render the interpretation of such experiments difficult. Nonetheless, the in vivo and in vitro evidence would point to the fact that these emulsions do interfere with IL-2 receptor interactions and we are currently examining whether or not the binding or release of other lymphokines such as gamma interferon are impaired in response to such stimuli as IL-2 or the OKT3 monoclonal antibody. If so, then this might indicate a general effect of these emulsions on lymphocyte receptor-ligand interactions. Such a finding would have important implications not only in oncology, but also for the nononcological septic patient who requires TPN because the early events in T-lymphocyte activation are common to other receptor-mediated activation systems such as activation of B cells by B-cell differentiation factor or growth factor (BCDF or BCGF). What then might be the mechanism whereby lipid emulsions interfere with IL-2/receptor binding at the cellular and subcellular level? In order to speculate about the potential mechanism, it is necessary to consider the general nature of the changes which occur during the alteration of the fatty acid profile of cell membranes and also the structure of the IL-2 receptor.

The lipid composition and architecture of the cell membrane play important roles in many aspects of cell physiology. It is considered that the lipid constituents of the cell membrane are in a fluid and homogeneous phase but free fatty acids can readily enter the cell membrane and influence the fluidity of the lipid bilayer (85). cis unsaturated fatty acids particularly can disorder the membrane interior and render the cell membrane more rigid (86). The function of certain cell surface receptors is dependent on their lateral mobility within the cell membrane. Consequently, any maneuvre which rigidifies the cell membrane prevents the lateral movement of these receptors or their components. Support for this contention arises from immunoglobulin capping experiments with murine B cells. In murine B lymphocytes, the incorporation of low concentrations of cis unsaturated fatty acids into the plasma membrane inhibits antibody capping by impairing the cross-linking of the surface immunoglobulin G (IgG) by anti-IgG antibodies (87). This finding has been confirmed using a number of different unsaturated fatty acid substitutions not only using fluorescence microscopy, but also with a flow cytometric technique for continuous monitoring of the lateral movement of B-cell membrane IgG (88). Interestingly, this phenomenon is seen only with unsaturated fatty acids and not following the incorporation of saturated fatty acids into the cell membrane. Clearly then, alteration of membrane fluidity by modifying the lipid composition of lymphocyte cell membranes with unsaturated fatty acids (present in high concentrations in the lipid emulsions used for TPN) can markedly influence receptor-ligand interactions.

The high-affinity IL-2 receptor is a two-chain (α and β) structure possessing external, transmembrane, and intracellular domains (89). Either the α or the β chain can separately bind IL-2 but cannot alone initiate the transmembrane signal. Thus, the α chain and/or the β chain may both represent the low-affinity receptor. When IL-2 is bound (at separate sites) by both the α and the β chains simultaneously, the high-affinity receptor is formed and in the presence of bound IL-2, endocytosis of the receptor-ligand complex occurs and the signal for intracellular T-cell activation is initiated.

If it is presumed that the apposition of the α and β chains depends on their lateral mobility in the cell membrane, any rigidification of the latter would presumably interfere with the aforementioned sequence of events. It is, therefore, possible that the incorporation of unsaturated fatty acids from the lipid emulsions, where they are present in relatively high concentrations, might provide an explanation for the interference with IL-2-mediated reactions described in the clinical and experimental studies described above. Thus, in the two clinical studies, elevated levels of IL-2 in supernatants from lectin-activated lymphocytes following lipid-based TPN might be explained by failure of apposition of the two chains of the IL-2 receptor. If lectin activation stimulates IL-2 production independently of initial receptor binding, then this failure to cobind IL-2 would ultimately lead to a diminished generation of new IL-2 receptor components and result in increased levels of IL-2 in the supernatants. Similarly, the failure of IL-2 to activate NK and LAK cells in the second clinical study might also be explained on the same basis. Finally, this hypothesis is an attractive explanation for the in vitro studies described above, the advantage conferred by the MCT solutions simply resulting from the fact that these solutions contain fewer of the long-chain unsaturated fatty acids. However, the in vitro findings with MCT have been confirmed in a further trial in which the MCT was found to be less suppressive of NK-cell activation with IL-2 (measured as LAK cytotoxicity) than a regimen containing either Intralipid or no lipid as the calorie source (see Fig. 6) (Sedman, Somers, Ramsden, Brennan & Guillou, 1991).

Much of the above hypothesis is, of course, speculative. Its validity hinges on at least two premises: First, that the unsaturated fatty acids present in the lipid emulsions are incorporated into the lymphocyte cell membranes under the conditions described, and second that even if incorporated, they do increase the rigidity of the plasma membrane, an fact that is by no means undisputed (90). Few studies are available which indicate whether or not the unsaturated fatty acids present in lipid emulsions are incorporated into the cell membranes. Most of the fatty acids in these emulsions are present as the unsaturated fatty acids, linoleic (C18:2, 48%), oleic (C18:1, 26%), and linolenic (C18:3, 8%), with the saturated fatty acids, palmitic and stearic, constituting 12 and 4%, respectively, of the remaining triglyceride-derived fatty acid pattern. One study has suggested that the concentration of linoleic acid in lymphocyte phospholipids was increased in four newborns fed relatively low doses of Intralipid over 1 month (91). We are currently examining lymphocyte membrane lipid profiles of cells activated in vitro in the presence of the various lipid emulsions and in TPN-treated patients in an endeavour to verify this. However, the binding of other growth factors such as transferrin to their receptors is also important for lymphocyte proliferation. Cascade phenomena dominate lymphocyte activation and the binding of this molecule to its receptors, which also consists of two subunits, may equally be influenced by membrane rigidification and merits investigation. Although it is possible to assume that a primary effect of lipids would be mediated through effects on accessibility of substrates to the cyclo-oxygenase and lipoxygenase enzyme systems, recent studies of Santoli and Zurier (92) and those discussed previously (66,80) clearly indicate that suppression, in particular of IL-2 production (92) generated by fatty acids, is actually independent of changes in cyclo-oxygenase products.

CONCLUSIONS

Biological Implications

The opportunity to investigate the effects of lymphocyte function of lipid emulsions administered to both malnourished and nonmalnourished patients has provided us with the impetus to learn more about the complex relationship between the cell membrane lipid profile and its function. Most of the above discussion has centered on the effects of incorporation of unsaturated fatty acids into membrane phospholipids and has at least provided us with a working explanation of our observations and the way in which plasmalemmal lipids may be involved in the control of cellular activation. This hypothesis would fit with the elegant concept of receptor capping described by Klausner et al. (86). Whether or not it proves to be correct awaits further investigation. However, it is becoming clear that phospholipids and cholesterol may also be of considerable importance in determining, for example, the resistance or susceptibility of target cells to humoral or cell-mediated lysis (65,93,94). Modification of the lipid components of the lymphocyte membrane may also imbue different lymphocytes with a number of other different properties. For example, the treatment of lymphoid cells with phospholipases also influences the mechanism of lymphocyte traffic in murine systems, again implying that the lipid components of the lymphocyte membrane are important for the cell-to-cell interactions involved in regulating cell migration (95).

The events which result in the sequence of activation of lymphocytes may be common to other lymphocyte/growth factor interactions. Thus, not only T-cell and NK cell interactions may be modified by fatty acids, but also those of B cells with BCDF and IL-4. Furthermore, although we report a direct interference of lipid emulsion with the binding of IL-2 to its receptor, it may be that some of the suppression of lymphocyte proliferation by polyunsaturated fatty acids is mediated via inhibition of accessory cell function. Good evidence exists to support the contention that lipid emulsions impair monocyte function, but an important question is whether or not interleukin 1 production is diminished. This remains to be seen, but the opportunity to modify cell membrane lipids both in vivo and in vitro continues to excite considerable interest and provide important insights into lymphoreticular physiology at the cellular and molecular levels.

CONCLUSIONS

Clinical Implications

Perhaps the most important clinical implication to be derived from the observations described in this review is that the standard lipid emulsions should not be administered to patients being considered for adoptive cellular immunotherapy with autologous lymphokine-activated killer cells. As yet, we are unsure as to whether non lipid-based TPN, which has its own effects on plasma triglycerides, induces changes in lymphocyte function in vivo. In the clinical trial cited above, lymphocyte responses were studied in patients randomized to receive no lipid, or a standard lipid emulsion or MCT as their lipid source. Accepting the necessity for at least some fat in the regimen, we were particularly interested to see the results with the MCT (Fig. 6) in view of the in vitro results we have obtained with this material. Similarly, whether or not MCT influences monocyte and polymorph function as adversely as do the standard lipid emulsions is currently under investigation in our laboratory.

Whether or not lipid emulsions change circulating levels of plasma lipoproteins is unclear. Plasma lipoproteins are immunosuppressive but, in vitro at least, the suppressive influences of plasma lipoprotein are negated by transferrin when present at levels close to those normally found in plasma (3). However, since plasma transferrin is often diminished in malnutrition, a complex state of affairs may exist in vivo.

The suggestion that TPN in the cancer patient impairs cellular cytotoxic mechanisms which normally act to scavenge micrometastatic tumor cells would support recently expressed views that wherever possible TPN should be avoided altogether in such patients. Other data exist which obliquely fit with this contention. Attempts to diminish fatal atherosclerotic events by taking a diet rich in polyunsaturated fat reduced the death rate from arterial disease compared with that in controls, but unfortunately the total mortality in the two groups was identical because of a statistically significant increase in the incidence of fatal cancer in the men taking the polyunsaturated fat diet (96). A tempting explanation for this finding is that the diet might have impaired the capacity to generate normal levels of cytotoxic antitumor cell activity. Dietary lipid can certainly modulate the effects of other biological response modifiers in experimental tumor models (97), and thus such a suggestion might be less naive than appears at first sight. On the other hand, manipulation of membrane fatty acid composition can alter lymphocyte localization in vivo (95,99), and this could perhaps be exploited for directing activated killer cells to sites of preference for metastasis such as the liver and lungs.

The availability of lipid emulsions for therapeutic administration has raised new questions and opened numerous avenues for their exploitation as biological response modifiers. Much of the available data are, however, contradictory and more detailed work with defined reagents is required at the cellular, molecular, and clinical levels before these studies can be placed in their proper perspective.

REFERENCES

1. Curtis ASG, Campbell J, Shaw FM (1975). Cell surface lipids and adhesion. I. The effects of lysophosphatidyl compounds, phospholipase A2 and aggregation-inhibiting protein. J Cell Sci 18:347.
2. Curtis ASG, Shaw FM, Spires VMC (1975). Cell surface lipids and adhesion. II. The turnover of lipid components of the plasmalemma in relation to cell adhesion. J Cell Sci 18:357.
3. Harmony JAK, Akeson AL, McCarthy BM, Morris RE, Scupham DW, Grupp SA (1986). Immunoregulation by plasma lipoproteins. In: Biochemistry and Biology of Plasma Lipoproteins. AM Scanu, AA Spector, eds. Marcell Dekker New York.
4. Foegh ML, Thomas G, Ramwell PW (1990). Free radicals, arachidonic acid metabolites, and nutrition. J Parenter Enter Nutr 14:244S.
5. Sedman PC, Monson JRT, Ramsden CW, Giles GR, Brennan TG, Guillou PJ (1987). Malnutrition adversely affects non-specific immunity but not tumor-directed cellular cytotoxicity in patients with gastrointestinal cancer (abstract). Br J Surg 74:1147.
6. Anderson CE, Lionnroth IC, Gelin LJ, Moldawer LL, Lundholm KG (1991). Pretranscriptional regulation of albumin synthesis in tumor-bearing mice. The role of anorexia and malnutrition. Gastroenterology 100:938.
7. Knox LS, Crosby LO, Feurer ID, Buzby GP, Miller CL, Mullen JL (1983). Energy expenditure in malnourished cancer patients. Ann Surg 197:152.
8. Chadwick SJD, Sim AJW, Dudley HAF (1986). Changes in plasma fibronectin during acute nutritional deprivation in healthy human subjects. Br J Nutr 55:7.
9. Dowd PS, Kelleher J, Walker BE, Guillou PJ (1986). Nutrition and cellular immunity in hospital patients. Br J Nutr 55:515.
10. Meakins JL, Pietsch JB, Bubenick O, et al. (1977). Delayed hypersensitivity: Indicator of acquired failure of host defenses in sepsis and trauma. Ann Surg 186:241.
11. Christou NV, Superina R, Broadhead M, Meakins JL (1982). Postoperative depression of host resistance: determinants and effect of peripheral protein-sparing therapy. Surgery 92:786.
12. Christou N (1990). Perioperative nutritional support: Immunologic defects. J Parenter Enteral Nutr 14:186S.
13. Copeland EM, MacFayden BV, Dudrick SJ (1976). Effects of intravenous hyperalimentation on established delayed hypersensitivity in the cancer patient. Ann Surg 184:60.
14. Haffejee AA, Angorn IB (1979). Nutritional status and the nonspecific cellular and humoral immune response in esophageal carcinoma. Ann Surg 189:475.
15. Copeland EM, Daley JM, Ota DM, Dudrick SJ (1979). Nutrition, cancer and intravenous hyperalimentation. Cancer 43:2108.
16. Muller JM, Brenner U, Dienst C, Pichlmaier H (1982). Preoperative parenteral feeding in patients with gastrointestinal carcinoma. Lancet 1:68.
17. Klein S, Simes J, Blackburn GL (1986). Total parenteral nutrition and cancer clinical trails. Cancer 58:1378.
18. Reynolds JV, Daly JM, Shou J, Sigel R, Ziegler MM, Naji A (1990). Immunologic effects of arginine supplementation in tumor-bearing and non tumor bearing hosts. Ann Surg 211:202.

19. Daly JM, Reynolds J, Sigel RK, Shou J, Liberman MD (1990). Effect of dietary protein and amino acids on immune function. Crit Care Med 18:586.
20. Nordenstrom J, Askanazi J, Elwyn DH et al. (1983). Nitrogen balance during total parenteral nutrition. Ann Surg 197:27.
21. MacFayden BV, Dudrick SJ, Tagudar EP, Maynard AT, Law DK, Rhoads JE (1973). Triglyceride and free fatty acid clearances in patients receiving complete parenteral nutrition using a ten percent soybean oil emulsion. SGO 137:813.
22. Press M, Kikuchi H, Shimoyama T, Thompson GR (1974). Diagnosis of essential fatty acid deficiency in man. Br Med J 2:247.
23. Tweedle DEF (1978). The use of fat emulsions in parenteral nutrition. In: Advances in Parenteral Nutrition. IDA Johnston, ed, MTP Press, Lancaster, England.
24. Freund U, Krausz Y, Levij IS, Eliakim M (1975). Introgenic lipidosis following prolonged intravenous hyperalimentation. Am J Clin Nutr 28:1156.
25. Berken A, Benacerraf B (1968). Depression of reticuloendothelial phagocytic function by ingested lipids. Proc Soc Exp Biol Med 128:793.
26. Mertin J, Hughes D (1975). Specific inhibitory action of polyunsaturated fatty acids on lymphocyte transformation induced by PHA and PPD. Int Archs Allergy Appl Immunol 48:203.
27. Mandel G, Shimizu S, Gill R, Clark W (1978). Alteration of the fatty acid composition of membrane phospholipids in mouse lymphoid cells. J Immunol 120:1631.
28. Mandel G, Clark W (1978). Functional properties of EL-4 tumor cells with lipid-altered membranes. J Immunol 120:1637.
29. Ota DM, Copeland EM, Corriere JN, Richie EK, Jacobson K, Dudrick SJ (1978). The effects of a 70% Soybean emulsion on lymphocyte transformation. J Parenter Enter Nutr 2:112.
30. Nordenstrom, J, Jarstrand C, Wiernik A (1979). Decreased chemotactic and random migration of leukocytes during intralipid infusion. Am J Clin Nutr 32:2416.
31. Hawley HP, Gordon GB (1976). The effects of long-chain free fatty acids on human neutrophil function and structure. Lab Invest 34:216.
32. Cleary TG, Pickering LK (1983). Mechanisms of intralipid effect on polymorphonuclear leukocytes. J Clin Lab Immunol 11:21.
33. Fraser I, Neoptolemos J, Woods P, Bowry V, Bell PRF (1983). The effect of intralipid on human lymphocyte and monocyte function. Clin Nutr 2:37.
34. Fraser I, Neoptolemos J, Darby H, Bell PRF (1984). The effects of Intralipid and Heparin on human monocyte and lymphocyte function. J Parenter Enter Nutr 8:381.
35. Fisher GW, Hunter KW, Wilson SR, Mease AD (1980). Diminished bacterial defences with intralipid. Lancet 2:819.
36. Spratt MG, Kratzing CC (1975). Oleic acid as a depressant of reticuloendothelial activity in rats and mice. J Reticuloendoth. Soc 17:135.
37. Palmblad J, Brostrom O, Lahnborg G, Uden AM, Venizelos N (1982). Neutrophil functions during total parenteral nutrition and intralipid infusion. Am J Clin Nutr 35:1430.
38. Ota DM, Jessup JM, Babcock GF, Kirschbaum L, Mountain CF, McMurtrey MJ, Copeland, EM (1985). Immune function during intravenous administration of a soybean oil emulsion. J Parenter Enter Nutr 9:23.
39. Gillis S, Ferns MM, Ou W, Smith KA (1978). T-cell growth factor: Parameters of production and a quantitative microassay for activity. J Immunol 120:2027.
40. Monson JRT, Ramsden CW, MacFie J, Brennan TG, Guillou PJ (1986). Immunorestorative effect of lipid emulsions during total parenteral nutrition. Br J Surg 73:843.
41. Guillou PJ (1987). Potential impact of immunobiotechnology on cancer therapy. Br J Surg 74:705.
42. Lotze M, Grimm EA, Mazumder A, Strausser JL, Rosenberg SA (1981). Lysis of fresh and cultured autologous tumor by human lymphocytes cultured in T-cell growth factor. Cancer Res 41:4420.

43. Grimm EA, Mazumder A, Zhang HZ, Rosenberg SA (1982). Lymphokine-activated killer cell phenomenon. Lysis of NK resistant fresh solid tumor cells by IL-2 activated human peripheral blood lymphocytes. J Exp Med 155:1823.
44. Rosenberg SA, Lotze MT, Muul LM, Chang AE, Avis FP, Leitman S, Linchan WM, Robertson CN, Lee RE, Rubin JT, Seipp CA, Simpson CG and White DE (1987). A progress report on the treatment of 157 patients with advanced cancer using lymphokine-activated killer cells and interleukin 2 or high dose interleukin 2 alone. N Engl J Med 316:889.
45. West WH, Tauer KW, Yannelli JR, Marshall GD, Orr DW, Thurman GB, Oldham RK (1987). Constant infusion recombinant interleukin-2 in adoptive immunotherapy of advanced cancer. N Engl J Med 316:895.
46. Eberlein TJ, Rosenstein M, Rosenberg SA (1982). Regression of a disseminated syngeneic solid tumor by systemic transfer of lymphoid cells expanded in interleukin 2. J Exp Med 156:385.
47. Lafreniere R, Rosenberg SA (1985). Successful immunotherapy of murine experimental metastases with lymphokine-activated killer cells and recombinant interleukin-2. Cancer Res 45:3735.
48. Papa MZ, Mule JJ, Rosenberg SA (1986). Antitumour efficacy of lymphokine-activated killer cells and recombinant interleukin-2 in vivo. Successful immunotherapy of established pulmonary metastases from weakly immunogenic and non-immunogenic murine tumours of three distinct histological types. Cancer Res 46:4973.
49. Mule JJ, Yang J, Shu S, Rosenberg SA (1986). The anti-tumour efficacy of lymphokine-activated killer cells and recombinant interleukin 2 in vivo. Direct correlation between reductions of established metastases and cytolytic activity of lymphokine-activated killer cells. J Immunol 136:3899.
50. Guillou PJ, Brennan TG, Giles GR (1973). PHA-stimulative transformation of peripheral and lymph node lymphocytes in patients with gastrointestinal cancer. Br J Surg 60:745.
51. Guillou PJ, Brennan TG, Giles GR (1975). A study of lymph nodes draining colorectal cancer using a two stage inhibition of migration technique. Gut 16:290.
52. Monson JRT, Ramsden CW, Guillou PJ (1986). Decreased interleukin 2 production in patients with gastrointestinal cancer. Br J Surg 73:483.
53. Monson JRT, Ramsden CW, Giles GR, Brennan TG, Guillou PJ (1987). Lymphokine activated killer (LAK) cells in patients with gastrointestinal cancer. Gut 28:1420.
54. Balch CM, Tilden AB, Dougherty PA, Cloud GA, Abo T (1984). Heterogeneity of natural killer lymphocyte abnormalities in colon cancer patients. Surgery 95:63.
55. Ortaldo JR, Mason A, Overton R (1986). Lymphokine activated killer cells. Analysis of progenitors and effectors. J Exp Med 164:1193.
56. Phillips JH, Lanier LL (1986). Dissection of the lymphokine-activated killer phenomenon. Relative contribution of peripheral blood natural killer cells and T lymphocytes to cytolysis. J Exp Med 164:814.
57. Sedman PC, Giles GR, Brennan TG, Ramsden CW, Guillou PJ (1988). Augmentation of lymphokine activated killer cell activity inpatients with gastrointestinal cancer. Br J Surg 75:591-594.
58. Mcleod GRC, Thomson DB, Hersey P (1987). Recombinant interferon alfa-2a in advanced malignant melanoma. A phase I-II study in combination with DTIC. Int J Cancer (Suppl. 1):31.
59. Guillou PJ, Sedman PC (1987). The use of recombinant interferon alfa-2a in combination with decarbazine in patients with advanced malignant melanoma. Interferons, Today Tomorrow 4:4.
60. Monson JRT, Sedman PC, Ramsden CW, Brennan TG, Guillou PJ (1988). Total parenteral nutrition adversely influences tumour-directed cellular cytotoxic responses in patients with gastrointestinal cancer. Eur J Surg Oncol 14:435.
61. Barone J, Herbert JR, Reddy MM (1989). Dietary fat and natural killer cell activity. Am J Clin Nutr 50:861.

62. Herbert JR, Barone J, Reddy MM, Backlund JY (1990). Natural killer cell activity in a longitudinal dietary fat intervention trial. Clin Immunol Immunopathol 54:103.
63. Rice C, Hudig D, Newton RS, Mendelsohn J (1981). Effect of unsaturated fatty acids on human lymphocytes: Disparate influences of oleic and linoleic acids on natural cytotoxicity. Clin Immunol Immunopathol 20:389.
64. Roozemond RC, Bonavida B (1985). Effect of altered membrane fluidity on NK-mediated cytotoxicity I. Selective inhibition of the recognition or post-recognition events in the cytolytic pathway of NK cells. J Immunol 134:2209.
65. Roozemond RC, Mevissen M, Urli DC, Bonavida B (1987). Effect of altered membrane fluidity on NK mediated cytotoxicity. III. Decreased susceptibility to natural killer cytotoxic factor (NKCF) and suppression of NKCF release by membrane rigidification. J Immunol 139:1739.
66. Meydani SN, Endres S, Woods MM, Goldin BR, Soo C, Morrill-Labrode A, Dinarello CA, Gorbach SC (1991). Oral (n-3) fatty acid supplementation suppresses cytokine production and lymphocyte proliferation: Comparison between young and older women. J Nutri 121:547.
67. Heatley RV, Williams RHP, Lewis MH (1979). Preoperative intravenous feeding—a controlled clinical trial. Postgrad Med J 55:541.
68. Copeland EM, Daley JM, Dudrick SJ (1977). Nutrition as an adjunct to cancer treatment in the adult. Cancer Res 37:2451.
69. Nixon DW, Moffit S, Lawson DH et al. (1981). Total parenteral nutrition as an adjunct to chemotherapy of metastatic colorecal cancer. Cancer Treat Rep 65:121.
70. Shamberger RC, Brennan MF, Goodman JT, et al. A prospective randomized study of adjuvant parenteral nutrition in the treatment of sarcomas: results of metabolic and survival studies. Surgery 1984, 96:1.
71. Perez RV, Manda R, Alexander JW (1988). Dietary immunoregulation of transfusion-induced immunosuppression. Transplant 45:614.
72. Fischer JE (1984). Adjuvant parenteral nutrition in the patient with cancer. Surgery 96:578.
73. Koretz RL (1984). Parenteral nutrition: Is it oncologically logical? J Clin Oncol 2:534.
74. Buzby GP, Mullen JL, Stein TP, Miller EE, Hobbs CL, Rosato EF (1980). Host-tumour: interaction and nutrient supply. Cancer 45:2940.
75. Popp MB, Wagner SC, Brito OJ (1983). Host and tumor responses to increasing levels of intravenous nutritional support. Surgery 94:300.
76. Popp MB, Kirkemo AK, Morrison SD, Brennan MF (1984). Tumour and host carcass changes during total parenteral nutrition in an anorectic rat tumour system. Ann Surg 199:205.
77. Gelin J, Moldawer LL, Lionnroth C, Sherry E, Chizzonite R, Lundholm L (1991). Role of endogenous tumor necrosis factor and interleukin 1 for experimental tumor growth and the development of cancer cachexia. Can Res 51:415.
78. Hanna N, Fidler IJ (1980). Role of natural killer cells in destruction of circulating tumour emboli. J Natl Cancer Inst 65:801.
79. Wiltrout RH, Herberman RB, Zhang SR, Chirigios MA et al. (1985). Role of organ-associated NK cells in decreased formation of experimental metastases in lung and liver. J Immunol 134:4267.
80. Domzig W, Stadler BM, Herberman RB (1983). Interleukin 2 dependence of human natural killer (NK) cell activity. J Immunol 130:1970.
81. Endres S, Ghorbani R, Kelley VE, Greorgilis K, Lonnemann G, Van Der Meer JWM, Gannon JG, Rogers TS, Klempner MS, Weber PC, Schaefer EJ, Wolff SM, Dinarello CA (1989). The effect of dietary supplementation with N-3 polyunsaturated fatty acids on the synthesis of interleukin-1 and tumor necrosis factor by mononuclear cells. N Engl J Med 320:265.

82. Eckart J, Adolph M, Van der Muhlen U, Naab V (1980). Fat emulsions containing medium chain triglycerides in parenteral nutrition of intensive care patients. J Parenter Enter Nutr 4:360.
83. Kolb S, Sailer D (1984). Effect of fat emulsions containing medium-chain triglycerides and glucose on ketone body production and excretion. J Parenter Enter Nutr 8:281.
84. Kelley DS, Branch LB, Love JE, Tayler PC, Rivera YM, Iacona JM (1991). Dietary alpha-lenolenic acid and immunocompetence in humans. Am J Clin Nutr 53:40.
85. Stubbs CD, Tsang W, Belin J, Smith AD, Johnson SM (1980). Incubation of exogenous fatty acids with lymphocytes. Changes in fatty acid composition and effects on the rotational relaxation time of 1,6-Diphenyl-1,3,5-Hexatriene. Biochemistry 19:2756.
86. Klausner RD, Kleinfeld AM, Hoover RL, Karnovsky MJ (1980). Lipid domains in membranes. Evidence derived from structural perturbations induced by free fatty acids and lifetime heterogeneity analysis. J Biol Chem 255:1286.
87. Klausner RD, Bhalla DK, Dragsten P, Hoover RL, Karnovsky MJ (1980). Model for capping derived from inhibition of surface receptor capping by free fatty acids. Proc Natl Acad Sci USA 77:437.
88. Wang Yang, M-C, Cuchens MA, Buttke TM (1986). Kinetics of membrane immunoglobulin capping on murine B-lymphocytes. Effects of phospholipid fatty acid replacement. J Biol Chem 261:3320.
89. Green WC (1987). An overview of the human interleukin-2 receptor: Molecular, biochemical and functional properties. Cancer Invest 5:369.
89a. Sedman PC, Somers SS, Ramsden CW, Brennan TG, Guillon PJ (1991). Effects of different lipid emulsions on lymphocyte function during total parenteral nutrition. Br J Surg 78:1396.
90. McVey E, Yguerabide J, Hanson DC, Clark WR (1981). The relationship between plasma membrane lipid composition and physico-chemical properties. I. Fluorescence polarization studies of fatty acid altered EL-4 tumor cell membranes. Biochim Biophys Acta: 642: 106.
91. Andersen GE, Christiensen NC, Johansen KB (1985). Fatty acid changes in plasmal lipids and lymphocyte phospholipids after infusion of intralipid to newborns. J Parenter Enter Nutr 9:691.
92. Santoli D and Zurier RB (1989). Prostaglandin E precursor FAs inhibit human IL-2 production by a prostaglandin E — independent mechanism. J Immunol 143:1303.
93. Schlager SI, Ohanian SH (1980). Tumour cell lipid composition and sensitivity to humoral immune killing. I. Modification of cellular lipid and fatty acid content by metabolic inhibitors and hormones. J Immunol 124:626.
94. Yoo T-J, Kuo C-Y, Spector AA, Denning GM et al. (1982). Effect of fatty acid modification of cultured hepatoma cells on susceptibility to natural killer cells. Cancer Res. 42: 3596.
95. Freitas AA, de Sousa M (1976). Control mechanism of lymphocyte traffic. Altered migration of 51Cr-labelled mouse lymph node cells pre-treated in vitro with phospholipases. Eur J Immunol 6:703.
96. Pearce ML, Dayton S (1971). Incidence of cancer in men on a diet high in polyunsaturated fat. Lancet 1:464.
97. Boeryd B, Hallgren B (1985). The fat composition of a mouse diet modifies the effects of levamisol on growth and spread of a murine tumour. Acta Pathol Microbiol Immunol Scand 93:99.
98. Novo C, Fonseca E, Freitas AA (1987). Altered fatty-acid membrane composition modifies lymphocyte localization in vivo. Cell Immunol 106:387.

24
Acquired Zinc Deficiency and Immune Dysfunction in Sickle Cell Anemia

Ananda S. Prasad
*Wayne State University School of Medicine,
Detroit, Michigan*

INTRODUCTION

Certain dietary components have now been shown to alter immune single system outcome beyond the level of preventing or correcting a deficiency. The use of therapeutic nutritional support is currently evolving with the recognition that the clinical outcome can be significantly affected (1,2). Work described here was initiated over 15 years ago, and provides an example of nutritional intervention in a complex clinical setting.

In this chapter, evidence supporting the conclusion that zinc deficiency occurs in sickle cell anemia (SCA) patients is presented, and also the effects of zinc supplementation on clinical, biochemical, and immunological parameters in these patients will be described. Recent studies have shown that zinc deficiency in humans may result in abnormalities of cellular immunity (3-5) and that a key thymic factor, thymulis, is zinc dependent (6). In this chapter, a summary of immune abnormalities in SCA related to zinc deficiency is also provided and a presentation of the effects of zinc supplementation (7) is discussed.

Clinical Similarities Between SCA Patients and Zinc-Deficient Subjects as Described from the Middle East

Certain clinical features are common to some SCA patients and zinc-deficient subjects, the latter reported from the Middle East Prasad et al 1975 (8). These features include delayed onset of puberty and hypogonadism in the males, characterized by decreased facial, pubic, and axillary hair, short stature and low body weight, rough skin, and poor appetite.

The presence of chronic leg ulcers which usually present problems in healing may also be a feature of zinc deficiency in SCA subjects. Inasmuch as zinc is an important constituent of erythrocytes, it appeared possible that long continued hemolysis in patients with SCA might lead to a zinc-deficient state by increasing both zinc loss and daily zinc requirement. Patients from the Harper-Grace Hospitals (Detroit Medical Center) Sickle Cell Adult Clinic were studied. Thirty-eight men and 46 women were included in this study. The diagnosis of SCA was established by history, physical examination, and hematological studies, which included electrophoresis of hemoglobin on cellulose acetate and quantitative determination of A_2, fetal (F), and S hemoglobins. Hemoglobin electrophoresis revealed the S-S pattern; quantitation of A_2 hemoglobin gave normal values and F hemoglobin was less than 20% in all our cases.

Height was retarded (less than 3 SD from the normal mean) in six men and five women. Sixty-seven of the SCA patients in this sample were below the fiftieth percentile from the normal mean for weight. Twenty-eight men showed a lack of facial and body hair, and five additional subjects showed only scanty facial hair.

Although the majority of our patients (31 of 84) were between the ages of 16 and 20 years, four subjects were more than 50 years old and seven were between 40 and 70 years old.

Chronically active leg ulcers were present in seven patients. The majority of our subjects had rough skin, and they gave a history of poor appetite.

ZINC LEVELS IN PLASMA, RED BLOOD CELLS, HAIR, NEUTROPHILS, AND URINE IN SCA PATIENTS

The results of zinc analysis have been presented in detail elsewhere (8,9). As such, only a brief summary will be provided here. In a larger study in 84 SCA subjects, plasma and red cell zinc were (mean ± SD) 104 ± 10.5 μg/dl and 34.0 ± 7.0 μg/g Hb in comparison to 70 controls, who were 113 ± 13.6 μg/dl and 40.0 ± 4.0 μg/g Hb, respectively. The differences between the two groups were highly significant statistically ($p < 0.001$). Likewise, hair zinc in SCA patients was 121 ± 30 μg/g in comparison to controls, who were 190 ± 17 μg/g ($p < 0.001$). We also documented hyperzincuria in SCA patients in an earlier study (8-10).

ACTIVITY OF ZINC-DEPENDENT ENZYMES IN SCA

We have so far investigated the activities of plasma ribonuclease (RNase), leukocyte alkaline phosphatase, deoxythymidine kinase in newly synthesized collagen tissue, and the carbonic anhydrase content of red cells in SCA patients.

Zinc is an inhibitor of RNase activity and its activity is known to increase in zinc-deficient tissue (8). We have reported earlier that the activity of plasma RNase in SCA patients is increased in comparison to the controls (0.435 ± 0.002 vs 0.31 ± 0.001 $\triangle$OD/min/ml, $p < 0.001$).

Neutrophil alkaline phosphatase in human subjects is a zinc metalloenzyme (10, 11). Neutrophil alkaline phosphatase activity in SCA patients is decreased significantly in comparison to the controls (12). On zinc supplementation, the activity of neutrophil alkaline phosphatase increased; and when the zinc supplementation was discontinued, the activity declined. This suggests that measurement of neutrophil alkaline phosphatase activity may provide a good assessment of body zinc status. Zinc supplementation in our subjects, however, did not result in restoration of neutrophil alkaline phosphatase activity to completely normal levels. This may have been due to inadequate zinc supplementation or poor compliance in some of our subjects.

The conversion of deoxythymidine to deoxythymidine 5'-monophosphate (dTMP), a precursor of thymidine triphosphate (TTP), is dependent on deoxythymidine kinase (DTHD kinase). Our previous studies in experimental animals have shown that as early as 6 days on the zinc-deficient diet, the activity of DTHD kinase was considerably reduced in the implanted sponge connective tissue, and this reduced activity was accompanied by decreased protein and collagen synthesis in the rats (13).

Following local anesthesia, one polyvinyl sponge measuring approximately 4 cm × 3 cm × 3 mm was implanted subcutaneously on the lateral wall of the chest in four SCA subjects. Twenty-one days after implantation, the sponges were isolated by blunt dissection, and the capsules surrounding the sponge were collected for study (14). In SCA subjects, DTHD kinase activity was not measurable, and RNA/DNA, total collagen, and total protein contents were significantly decreased as compared to normal controls.

Carbonic anhydrase is a zinc metalloenzyme. We measured red cell carbonic anhydrase protein and its isozymes I and II by a radioimmunosorbent technique (8) in patients with SCA and controls. Our results showed a significant correlation ($r = 0.94$, $p < 0.001$) between carbonic anhydrase and red cell zinc. Carbonic anhydrase and red cell zinc were both decreased in SCA subjects. Thus, the results of assays of zinc-dependent enzymes such as plasma RNase, leukocyte alkaline phosphatase, deoxythymidine kinase in newly synthesized connective tissue, and carbonic anhydrase in red cells supported our conclusion that zinc deficiency existed in SCA adult patients.

EFFECTS OF ZINC SUPPLEMENTATION ON ENDOCRINOLOGICAL FUNCTIONS IN SCA PATIENTS

Ambulatory stable male patients between the ages of 16 to 28 years with homozygous sickle cell disease were included in this study (14a). In the first experiment, four patients received placebo for 12 months, following which zinc (15 mg t.i.d. as zinc acetate) was administered orally for 12 months in a double-blind fashion. The endocrinologist (Dr. A.A. Abbasi) and the patients were blinded as to the type of supplementation being given. Likewise, the laboratory personnel involved with the hormone and zinc assays were not aware of the treatment plan.

Besides routine hematological studies, special tests included zinc determination in the plasma and neutrophils, alkaline phosphatase activity measured quantitatively in the neutrophils, basal serum follicle-stimulating hormone (FSH), luteinizing hormone (LH), testosterone, and dihydrotestosterone levels, which were carried out every 12 weeks.

Every 24 weeks, the hormones were assayed following IV administration of gonadotropin-releasing hormone (GnRH). Blood samples were drawn between 8 and 9 a.m. for the determination of serum testosterone, FSH, and LH. Synthetic GnRH, 0.2 mg (luteinizing hormone-releasing hormone) was injected IV over a 30-sec period, and blood samples were drawn from an indwelling intravenous catheter using a throughway stopcock, before the administration of GnRH and 15, 30, 60, 120, 180, and 240 min later, for the determination of serum FSH and LH levels. Serum testosterone levels were also measured before the injection of GnRh and 60, 120, 180, and 240 min later. For each test, the average of all five serum testosterone values was determined first and then group evaluation was made. Blood samples were refrigerated and centrifuged at the end of each test. Serum was separated and frozen at $-10\,°C$. Serum LH, FSH, and testosterone were measured by radioimmunoassay techniques (15-17).

In the second experiment, 14 patients were divided into two groups. Seven patients received placebo (group A) orally and seven received oral zinc (group B), 15 mg, three times a day as acetate. Both groups were age matched and the study was conducted in a double-blind fashion.

The first three patients in both groups received the supplementation for 12 months. The other three pairs of patients were supplemented for 6 months and one pair received the supplementation for 18 months. The periods for supplementation were varied in order to determine the length of time necessary for the supplementation to produce its maximum effects on serum testosterone levels.

In the second experiment, basal serum testosterone and dihydrotestosterone, plasma zinc, neutrophil zinc, and neutrophil alkaline phosphatase activity were assayed every 8 weeks. Following intravenous administration of GnRH, serum testosterone and dihydrotestosterone were measured at 0, 60, 120, 180 and 240 mins. This test was done every 12 weeks. In three group B patients, zinc supplementation was discontinued for 6 months and its effect on the above parameters were reassessed.

The controls for these studies were healthy age-matched individuals of both races. We have not observed any significant difference between the black and white individuals with respect to zinc and hormone levels in our previous study (18).

The data were analyzed by a simple t test and paired t test by the methods of Snedecor and Cochran (19).

In the *first* experiment, plasma zinc, neutrophil zinc, and neutrophil alkaline phosphatase activity increased significantly following zinc supplementation in comparison to the results obtained during placebo administration. Similarly, basal serum testosterone and mean serum testosterone level following administration of GnRH also increased following supplementation with zinc. In general, in response to GnRH administration, plasma levels of LH and FSH decreased following zinc supplementation in comparison to the values obtained during placebo administration.

Three out of four patients had 2+ to 3+ growth of pubic hair during placebo administration. One patient had normal pubic hair growth (4+). Following supplementation with zinc, for 1 year all three showed an increase in growth of pubic hair. Three patients who were tall and eunuchoid showed no effect in height, but one, who was 164.5 cm tall during placebo administration, grew 5.5 cm on zinc supplementation for 1 year. Weight gain (mean ± SD) during placebo treatment was 1.0 ± 1.13 kg, whereas following zinc supplementation, the gain in weight was 5.03 ± 1.5 kg ($p < 0.01$).

In the *second* experiment in which 14 subjects were involved, the effect of zinc supplementation appeared to be maximal at the end of 6 months with respect to basal testosterone, DHT, plasma zinc, neutrophil zinc, and neutrophil alkaline phosphatase activity; as such the data for 6, 12, and 18 months were combined for statistical evaluation. Zinc supplementation resulted in a significant increase in the serum testosterone level, plasma zinc, neutrophil zinc, and neutrophil alkaline phosphatase activity. The maximum level of serum testosterone and mean serum testosterone level following GnRH administration also showed a significant increase following zinc supplementation. In three patients (group B), zinc supplementation was discontinued for six months and additional follow up data were obtained. This resulted in a significant decrease in serum testosterone, neutrophil zinc and neutrophil alkaline phosphatase activity. The maximum level of serum testosterone and mean serum testosterone level following GnRH use also declined as a result of discontinuation of zinc.

Zinc deficiency is known to affect testicular function adversely in animals and humans (10,11). Supplementation with zinc to zinc-deficient patients such as those with chronic uremia (20) and in those in whom a mild zinc-deficient state was induced by dietary means (21) has been reported to improve testicular functions. Thus, our results in sickle cell anemia patients further confirm the important role of zinc on testicular functions.

The mechanism by which zinc affects the testosterone level in zinc-deficient subjects is not well understood. Zinc is essential for the function of many enzymes (10, 11). It is possible that a zinc-dependent enzyme or enzymes may be involved in sex hormone steroidogenesis. The other possibility is that the main effect of zinc may be on the testicular size; and, inasmuch as it is known that testis size is decreased owing to zinc deficiency, testosterone production may also be affected adversely. Zinc is required for cell division in general, but the testis appears to be a very sensitive organ and is known to atrophy as a result of lack of zinc (10,11).

EFFECT OF ZINC ON HYPERAMMONEMIA IN SCA PATIENTS

Recently, we have observed an increase in the plasma ammonia level in human volunteers as a result of restricted zinc intake (21a). After oral supplementation with zinc, the plasma ammonia concentration returned to normal levels. This was an unexpected finding, and to that time hyperammonemia had not been related to zinc deficiency either in humans or experimental animals. We, therefore, investigated this problem in zinc-deficient rats. An increased level of plasma ammonia and a decreased activity of the hepatic ornithine carbamoyltransferase (OCT), an enzyme required for urea synthesis, were noted in deficient animals as compared to the pair-fed controls (22).

Ammonia is highly neurotoxic and, along with other factors, undoubtedly contributes to the development of encephalopathy and coma, a terminal event in patients with severe liver disease. Inasmuch as zinc deficiency has been observed in patients with SCA, it was considered desirable to measure plasma ammonia levels in these patients (23).

Six patients were assayed for plasma zinc and ammonia levels prior to zinc therapy. They then received 25 mg of zinc as acetate orally three times a day for varying periods (16, 14, 14, 12, 7, and 4 months, respectively), at the end of which they were rechecked for plasma zinc and ammonia levels. In five patients, zinc was discontinued for a period ranging from 3 to 8 months (3, 4, 6, 8, and 8 months, respectively), at the end of which plasma zinc and ammonia were reassayed. One patient received continuous zinc therapy because he had a chronic leg ulcer; and, therefore, it was decided not to discontinue therapy with zinc. Plasma zinc and ammonia levels (mean ± SD) for the three periods (pre-zinc therapy, on zinc, and off zinc) were calculated, and the Student t-test was done to determine the statistical significance of zinc therapy on ammonia levels.

Patients with SCA had a significantly increased plasma ammonia, decreased plasma zinc, and decreased level of plasma urea nitrogen. Following zinc supplementation, the plasma ammonia levels in SCA patients declined significantly ($p < 0.001$). Once the supplementation with zinc was discontinued, plasma ammonia increased significantly ($p < 0.01$); thus establishing the effect of zinc on plasma ammonia levels in SCA patients. Plasma urea nitrogen increased significantly following zinc supplementation and decreased when zinc administration was discontinued in SCA patients.

The mechanism by which deficiency of zinc may cause hyperammonemia is not known at present. Our studies in experimental animals revealed that zinc deficiency decreased the activity of hepatic ornithine carbamoyltransferase (22), an enzyme known to be important in the urea cycle. Ammonia is utilized for the biosynthesis of glutamic acid, glutamine, and carbamoyl phosphate. Although the liver is undoubtedly the most important organ in the maintenance of physiological blood ammonia levels in normal human subjects, skeletal muscle contains glutamine synthetase, and thus may also play a role in ammonia homeostasis under certain conditions. Zinc is known to regulate activities of a large number of enzymes; thus, it is possible that the activity of muscle glutamine synthetase may be affected such that hyperammonemia results in zinc deficiency. Clearly, more studies are needed to establish the enzymatic role of zinc on urea and glutamine synthesis if we are to understand the mechanism by which hyperammonemia results in a zinc-deficient state.

Zinc administration also resulted in an increase in plasma urea nitrogen concentration in SCA patients, and this effect was reversed following discontinuation of zinc therapy. This observation may be suggestive of a role of zinc in urea synthesis, but further work is needed to document this conclusively.

Brady et al. (23a) have demonstrated an increased activity of muscle adenosine monophosphate (AMP) deaminase, an enzyme of the purine nucleotide cycle, in zinc-deficient rat muscle. This finding is consistent with the observation that plasma aspartic acid levels are reduced and plasma ammonia levels are increased owing to deficiency of zinc, inasmuch as the purine nucleotide cycle results in the net production of ammonia from aspartic acid. Yoshino et al. (24) have observed that AMP deaminase is inhibited by zinc with a remarkable high affinity; thus, in zinc deficiency reversal of zinc inhibition of the enzyme may contribute to the recently observed increase in ammonia and the decrease in aspartate in the blood of zinc-deficient animals.

Hyperammonemia is known to complicate severe liver disease. There is no evidence to suggest, however, that patients with SCA have severe liver disease, although minor morphological changes in the liver have been observed (23). In our patients, transaminases, serum proteins, and prothrombin times were within normal limits. Inasmuch as zinc supplementation seems to correct the plasma ammonia levels, we conclude that hyperammonemia in SCA patients is a result of zinc deficiency.

EFFECT OF ZINC SUPPLEMENTATION ON DARK ADAPTATION IN SCA

We have recently studied dark adaptation in SCA subjects and have reported that a significant number of our patients had abnormal dark adaptation (25). Retinal reductase, a zinc-dependent enzyme, is required for the regeneration of rhodopsin from retinol. This reaction is essential for normal rod function, which is responsible for dark adaptation in patients with homozygous SCA. Of 13 studied, 6 had prolonged dark adaptation responses. This group had reduced plasma and neutrophil zinc when compared to the seven patients whose dark adaptation was normal. Three of the zinc-deficient patients were treated with oral zinc with improvement in their dark adaptation. We conclude that patients with SCA may show a decreased ability to dark adapt, which is correctable with zinc supplementation.

ZINC DEFICIENCY AND GROWTH RETARDATION IN SCA

Growth retardation in SCA is a well-known clinical entity (26,27). The rate of growth is decreased and many fail to attain normal stature. Our studies in two sets of experiments establish a beneficial role of zinc on growth and development of adult SCA patients.

For the supplementation study we selected only male patients, inasmuch as we were interested in observing the effects of zinc supplementation on both growth and testicular development (28). Although ovaries do not appear to be sensitive target tissues for zinc, female dwarfs responsive to zinc therapy have been reported from Iran and Turkey (11).

In the first experiment, 10 growth-retarded male SCA patients between the ages of 14 and 17 were subdivided randomly into two groups. Five patients received placebo twice a day, and the other five received 15 mg of zinc supplementation as acetate twice a day for 1 year. Height and body weight were carefully recorded initially and at 3-month intervals throughout the study. Bone age was determined radiographically twice—initially and at the end of the 1-year treatment period.

In the second experiment, six growth-retarded male patients between the ages of 14 to 18 years were supplemented with zinc (15 mg twice a day as acetate) for 1 year. Prior to supplementation with zinc, they received a placebo for 1 year. Thus, the patients on zinc supplementation served as their own controls.

In Experiment I, the mean plasma and erythrocyte zinc (mean ± SD) in the placebo- and zinc-treated groups at the end of 1 year were as follows: plasma zinc 90 ± 0.8 versus 124 ± 9 μg/dl, ($p < 0.001$); erythrocyte zinc, 29.0 ± 2.0 versus 36.37 ± 5.7 μg/g Hb, ($p < 0.02$). The increase (mean ± SD) in height (2.2 ± 0.3 versus 6.3 ± 1.7 cm/year, $p < 0.001$), body weight (0.92 ± 0.72 versus 4.4 ± 1.4 kg/year, $p < 0.001$), and bone age ($p < 0.001$) was significantly greater in the zinc-treated group. Increased activities of neutrophil alkaline phosphatase and erythrocyte nucleoside phosphorylase and higher level of serum testosterone in zinc supplemented subjects were observed.

In Experiment II, the gain (mean ± SD) in height (1.8 ± 0.96 versus 4.6 ± 0.46 cm/year, $p < 0.005$), body weight (1.7 ± 0.88 versus 3.97 ± 0.65 kg/year, $p < 0.0005$), and bone age was significantly greater when subjects were switched to zinc treatment. Serum testosterone also increased significantly following zinc supplementation. Zinc levels (mean ± SD) in the plasma, erythrocytes, and neutrophils during placebo and zinc supplementation, respectively, were as follows: Plasma 89.3 ± 5.2 versus 121.7 ± 11.5 μg/dl ($p < 0.005$); erythrocytes 31.0 ± 5.4 versus 35.4 ± 3.7 μg/g Hb ($p < 0.02$); neutrophils* 82.2 ± 10.6 versus 115.6 ± 5.8 μg/10^{10} cells ($p < 0.001$). The

---

*In this study, no attempt was made to remove the platelets from neutrophils. Platelets are usually present in the neutrophil fractions as contaminants, and as a result zinc levels are higher in the neutrophils by this procedure in comparison to the technique in which the platelets are removed from the neutrophils prior to assay.

activities of neutrophil alkaline phosphatase and erythrocyte nucleoside phosphorylase (mean ± SD) in placebo and zinc treated periods were as follows: 5.47 ± 1.9 versus 10.4 ± 3.5 sigma units/mg protein, (p <0.005); and 8.3 ± 1.07 versus 11.8 ±1.1 △OD/hr/mg Hb (p <0.008).

ZINC DEFICIENCY AND IMMUNE FUNCTION IN SCA

It has been known for many years that zinc deficiency in experimental animals resulted in atrophy of thymic and lymphoid tissue (29). These changes are associated with a variety of functional abnormalities. For example, young adult mice maintained on diets deficient in zinc for a 28-day period were found to rapidly develop atrophy of the thymus with preferential involution of the cortex, reductions in the absolute numbers of splenocytes, and greatly depressed responses to both T-cell-dependent (TD) and T-cell-independent antigens (30-33). Some of these abnormalities were shown to be related to defects in T-helper cell function. Zinc deficiency in mice has also been shown to result in impaired in vivo generation of tumor-specific cytotoxic T-killer cells (30), reduced natural killer (NK) cell activity, and impaired development of delayed skin test reactivity following cutaneous sensitization (34).

Abnormalities of cellular immunity have also been observed in zinc-deficient humans. An extreme example of the effects of zinc deficiency on the human immune system is acrodermatitis enteropathica, a genetic disorder of zinc malabsorption (35). This condition is characterized by mucocutaneous lesions, diarrhea, failure to thrive, and frequent severe infections with fungi, viruses, and bacteria. Affected patients have thymic atrophy, anergy, reduced lymphocyte proliferation response to mitogens, a selective decrease in T_4^+-helper cells, and deficient thymic hormone activity (36). All of these changes are corrected by zinc supplementation (36,37). Less severe cellular immune defects have been observed in patients who become zinc deficient while receiving total parenteral nutrition. These abnormalities, which include lymphopenia, decreased ratios of T-helper and T-suppressor cells, decreased NK activity, and increased monocyte cytotoxicity, are readily corrected by zinc supplementation (38). Similarly, Cunningham-Rundles et al. (39) have observed zinc deficiency in primary immunodeficiency.

Further evidence of a relationship between zinc deficiency and immune dysfunction in humans comes from studies of two groups known to have a high incidence of mild to moderate zinc deficiency—uremic patients on hemodialysis and the elderly. In one study, delayed hypersensitivity skin tests to mumps antigen were carried out in 25 apparently well-nourished men who gave a prior history of mumps infection and were receiving regular hemodialysis because of end-stage renal disease (40). Nine patients were receiving zinc in their dialysis bath for the treatment of hypogonadism. Only one patient in the zinc-treated group was anergic to mumps. In contrast, anergy to mumps and other antigens was observed in 11 of 16 untreated patients. Skin sensitivity test was restored to normal in three of four anergic patients treated with zinc. In another study, 15 institutionalized, apparently healthy persons aged 81 ± 5 years were given 100 mg zinc daily for 1 month, whereas 15 control subjects, aged 79.6 ± 4.2 years, were given placebo (41). The group receiving zinc displayed an increased percentage of circulating T lymphocytes, an increased frequency and magnitude of delayed hypersensitivity skin reactions to purified proteins, and a greater immunoglobulin G (IgG) antibody response to tetanus toxoid. Although the results clearly suggest that some defects in cellular immunity in these two groups are related to zinc deficiency, the findings are not definitive, since zinc status was not evaluated prior to the treatment.

INFECTIONS IN SCA

Infection is the most common cause of death in children with SCA according to some investigators. In one study, it was noted that the risk of bacterial infection reduced markedly after age 3, and proven pneumococcal infection was not seen unless the children experienced previous pneumococcal infection (42). Survival past the age of 3 without prior recognized bacterial infection implied a definite reduced risk to subsequent bacterial infections except for infections due to coliform bacteria. Although in the study reported by Barrett-Conner (42), increased incidence of salmonellal infection and increased mortality and morbidity due to tuberculosis in patients with sickle cell disease were not observed, other reports have observed such associations.

The risk of salmonella osteomyelitis is several hundred times greater in patients with SCA as compared to the normal population (43). An increased incidence of urinary tract infections, with clinical pyelonephritis in up to 25% of adults with SCA due to *Escherichia coli*, have been observed (42). These patients also appear to be susceptible to *Enterobacter-Klebsiella* infection. Our own clinical impression is that a large number (three out of four patients) of our adult SCA patients who are admitted to the hospital give suggestive evidences for upper respiratory tract infection, probably viral in etiology, and/or urinary tract infection prior to the onset of pain crisis.

One review suggests that an overwhelming infection caused by encapsulated bacteria, *Salmonella* spp., and *Plasmodium falciparum* (in malarious areas) are important causes of morbidity and death in patients with SCA (44). Although contributing factors to increased susceptibility to infections in patients with SCA may include a state of functional asplenia, an opsonophagocytic defect due to an abnormality of the alternative complement pathway, and a deficiency of specific circulating antibodies, the role of lymphocytes in cell-mediated immunity in this disease remains to be established.

Some investigators have observed that patients with SCA are unusually susceptible to *Mycoplasma* pneumonia infection, often manifesting unusual clinical features (45,46). Although proven examples of viral hepatitis in SCA patients do not suggest an increased incidence of this infection, a 20-40% prevalence of macronodular cirrhosis among adult subjects has been reported. It has been shown that primary infection with a novel parvoviruslike agent (PVLA) is the major cause of aplastic crises in children with SCA (47). Cryptococcal pneumonia and pneumonia due to cytomegalovirus in patients with SCA have also been reported (48,49).

Cellular immune responses of which delayed hypersensitivity reactions are a prototype are of paramount importance in the defense against a number of obligate or facultative intracellular parasites such as viruses, rickettsiae, mycobacteria, *Listeria monocytogenes, Brucella abortus, Salmonella typhosa*, and certain protozoa. In patients with acquired immunodeficiency syndrome (AIDS), an extreme example of impaired cellular immune function affecting T cells, *Pneumocystis carinii* pneumonia, candidiasis, cytomegalovirus (CMV) infection, perirectal herpes simplex virus (HSV) infection, *Mycobacterium avium intracellular* complex infection, cryptococcosis, cryptosporidiosis, toxoplasmosis, *Salmonella bacterieum*, and aspergillosis have been observed (50). Multiple infections were common and overall mortality was 97.3% in 12 months. Clearly, we are not dealing with a severe T-cell disorder in SCA; nonetheless it appears that these patients do have problems of cell-mediated immunity. Although zinc deficiency also occurs in HIV disease and AIDS, the relationship to disease progress has not been established, and in any event is not primary.

STUDIES IN PATIENTS WITH SCA

Anergy

To examine the relationship between zinc status and in vivo cell-mediated immunity in SCA, we measured delayed skin test responsiveness in 26 adult SCA patients (51). There were 16 men and 10 women, with a mean age of 25.8 years. All patients were evaluated when they were without pain. No patient was admitted to the study within 3 weeks of a crisis or infection, or within 3 months of a blood transfusion. Six patients who had proven zinc deficiency had been receiving an oral zinc supplement (zinc acetate, 45 mg/day) for a minimum of 1 year. Eleven healthy, age- and sex-matched persons, including seven blacks and four whites, were recruited as controls. The zinc levels and results of skin tests with four antigens (PPD, SKSD, *candida*, and mumps) were recorded. An area of induration of 5 mm or more was recorded as a positive reaction.

Six patients were anergic, with negative responses to all four antigens. Four patients had only one positive test result. The remaining 16 patients had two or more postive reactions. Ten of the eleven controls also had two or more positive reactions. For the purpose of comparison, patients were grouped according to the delayed hypersensitivity reaction responses. Group A included patients who were anergic or had only one positive test, whereas all patients in group B had two or more positive tests. Patients in group C, those receiving oral zinc supplements, were analyzed separately. When compared to groups B and C and the controls, patients in group A were found to have significantly lower neutrophil zinc concentrations and PNP activity ($p < 0.001$) and decreased levels of plasma and erythrocyte zinc ($p < 0.01$). No significant difference in zinc levels or PNP activity were found in group A between anergic patients and patients with one positive test. There were no significant differences in zinc levels or PNP activity in groups B and C and the controls except for higher plasma zinc levels in patients receiving an oral zinc supplement (group C). There were no significant differences in the activity of adenosine deaminase in the various groups.

The correlation between neutrophil zinc (one of the best indicators of tissue zinc status) and the activity of erythrocyte PNP in 21 patients, with both measurements done simultaneously, was highly significant ($r = 0.716$, $p < 0.0001$). All patients in group A (with one exception) had levels of neutrophil zinc and PNP activity lower than the controls.

Three anergic patients from group A entered a trial of oral zinc supplementation (zinc acetate, 45 mg/day) and were reevaluated 6 months later. All three patients showed a correction of neutrophil zinc levels and normal or significantly improved PNP activity. On repeat skin tests, one patient had a positive response to two tests, and the remaining two patients had positive responses to one test each.

Taken together, these findings indicate that in patients with SCA, anergy is associated with zinc deficiency. The improvement in skin test responses of some, but not all, zinc-deficient patients following zinc treatment suggests that in these subjects zinc deficiency may be directly responsible for their anergy. Longer periods of supplementation or higher doses of zinc may be necessary to restore normal tissue zinc stores in others.

The correlation of decreased zinc levels with decreased activity of PNP is of interest because the congenital deficiency of this enzyme in humans induces severe defects in cell-mediated immunity (52). Our patients with SCA with zinc deficiency and impaired delayed hypersensitivity reactions had a mean PNP activity of 59% of that of normal controls. Heterozygotes for congenital PNP deficiency with comparable decreases in PNP activity have been reported to be clinically unaffected, suggesting that the occurrence of decreased PNP activity may not be sufficient to explain our findings. The role played by decreased nucleoside phosphorylase activity, however, needs further evaluation, inasmuch as a chronic accumulation of toxic nucleotides as a result of PNP deficiency in lymphocytes may ultimately be harmful.

Decreased Natural Killer Cell Activity in SCA Patients with Zinc Deficiency

Because natural killer (NK) cells are known to be important in host defense against viruses, we compared the NK activity of eight zinc-deficient SCA patients (group 1) with that of eight SCA patients with normal zinc status (group 2), five SCA patients who were receiving zinc therapy because of previously diagnosed zinc deficiency (group 3), and 12 healthy age- and sex-matched adults (nine men and three women, seven blacks and five whites) who served as controls (53). None of the SCA patients participated within 3 weeks of a crisis or infection, or within 3 months of a blood transfusion. The three groups of SCA patients had no significant differences in hemoglobin levels, hematocrit values, mean corpuscular volume, and erythrocyte, reticulocyte, and leukocyte counts. Hemoglobinopathy was ruled out in black controls by hemoglobin electrophoresis. We also studied two male volunteers, aged 48 (patient 1) and 33 (patient 2) years who were inpatients on a metabolic ward where their dietary zinc intake was restricted to 3 mg/day for 20 weeks. These volunteers were screened thoroughly before inclusion. They were free of any disease, and their zinc status was normal as judged by zinc assay in plasma, erythrocyte, hair, neutrophils, and urine, and by metabolic zinc balance data. These subjects were tested for NK activity and plasma zinc concentration at baseline, during dietary zinc restriction, and after zinc repletion with a dietary zinc intake of 30 mg/day for 14 weeks.

Zinc-deficient SCA patients (group 1) had significantly lower NK activity than the patients in groups 2 and 3 and the normal controls.

These findings suggest that zinc deficiency in SCA patients is associated with diminished NK activity. This defect in NK activity is likely due to zinc deficiency per se rather than to some associated condition, since a decline in NK activity was observed in zinc-restricted volunteers. In support of this conclusion, it may be noted that Cunningham-Rundles et al. (54) found that zinc depletion associated with chelation therapy was associated with depressed NK activity.

Interleukin 2 Production

In addition to its critical role in T-cell proliferation, interleukin 2 (IL-2) is a major in vivo activator of NK activity. Could the impairments of both T-cell proliferation and NK activity associated with zinc deficiency result from an underlying defect of IL-2 production? The results of our preliminary study are consistent with this possibility. Supernatants of peripheral blood lymphocytes stimulated for 48 hr with phytohemagglutinin (PHA) were assayed for IL-2 activity in a murine thymocyte proliferation assay.

Production of IL-2 by zinc-deficient SCA patients (plasma zinc < 100 μg/dl) was significantly lower ($p < 0.05$) than that of SCA patients with normal zinc levels and control subjects. Our results suggest that diminished IL-2 production may be responsible for impaired T-cell proliferation and NK activity in zinc-deficient subjects.

Lymphocyte Subpopulation Abnormalities in SCA

In this study, we evaluated lymphocyte subpopulation in 23 adults with SCA (55). When compared to controls, SCA patients had higher lymphocyte counts with normal numbers of $T101^+$ cells (T lymphocytes) and $T4^+$ cells. T8 cells were significantly increased in SCA patients in comparison to controls (1684 ± 243 vs 980 ± 367, $p < 0.001$). This increment was largely dependent on a $T101^-$, $T8^+$ cell population. The SCA patients as a group had a significantly decreased T4/T8 ratio ($p < 0.0001$). The SCA patients with a history of blood transfusions had a higher $T4^+$ cell numbers and a higher T4/T8 ratio, but no other significant differences from nontransfused patients were noted. Thus, in our study, a distinct pattern of abnormalities was seen in lymphocyte subpopulations of adult SCA patients.

Serum Thymulin in SCA Patients

Thymulin (formerly called serum thymic factor) is a well-defined thymic hormone with the following amino acid sequence: < Glu-Ala-Lys-Ser-Gln-Gly-Gly-Ser-Asn-OH (56). Since its initial isolation from pig serum, a number of actions of thymulin on the immune system have been recognized. Dardenne et al. (57) showed previously that thymulin required the presence of zinc to express its biological activity. Recent studies indicate the existence of two forms of the hormone: the first one deprived of zinc and biologically inactive, the second one containing zinc and biologically active.

The zinc/thymulin relationship was previously investigated using two models of in vivo zinc deficiency (58,59). In the first model, active thymulin levels in sera from mice subjected to a long-term marginally zinc-deficient diet was studied. In spite of the absence of thymic atrophy, it was observed that the serum levels of thymulin decreased as early as 2 months after beginning the diet. However, these levels could be consistently restored after in vitro addition of zinc.

Similar observations were made with sera from children suffering from nephrotic syndrome with zinc deficiency (the second model), a disease in which a low level of thymulin activity was observed that could be restored to normal after in vitro serum chelation and incubation with zinc. These results confirm the presence of the inactive hormone in the serum of zinc-deficient individuals and its potential activation following zinc addition. The specificity of these results was confirmed by the lack of activation in experiments performed with sera from thymectomized mice or patients with DiGeorge's syndrome in whom the hormone is nonexistent.

Six zinc-deficient homozygous male SCA patients were included in our recent study (60). Their ages ranged from 17 to 33 years. They were ambulatory, had no neurological or psychiatric deficits, were not dependent on drugs, and no other hemoglobinopathies such as α-thalassemia, β-thalassemia, Hb C disease, etc., were associated in these cases. These patients have been followed regularly in the adult sickle cell clinic of the University Health Clinic of Wayne State University, Detroit Medical Center. They had received no blood transfusions, at least during the 6 months prior to this study. Prior to selection of these patients for our study, zinc was assayed in lymphocytes, granulocytes, and platelets by flameless atomic absorption spectrophotometry. In this study, care was taken to remove platelets from granulocytes and lymphocyte fractions prior to assay. Plasma zinc levels ranged from 98 to 118 µg/dl and were considered to be within the normal range.

The serum level of biologically active thymulin was evaluted by a rosette assay described in detail elsewhere, and shown by us and several other investigators to be strictly thymus specific. The assay analyses the converstion of relatively azathioprine (Az)-resistant spleen of adult thymectomized mice to theta-positive rosette-forming cells that are more sensitive to Az. In the presence of thymulin-containing sera, rosette formation was inhibited by Az. The results were expressed as the log 2 of reciprocal highest serum dilution conferring sensitivity to Az inhibition upon spleen cells from adult Tx (ATx) mice. To confirm the specificity of the biological activity measured, all the determinations were repeated after preincubation of the sera under study with an antithymulin monoclonal antibody (MAb) or a specific antithymulin immunoabsorbent.

Sera (100 µl) from patients and control subjects were incubated for 30 min at room temperature with an equal volume of Chelex 100 at 50 mg/ml in distilled water. At the end of the incubation, the mixture was centrifuged at 12000 × g for 2 min to eliminate the chelating resin and the biological activity in the supernatant of Chelex 100-treated serum was measured. Ten micrograms of $ZnCl_2$ was then added to 100 µl of Chelex-treated serum. The mixture was then incubated for 15 min at room temperature and its biological activity was measured by the rosette assay.

Abnormally low levels of active thymulin in the sera were found in zinc-deficient SCA patients as compared to age-matched healthy individuals. This was correctable following in vitro addition of zinc. Following supplementation with 50 mg of zinc (as acetate) orally in two divided doses daily for 3-8 months, the serum thymulin activity (mean ± SD) became normal (before 2.49 ± 0.81 versus after 4.44 ± 0.65 log 2, $p < 0.0001$). Zinc levels (mean ± SD) in granulocytes, lymphocytes, and platelets ($µg/10^{10}$ cells) before and after supplementation were: granulocytes 35.6 ± 4.2 versus 42.8 ± 3.37 $p < 0.01$, lymphocytes 51.8 ± 4.6 versus 61.4 ± 5.5 $p < 0.01$, platelets 1.35 ± 0.26 versus 2.24 ± 0.71, $p < 0.03$.

PROBABLE MECHANISMS OF ZINC ACTION ON CELL-MEDIATED IMMUNITY

Although the mechanism underlying zinc deficiency-related abnormalities of cellular immunity remain to be determined, some are almost certainly related to the deleterious effects of zinc deficiency on lymphocyte proliferative responses. Zinc probably operates at several different levels to influence lymphocyte proliferation. Zinc deficiency can impair DNA synthesis in general, since zinc is critical for the activity of many enzymes active in DNA synthesis. Dexoythymidine kinase is an example of a zinc-dependent enzyme which is extremely sensitive, such that even a mild state of zinc deficiency may significantly affect its activity adversely.

A congenital deficiency of the purine enzyme PNP is associated with a severe T-cell immune deficiency and a congenital deficiency of adenosine deaminase result in an impaired T- and B-cell development (51). Our recent studies in experimental animals and humans indicate that PNP may be zinc dependent. Thus, a decreased activity of PNP may additionally account for T-cell dysfunction in zinc deficiency. The regulation of expression of three purine-metabolizing enzymes, adenosine deaminase (ADA), PNP and 5'-ecto-nucleotidase (5'NT), and TdT (terminal deoxyribonucleotidyl transferase) are considered to be important for homeostatic T-cell development. Ma et al. (61) have suggested that the high ADA vs low PNP and 5'NT and a sudden fall of TdT activities in cortical thymocytes is a lethal combination. The preferential substrate of TdT is dGTP and dATP, so TdT may buildup "nonsense" DNA polymers, which in turn protect the cells from the accumulation of potentially toxic-free purine nucleotides. The toxic effect of high intracellular dGTP and dATP is explained by their inhibitory effects on essential methylation of RNA, DNA, and proteins via S-adenosyl-homocysteine hydrolase. A deficiency of PNP also results in accumulation of GTP in lymphocytes. It has been shown that GTP accumulation also has a marked inhibitory effect on cell growth and is associated with ATP depletion (62). The exact role of increased GTP levels in inhibiting lymphocyte growth is not understood at present. It is very likely that several of these mechanisms are operative and that no one single factor is solely responsible for the effects seen on lymphocytes as a result of zinc deficiency (63).

The ectoenzyme 5'-nucleotidase (5'NT) catalyzes the dephosphorylation of nucleoside 5'-monophosphates to yield the corresponding nucleoside. Lymphocytes are in general incapable of synthesizing purine de novo; hence, it has been postulated that 5'NT provides necessary nucleic acid metabolites that can be transported across the cell membrane. A deficiency in this enzyme, which is known to be zinc dependent, may predispose to an immunodeficient state secondary to an arrest in lymphocyte differentiation and proliferation.

T-helper cell activity is depressed in zinc-deficient animals. T-helper cells produce interleukin 2, a lymphokine that, in addition to triggering T-cell proliferation, augments NK activity. Thus, impaired T-helper activity in zinc deficiency could cause an in vivo deficiency of IL-2, which in turn could result in diminished in vivo activation of NK cells.

Low NK activity has been detected in association with a variety of clinical conditions, including malignancies, inflammatory bowel diseases, chronic renal failure, and systemic lupus erythematosus. Our results raise the possibility that zinc deficiency which occurs frequently in these disorders and in SCA, may contribute significantly to the decreased NK activity in these conditions. Recent reports support this possibility. According to some investigators, NK cells play an important role in host defense against viral infections. The observation that neonates, who are uniquely susceptible to certain viral infections, have low NK activity is consistent with this.

Defective production or responsiveness to IL-2 may be another mechanism contributing to some of the immune abnormalities associated with zinc deficiency (60). Interleukin 2 is a lymphokine produced primarily by $T4^+$ helper cells which plays a crucial role in T-cell proliferation, generation of cytotoxic T cells, and activation of NK lytic activity. The results of preliminary studies suggest that IL-2 production in zinc-deficient SCA subjects may be impaired. In addition, since IL-2 production is known to depend on adequate production and activity of IL-2, the possibility that IL-1 production in zinc-deficient SCA patients is decreased needs to be investigated.

Although several polypeptides have been extracted from the thymus, and a number of them have been characterized chemically from the physiological point of view, only two of these are true thymic hormones actually produced by the thymus and biologically active on T cells. These are thymopoeitin and thymulin. Recent studies show that thymulin binds to high-affinity receptors, induces several T-cell markers, and promotes T-cell function, including allogenic cytotoxicity, suppressor function, and interleukin 2 production.

For the first time, our study has provided evidence that zinc deficiency in SCA adversely affects serum thymulin activity. Interestingly, not only oral zinc supplementation in vivo corrected serum thymulin activity in all zinc-deficient SCA patients in this study, a correction of thymulin activity was also achieved with the addition of zinc in vitro.

CONCLUSIONS

It is clear from the above discussion that the effects of zinc deficiency on cell-mediated immune function in SCA are multifactorial. It appears that a decreased serum thymulin activity as a result of zinc deficiency may play a crucial role in the overall picture accounting for T-cell disorders in SCA. Clearly, further investigations and controlled zinc supplementation trials must be carried out in the future in order to understand the mechanism of immune dysfunction in SCA.

ACKNOWLEDGMENTS

Supported in part by VA Medical Research Funds, Allen Park, Michigan; a grant from NIH/NIDDK No. DK 31401, and a grant from Food and Drug Administration No. FDA-U-000457.

REFERENCES

1. Alexander JW, Peck MD (1990). Future prospects for adjunctive therapy: Pharmacologic and nutritional approaches to immune system modulation. Crit Care Med 18:5159.
2. Spallholtz JE, Stewart JR (1989). Advances in the role of minerals in immunobiol. Biol Trace Element Res 19:129.
3. Chandra RK (1989). Nutritional regulation of immunity and risk of illness. Ind J Ped 56:607.
4. Fenwick PK, Aggett PJ, Macdonald D, Huber C, Wakelin D (1990). Zinc deficiency and zinc repletion: Effect on the response of rats to infection with trichinella spiralis. Am J Clin Nutr 52:166.
5. Bogden JD, Oleske JM, Lavenhar MA, Munves EM, Kemp FW, Bruening KS, Holding KJ, Denny TN, Guarino MA, Holland BK (1990). Effects of one year supplementation with zinc and other micronutrients on cellular immunity in the elderly. J Am Coll Nutr 9:214.
6. Bach JF, Dardenne M (1989). Thymulin, a zinc dependent hormone. Med Oncol Tumor Pharmacol 6:25.
7. Prasad AS, Kaplan J, Brewer GJ, Dardenne M (1989). Immunological effects of zinc deficiency in sickle cell anemia. Prog Clin Biol Res 319:629.
8. Prasad AS, Schoomaker EB, Ortega J, Brewer GJ, Oberleas D, Oelshlegel FJ (1975). Zinc deficiency in sickle cell disease. Clin Chem 21:582.
9. Prasad AS, Ortega J, Brewer GJ, Oberleas D (1976). Trace elements in sickle cell disease. JAMA 235:2396.

10. Prasad AS (1976). Deficiency of zinc in man and its toxicity. In Prasad AS (ed): Trace Elements in Human Health and Disease. Vol I. New York: Academic Press, p 1.
11. Prasad AS (1978). Trace Elements and Iron in Human Metabolism. New York: Plenum, p 251.
12. Prasad AD (1984). Zinc deficiency and effects of zinc supplementation on sickle cell anemia subjects. In Brewer GJ (ed): The Red Cell: Fifth Ann Arbor Conference. New York: Liss, p 99.
13. Prasad AS, Oberleas D (1974). Thymidine kinase activity and incorporation of thymidine into DNA in zind-deficient tissue. J Lab Clin Med 83:634.
14. Prasad AS, Fernandez-Madrid F, Ryan JR (1979). Deoxythymidine kinase activity of human implanted sponge connective tissue in zinc deficiency. Am J Physiol 236:E272.
14a. Prasad AS (1981). Zinc deficiency in sickle cell disease. In Brewer GF (ed): The Red Cell: Sixth Ann Arbor Conference. New York: Liss, p 49.
15. Midgley AR Jr, Jaffe RB (1966). Human luteinizing hormone in serum during the menstrual cycle: Determination by radioimmunoassay. J Clin Endocrinol Metab 26:1375.
16. Midgley AR Jr (1967). Radioimmunoassay for human follicle stimulating hormone. J Clin Endrocrinol Metab 27:295.
17. Aulette FJ, Caldwell BZ, Hamilton GL (1975). Androgen testosterone and dihydrotestosterone. In Jamme BM, Behrman HR (eds): Methods of Radio Immunoassay. New York: Academic Press, p 359.
18. Abbasi AA, Prasad AS, Ortega J, Congco E, Oberleas D (1976). Gonadal function abnormalities in sickle cell anemia: Studies in adult male patients. Ann Int Med 85:601.
19. Snedecor GW, Cochran WG (1967). Statistical Methods. 6th ed. Ames, Iowa: Iowa State University Press.
20. Mahajan SK, Abbasi AA, Prasad AS, Rabbani P, Briggs WA, McDonald FD (1982). Effect of oral zinc therapy on gonadol function in hemodialysis patients. Ann Int Med 97:357.
21. Abbasi AA, Prasad AS, Rabbani P, DuMouchelle E (1980). Experimental zinc deficiency in man: Effect on testicular function. J Lab Clin Med 96(3):544.
21a. Prasad AS, Rabbani P, Abbasi A, Bowersox E, Fox MRS (1978). Experimental zinc deficiency in humans. Ann Int Med 89:483.
22. Rabbani P, Prasad AS (1978). Plasma ammonia and liver ornithine transcarbamoylase activity in zinc deficient rats. Am J Physiol 235:E203.
23. Prasad AS, Rabbani P, Warth JA (1979). Effect of zinc on hyperammonemia in sickle cell anemia subjects. Am J Hematol 7:323.
23a. Brady MS, Steinberg JR, Svinger BA, Luecke RE (1977). Increased purine nucleotide cycle activity associated with dietary zinc deficiency. Biochem Biophys Res Commun 78:144.
24. Yoshino M, Murakami K, Tusushima K (1978). Inhibition of AMP deaminase by zinc ions. Biochem Pharmacol 27:2651.
25. Warth JA, Prasad AS, Zwas F, Frank RN (1981). Abnormal dark adaptation in sickle cell anemia. J Lab Clin Med 98(2):189.
26. Daeschner III CW, Matustik MC, Carpentieri R, Haggard ME (1981). Zinc and growth in patients with sickle cell anemia. J Pediatr 98:778.
27. Olambiwonnu NO, Penny R, Frasier SD (1975). Sexual maturation in subjects with sickle cell anemia: Studies of serum gonadotropin concentration, height, weight, and skeletal age. J Pediatr 87:459.
28. Prasad AS, Cossack ZT (1984). Zinc supplementation and growth in sickle cell disease. Ann Int Med 100:367.
29. Prasad AS (1984). Discovery and importance of zinc in human nutrition. Fed Proc 43:2829.
30. Fraker PJ, Haas S, Luecke RW (1977). Effect of zinc deficiency on the immune response of the young adult A/jax mouse. J Nutr 107:1889.

31. Fraker PJ, DePasquale-Jardieu P, Zwickl CM, Leucke RW (1978). Regeneration of T cell helper function in zinc-deficient adult mice. Proc Natl Acad Sci USA 75:5660.
32. Fernandes G, Nair M, Onoe K, Tanaka T, Floyd R, Good RA (1977). Impairment of cell-mediated immunity by dietary zinc deficiency in mice. J Nutr 107:1889.
33. Fraker PJ (1983). Zinc deficiency: A common immunodeficiency state. Surv Immunol Res 2:155.
34. Fraker PJ, Zwickl CM, Luecke RW (1982). Delayed type hypersensitivity in zinc deficient adult mice: Impairment and restoration of responsivity to dinitrofluorobenzene. J Nutr 112:309.
35. Oleske JM, Westphal ML, Shore S, Gorden D, Bogden JD, Nahmias A (1979). Zinc therapy of depressed cellular immunity in acrodermatitis enteropathica. Am J Dis Child 133:915.
36. Chandra RK, Dayton DH (1982). Trace element regulation of immunity and infection. Nutr Res 2:721.
37. Good RA, Fernandes G, Garofalo JA, Cunningham-Rundles C, Iwata T, West A (1982). Zinc and immunity. In Prasad AS (ed): Clinical, Biochemical, and Nutritional Aspects of Trace Elements. New York: Liss, p 189.
38. Allen JI, Perri RT, McClain CJ, Kay NE (1983). Alterations in human natural killer cell activity and monocyte cytotoxicity induced by zinc deficiency. J Lab Clin Med 102:577.
39. Cunningham-Rundles S, Cunningham-Rundles WF (1988). Zinc Modulation of Immune Response. In Chandra R (ed): Nutrition and Immunology. New York: Liss, p 197.
40. Antoniou LD, Shalhoub RJ, Schechter GP (1981). The effect of zinc on cellular immunity in chronic uremia. Am J Clin Nutr 34:1912.
41. Duchateu J, Delepesee G, Virgens R, Collet HJ (1981). Beneficial effects of oral zinc supplementation on the immune response of old people. Am J Med 70:1001.
42. Barrett-Conner E (1971). Bacterial infection and sickle cell anemia. Medicine 50:97.
43. Golding JSR, MacIver JE, Went LH (1959). The bone changes in sickle cell anemia and its genetic variants. J Bone Joint Surg 41B:711.
44. Onwubalili JK (1983). Sickle cell disease and infection. J Infect 7:2.
45. Shulman ST, Bartlett J, Clyde WA, Ayoub EM (1972). The unusual severity of mycoplasma pneumonia in children with sickle cell disease. N Engl J Med 287:164.
46. Mann JR, Cotter KP, Walker RA, Bird GWG, Stuart J (1975). Anemia crisis on sickle cell disease. J Clin Pathol 28:341.
47. Sergeant GR, Topley JM, Mason K, Sergeant BE, Pattison SE, Mohamed R (1981). Outbreak of aplastic crisis in sickle cell anemia associated with parvovirus like agent. Lancet 11:595.
48. Hardy RE, Cummings C, Thomas F, Harrison D (1986). Cryptococcal pneumonia in a patient with sickle cell disease. Chest 89:892.
49. Haddad JD, John JF, Pappas AA (1984). Cytomegalovirus pneumonia in sickle cell disease. Chest 86:265.
50. Douglas Jr RG, Roberts RB, Romano P, Metroka C, Amberson J, Soave R, Stover D (1984). In Gottlieb MS, Groopmen JE (eds): Acquired Immune Deficiency Syndrome. New York: Liss, p 321.
51. Ballester OF, Prasad AS (1983). Anergy, zinc deficiency and decreased nucleoside phosphorylase activity in patients with sickle cell anemia. Ann Int Med 98:180.
52. Giblett ER, Ammann AJ, Wara DW, Sandman R, Diamond LK (1975). Nucleoside phosphorylase deficiency in a child with severely defective T-cell immunity and normal B-cell immunity. Lancet 1:1010.
53. Tapazoglou E, Prasad AS, Hill G, Brewer GJ, Kaplan J (1985). Decreased natural killer cell activity in zinc deficient subjects with sickle cell. J Lab Clin Med 105:19.
54. Cunningham-Rundles S, Bockman RB, Lin A, Giardina PV, Hilgartner MW, Calwell-Brown D, Carter DM (1990). Ann NY Acad Sci 587:113.
55. Ballester OF, Abdallah JM, Prasad AS (1986). Lymphocyte subpopulation abnormalities in sickle cell anemia. Am J Hematol 21:23.

56. Bach JF, Dardenne M, Pleau JM, Rosa J (1977). Biochemical characterization of a serum thymic hormone. Nature 266:55.
57. Dardenne M, Pleau JM, Nabarra B, Lefrancier P, Derrien M, Choay J, Bach JF (1982). Contribution of zinc and other metals to the biological activity of the serum thymic factor. Proc Natl Acad Sci USA 79:5370.
58. Dardenne M, Savino W, Wade S, Kaiserlian D, Lemonnier D, Bach JF (1984). In vivo and in vitro studies of thymulin in marginally zinc-deficient mice. Eur J Immunol 14:454.
59. Bensman A, Dardenne M, Morgant G, Vesmant D, Bach JF (1985). Decrease of biological activity of serum thymic factor in children with nephrotic syndrome. Int J Paediatr Nephrol 5:201.
60. Prasad AS, Meftah S, Abdallah J, Kaplan J, Brewer GJ, Bach JF, Dardenne M (1988). Serum thymulin in human zinc deficiency. J Clin Invest 82:1202.
61. Ma DDF, Sylwestrowicz T, Janossy G, Hoffbrand AV (1983). The role of purine metabolic enzymes and terminal deoxynucleotidyl transferase in intrathymic T cell differentiation. Immunol Today 4:65.
62. Mitchell BS, Sidi Y (1985). Differential metabolism of guanine nucleosides by human lymphoid cell lines. Proc Soc Exp Biol and Med 179:427.
63. Prasad AS (1991). Discovery of human zinc deficiency and studies in an experimental human model. Am J Clin Nutr 53:403.

25
Effect of Therapeutic Chelation on Immune Response in Transfusion Dependent Thalassemia

Susanna Cunningham-Rundles, Patricia J. Giardina, and Margaret W. Hilgartner
The New York Hospital, Cornell University Medical Center, New York, New York

John Thomas Pinto
Memorial Sloan-Kettering Cancer Center, New York, New York

INTRODUCTION

The interaction of metals with the immune system appears to constitute a unique class of modulatory effects affecting reactions at several levels. In addition to being essential for the activity of key enzymes and hormones, some metals may exert effects at the cell surface and affect signaling either at the level of receptors or cytokines in processes which can involve gene activation, as discussed in several chapters in this volume.

Dietary deficiency of certain metals such as iron, zinc, copper, manganese, selenium, and magnesium have been associated with significant impairment of the immune response (1-4). Also, the toxic effects of metals such as lead, cadmium, arsenic, and mercury have been found to be mediated by increasing susceptibility to bacterial endotoxin (5-7). Lead has been found to reduce viral resistance through impairing the generation of interferon without affecting the response to interferon itself (7). Interestingly, concentrations of certain toxic metals, such as lead, at a level that would not cause metabolic problems per se have been found to produce highly significant susceptibility to endotoxin challenge and to heat-killed *Escherichia coli* (8). It seems likely that there is no single mechanism for these effects. For example, the lethality induced by lead, but not by cadmium, has been observed to be preventable with glucocorticoid (8). Mechanisms that have been identified as taking part in these toxic effects on the immune system include reduced phagocytic function, involving both reduced antigen processing and presentation, and reduced antibody synthesis.

The effects of metals in immune reactions seem to be highly dependent upon concentration, timing, and the presence of other activating pathogens or microbes in the host. Even the effect of arsenicals can apparently be positive and growth promoting in low doses which stimulate rather than suppress the interferon system (9). The interactions of metals with each other has marked influence on the observed net effect. For example, some of the toxic effects of cadmium and lead appear to be mediated through adverse effects on zinc metalloenzymes (10). The toxicity of mercury for the immune system, which blocks the primary antibody response (11), can be ameliorated by selenium (12). Metals also compete for binding sites in ways which profoundly modify the results of dietary intake (10). In studies of specific metals such as zinc, we as well as others have observed that the effects of deficiency are highly associated with specific settings in which they are found (13-16). In assessing the effect of zinc deficiency in patients with primary immunodeficiency, we found a close relationship between impaired proliferative response in vitro and low serum zinc and reduced levels of thymic hormone, whereas among healthy persons there was no direct relationship between level of in vitro response to T-cell activators and serum zinc levels despite the wide variation in both within the normal range (17). Although this lack of correlation may be based in part on the relatively insensitive methods used to measure zinc nutriture and the internally compensatory nature of the immune response, it seems likely that metals act as sensitizing agents in the context of signals present in the system such that subtle losses or excesses are strongly active in the context of specific antigen presence or signal encounter. Alternatively, this relative weak correlation between levels of metals and immune response over a range of physiological concentrations in the healthy person could be viewed as evidence that other unrecognized changes in metabolism associated with disease states are really responsible for the effects seen. However, in light of the fact that metals can directly activate the immune system, serve as biological response modifiers, and potentiate response to other activators in in vitro systems with normal cells, it seems more probable that metals are critically determinative elements in immune reactions and do interact to generate key regulatory signals (15,18,19) in ways which require further clarification.

In the studies described here, we assessed the effects of iron chelation on immune response in iron overload and found evidence for acute effects on cell surface antigen expression and cytotoxic effector cell function that could be related to the removal of zinc as well as iron, and also reflected differences in the patient group potentially related to metal metabolism.

BIOLOGICAL EFFECTS OF DEFERIOXAMINE

Metal Metabolism

Deferioxamine (DF) is a polyhydroxamic acid siderophore produced naturally by *Streptococcus pilosus* which functions to secure iron from the environment (20). The complex formed by DF with ferric ion is quite stable, so that DF has been widely used theraputically to reduce iron overload both in acute iron poisoning and, more extensively, in the treatment of patients with transfusional iron overload (21-24). Deferoxamine has a half-life of 5-10 min in peripheral blood, since it penetrates cells and combines with intracellular free iron to form ferrioxamine or is excreted by the kidneys.

Chronic transfusion with red blood cells in thalassemia and in severe sickle cell anemia can lead to the addition of more than 7 g of iron each year to the total iron body pool, and therefore to iron accumulation in major organs (25). In the absence of iron removal, the development of severe endocrinpathies and liver and cardiac complications result and become a cause of morbidity and mortality (26-28). Experience over the past 2 decades has shown that thalassemia patients who do comply with daily subcutaneous chelation with DF have fewer cardiac arrhythmias and less heart failure, which is associated with increased survival (26,29). However, delayed growth rate and sexual maturation have continued as major clinical problems (30-32). In addition, DF appears to have significant neurotoxicity, as reflected specifically in ear and eye abnormalities (33-35). Some of the visual deficits observed, for example, defective dark adaptation, are similar to those reported by Prasad in zinc-deficient sickle cell anemia patients (36) (see also Chap 24). The growth retardation and delayed sexual maturation are also reminiscent of conditioned zinc deficiency secondary to a high intake of dietary phytate; also reported by Prasad (37). Since these phenomena were observed originally in thalassemia patients in the context of high-dose chelation therapy and relatively lower levels of iron stores, it has been suggested that chelation of other trace metals, copper, or zinc (38,39) might be responsible. However, some recent studies have shown that these changes may take place without evidence that the dose of DF was inappropriately high (40).

While there is considerable debate as to the incidence rate of these neurotoxic effects, there is little doubt that the changes are actually related to DF, since similar effects have been seen in arthritis patients with normal iron levels receiving DF for potential anti-inflamatory effects (41). Recent studies in our laboratory (19) discussed subsequently have shown that about one-half of thalassemia patients, all of whom undergo regular DF chelation, have low serum zinc. Although the basis of this is not entirely established, DF appears to be strongly implicated.

Reduced zinc has been suggested as a potential basis for the growth retardation seen in thalassemia patients in whom treatment was started before the age of 3 (38). In these studies, De Virgiliis et al found low hair and plasma zinc and reduced leukocyte alkaline phosphatase activity among those patients with apparent DF-related lowered longitudinal growth. Recently, we reported bone dysplasia associated with DF therapy that improved with dose reduction, but we did not find low serum zinc in the affected patients (42). This lack of correlation in our study may indicate that serum zinc is a relatively insensitive indicator of zinc level, as has been suggested by others (43), especially in a growing child whose needs may be greater, or reflect other effects of DF unrelated to zinc.

Effects at the Cellular Level

Since cells require iron for cell division, reduction of iron can affect cell growth. Cells acquire iron from tranferrin by a process of receptor-mediated endocytosis and in association with this produce upregulation of transferrin receptors during growth. Bomford et al. have shown that DF causes an increase in transferrin receptor number (44) in growing cells. Iron uptake was not impeded by DF, but it appeared likely that intracellular iron was made unavailable by DF which had crossed the cell membrane.

Low concentrations of DF (20-50μg) have been shown to arrest some established tumor cell lines in the S phase (44) without inhibition of DNA synthesis. At higher concentrations, DNA synthesis was also blocked, and in recent times there has been interest in the use of DF in combination iron-depletion therapy against tumor growth (45,46).

In contrast, low concentrations of DF have been found to block the entry of mitogen-stimulated T lymphocytes at the G_0/G_1 interface (47) through inhibiting DNA synthesis catalyzed by ribonucleotide reductase (45). These effects were observed to be readily reversible and to spare RNA and protein synthesis. The discovery that DF could inhibit the generation of cytotoxic T lymphocytes and control graft injection has lead to the consideration of DF as a therapeutic agent in transplantation. Studies by Carotenuto (48) have shown that at the level of 100 μM, DF could block interleukin 2 (IL-2) receptor expression of human T lymphocytes, whereas the expression of 4F2 antigen and Ia antigens was not affected. Production of Il-2 was not affected. These data suggested strongly that DF might be acting as an immunomodulating agent through effects on metals.

The studies described in the following section may be considered in light of other studies in this book on individual metals, and suggest that it is the interaction of particular metals together that may constitute a means whereby cell surfaces can be modulated to express receptors and consequently to respond to stimulii and cytokines.

EFFECT OF CHELATION *IN VIVO* ON CYTOTOXIC EFFECTOR FUNCTION *IN VITRO*

The effect of altered trace element metabolism on immune response, particularly in the chronically transfused patient, is currently under investigation in our laboratory as a possible cofactor in the iron-associated morbidity of the thalassemia patient. As discussed elsewhere in this volume, iron excess has been implicated in downregulation of immune response (Chapter 7). Furthermore, it has seemed likely that impaired immune response in patients who frequently also acquire infections such as hepatitis viruses through transfusions could contribute significantly to morbidity. The question arises as to the possible sensitizing effect of metal imbalance on immune cell function. Approximately 10% of our patients have also acquired the human immunodeficiency virus (HIV), but studies on this subgroup are not included in the findings discussed here, since the direct effects of HIV on the immune system make interpretation of observations on the effect of chelation uncertain.

Initial studies in 33 patients (49) showed no significant difference from that of controls studied in parallel in assay of the lymphocyte proliferative response in vitro to phytohemagglutinin (PHA) or pokeweed mitogen (PWM) when lymphocytes were isolated from peripheral blood and cultured at a standardized concentration in medium supplemented with pooled normal human serum (PNHS), although a subset of the patient group had a markedly reduced response. However, natural killer (NK) cell activity against the K562 erythroleukemia tumor target in vitro in PNHS-supplemented media was quite significantly reduced in thalassemia patients compared to controls (19), as shown in Figure 1 ($p < 0.001$).

Since it seemed probable that low NK activity might parallel iron overload, comparison with serum ferritin was attempted, but no correlation was found despite the fact that patients with more lifetime transfusions (more than 450) tended to have lower NK function than patients with fewer (less than 450). Since these patients were regular recipients of chelation therapy with DF, which chelates iron but also other

Therapeutic Chelation of Immune Response in Thalassemia

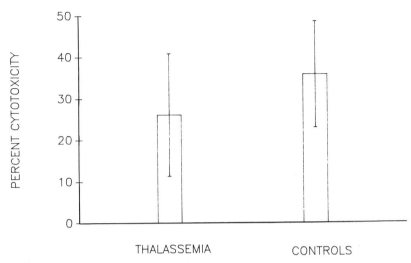

Figure 1 Natural killer cell activity toward K562 in thalassemia compared to controls. Data are given as mean cytotoxic activity at an effector/target ratio of 100:1 in the 4-hr ^{51}chromium release assay.

metals including, zinc, where deficiency has been linked to reduced NK cell activity (50), the relationship to zinc was also studied. Comparison showed that low NK activity was closely correlated with a low serum zinc level. Patients fell naturally into two groups with significantly different serum zinc levels (19). Of 42 patients, 21 had serum zinc levels below the normal range (71 to 142 μg/dl) with a mean level of 57.2 μg in comparison with the other half of the patient group who had a mean serum zinc level of 87.7 μg/dl ($p < 0.001$). The NK activity was significantly lower in the group with low serum zinc compared to the group with normal serum zinc, as shown in Figure 2. ($p < 0.001$).

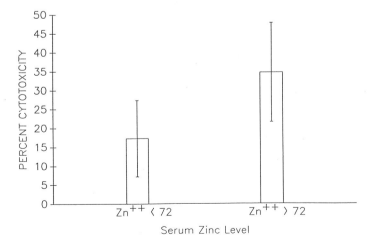

Figure 2 The relationship between NK activity in vitro and serum zinc level in vivo. Data show the mean cytotoxic activity against K562 as described in Figure 1 in patients with normal or abnormal serum zinc as described further in the text.

Table 1 Serum Copper Levels in Thalassemia Patients with Low Serum Zinc

Case	Zn^{2+}	Cu^{2+}
1	41	133
2	45	140
3	52	151
4	52	154
5	54	148
6	55	134
7	61	142
8	65	122

Despite the fact that the stability constant of DF for Cu^{2+} is 10^{14} compared to 10^{11} for Zn^{2+}, and that other studies have shown increased copper excretion during DF infusions, low serum zinc was not associated with low serum copper, as shown in Table 1, for eight of the cases with the lowest serum zinc.

Patients also showed a variation in their compliance with self-administrated chelation therapy, which was designed to supply approximately 40 mg/kg DF subcutaneously. Lack of compliance was determined by failure to show stable or decreasing serum ferritin levels. In order to compensate for ineffective iron removal occurring either because of low compliance or due to other unknown factors, such as increased dietary iron absorption, patients were placed on intravenous DF for 8-hour cycles. This made possible direct studies of the relationship between trace element changes in vivo and the immune response in vitro. Since DF is cleared rapidly from peripheral blood, the results obtained could not be ascribed to any direct effects of DF per se.

When NK activity was compared before and after successive cycles of DF chelation therapy in 34 patients, significantly reduced cytotoxicity toward K562 was seen in approximately 70% of cases ($p < 0.01$), whereas some degree of increase was seen in 30%. The increases in these 11 patients were not significantly different than baseline ($p = 0.058$), although in 4 cases the augmentation was 50% greater compared to the preinfusion level.

In the study shown in Figure 3, where zinc levels were measured before and after chelation, decreasing zinc was associated with a drop in NK activity.

However, the long-term consequences of chelation therapy on NK activity were not equally suppressing and were even augmenting in some cases, as shown in Table 2.

Since the lymphocyte subsets associated with spontaneously occurring, non-major histocompatibility complex-restricted cytotoxicity may be partially defined as CD8, Leu7 (HNK-1), and CD16, we also examined changes in these subsets during chelation. While there was no statistically significant difference between pre- and postchelation percentage of $CD8^+$ T cells in 29 patients as a whole, 6 patients showed an increase in percentage of lymphocytes expressing $CD8^+$ in contrast to 23 patients who showed a decrease. Whereas the two groups had similar mean level of $CD8^+$ cells prechelation (19.0 versus 16.0%), after chelation, there was a significant difference (25.0 versus 11.0%; $p < 0.04$) The decrease in CD8 expression following chelation was significant in this subgroup ($p < 0.03$).

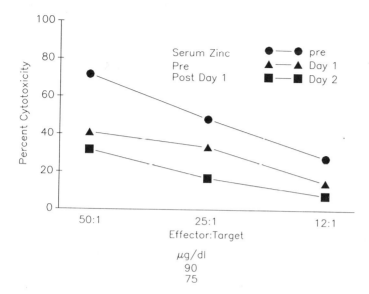

Figure 3 Effect of chelation on NK activity on relationship to serum zinc in thalassemia. Data show changes in cytotoxicity against the K562 target cell at effector/target ratios 50:1, 25:1, and 12.5:1 following a single cycle of chelation and serum zinc level assayed in parallel.

Table 2 Acute and Long-Term Effects of Iron Chelation on Natural Killer Cell Activity in Thalassemia[a]

Case	Pre	End of infusion period[b]	Post therapy[c]
1	34.5	3.6	45.9
2	47.7	12.3	29.3
3	32.0	9.0	32.6
4	34.7	7.7	28.5
5	18.7	11.2	23.9
6	8.9	2.3	13.0

[a]Percent release at ET 100:1 against K562.
[b]First or second cycle.
[c]3 weeks after final infusion.

There was no relationship between depressed NK activity in the patients who showed this effect and change in percentage of cells expressing NK-associated surface antigens, HNK-1 (Leu7), or CD16 (Leu11). As shown in Table 3, the population of cells theoretically able to mediate NK activity actually increased during chelation. However, there was a possible relationship as suggested by the data between expression of the transferrin receptor and NK activity, as shown in Table 4.

These observations on the changes in lymphocyte functional response following chelation suggest that profound alterations presumably initiated at the cell surface level affect at least the short-term capabilities of the NK system, and possibly other as yet unstudied aspects of the immune system. In other studies, we have shown that

Table 3 Relationship Between NK Activity and Lymphocyte Subset Changes During Iron Chelation Therapy

Case	Time	100:1	50:1	25:1	CD8	Leu 7	CD16
1	Pre	34.7	29.0	27.0	23.3	19.0	8.7
1	Day 1	7.7	7.3	2.9	26.8	23.9	7.8
1	Day 3	7.9	3.4	2.9	19.0	16.1	6.4
1	Day 6	11.6	12.6	6.3	19.8	19.9	6.0
2	Pre	32.0	34.7	28.6	17.9	5.9	5.8
2	Day 1	9.0	3.2	4.2	23.8	11.7	6.4
2	Day 3	8.9	6.9	4.7	10.9	3.2	5.7
2	Day 6	14.3	9.7	7.4	22.3	11.3	5.5

Table 4 Lymphocyte Surface Antigen Expression During Chelation

Case	Time	Lymphocyte Markers			NK Activity[b]	
		CD8	LEU 7	TR[a]	100:1	50:1
1	Pre	15.9	6.9	5.9	29.0	16.9
1	Post	19.5	9.5	1.2	15.0	8.2
2	Pre	20.7	12.5	12.6	43.3	31.5
2	Post	20.4	12.7	17.5	56.3	45.5

[a]Transferrin receptor.
[b]Percent cytotoxicity at the noted effector-target ratios.

zinc may bind to the Fc receptor type III (19). In related work, we have shown that under soluble conditions, 3G8, a monoclonal antibody recognizing FcRIII and other molecules which bind to the FcRIII can trigger gamma interferon (INF-γ) production (51). Thus, it is possible that zinc normally has a positive regulatory effect on NK activity through inducing INF-γ synthesis. If so, this would constitute a primary mechanism for metal regulation of the immune response. These studies suggest that metal processing elicits immediate effects on immune function and that these changes may have the potential for long-term consequences.

ACKNOWLEDGMENTS

These studies were supported in part by National Institutes of Health, National Cancer Institute grant PO1CA29502, New York State grant MCJ363023, the Helena Rubenstein Foundation, and the Children's Blood Foundation, New York, New York.
    The authors thank Joyce O'Flaherty, Christina Milburn, Desiree Ehleiter, Theresa Manalo, and Mahasti Hassani for expert technical assistance.

REFERENCES

1. Dallman PR (1987). Iron deficiency and the immune response. Am J Clin Nutr 46P:329-334.
2. Prasad AS (1979). Trace elements: Biochemical and clinical effects of zinc and copper. Am J Hematol 6:77-87.

3. Nalder BN, Mahoney AW, Ramakrishnan R, Hendricks DG (1972). Sensitivity of the immunological reactivity to the nutritional status of rats. J Nutri 102:535-541.
4. Elin RS (1975). The effect of magnesium deficiency in mice or serum immunoglobulin concentrations and antibody plaque forming cells. Proc Soc Exp Biol Med 148:620-622.
5. Koller LD, Exon JH, Roan JG (1976). Humoral antibody response in mice after single dose exposure to lead or cadmium. Proc Soc Exp Biol Med 151:339-347.
6. Koller LD, Vos JG (1981). Immunologic effects of metals. In: Immunologic Considerations in Toxicology. RP Sharma (ed). Boca Raton, Florida, CRC Press, pp 67-78.
7. Cook JA, Hoffman EO, Diluzio RN (1975). Influence of lead and cadmium on the susceptibility of rats to bacterial challenge. Proc Soc Exp Biol Med 150:741-746.
8. Cook JA, Hoffman EO, Diluzio RN (1975). Factors modifying susceptibility to bacterial endotoxin. The effect of lead and cadmium. CRC Crit Rev Toxicol 3:201-215.
9. Gainer JH, Pry TW (1972). Effects of arsenicals on viral infections in mice. Am J Vet Res 33:2299.
10. Prasad AS (ed) (1976). Trace Elements in Human Health and Disease. New York, Academic Press.
11. Koller LD, Exon JH, Arbogast B (1977). Methyl mercury: Effect on serum enzymes and humoral antibody. J Toxicol Environ Health 2:1115-1111.
12. Ganther HE, Hafeman DG, Lawrence RA, Serfass RE, Hoekstra WG (1976). Selenium and glutathione peroxidase in health and disease—A review. In: Trace Elements in Human Health and Disease. AS Prasad (ed). New York, Academic Press, p. 281.
13. Garofalo JA, Cunningham-Rundles S, Braun DW, Good RA (1980). In vitro effect of Zn^{++} on peripheral blood lymphocytes in patients with cancer. Int J Immunopharmacol 1:60-68.
14. Good RA, Fernandes G, Cunningham-Rundles C, Cunningham-Rundles S, Garofalo JA, Roos MK, Incefy GS, Iwata T (1980). The relation of zinc deficiency to immunologic function in animals and man. INSERM Symposium 16: Primary Immunodeficiencies. Seligman M and Hitzig WH (eds). Amsterdam, Elsevier/North Holland Biomedical Press, pp 223-234.
15. Cunningham-Rundles S, Cunningham-Rundles C, Dupont B, Good RA (1980). Zinc induced activation of human B lymphocytes. Clin Immunol Immunopathol 16:115-122.
16. Iwata T, Incefy GS, Cunningham-Rundles S, Cunningham-Rundles C, Smithwick E, Geller N, O'Reilly RJ, Good RA (1981). Circulating thymic hormone activity (FTS) in patients with primary and secondary immunodeficiency diseases. Am J Med 71:385-394.
17. Cunningham-Rundles C, Cunningham-Rundles S, Iwata T, Incefy G, Garofalo J, Menendez-Botet C, Lewis V, Twomey JJ, Good RA (1981). Zinc deficiency depressed thymic hormones and T lymphocyte dysfunction in patients with hypogammaglobulinemia. Clin Immunol Exp Pathol 21:387-396.
18. Cunningham-Rundles S, Cunningham-Rundles WF (1988). Zinc modulation of immune response. In: Nutrition and Immunology. Chandra R (ed). Liss, New York, pp 197-214.
19. Cunningham-Rundles S, Bockman RS, Lin A, Giardina PV, Hilgartner MW, Caldwell-Brown D, Carter DM (1990). Physiological and pharmacological effects of Zinc on immune response. Ann NY Acad Sci 587:113-122.
20. Keberle H (1964). The biochemistry of desferrioxamine and its relation to iron metabolism. Ann NY Acad Sci 119:758-768.
21. Wolman L (1964). Transfusion therapy in Cooley's anemia: Growth and health as related to lung range hemaglobin levels. A progress report. Ann NY Acad Sci 119:736.
22. Barry M, Flynn DM, Letsky et al. (1974). Long term chelation therapy in thalassemia major: Effect on liver iron concentration, liver histology and clinical progress. Br MJ Clin Res 2:16-20.
23. Propper RD, Cooper B, Rufo BL et al. (1977). Continuous subcutaneous administration of deferrioxamine in patients with iron overload. N Engl J Med 297:418-423.

24. Pippard MJ, Callender ST, Weatherall DJ (1978). Intensive iron chelation therapy with desferrioxamine in iron-loading anaemias Clin Sci 54:99-106.
25. Cairo MS (1990). Clinical spectrum of iron overload, novel uses of iron chelators and potential treatment of pediatric anemias with erythropoietin. Am J Pediatr Hematol Oncol 12:1-3.
26. Kaye SB, Owen M (1978). Cardiac arrhythmias in thalassemia major: Evaluation of chelation treatment using ambulatory monitoring. Br Med J 1:342-346.
27. Modell E, Letsky EA, Flynn DM et al. (1982). Survival and desferrioxamine in thalassemia major Br Med J 284:1081-1084.
28. Zurlo MG, DeStefano P, Borgina-Pignatt C et al. (1989). Survival and causes of death in thalassemia major. Lancet 2:27-30.
29. Wolfe L, Oliveri N, Sallan D et al. (1985). Prevention of cardiac disease by subcutaneous deferioxamine in patients with thalassemia major. N Engl J Med 312:1600-1603.
30. Maurer HS, Lloyd-Still JD, Ingrisano C, Gonzolez-Frussi F, Hong GR (1988). A prospective evaluation of iron chelation therapy in children with severe B-thalassemia. Am J Dis Child 142:287-292.
31. Modell B (1979). Advances in the use of iron chelating agents for the treatment of iron overload. Prog Hematol 11:267-312.
32. Cohen A (1990). Current status of iron chelation therapy with deferoxamine. Semin Hematol 27:86-90.
33. Davies SC, Hungerford JL, Arden GB, Marcus RE, Miller MH, Huehms ER (1983). Ocular toxicity of high dose intravenous desferrioxamine. Lancet 2:181-184.
34. Guerin A, London G, Marchais S, Metivier F, Pelisse J (1985). Acute deafness and desferrioxamine. Lancet 2:39-40.
35. Oliveri NF, Buncic JR, Chew E (1986). Visual and auditory neurotoxicity in patients receiving subcutaneous deferioxamine infusions. N Engl J Med 314:869-873.
36. Warth JA, Prasad AS, Zwas F, Frank RN (1981). Abnormal dark adaptation in sickle cell anemia. J Lab Clin Med 96:189-192.
37. Prasad AS, Niale A, Farid S et al. (1963). Zinc metabolism in normals and patients with the syndrome of iron deficiency anemia, hypogonadism and dwarfism. J Lab Clin Med 73:486-490.
38. DeVirgilis S, Congia M, Fra F, Argiolu F, Diana G, Cuc AI, Varsi A, Sanna G, Padd G, Fodde M, Franco-Pirastu G, Cao A (1988). Deferoxamine—Induced growth retardation in patients with thalassemia major. J Pediatr 113:661-669.
39. Hall H, DeVirgilis S, Congia M, Turio MD et al. (1988). Depletion of trace elements and acute ocular toxicity induced by desferrioxamine in patients with thalassemia. Arch Dis Child 63:250-255.
40. Cohen A, Martin M, Mizanin J, Kankle DF, Schwartz E (1990). Vision and hearing during deferoxamine therapy. J Pediatr 117:326-330.
41. Hall H, Blake DR, Winguard P et al. (1989). Ocular toxicity of desferrioxamine: An example of copper, promoted auto-oxidative damage? Br J Opthalmol 73:42-47.
42. Brill PW, Winchester P, Giardina PV, Cunningham-Rundles S (1990). Deferoxamine—Induced bone dysplasia in patients with thalassemia major. Am J Roentgenol 156:561-565.
43. Whitehouse BC, Prasad AS, Rabbani PI, Cossack ZT (1982). Determination of zinc in plasma, neutrophils, lymphocytes, and erythrocytes by flameless atomic absorption spectrophotometry. Clin Chem 28:475-481.
44. Bomford A, Isaac J, Roberts S, Edwards A, Young S, Williams R (1986). The effect of deseferrioxamine on transferrin receptors. The cell cycle and growth rates of human leukaemic cells. Biochem J 236:243-249.
45. Estrov Z, Tawa A, Wang XH et al. (1987). In vitro and in vivo effects of deferoxamine in neonatal acute leukemia. Blood 69:757-761.

46. Taetle R, Honeysett JM, Bergeron R (1989). Combination iron depletion therapy. J Natl Can Inst 81:1229-1235.
47. Lederman HM, Cohen A, Lee JWW, Freedman MH, Gelfand EW (1984). Deferoxamine a reversible S-phase inhibitor of human lymphocyte proliteration. Blood 64:748-753.
48. Carotenuto P, Dontessilli G, Cambier JC, Hayward AR (1986). Desferoxamine blocks IL-2 receptor expression an human T lymphocytes. J Immunol 136:2342-2347.
49. Cunningham-Rundles S, Pinto J, Giardina PV, Hilgartner MW (1991). Modulation of immune function by deferoxamine (submitted).
50. Fernandes G, Nair M, Onoe K, Tanoka T, Floyd R, Good RA (1979). Impairment of cell mediated function in zinc-deficient adult mice. Proc Natl Acad Sci USA 76:45-51.
51. Cunningham-Rundles S, Pearson FP (1990). Imuvert activation of natural killer cytotoxicity and interferon gamma production via CD16 triggering. Int J Immunopharmacol 6:589-598.

26
Stimulation of Breast Cancer-Specific Cellular Immunity by High-Dose Vitamin E and Vitamin A: Adjuvant Therapeutic Implications

Maurice M. Black and Reinhard E. Zachrau
New York Medical College, Valhalla, New York

INTRODUCTION

The adverse behavior of cancers in general and of breast cancer in particular is expressed in the clinically evident dissemination and progression of the disease. Such behavior reflects an interaction between the intrinsic aggressiveness of the cancer and the tumor-retarding potential of the host (1-3).

The aggressiveness of a cancer correlates inversely with the degree of nuclear differentiation of the cancer cells, expressed as nuclear grade (NG) (4). So powerful is NG as a prognostic feature that the 5-year postoperative survival can be shown to correlate markedly when this is the only considered variable, i.e., approximately 45, 65, and 90% for NG I (undifferentiated), NG II (moderately differentiated), and NG III (highly differentiated) breast cancers, respectively (5). Therefore, this relationship can be specifically useful in the evaluation of the effects of putative therapeutic agents, whether surgical, radiological, chemical, hormonal or immunological. In addition, there appear to be distinctive associations between NG and the effects of cytotoxic agents used in adjuvant therapy (6,7).

The aggressive potential of breast cancer in individual patients is also influenced by specific antitumor cell-mediated immunity (CMI) of the host. The expression of such reactivity is in turn dependent on specific antigenicity of the cancer cells. The striking influence of the interactions between tumor aggressiveness and host CMI on the biological behavior of breast cancer has been shown in previous publications (1,8,9). These data demonstrate that a system of prognostic classification can be constructed on the basis of NG and specific CMI, without regard to variables comprising the TNM classification. Our studies also indicate that specific CMI is a significant deterrent to the development of metachronous second primary breast cancers (5,8). Thus, the risk of metastases and second primary breast cancers might be reduced if one could maintain spontaneously occurring specific CMI or reduce a negative-to-positive change in CMI against autologous breast cancer (3,5).

Before evaluating the prognostic significance of putative immunotherapeutic agents, it is necessary to demonstrate that such agents can augment specific CMI. It was, therefore, of interest that a number of investigators had reported that high doses of vitamin E (VE) and vitamin A (VA) could enhance immune responses to recall antigens and, when used as adjuvants, could augment primary responses to neoantigens (10-13). It was of particular interest to us that these agents were reported to augment CMI as well as humoral immunity. The possibility that readily available, minimally toxic, and relatively inexpensive agents could apparently increase CMI, led to the present investigation of whether these agents could induce and/or maintain specific CMI in breast cancer patients. If so, it would then be appropriate to determine whether such induced reactivity had the same prognostic significance as spontaneous reactivity to antigens expressed on breast cancers.

We and others have shown that specific CMI can be monitored by means of leukocyte migration inhibition, blastogenesis, and skin test assays (14-17). In our hands, the skin window (SW) test has proven to be a particularly valuable indicator of spontaneously occurring, prognostically significant CMI (8,9). Analogous, albeit more limited, observations have also been made by Jansa et al. (18). The SW procedure is less costly than in vitro techniques and has the special advantage of yielding permanent preparations which can be reexamined at will and compared seriatim.

Microscopic studies as well as studies using leukocyte migration inhibition and SW tests demonstrated prognostically significant CMI responses to an antigen(s), operationally defined as "CMI determinant," that was more frequently expressed in preinvasive rather than invasive breast cancers (5,19-21). It further appears that this CMI determinant is analogous to a determinant of RIII-gp55, the major envelope glycoprotein of the RIII-murine mammary tumor virus (5,9,22). Therefore, gp55 can be used as a reference antigen in the SW test. Moreover, SW reactivity against autologous breast cancer was found to be directly associated with reactivity against gp55. However, the gp55-like CMI determinant is not demonstrable in approximately one-quarter to one-third of invasive breast cancers. In the absence of this determinant, there is a consequent absence of potentially protective reactivity against the autologous cancer despite the presence of specific host immunity. Therefore, we have used SW reactivity against both gp55 and autologous breast cancer as endpoints in the evaluation of the ability of high-dose vitamin therapy to augment specific CMI. Our earlier studies indicated that such treatment did favor negative-to-positive changes in reactivity against the gp55-like CMI determinant of breast cancer (23,24). We now present an expanded series of observations with particular reference to the clinical implications of reactivity associated with high-dose VE and/or VA therapy.

STUDY DESIGN

Patient Population

Breast cancer patients who were participants in our program for monitoring specific immunity were offered an opportunity to enroll in a study of the influence of high doses of VE and/or VA on such immunity. All patients were classified according to the NG of their breast cancers and the presence or absence of morphological evidence of immune reactivity against their cancers. In addition, the more conventional variables, such as histological type and stage of the disease, were recorded. The postoperative intervals at which the patients entered the study ranged from 2 months to more than 10 years. With one exception, all patients in this study had at least one and usually two or more negative SW tests against autologous breast cancer and/or gp55 prior to the initiation of high-dose vitamin therapy. Approximately one-third of the patients who were nonreactive before vitamin therapy had shown spontaneous SW reactivity against these targets in earlier time periods. *All patients were clinically free of recurrent disease and second primary cancers of the breast and other sites at the time of testing and classification of the SW responses.*

The Skin Window Technique

The salient feature of the SW test procedure is exposure to the target material, mounted on a glass coverslip, to an abraded area of skin for 28 to 32 hr. As described previously, the target materials are either 15-μ thick sections of autologous breast cancer tissue or 2 μg of purified gp55 (8,9,14). The purified preparations of gp55 were provided by Dr. Arnold S. Dion, Center for Molecular Medicine and Immunology, Newark, New Jersey. The isolation procedure for gp55 from RIII-murine mammary tumor virus has been described in detail elsewhere (25). After removal, the test coverslips are air dried, Wright-stained, and examined microscopically for the presence and prominence of distinctive patterns of mononuclear cell aggregates.

The Skin Window Response

Positive Response

Several distinctive types of SW responses are recognizable and have been found to correlate with a favorable prognosis (9,14). They include (a) aggregates of lymphoblastoid cells; (b) aggregates of histiocytic cells in mono- and/or multilayered arrangements; (c) aggregates of hypertrophied epithelioid-type cells, some of which may be multinucleated and resemble Langhans-type giant cells; and (d) focal aggregates of lymphoblastoid cells admixed with neutro-, baso-, and eosinophilic leukocytes, suggestive of a Jones-Mote-type response. Infrequently, a response pattern occurs, designated as "stellate," which involves elongated and star-shaped histiocytic cells resembling fibroblasts in tissue culture. In this chapter, the designation "positive," or "SW-3," is used collectively for any of these types of responses, as long as the size of the respective aggregates was at least one-half of a low-power microscopic field.

Negative and Intermediate Responses

Each of the positive types of cellular exudates has been found to have a degenerative counterpart, which is characterized by cytoplasmic vacuolization and cytonecrosis and typically associated with an admixture of intact and degenerating polymorphonuclear leukocytes. Such degenerative responses are classified as "negative." Exudates consisting of scattered macrophages, as commonly seen in tests with blank coverslips, as well as hypocellular exudates and exudates, consisting of a mixture of acute and chronic inflammatory cells, were also classified as "negative." Exudates with the qualitative characteristics of "positive" responses but of a lesser quantity (one-quarter to less than one-half of a low-power microscopic field) were designated as "intermediate," or "SW-2," responses.

Vitamin Regimen

In these studies, courses of VE therapy consisted of daily doses of 1200-2000 IU, whereas courses of VA therapy consisted of the daily intake of 200,000-300,000 IU, both for 21-35 days. In VE/VA combination treatment, the same doses as those used in single-agent therapy were prescribed.

Our earlier observation that VE and VA had similar capabilities with regard to immune augmentation led us to the use of VE as the initial agent, since there have been no adverse effects. Patients who failed to demonstrate increased reactivity after VE treatment were given VA. If the latter approach failed to augment SW reactivity, VE and VA were used in combination. In this study, we attempted to maintain reactivity by repeated therapy courses with one or both agents. The symbol VE/VA is used to indicate treatment with either or both of these agents.

CLINICAL EFFECTS OF VITAMIN E AND VITAMIN A

General

All patients who participated in this study were regularly questioned about possible adverse effects of the treatments and, initially, their chemistry profiles (SMAC) were monitored. For VE-treated patients, coagulation status screens were also monitored. No clinical complaints were reported by any of our patients treated with VE except for occasional reports of flatulence. There was no evidence of abnormal bleeding, thrombosis, impaired wound healing, or hypertension.

Approximately one-third of VA-treated patients reported mild to moderate dryness of the mouth and some itchiness of the skin while taking 300,000 IU VA/day. These symptoms subsided in all instances within days after termination of the VA administration. Occasionally, the mucosal dryness was so pronounced that the daily VA dosage was reduced to 200,000 IU, which caused only mild dryness during the remainder of the treatment course. None of our patients reported blurred vision, nausea, hair loss, conjunctival irritation, skin sores, or bone pain. Three patients experienced recurrent transient headaches while on VA therapy. None of these patients showed any abnormalities in repeated clinical chemistry profiles. One patient who reported no clinical complaints presented with a transient elevation of liver enzyme levels after 28 days of VA therapy. All values returned to normal range within 10-30 days after cessation of the VA intake. It is our current practice to evaluate the liver enzyme levels prior to the first and after completion of each VA therapy course.

Because of reports linking high-dose VA intake to an increased risk of birth defects (26), pregnant women are considered noneligible for participation in the VA program, and women of child-bearing age were advised to practice contraception during and for at least 3 months after cessation of VA therapy.

Changes in SW Reactivity in the Absence of Vitamin Therapy

Of those breast cancer patients who did not receive VE/VA therapy, approximately one-fourth showed positive SW responses to autologous breast cancer during the first postoperative year. As shown in Table 1, this reactivity did not vary significantly with the NG of the cancer. During the succeeding year, striking differences in SW reactivity were found in relation to the reactivity during the preceding interval. Pa-

Table 1 Spontaneous (Naturally Occurring) Skin Window Reactivity

Interval Prior SW Reactivity	Nuclear grade[a]			
	I	II	III	Total
1-12 mpo[b]				
no prior test	18/91(20)[d]	23/97(24)	16/49(33)	57/237(24)[e]
13-24 mpo				
prior SW − 3[c]	3/ 5(60)	4/ 9(44)	6/ 7(86)	13/ 21(62)[f]
prior SW < 3[c]	5/23(22)	5/20(25)	8/19(42)	18/ 62(29)[f]
total	8/28(29)	9/29(31)	14/26(54)	31/ 83(37)[e]
25-36 mpo				
prior SW − 3[h]/SW − 3[i]	1/ 1	2/ 3	2/ 4	5/ 8(63)
prior SW < 3/SW − 3	1/ 1	2/ 4	3/ 4	6/ 9(67)
Subtotal	2/ 2	4/ 7	5/ 8	11/ 17(65)[g]
prior SW − 3/SW < 3	0	1/ 3	0	1/ 3(33)
prior SW < 3/SW < 3	1/ 4	0/ 8	1/ 6	2/ 18(11)
Subtotal	1/ 4	1/11	1/ 6	3/ 21(14)[g]
Total	3/ 6(50)	5/18(28)	6/14(43)	14/ 38(37)

Spontaneous skin window (SW) reactivity against autologous breast cancer at successive postoperative intervals; maximal reactivity per interval of patients who were not treated with vitamin E/vitamin A; all patients clinically free of recurrent disease at the time of testing.
[a]Nuclear grades I, II, and III represent low, moderate, and high degree of nuclear differentiation, respectively.
[b]Months postoperatively.
[c]SW − 3, positive, and SW < 3, negative or intermediate reactivity.
[d]Number with SW-3/total number tested; percentage in parenthesis.
[e]$p < 0.05$.
[f]$p < 0.02$.
[g]$p < 0.005$.
[h]Refers to reactivity, 1-12 mpo.
[i]Refers to reactivity, 13-24 mpo.

tients with positive reactivity 1-12 months postoperatively had positive reactivity more frequently during the subsequent year than patients who were nonreactive during the first postoperative year; i.e., 62 and 29%, respectively ($p < 0.02$). There was also a modest but significant increase in the overall proportion of patients with positive reactivity ($p < 0.05$). A similar relationship was observed between SW reactivity during the 13-24-month period and that during the 25-36-month period. That is, patients who were either responsive during the first *and* second postoperative year, or those who became responsive during the second postoperative year, were more frequently responsive during the third postoperative year compared to patients who had either never responded in the prior intervals or who lost reactivity during the second year. Thus, 65% of patients who were reactive in the second year were also reactive in the third year compared to only 14% of patients who were nonreactive in the second year ($p < 0.005$). Thus, positive reactivity is commonly maintained during succeeding time intervals, whereas only a minority of nonreactive patients subsequently became reactive spontaneously. These observations provided the reference for the evaluation of the influence of VE/VA adjuvant therapy on specific immunity.

Vitamin-Associated SW Reactivity

Prototypic Observations

Table 2 lists some representative observations on the ability of VE and VA, singly and in combination, to induce negative-to-positive changes in reactivity against gp55. The data indicate that each of these treatment modalities can augment SW reactivity against gp55. It is noteworthy that some patients who did not become reactive after treatment with VE and VA alone did so after treatment with VE and VA in combination.

While the duration of therapy-associated reactivity was usually limited to a few months, a minority of patients maintained such reactivity for more than 12 months after completion of a treatment course. Moreover, in a high proportion of patients, reactivity could be restored repeatedly by subsequent therapy courses. Such treatment-related repetitive changes in SW reactivity are exemplified in Figures 1a-1d. In this patient, treatment with VE led to a SW response to gp55, which was characterized by aggregates of epithelioid-type cells in a tubercle-like arrangement (Fig. 1b). Although the pretreatment negative response did involve aggregation of mononuclear cells, these cells showed extensive cytoplasmic vacuolization, phagocytosis, and cytonecrosis. In addition, there were prominent accumulations of intact and degenerating polymorphonuclear cells among the mononuclear cell aggregates (Fig. 1a). This type of degenerative response reappeared after VE treatment was halted for 4 months (Fig. 1c). After repeat treatment with VE, the SW once again showed an intact tubercle-like pattern as well as foci of lymphoblastoid cells (Fig. 1d). Such repeated augmentation of SW reactivity against gp55 has been observed in the majority of patients who showed an initial negative-to-positive change in reactivity after treatment with VE and/or VA.

Augmented Reactivity Against Autologous Invasive Breast Cancer and GP55

Table 3 lists the specific SW responses to autologous invasive breast cancer and to gp55 in individual patients, unselected as to stage, 1-24 months before and after

Table 2 Effect of Vitamin Adjuvant Therapy on Skin Window Reactivity

Type of therapy[a]	Postoperative interval before vitamin therapy		
	≤24 months	25-120 months	total
VE only	14/24 (58)[b,c]	16/22 (73)	30/46 (65)
VA only	5/12 (42)	11/18 (61)	16/30 (53)
VE plus VA	7/11 (64)	7/ 9 (78)	14/20 (70)

Relative frequency of negative-to-positive conversion of skin window reactivity against gp55 among breast cancer patients, following adjuvant therapy with high-dose vitamin E (VE) and/or vitamin A (VA); maximal reactivity change per patient per postoperative interval during which therapy was begun.
[a]For therapy schedules, see study design.
[b]Numbers of patients showing posttherapy negative-to-positive conversion of skin window reactivity/total numbers of patients treated; in parentheses, percentages.
[c]All patients clinically free of recurrent disease at the times of testing.

Table 3 SW Reactivity to Autologous Cancer and GP55

Pre-VE/VA therapy[a]	Post-VE/VA therapy[a]		
	SW−3	SW<3	total
SW Tests Against BCa			
SW−3	10	6	16 (30)[b,d]
SW<3	21 [55][c]	17	38 [100]
Total	31 (57)[d]	23	54 (100)[f]
SW Tests Against GP55			
SW−3	16	4	20 (36)[e]
SW<3	27 [75]	9	36 [100]
Total	43 (77)[e]	13	56 (100)[f]

Maximal skin window (SW) reactivity against autologous invasive breast cancer (BCa) and against gp55, 1-24 months before and 1-24 months after adjuvant therapy with vitamin E and/or vitamin A (VE/VA); 71 patients treated at postoperative intervals ranging from 3 months to more than 10 years.
[a]All patients clinically free of recurrent disease at the time of testing.
[b]In parentheses, percentages of totals in parentheses (100%).
[c]In brackets, percentages of bracketed totals [100%].
[d]$p < 0.01$.
[e]$p < 0.0001$.
[f]Thirty-nine patients had pre- and posttherapy SW tests against both, BCa *and* gp55; 15 patients had pre- and posttherapy tests against BCa only and 17 patients against gp55 only.

the start of VE/VA treatment. VE/VA treatments were initiated over a wide range of postoperative intervals.

Among our patients who were treated with VE/VA, approximately one-third showed pretreatment-positive (SW-3) responses to autologous breast cancer. This percentage was similar to that found in the reference series of patients who received no VE/VA therapy. Those VE/VA-treated patients who were reactive against autologous breast cancer prior to treatment, tended to maintain reactivity after treatment; i.e., 10/16 (63%), showing that VE/VA treatment did not negate pretreatment reactivity. This proportion of reactive patients is similar to that in the reference series (see Table 1).

After treatment with VE/VA, the overall proportion of patients with positive reactivity increased approximately twofold; i.e., from 30 to 57%, $p < 0.01$. This treatment-related increase in the proportion of reactive patients reflected negative-to-positive changes in reactivity. Thus, of 38 patients who were nonreactive (SW<3) before VE/VA therapy, 21 (55%) became reactive after treatment. As indicated in Table 1, spontaneous negative-to-positive changes in reactivity against autologous breast cancer in successive test intervals were significantly less common; i.e., 29% for the second and 14% for the third postoperative year, $p < 0.02$ and $p < 0.01$, respectively. These data indicate that negative-to-positive changes in CMI against autologous breast cancer were significantly associated with VE/VA treatment.

Since our prior studies indicated that spontaneous SW reactivity against autologous breast cancer is related to reactivity against gp55, VE/VA was expected to have similar effects on SW reactivity against both test antigens. The data in Table 3 show that this did occur. Further, the VE/VA-augmented reactivity against autologous breast cancer and against gp55 was not exclusively due to an increment in the

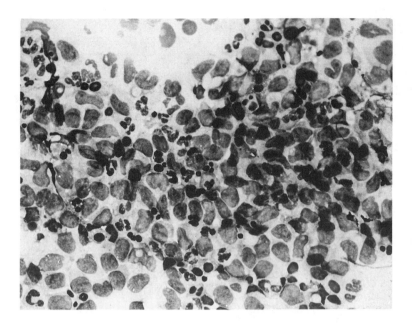

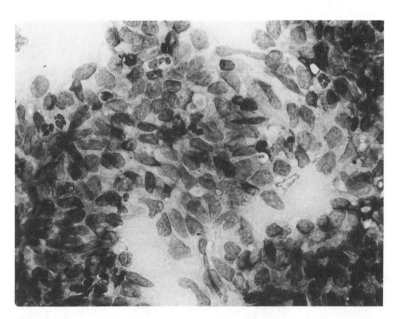

Figure 1 Skin window (SW) responses of a postoperative stage 0 breast cancer patient (Code No. 32) to gp55, in relation to VE therapy (Wright's stain × 475); this patient had six spontaneously positive SW tests, 1-22 months postoperatively (mpo), and was SW-negative, 25 and 27 mpo. (a) Prior to the first course of VE therapy (27 mpo): Aggregates of vacuolated histiocytic cells, showing phagocytosis and cytonecrosis, with intermingled polymorphonuclear leukocytes (*negative* response). (b) After 21 days of the first course of VE therapy: multilayered

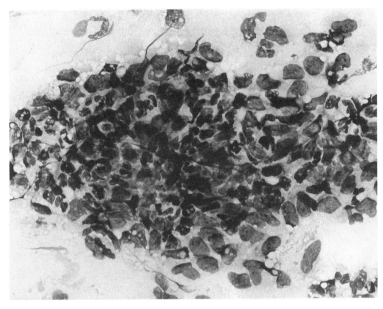

(c)

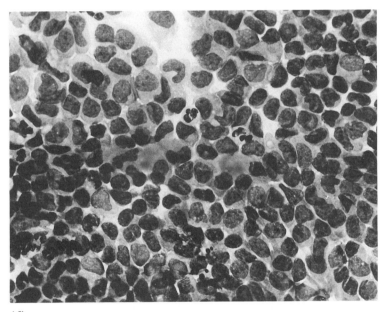

(d)

aggregates of epithelioid-type histiocytic cells in a tubercle-like arrangement (*positive* response). (c) 114 days after completion fo the first course of VE therapy: Small multilayered aggregates of phagocytic vacuolated histiocytic cells with intermingled polymorphonuclear leukocytes (*negative* response). (d) After repeat treatment with VE for 28 days: Aggregates of epithelioid-type histiocytic cells, similar to those seen in Figure 1b; in addition, foci of compact aggregates of large lymphoblastoid cells (*positive* response).

cellular exudate. In both instances, it frequently involved a change from the *degenerative* counterpart of a positive type of response to the *intact* positive type of cellular response, as exemplified in Figure 1.

SW Reactivity Against Autologous Breast Cancer in Relation to Reactivity Against GP55

Table 3 demonstrates that VE/VA treatment was associated with a significant increase in positive SW responses to autologous breast cancer and to gp55, separately. As noted earlier, SW reactivity against autologous breast cancer is closely associated with reactivity against gp55, presumably because of the expression of a gp55-like CMI determinant in the cancer tissue (9). Accordingly, it was pertinent to evaluate the persistence of this relationship in VE/VA-treated patients. The data in Table 4 indicate that before *and* after VE/VA treatment *SW reactivity against the autologous breast cancer was similarly closely associated with reactivity against gp55*. In short, this constitutes indirect evidence that VE/VA therapy of breast cancer patients augments CMI against a gp55-like determinant in the autologous cancer.

Prognostic Significance of Augmented Reactivity

Metastatic Progression

Our prior studies (8,9) and our current observations (Table 5) indicate that among patients with NG I and NG II breast cancers, the survival characteristics are related to SW reactivity against autologous breast cancer. Table 5 also indicates that this relationship continued to exist among patients with and without adjuvant therapy

Table 4 Relative Reactivity To Autologous Cancer and GP55

SW reactivity against GP55	SW reactivity against BCa		
	SW − 3	SW < 3	Total
Pre-VE/VA[a]			
SW − 3	10 (59)[b,c]	7	17 (100)
SW < 3	4 (14)[c]	25	29 (100)
Total	14 (30)	32	46 (100)[e]
Post-VE/VA[a]			
SW − 3	21 (64)[d]	12	33 (100)
SW < 3	2 (17)[d]	10	12 (100)
Total	23 (51)	22	45 (100)[e]

Relationship between skin window (SW) reactivity against gp55 and against autologous invasive breast cancer (BCa) before and after adjuvant therapy with vitamin E and/or vitamin A (VE/VA); intervals between BCa surgery and VE/VA therapy ranging from 3 months to >10 years.
[a]Pre-VE/VA = 1-24 months before, post-VE/VA = 1-24 months after initiation of VE/VA therapy; all patients clinically free of recurrent disease at the times of testing.
[b]In parentheses, percentages.
[c]$p < 0.005$.
[d]$p < 0.02$.
[e]Thirty-nine patients were tested against both targets pre- and post-VE/VA; seven patients, tested against both targets pre-VE/VA, were tested against only one target post-VE/VA; six patients, tested against both targets post-VE/VA, were tested against only one target pre-VE/VA.

Table 5 Skin Window Reactivity and Adjuvant Cytotoxic Chemotherapy

Reactivity against autologous BCa	Nuclear grades I and II[a]				Nuclear grade III[a]	
	No chemo-R_x		chemo-R_x[b]			
	control	VE/VA	control	VE/VA	control	VE/VA
SW − 3[c]	7/ 40 [0.18][d,e]	1/ 7 [0.14]	0/ 3	0/4	0/19	0/3
SW < 3[c]	51/ 61 [0.84][e]	3/ 7 [0.43]	13/ 9 [1.44]	1/1	2/24 [0.08]	0/1
Total	58/101 [0.57][f]	4/14 [0.29][f]	13/12 [1.08][g]	1/5 [0.20][g]	2/43 [0.05]	0/4

Skin window (SW) reactivity against nuclear grade-characterized autologous invasive breast cancer (BCa), spontaneous and 1-24 months after initiation of adjuvant therapy with vitamin E and/or vitamin A (VE/VA), administered between 3 and 24 months postoperatively; patients with and without prior adjuvant cytotoxic chemotherapy; relationship to postoperative survival characteristics.
[a]Nuclear grades I, II, and III represent low, moderate, and high degree of nuclear differentiation of the cancer cells, respectively.
[b]Chemo-R_x, postoperative adjuvant therapy with cytoxan, methotrexate, and 5-fluorouracil.
[c]SW − 3, positive reactivity; SW < 3, negative or intermediate reactivity.
[d]Numbers of patients with metastasis within 60 months/numbers of patients with recurrence-free survival for ≥60 months postoperatively; in brackets, ratios.
[e]$p < 0.0005$.
[f,g]not significant.

with CMF and/or VE/VA. In the series without adjuvant therapy, the ratios of patients with metastasis <60 months/patients without metastasis ≥60 months postoperatively were 0.18 and 0.84, respectively, for patients with and without positive SW reactivity, $p < 0.0005$. Analogous reactivity-related differences in survival ratios were maintained among patients with NG I and NG II breast cancers who received adjuvant therapy with CMF and/or VE/VA. However, probably because of smaller numbers of patients, the observed differences are below the level of statistical significance. In accord with our prior observations (8), metastases were infrequent among patients with NG III invasive breast cancers. This was the case even among patients who were nonreactive to autologous cancer. VE/VA-treated patients who responded showed the same survival characteristics. Thus, VE/VA therapy-induced responders had the same survival advantage as natural responders.

Considered together, the data of Tables 4 and 5 indicate that VE/VA treatment augments SW reactivity in a high proportion of breast cancer patients and that both specificity and prognostic characteristics are equivalent among the treated and the untreated responders. In all cases where reactivity against gp55 was not accompanied by reactivity against autologous breast cancer, it may be assumed that the cancer lacked the gp55-like CMI determinant. In such cases, CMI against gp55 would not be expected to impede metastatic progression.

Metachronous Second Primary Breast Cancers

Previous studies had suggested that SW reactivity against autologous breast cancer and/or gp55 was inversely related to the subsequent development of invasive breast cancers (5,8). Such an inverse relationship was *not* found in regard to the development of precursor lesions (in situ carcinoma and precancerous mastopathy).

To date, we have enrolled a total of 397 patients with in situ or invasive breast cancers in our SW study. Twenty-five of these patients have developed metachronous invasive breast cancers and 10 have developed metachronous precursor lesions over a wide range of postoperative intervals (12 to >120 months). In 13 of the patients

Table 6 Skin Window Reactivity and Metachronous Primary Invasive Cancer

Metachronous Second Primary Breast Lesion	Reactivity against autologous first BCa and/or GP55					
	SW – 3[a]			SW < 3[a]		
	total	control	VE/VA	total	control	VE/VA
Invasive BCa	1 (14)[c]	0	1	12 (92)[c]	10	2
Precursor[b]	6	2	4	1	1	0
Total	7 (100)	2	5	13 (100)	11	2

Relative frequency of metachronous primary invasive breast cancers, in relation to the maximal skin window (SW) reactivity against the autologous first primary breast cancer and/or gp55 within the 30 month preceding the diagnosis of a metachronous primary breast lesion; all patients clinically free of recurrence and metachronous primary cancer at the time of testing.
[a]SW – 3, positive, and SW < 3, negative or intermediate reactivity.
[b]Precursor category includes three precancerous mastopathies (one in the SW – 3 control series, two in the SW – 3 VE/VA series) and four in situ carcinomas.
[c]$p < 0.005$.

who developed metachronous invasive breast cancers, and in 7 of the patients who developed metachronous precursor lesions, we had performed one or more SW tests against autologous breast cancer and/or gp55 < 30 months before the proximate metachronous lesions became clinically evident.

As shown in Table 6, the proximate metachronous lesions were less likely to be invasive in patients who had positive (SW-3) responses to autologous breast cancer and/or gp55 than in those without such reactivity, $p < 0.0005$. It also appears that the relationships between SW reactivity and the types of proximate subsequent lesions are similar among patients with and without adjuvant VE/VA therapy.

The data in Table 6, coupled with those of Table 5, indicate that VE/VA-associated positive SW reactivity is equivalent to natural positive reactivity in the impeding effect on the progression of occult metastatic foci and the progression of in situ breast cancers.

VITAMIN THERAPY AND CMI

In general, *in vivo* CMI responses involve an antigen-induced, focalized accumulation of lymphoreticuloendothelial cells. The analogous cellular responses in the SWs also manifest focalized accumulations of lymphoid and/or epithelioid cells, as indicated under the description of "positive" responses. The distinctive features of CMI responses, both in tissues and on SWs, depend on a prior sensitizing exposure to the antigen in question, subsequent contact between the antigen and sensitized cells, and an intact capability of the sensitized cells to undergo changes consisting of a sequence of focalization and differentiation.

Our observations indicate that VE/VA-associated changes in SW reactivity against the gp55-like CMI determinant are not simply accomplished in an "off/on" fashion. On the contrary, there are duration as well as dose requirements that must be met in order to achieve negative-to-positive changes (23). These observations suggest that the augmented reactivity involves a significant change in the number and/or in the differentiation of circulating mononuclear cells that are responsive to the antigen in question. This interpretation is supported by the persistence of augmented reactivity after cessation of VE/VA therapy.

These studies indicate that a high proportion of *negative* responses are in the form of *degenerative variants of positive* responses, as judged by morphological features. Such negative responses are associated with aggregations of epithelioid and/or lymphoid cells. However, as indicated earlier, these cells show cytoplasmic vacuolar degeneration, phagocytosis, and cytonecrosis and are commonly associated with accumulations of neutrophilic polymorphonuclear leukocytes. Analogous degenerative epithelioid cellular responses have been observed in the sinusoids of lymph nodes that drain breast cancers (19,27). In both SW and lymph node responses antigens can apparently trigger degenerative as well as reactive changes. In both SW and lymph node responses aggregates of activated lymphoreticuloendothelial cells are prognostically favorable, whereas the degenerative counterparts are not. In both, the vacuolar degenerative changes apparently reflect a subverted type of response involving phagocytic changes or an ineffective transformation of differentiated cells. Our current study suggests that high-dose VE/VA therapy protects against degenerative transformations of prognostically favorable cellular responses and promotes restoration of positive responses. It is noteworthy in this regard that VE has been reported to exert protection against oxidative damage of T cells in particular (28,29), whereas VA is reported to be less effective. However, VA has been shown to upregulate interleukin-2 receptors on activated human thymocytes and to reduce the suppressive effects of corticosteroids and cytoxan on immune responses (30,31).

Since all of our patients were well nourished at the time of diagnosis, it is unlikely that the observed VE/VA-associated immune augmentation involved a correction of dietary inadequacy. Moreover, specific questioning disclosed that approximately one-third of our patients had been taking daily vitamin supplements for several years before the diagnosis of their breast cancers. The vitamin supplements commonly included VA (5000-10,000 IU daily) and/or VE (400-800 IU daily) with or without other vitamins.

In a related study of the influence of VA and VE on mammary carcinogenesis, Wald et al. examined plasma retinol, β-carotene and VE levels in a prospective study of a large population of women (32). A comparison of plasma levels of these constituents in a series of women who subsequently developed breast cancer with those in a series of control women revealed no significant differences in the retinol and β-carotene levels between the two series. There appeared to be some differences in the VE levels between the two series; namely, the lower the level, the higher the risk of a subsequent breast cancer. However, continued studies have not substantiated the latter findings, a conclusion also reached by Willett et al. (33). In the light of these observations as well as our own data, it does *not* seem likely that intervention in the form of *conventional* VE or VA supplementation is likely to induce specific tumor-retarding CMI in control individuals. Among 14 of our patients who had been taking vitamin supplements up until the diagnosis of their cancers, none showed spontaneous reactivity against gp55. However, after seven of these patients were given high-dose VE/VA therapy, six of them demonstrated SW reactivity against gp55 within 6 months postoperatively. These observations indicate that there are important differences in the effects of physiological and pharmacological doses of VE and VA on the immune system.

Our study on VE/VA-associated SW reactivity may provide a prototype for investigations of diverse types of putative immunostimulants. Of course, potentially favorable CMI, spontaneous or induced, is unlikely to be therapeutically effective if the cancer in question lacks the CMI determinant to which reactivity is tested (34). It is noteworthy in this context that Eccles et al. demonstrated that a retinoic acid analogue had the ability to inhibit the growth and metastasis of syngeneic transplantable tumors (35,36). This inhibition was apparently mediated by an augmented function of the host T lymphocytes *and* the expression of specific antigenicity by the tumor. These observations are analogous to our findings regarding the prognostic significance of spontaneous and VE/VA-associated specific immunoty against autologous breast cancer.

If induced negative-to-positive changes in specific CMI are prognostically favorable, then induced positive-to-negative changes would be prognostically unfavorable. The latter possibility warrants consideration in light of the increasing adjuvant use of cytotoxic radiation and chemotherapy. Our data suggest that the benefits and limitations of adjuvant cytotoxic therapy would be more adequately assessed if attention were paid to the nuclear differentiation of the cancers *and* to the specific CMI of the host.

Perhaps the most provocative of our observations is the inverse relationship between specific immunity and the proximate development of second primary invasive breast cancers. This relationship was found with spontaneous and VE/VA-associated reactivity. In both instances, the reduction in proximate second invasive breast cancers appeared to reflect an immunologically mediated impediment of the progression of in situ-to-invasive cancer. Such a relationship is critically pertinent to the potential development of immunoprophylaxis (5,34). It is, thus, of great interest that Shklar et al. have reported that the administration of VE inhibits the development of buccal carcinomas induced in hamsters by the local application of 7,12-dimethylbenz[a]anthracene (37). In this study, VE-treated animals showed malignant changes which were limited to dysplasias and degenerating in situ cancers associated with dense mononuclear cell infiltrates. The authors concluded that VE stimulated an immunological response which selectively destroyed the tumor cells *as they began to develop*. Hong et al. have reported on a series of patients with invasive cancers of the head and neck who were treated with high daily doses of isotretinoin (38). In these patients, there was a reduced incidence of second primary invasive cancers without apparent effect on the initial carcinoma. These latter observations as well as those of Shklar et al. are consistent with our prior view on the immunoprophylactic significance of in situ carcinoma-associated immunogenicity (5,21) and with our current observations on the VE/VA therapy-associated augmentation of specific immunity.

CONCLUSIONS

Investigations of the clinical benefits of putative stimulants of antitumor immunity should address the following questions:

1. Is there evidence of *spontaneously* occurring immunity against autologous cancer?
2. If so, are such *spontaneously* occurring responses prognostically favorable?
3. Can the putative stimulant induce a negative-to-positive change in the indices of spontaneously occurring prognostically favorable immunity?

Our prior studies provide ample documentation for affirmative answers to questions 1 and 2. Our current report supports an affirmative answer to question 3 for vitamin E and vitamin A, used singly or in combination at defined doses for defined periods of time. Accordingly, induced reactivity should be prognostically favorable. Thus, the adjuvant use of VE/VA should be clinically beneficial. While our data are consistent with this expectation, there is a need for observations on a larger series of patients over extended periods of time. We submit that the available data provide ample justification for such an expanded investigation.

ACKNOWLEDGMENTS

Supported in part by a grant from the Cancer Research Institute, Inc., New York, New York.

We thank Monique C. Katz, M.D., Associate Professor of Clinical Radiology, Columbia Presbyterian Hospital, New York, New York, for prompting us to examine the possibility that high doses of vitamin A would stimulate specific cell-mediated immunity in breast cancer patients. We also wish to thank Hemmige N. Bhagavan, M.D., Hoffmann-La Roche Inc., Nutley, New Jersey, for providing vitamin E and vitamin A for our patients during the early phases of this study.

REFERENCES

1. Black MM, Barclay THC, Hankey BF. Prognosis in breast cancer utilizing histologic characteristics of the primary tumor. Cancer 36:2048-2055, 1975.
2. Black MM, Zachrau RE. Antitumor immunity in breast cancer patients: Biologic and therapeutic implications. J Reprod Med 23:21-32, 1979.
3. Black MM, Zachrau RE. Immune mechanisms: Prognostic, therapeutic, and preventive significance. In: Breast Cancer: Diagnosis & Treatment (IM Ariel, JB Cleary, eds). McGraw-Hill, New York, 1986, pp 128-142.
4. Black MM, Speer FD. Nuclear structure in cancer tissues. Surg Gynecol Obstet 105:97-102, 1957.
5. Black MM, Zachrau RE. In situ carcinoma-associated immunogenicity: Therapeutic and prophylactic implications in breast cancer patients. In: Advances in Cancer Research. Vol. 56 (GF Vande Woude, G Klein, eds). Academic Press, New York, 1991, pp 105-131.
6. Black MM, Hankey BF, Barclay THC. Intrastage prognostic heterogeneity: Implications for adjuvant chemotherapy of breast cancer. J Natl Cancer Inst 68:445-447, 1982.
7. Fisher B, Fisher ER, Redmond C. Ten-year results from the National Surgical Adjuvant Breast and Bowel Project (NSABP) clinical trial evaluating the use of L-phenylalanine mustard (L-PAM) in the management of primary breast cancer. J Clin Oncol 4:929-941, 1986.
8. Black MM, Zachrau RE, Hankey BF, Wesley M. Skin window reactivity to autologous breast cancer: An index of prognostically significant cell-mediated immunity. Cancer 62:72-83, 1988.
9. Black MM, Zachrau RE, Ashikari RH, Hankey BF. Prognostic significance of cellular immunity to autologous breast carcinoma and glycoprotein 55. Arch Surg 124:202-206, 1989.
10. Dresser DW. Adjuvanticity of vitamin A. Nature 217:527-529, 1968.
11. Cohen BE, Cohen IK. Vitamin A: Adjuvant and steroid antagonist in the immune response. J Immunol 111:1376-1380, 1973.
12. Patek P, Collins JL, Yogeeswaran G, Dennert G. Anti-tumor potential of retinoic acid: Stimulation of immune-mediated effectors. Int J Cancer 24:624-628, 1979.
13. Tengerdy RP, Mathias MM, Nockels CF. Effect of vitamin E on immunity and disease resistance. In: Vitamins, Nutrition and Cancer (KN Prasad, ed). Karger, Basel, 1984, pp 123-133.

14. Black MM, Leis HP Jr. Human breast carcinoma. III. Cellular responses to autologous breast cancer: Skin window procedure. NY State J Med 70:2583-2587, 1970.
15. Black MM, Leis HP Jr, Shore B, Zachrau RE. Cellular hypersensitivity to breast cancer: Assessment by a leukocyte migration procedure. Cancer 33:952-958, 1974.
16. Akiyoski T, Nakamura Y, Kawaguchi M, Tsuji H. Cellular hypersensitivity to autologous tumor extracts in patients with breast carcinoma. Jpn J Surg 8:236-241, 1978.
17. Cannon GB, Dean JH, Herberman RB, Keets M, Alford C. Lymphoproliferative responses to tumor extracts as prognostic indicators in patients with resected breast cancer. Int J Cancer 27:131-138, 1981.
18. Jansa P, Podstata J. Cellular reaction to autologous tumor tissues followed by "skin window" technique in orofacial tumors. Neoplasma 25:197-201, 1978.
19. Black MM, Chabon AB. In situ carcinoma of the breast. Pathol Annu 4:185-210, 1969.
20. Black MM. Structural, antigenic and biological characteristics of precancerous mastopathy. Cancer Res 36:2596-2604, 1976.
21. Black MM, Zachrau RE. Stepwise mammary carcinogenesis: Immunological considerations. In: Advances in Early Detection and Treatment of Breast Cancer (J Zander, J Baltzer, eds). Springer, New York, 1985, pp 64-72.
22. Zachrau RE, Black MM, Dion AS, Shore B, Williams CJ, Leis HP Jr. Specificity of the simultaneous cell-mediated immune reactivity to RIII murine mammary tumor virus glycoprotein 55 and human breast cancer tissues. Cancer Res 38:3414-3420, 1978.
23. Black MM, Zachrau RE, Dion AS, Katz M. Stimulation of prognostically favorable cell-mediated immunity of breast cancer patients by high dose vitamin A and vitamin E. In: Vitamins, Nutrition and Cancer (KN Prasad, ed). Karger, Basel, 1984, pp 134-146.
24. Black MM, Zachrau RE, Katz MF. Adjuvant immunotherapy of breast cancer: Prototypic observations with alpha-tocopherol and retinol. In: Nutrients and Cancer Prevention (KN Prasad, FL Meyskens Jr, eds). Humana Press, Clifton, New Jersey, 1990, pp 319-328.
25. Dion AS, Williams CJ, Pomenti AA. The major structural proteins of murine mammary tumor virus: Techniques for isolation. Anal Biochem 82:18-28, 1977.
26. Geelen JAG. Hypervitaminosis A induced teratogenesis. CRC Rev Toxicol 6:351-375, 1979.
27. Hirschl S, Black MM, Kwon CS. Ultrastructural characteristics of sinus histiocytic reaction in lymph nodes draining various stages of breast cancer. Cancer 38:807-817, 1976.
28. Bendich A. Antioxidant micronutrients and immune responses. Ann NY Acad Sci 587:168-180, 1990.
29. Tengerdy RP. The role of vitamin E in immune response and disease resistance. Ann NY Acad Sci 587:24-33, 1990.
30. Sidell N, Ramsdell F. Retinoic acid upregulates interleukin-2 receptors on activated human thymocytes. Cell Immunol 115:299-309, 1988.
31. Nuwayri-Salti N, Murad T. Immunologic and anti-immunosuppressive effects of vitamin A. Pharmacology 30:181-187, 1985.
32. Wald NJ, Boreham J, Hayward JL, Bulbrook RD. Plasma retinol, beta-carotene and vitamin E levels in relation to the future risk of breast cancer. Br J Cancer 49:321-324, 1984.
33. Willett WC, Polk BF, Underwood BA, Stampfer MJ, Pressel S, Rosner B, Taylor JO, Schneider K, Hames CG. Relation of serum vitamins A and E and carotenoids to the risk of cancer. N Engl J Med 310:430-434, 1984.
34. Black MM, Zachrau RE. Immunotherapy of breast cancer? In: The Breast (HS Gallager, HP Leis Jr, RK Snyderman, JA Urban, eds). Mosby, St. Louis, 1978, pp 393-408.
35. Eccles SA, Barnett SC, Alexander P. Inhibition of growth and spontaneous metastasis of syngeneic transplantable tumours by an aromatic retinoic acid analogue: 1. Relationship between tumour immunogenicity and responsiveness. Cancer Immunol Immunother 19:109-114, 1985.

36. Eccles SA, Purvies HP, Barnett SC, Alexander P. Inhibition of growth and metastases of syngeneic transplantable tumours by an aromatic retinoic acid analogue: 2. T cell dependence of retinoid effects in vivo. Cancer Immunol Immunother 19:115-120, 1985.
37. Shklar G, Schwartz JL, Trickler DP, Reid S. Prevention of experimental cancer and immunostimulation by vitamin E (immunosurveillance). J Oral Pathol Med 19:60-64, 1990.
38. Hong WK, Lippman SM, Itri LM, Karp DD, Lee JS, Byers RM, Schantz SP, Kramer AM, Lotan R, Peters LJ, Dimery IW, Brown BW, Goepfert H. Prevention of second primary tumors with isotretinoin in squamous-cell carcinoma of the head and neck. N Engl J Med 323:795-801, 1990.

27
Malnutrition and Lymphocyte Subpopulation Responses in Humans

Sudhir Gupta
University of California, Irvine, California

INTRODUCTION

A well-balanced and optimal nutrition is a key to normal health. Therefore, both undernutrition and overnutrition could lead to an abnormal state of health. A number of these pathological effects of malnutrition appear to be mediated by the effect of the lack of or excess of various components of our daily diet on immune response. Although malnutrition comprises both overnutrition and undernutrition, only the immune respones associated with undernutrition will be discussed here. Changes in lymphocyte responses associated with protein, caloric, protein-caloric, vitamins, and trace element deficiencies in malnutrition will be considered.

LYMPHOCYTE SUBPOPULATIONS

During the past 10 years because of the development of a large number of monoclonal antibodies, it has been possible to subdivide major lymphocyte subpopulations of T and B lymphocytes into subcategories. A list of these lymphocyte subpopulations, according to recent nomenclature by the World Health Organization nomenclature committee, and their distribution is shown in Table 1 (and reviewed in Refs. 1-3). A few salient features warrant a brief description. It should be mentioned that to date we do not have a cell surface antigen, defined by currently available monoclonal antibodies, that is present exclusively on natural killer cells. In the T-cell lineage, CD1 genes are mapped on chromosome 1. CD1 antigen has been divided into three CD1a, CD1b, and CD1c clusters of p49, p45, and p43 molecular weight, respectively. CD1a molecules form intermolecular complexes with either CD1b or CD1c or CD8 molecules which are not present on malignant cell lines. The recently described antigen CD27 is present on mature T cells but is lacking in phytohemagglutinin (PHA)-acti-

Table 1 Surface Antigens of Lymphocyte Subpopulations

Antigen	Distribution
T-cell lineage	
CD1a	Thymocytes, Langerhans cells
CD1b	Thymocytes
CD1c	Thymocytes
CD2	Pan-T cell (sheep RBC receptor)
CD3	Pan-T cell
CD4	T subset (helper/inducer)
CD5	Pan-T cell
CD6	Pan-T cell
CD7	Pan-T cell
CD8	T subset (suppressor/cytotoxic)
CD25	Activated T and B (Tac antigen)
CD26	Activated T cells
CD28	Subset of CD8 (cytotoxic)
CDw29	Subset of CD4 (helper)
CD45R	Subset of CD4 (suppressor inducer), some B cells, granulocytes, and monocytes
B-cell lineage	
CD19	B-progenitors, Pan-B cell
CD20	Pan-peripheral B cell
CD21	Restricted B, follicular dendritic cells
CD22	Most peripheral B cells, cytoplasmic antigen in B progenitors
CD23	Most B cells, variable expression on follicular B cells
CD24	Pan-B cell, B progenitors, polymorphs (some)
CD37	Pan-peripheral B cells, weak reaction with other leucocytes
CD39	B cells and some macrophages
CDw40	Most B cells, linked with activation of B
CD45R	Subgroup of the family of common leukocyte antigens
CD5	Minor subset of B cells, most T cells
CD9	Different stages of B-cell lineage, monocytes, polymorphs, platelets, and other tissues
CD10	Common ALL antigen
CD38	Plasma cells +++, germinal center B cells ++, T cells +, leukocyte progenitors ++.

CD = cluster of differentiation antigens.

vated blasts and interleukin 2 (IL-2)-dependent cell lines. Some reactivity is present with B-chronic lymphocytic leukemia (CLL). CD28 is defined by a monoclonal antibody 9.3. $CD28^+CD8$ cells are cytotoxic, whereas $CD28^-CD8$ cells are suppressors. The CDw29 antigen is defined by 4B4 antibody and is present on the helper subpopulation of $CD4^+$ T cells. CDw29 antigen is also present on B cells. Antibody 2H4 defines CD45R antigen and reacts with a subset of $CD4^+$ T cells that is known to identify the suppressor/inducer subset of CD4 cells. The antigen recognized by 2H4 is a part of T200 (CD45) complex.

In the B-cell lineage, CD19 and CD24 and major histocompatibility complex (MHC) class II antigens are present on pan B plus B progenitors. CD19 defines a pan B antigen which is also expressed from the earliest stages of B-progenitor development (i.e., V_H rearrangement). The prototype of this group is B4 antibody. The prototype of CD24 is BA-1 antibody. CD24 expression occurs at terminal differentiation. CD24 antibody reacts with neutrophils but does not react with peripheral T cells and T-cell lines. CD20 and CD37 are present on all B lymphocytes but are lacking from the B progenitors. The prototype antibody for CD20 is B1. It is completely lacking from non-B leukocytes. CD37 is strongly expressed on all peripheral B cells and lost during B-cell maturation to plasma cells. Antibodies defining CD37 antigen react weakly with T cells, neutrophils, and monocytes. CD22, CD45R, CD39, CD23, CD9, CD10, and CD5 antigens have restricted B-cell distribution. Antibodies defining these antigens reacts with other cell types as well. The CD38 antigen is present on plasma cells; however, the antibodies defining this cluster also react weakly with thymocytes and activated T cells. CD5 antigen is strongly present on thymocytes and

Table 2 Functional Properties of T and B Lymphocytes

Functions	T lymphocytes	B lymphocytes
DNA synthesis		
soluble antigens	+	−
Epstein-Barr virus	−	+
Anti-Ig	−	+
allogeneic MLR (R)	+	−
allogeneic MLR (S)	−	+
AMLR (R)	+	−
AMLR (S)	−	+
Cytotoxic functions		
CTL	+	−
ADCC	+S	−
LAK	+	−
NK	+S	−
LDCC	+	?
Cytokine production		
IL-1	−	+
IL-2	+	−
IL-4	+	−
IL-5	+	−
IL-6	+	+
TNF	+	−
TGF	+	−
Immunoregulatory functions		
helper	+	−
suppressor inducers	+	−
suppressors	+	−
Antibody production	−	+

Abbreviations: S = subset; AMLR = autologous mixed lymphocyte reaction; CTL = cytotoxic T lymphocytes; NK = natural killer; ADCC = antibody-dependent cellular cytotoxicity; LDCC = lectin-dependent cellular cytotoxicity; TGF = transforming growth factor; R = responder; S = stimulator; TNF = tumor necrosis factor.

Table 3 Functional Properties of Human T-Cell Subpopulations

Functions	CD4$^+$ T Cells	CD8$^+$ T Cells
DNA Synthesis		
soluble antigens	+	−
allogeneic MLR	+	+
AMLR (T-non T)	+	−
AMLR (T-T)	+	−
Cytokine production		
IL-2	+	±
IL-4	+	±
IL-6	+	±
gamma interferon	±	+
Cytotoxic functions		
MHC class I specific	−	+
MHC class II specific	+	−
Regulatory functions		
helper		
T-B interaction	+	−
T-T interaction	+	−
T-macrophage interaction	+	−
Suppressor		
T-B interaction	+S	+S
T-T interaction	+S	+S

S = subset.

peripheral T cells. But this antigen is also present on most of B-CLL cells, centrocytic lymphoma, a minor subset of follicular cells, and a very small subset of peripheral B lymphocytes. CD5$^+$ peripheral blood B cells have shown to produce autoantibodies (i.e., the rheumatoid factor in patients with rheumatoid arthritis) and quantitative increases of this population have been found in certain autoimmune disease states. It is not clear, however, whether this subset is under the genetic control of the MHC. There appears to be a heterogeneity in recently described lymphokine-activated killer (LAK) cells. This subset of lymphocytes expresses surface antigens shared by T cells as well as non-T, non-B cells and is responsible for the killing of the tumor cells that are resistant to NK cell killing. This subset has been used in the adoptive immunotherapy of malignancy.

The use of monoclonal antibodies and the fluorescence-activated cell sorter have been instrumental in defining the functions of various subsets of lymphocytes. A list of functions of T and B lymphocytes is given in Table 2 and the functions of T-cell subsets is shown in Table 3. (These functions have been reviewed in Refs. 3-5.)

T-CELL–MEDIATED IMMUNITY IN MALNUTRITION

Thymus in Malnutrition

Thymus is the central organ in the differentiation and maturation of T lymphocytes and their subsets. This process takes place as a result of an interaction between thymic epithelium and thymic factors with precursor T cells. Abnormal thymus morphology is present in a variety of primary and secondary immunodeficiency disorders that are characterized by T cell-mediated immunity. Borysenko and Lewis (6) observed profound atrophy of the thymus gland in an experimental model of protein-energy malnutrition (PEM). In human malnutrition, the thymus gland is depleted of thymocytes, thymic epithelial cell mass is reduced, and the differentiation between cortex and medulla is lost. This subject is further discussed in chapter 18. In contrast to the morphology of the thymus gland in acquired immunodeficiency syndrome (AIDS) where thymic architecture is obliterated and Hassall's corpuscles are lost. Hassall's corpuscles are present and cystically dilated in PEM (7). It is likely that the abnormal expression of MHC antigens or the absence of certain differentiation antigens on thymic epithelial cells could prime the thymus to intrathymic immunological insult. Wade et al. (8) examined the plasma levels of thymulin (Zn-FTS, Zinc, facteur thymique serique), one of the thymic factors, in Senegalese children suffering with PEM. The specific thymulin activity (total plasma thymulin activity minus the activity measured following adsorption of the plasma with an antithymulin monoclonal antibody) was almost undetectable in malnourished children with concurrent infections. It appears likely that infections/infestations play at least a contributory role in thymic dysfunction in PEM. Schonland et al. (9) reported elevated levels of plasma corticosteroids in PEM, which could be responsible for some of the morphological changes observed in the thymus in PEM. In summary, changes in thymus and thymic factors in PEM appear to be due to multiple factors, including infections, as discussed in chapters 18 and 30.

T Lymphocytes and Their Subsets

Lymphopenia, which is often very severe, is observed in a subset of patients with malnutrition. Earlier studies showed reduction in the circulating levels of T cells as measured by their capacity to form spontaneous rosettes with sheep erythrocytes (E-RFC). A number of factors, including circulating immune complexes, C-reactive protein, and other plasma inhibitory factors have been implicated for the reduced number of T cells in PEM. Cruz et al. (10) demonstrated the E-RFC increased following nutritional therapy in acutely malnourished children; however, the changes were not statistically significant and the thymosin fraction V responsive-E-RFC persisted. Therefore, in acute malnutrition, the proportion of E-RFC- and thymosin-responsive (relatively immature) T cells does not correlate with anthromorphic measurements of nutritional status. This would suggest that other factors might be responsible for the changes in T cells observed in acute malnutrition.

Prior to the definition of monoclonal antibody-defined T-cell subsets, functionally distinct T-cell subsets were defined by the presence of receptors for immunoglobulin M (Tμ) or IgG (Tγ) as helper/inducers and suppressor/cytotoxic, respectively (11). Chandra (12) reported a quantitative decrease in Tμ cells and an increased number of Tγ cells resulting in abnormally low ratios of Tμ/Tγ cells. However, no functional studies were performed. Therefore, it could not be ascertained whether the quantitative changes reflected functional changes.

In fact, Woodward et al. (13) have recently reported that depression of cellular immunity (thymus dependent) in wasting protein energy malnutrition does not depend upon altered T lymphocyte subpopulation ratios or even upon a generalized atrophy of T cells relative to B cells. However, this was an animal model, so the conclusions may not be directly applicable to humans. Some studies of lymphocyte subsets in human PEM have also utilized monoclonal antibodies. Chandra et al. (14)

reported quantitative and qualitative deficiency of $CD4^+$ T cells, whereas $CD8^+$ were not significantly affected.

Abbott et al. (15) observed significant depression of CD3, CD4, and $CD8^+$ T cells in adult patients with kwashiorkor-like hypoalbuminemic malnutrition, but no decrease in adult patients with marasmus. No significant effect of nutritional therapy on any lymphocyte subsets was observed. This study stresses the need for the evaluation of coexistence of kwashiorkor-like hypoalbuminemic state when evaluating the immune functions in malnutrition.

Roussel et al. (16) observed decreased proportions of $CD2^+$ and $CD4^+$ T cells in malnourished patients with gastrointestinal neoplasia when compared to well-nourished patients with gastrointestinal neoplasia. They observed a direct correlation between decreased $CD4^+$ T cells and PHA-induced DNA synthesis.

Garraud et al. (17) and Joffe et al. (18) observed a quantitative decrease in all $CD3^+$, $CD4^+$, and $CD8^+$ T cells. Approximately 5% of the T cells showed activation markers (17). However, analysis was not done to demonstrate which subset of T cells had activation markers. It is likely that the activation of T-cell subsets is due to secondary factor(s) like infection.

Dagan et al. (19) showed a significant reduction in $CD4^+$ T cells resulting in abnormally low ratios of $CD4^+/CD8^+$ T cells in children with acute measles. The malnourished children with acute measles had greater decrease in both $CD4^+$ and $CD8^+$ T cells during the acute phase than in well-nourished children with acute measles. This would suggest that infection (as a cofactor) plays a role in malnutrition associated changes in lymphocyte subsets.

There is no study reported at the time of this writing that has analyzed further $CD4^+$ T cells (into helpers and inducers of suppressors) and $CD8^+$ T cells (into suppressor and cytotoxic cells) in human PEM using monoclonal antibodies. Chandra (20,21) has shown evidence for decreased helper function in PEM using total T cells cocultured with B cells.

Patients with PEM show poor DNA synthesis by mononuclear cells in response to mitogens (22-24). The mechanisms for poor proliferative response of T cells include plasma inhibitory factor(s) (23,25) or lack of growth supporting factors (24). It is also likely that the T lymphocytes from malnourished patients are more sensitive to suppressive influence of inhibitory factors as discussed in chapter 22. Interestingly, Murphy (26) has shown an enhanced inhibitory effect of UV exposure on cell-cycle progression of lymphocytes from malnourished children. Roussel (16) reported a direct correlation between decreased proportions of $CD4^+$ cells and PHA-induced DNA synthesis in malnourished patients with gastrointestinal neoplasia. The production of or in vitro effect of interleukin 2 (IL-2) was not examined in any of these studied. Bhaskaram and Shivkumar (27) reported decreased production of IL-1 by macrophages from children with severe malnutrition. Since IL—1 activates T cells to produce IL-2 and express IL-2 receptors (28), it is likely that the decreased proliferation of T cells is a consequence of the defect in IL-2 autocrine pathway in malnutrition. Further, Chandra has reported reduced IL-2 and gamma interferon production in PEM (21). The delayed type cutaneous hypersensitivity to recall antigens is also depressed in patients with PEM (29). Toss and Symreng (30) reported decreased delayed cutaneous hypersensitivity response to recall antigens (Candida, mumps, PPD, Trycophyton, and varidase) in subjects with vitamin D deficiency. Therefore, a role of vitamin D in depressed delayed hypersensitivity in PEM must be considered.

B-CELL–MEDIATED IMMUNITY IN MALNUTRITION
B Lymphocytes and Their Functions

Chandra (12) reported normal proportions and absolute numbers of surface Ig$^+$ B lymphocytes in PEM. However, recent studies using monoclonal antibodies show decreased proportions and numbers of CD20$^+$ B lymphocytes (17). Roussel (16) observed decreased proportions of CD20$^+$ B cells in malnourished patients with gastrointestinal neoplasia when compared with well-nourished patients with gastrointestinal neoplasia. This discrepancy in the data could be as a result of an over estimate of B cells in an earlier study (12) due to cytophilically attached serum Ig on non T non B lymphocytes. Studies are needed to examine B lymphocytes with a panel of monoclonal antibodies that define surface antigens present on various stages of B-cell differentiation.

Serum immunoglobulin levels in PEM are elevated, normal, or depressed. The age of the patient at the time of PEM appears to be important. In adults and older children, polyclonal hyperimmunoglobulinemia is frequent. This is often associated with frequent bacterial infection and/or parasitic infestation. In patients with anorexia nervosa, which comprise a small fraction of patients with PEM, IgM and IgG levels are frequently decreased which return to normal following nutritional replenishment (31). Children affected with PEM before 7 months of age show profound panhypogammaglobulinemia. Serum IgA and IgG levels recover with adequate nutritional supplementation; however, the levels of IgM are still depressed as late as 6 months following recovery from PEM (32). It remains to be determined whether this represents a permanent effect of PEM on IgM response or simply a profound delay in the return of IgM synthesis. In children, the secretory levels of IgA are also low and IgA antibody response to viral vaccine is reduced (32,33). The levels of free secretory components and secretory IgA in tears are decreased in severely malnourished patients, whereas in moderately severe malnourished patients, secretory IgA is decreased, but the free secretory components are comparable to controls (34). This would suggest that the decrease in secretory IgA levels in PEM is not due to the failure to secrete free secretory components but rather the decrease could be due to a defect in the transport and/or an assembly of free secretory component with secretory IgA. The role of parasitic infestation or bacterial/viral infection of the gastrointestinal tract remains to be evaluated; however increased binding of bacteria to epithelial cells has been observed (35). The affinity of specific antibodies produced in response to immunization is markedly diminished in children with PEM as compared to well-nourished control children. Protein-energy malnutrition markedly affects high-affinity IgG antibodies to T-dependent antigens (36). This could represent an abnormality in T-B cell cooperation (especially a functional defect of T-helper cells) and/or defect in macrophage-T helper cell interaction (antigen processing and presentation by the macrophages to T-helper cells).

ROLE OF OTHER NUTRIENTS ON IMMUNE DYSFUNCTIONS ASSOCIATED WITH MALNUTRITION

A number of nutrients, including vitamins and minerals, influence the immune response. (For detailed reviews, see Refs. 37–40.) Many of the changes observed may operate through altered lymphocyte subsets.

Proteins

Both the quality and the quantity of protein intake influence the specific antibody response; the T-cell responses are minimally affected (41). In addition a number of essential amino acids in particular arginine appear to influence immune functions (see Chap. 3). Tryptophan and phenylalanine appears to be necessary for an optimal specific antibody response. In experimental animals, a deficiency of branched chain and sulfur-containing amino acids produce changes in the thymus and other peripheral lymphoid tissues (32,42).

Vitamins

Although many vitamins are known to influence the phagocytic cell system, only a few have been shown to have a role in modulating specific immune response in humans. Almost all of the B series vitamins activate cyclic guanosine monophosphate, which is a positive regulator of lymphocyte functions. Therefore, theoretically a severe deficiency of any of these vitamins could lead to lymphocyte dysfunctions, but only few of them have been shown conclusively to influence lymphocyte functions in humans. In humans, the role of niacin, nicotinic acid, nicotinamide, pantothenic acid, thymine, or riboflavin in immune response has not been documented.

Biotin

An inborn error of metabolism involving biotin in humans is associated with combined T- and B-cell deficiency (43); however, a similar deficiency of biotin without immune dysfunction has also been reported (44). It is not known whether any of the immune depression associated with PEM is due to a deficiency (if any) of biotin.

Pyridoxine

Pyridoxine, a vitamin B_6, is essential for RNA and DNA synthesis. Deficiency of pyridoxine arises secondary to malabsorption or is due to the intake of drugs that interact with the vitamin. Pyridoxine deficiency is a common hypovitaminosis in hospitalized patients. To what degree the deficiency of pyridoxine exists in PEM is unclear. In experimental animals, deficiency of pyridoxine results in the atrophy of the thymus and decreased cellularity of the peripheral lymphoid tissues (47). As a consequence both cell-mediated and antibody-mediated immunity are effected (42,48). In human volunteers, pyridoxine deficiency produced only a mild decrease in specific antibody response to tetanus toxoid and typhoid vaccine; however, additional pantothenic acid deficiency (pantothenic acid deficiency alone has no effect on immune response) resulted in almost complete lack of specific antibody response (49,50). In contrast in a controlled study of healthy elderly volunteers (45) Meydani et al. found that B_6 depletion was associated with decreased lymphocyte numbers and impaired immune response. Further, Charance et al. found reduced CD4+ and CD5+ lymphocytes among elderly persons with B_6 deficiency (46). In pyridoxine deficiency, impaired cytotoxicity, depressed lymphocyte proliferation, and decreased levels of serum thymic hormone have been reported (51–53).

Vitamin B_{12}

The role of vitamin B_{12} is limited to the studies in humans and in particular to the patients with pernicious anemia. In pernicious anemia, the number of T and B lymphocytes are normal; however, the number of $CD8^+$ T cells is decreased. This defect of CD8$^+$ T cells is corrected by B$_{12}$ replacement treatment (54,55). There is an increased association between pernicious anemia and selective IgA deficiency. IgA deficiency appears to be due to a primary B-cell defect rather than the presence of anti-IgA antibodies (56). Hypogammaglobulinemia may also occur in pernicious anemia, but it appears to be unrelated to vitamin B$_{12}$ deficiency, as the treatment with B$_{12}$ corrects the anemia but not the hypogammaglobulinemia. Congenital deficiency of transcobalamin II is associated with hypogammaglobulinemia and impaired bactericidal activity, but normal cell-mediated immunity (57). Treatment of this disorder with a combination of B$_{12}$ and leucovorin corrected the bactericidal defect and hypogammaglobulinemia (50), suggesting a role for these two vitamins in antibody production. Because in humans there is remarkably prolonged storage of vitamin B$_{12}$, it is unlikely that in PEM there is a deficiency of vitamin B$_{12}$; however, it very severe and prolonged PEM this possibility cannot be excluded.

Folic Acid

Folic acid deficiency is associated with both cell-mediated and antibody-mediated immunity (42). Patients with PEM who show severe deficiency of folic acid have worse impairment of phagocytosis and bactericidal activities. Supplementation of folic acids correct these defects (58). Folic acid deficiency is also associated with a decreased cell-mediated immune response; namely, delayed-type hypersensitivity reaction to recall antigens and the proliferative response to mitogens is depressed (32, 42-59). These functions recovered following treatment with folic acid. Because of the very limited stores of folic acid in humans, the deficiency of folic acid in PEM is very likely.

Vitamin C

In experimental animals, vitamin C deficiency is associated with a decreased production of thymic hormone and a decreased immune response to allograft (42). However, there is no clear evidence that vitamin C deficiency in humans is associated with any significant changes in cell-mediated or antibody-mediated immunity. Vitamin C deficiency in humans is associated with an abnormality of the phagocytic cell system and an impairment of complement activity (observed only in severe deficiency of vitamin C). The relationship of vitamin C to phagocytosis is discussed in chapter 5, and to lymphocyte activation in chapter 6.

Vitamin D

Vitamin D is hydroxylated in the liver and kidney to 1,25-dihydroxycholecalciferol (vitamin D$_3$), which is the active metabolite of vitamin D. Vitamin D$_3$ induces differentiation and maturation of monocytes and macrophages (60). It induces the production of the tumor necrosis factor (TNF) and the granulocyte-monocyte colony-stimulating factor (GM-CSF) from human monocytes and macrophages and enhances their cytotoxic capacity against *Mycobacterium avium complex* (61). In T cells, vitamin D$_3$ inhibits lymphocyte transformation to mitogens, which appears to be due to an inhibition of IL-2 production and IL-2 receptor expression (62). These issues are discussed further in Chapter 1. Toss and Smyrang (30) observed a correlation between low serum vitamin D levels and anergy or hypoanergy on delayed cutaneous hypersensitivity testing against five recall antigens. Although depressed phagocytic cell functions and increased susceptibility to infections has been reported in children with vitamin D-deficient rickets, no study has been done of specific immune response using contemporary immunological techniques. We have shown that vitamin D_3 inhibits human B-cell differentiation to immunoglobulin-secreting cells, and this inhibition appears to be mediated by its effect on interleukin 1 production (63).

Vitamin A

Vitamin A deficiency is one of the most common vitamin deficiency in Third World countries. In the industrialized nations, deficiency of vitamin A is observed in association with malabsorption, malnutrition, and chronic illness. In one study, supplementation of preoperative subjects with high daily doses of vitamin A resulted in the improvement of both lymphopenia and the decreased response to allogeneic cells in vitro observed in the untreated group (57). In one animal model, vitamin A deficiency has been associated with deficient NK cell function (65). Currently, retinoids are being used as immunopotentiators or adjuvants in the management of patients with neoplasms. The possible use of vitamin A in cancer therapy is described in Chapter 26. Retinoids appear to influence the differentiation and maturation of B lymphocytes. β-Carotene supplementation in older human volunteers has been reported to be associated with increased expression of IL-2 receptors and NK cells (66). Studies of specific immune response using current technical approaches to the study of immune response and involving interactions between cells of the immune system and cytokines are needed to define the in vivo role of vitamin A in the immune response and the consequences of its deficiency. Studies of this nature are described in Chapter 3.

Vitamin E

The role of vitamin E or the consequence of vitamin E deficiency on the immune response in humans is poorly understood, although a reduced level of vitamin E has been noted in elderly persons with increased infections (46). In normal healthy individuals, administration of vitamin E resulted in depressed bactericidal activity of leukocytes and depressed proliferative response to PHA (67). Recent studies suggest that both antioxidant effects and effects on the cyclooxegenase pathway may underly these observations (see Chap. 14).

Minerals

A number of minerals appear to influence the immune response. It is, however, difficult to dissociate the effect of one mineral from the other because of the complex deficiency of several minerals in PEM. Of all the minerals, zinc is best studied because of the experimental model of isolated zinc deficiency and several clinical trials in humans (see Chaps. 24 and 33). Since zinc is required for the biological activity of the thymic hormone (thymulin), there is a direct effect of zinc deficiency upon T-cell differentiation. Interestingly, thymic atrophy per se in association with iron deficiency has been found to produce overall loss of thymocytes but not T cells in the thymus (68), suggesting a highly specific interaction rather than a general effect. Similarly, experimental copper deficiency (see Chap. 15) causes loss of T cells and relative increase of B cells in the spleen (69), but this effect is limited mainly to male and not female rats.

Selenium is an integral component of glutathione peroxidase. The deficiency of selenium is corrected with vitamin E, suggesting close interactions between these two nutrients. T-Cell activation is dependent on adequate amounts of selenium (70). In experimental animals, selenium deficiency is associated with an impaired T cell-dependent antibody response, especially in the presence of vitamin E deficiency. In humans, the significance of selenium deficiency in relation to specific immune response is unclear.

Although no well-defined changes in immune response have been noted in magnesium deficiency in humans, in experimental animals thymic hyperplasia is accompanied with paradoxical abnormal cell-mediated immunity and impaired antibody responses (42).

In summary, both a deficiency and an excess of minerals and vitamins are associated with an abnormal immune response; only a few of these are well documented in humans. In PEM, there is usually simultaneous deficiency of several vitamins and minerals, and it is difficult, if not impossible, to determine the contribution of individual nutrients on the observed abnormal immune response associated with PEM. Therefore, the need to develop appropriate systems which could provide sufficient complexity to reflect in vivo physiology and yet be effectively focused to permit the study of the mechanism is critical. Other chapters in this volume suggest that such studies are now feasible and indeed underway.

CONCLUSIONS

Although malnutrition is associated with a wide range of immunological abnormalities, it is difficult to assign all the abnormalities to malnutrition because of the concommitant presence of infections and/or infestations, elevated levels of plasma corticosteroids, and the difference in age of subjects in which these studies are carried out. It is likely that the effects of malnutrition are amplified in the presence of infection and/or infestation. Age (immaturity and aging) also influences the degree of immunological insult due to malnutrition. It is crucial that prospective longitudinal studies are done in which the effects of infection/infestation, age, and sex on malnutrition-associated immunological deficiencies are better defined. It has become increasingly clear that there is close interaction between the immune system, endocrine system, and the neurological systems. Therefore, it is imperative that we study and interpret any data on immune responses associated with malnutrition in relation to endocrine status and any associated abnormality of neuropeptides and neurotransmitters, since the latter appear to have a profound influence on the immune response. Last, studies in malnutrition should be done for the role of various recently discovered cytokines and their interactions with lymphocytes and macrophages utilizing most contemporary immunological tools.

ACKNOWLEDGMENT

This work was supported in part by grants from USPHS AI-23456 and GM-21808.

REFERENCES

1. Ling NR, Maclennan ICM, Mason DY. B cell and plasma cell antigens: New and previously defined clusters. In: Leucocyte Typing III (AJ McMichael, ed). Oxford Press, Oxford, England, 1987, pp 302-335.
2. McMichael AJ, Gotch FM. T cell antigens: New and previously defined clusters. In: Leucocyte Typing III (AJ McMichael, ed). Oxford Press, Oxford, England, 1987 pp 31-62.

3. Knapp W, Rieber P, Dorken B, Schmidt RE, Stein H, Borne A. Towards a better definition of human leucocyte surface molecules. Immunol Today 10:253, 1989.
4. Gupta S. Cell-mediated immune response in insulin-dependent (Type I) diabetes mellitus. In: Immunology of Clinical and Experimental Diabetes (S Gupta, ed). Plenum Press, New York, 1984, pp 329-349.
5. Gupta S. Lymphocyte subpopulations. Phenotypic expression and functions in health and rheumatic diseases. In: Immunology of Rheumatic Diseases (S Gupta, N Talal, eds). Plenum Press, New York, 1985, pp 21-83.
6. Borysenko M, Lewis S. The effect of nutrition on immunocompetence and whole body resistance to infection in Chelydra serpentian. Dev Compar Immunol 3:89-100, 1979.
7. Linder J. The thymus gland in secondary immunodeficiency. Arch Pathol Lab Med 111: 1118-1122, 1987.
8. Wade S, Parent G, Bleiberg-Daniel F, Maire B, Fall M, Schnieder D, Le Moullac B, Dardenne M. Thymulin (Zn-FTS) activity in protein-energy malnutrition: New evidence for interaction between malnutrition and infection on thymic function. Am J Clin Nutr 47: 305-311, 1988.
9. Schonland MM, Shanley BC, Loening WE, Parent MA, Coovadia HM. Plasma cortisol and immunosuppression in protein-caloric malnutrition. Lancet 2:435, 1972.
10. Cruz JR, Chew F, Fernandez RA, Torun B, Goldstein AL, Keusch GT. Effect of nutritional recuperation on E-rosette-forming lymphocytes and in vitro response to thymosin in malnourished children. J Pediatr Gastroenterol Nutr 6:387-291, 1987.
11. Gupta S, Good RA. Subpopulations of human T lymphocytes. Laboratory and Clinical studies. Immunol Rev 56:89-111, 1981.
12. Chandra RK. T and B lymphocyte subpopulations and leukocyte terminal deoxynucleotidyl transferase in energy protein undernutrition. Acta Pediat Scand 68:841-845, 1979.
13. Woodword BD, Miller RG. Depression of thymus dependent immunity in wasting protein energy malnutrition does not depend on an altered ratio of helper (CD_4^+) to suppressor (CD_8^+) T cells or on a disproportionately large atrophy of the T cell relative to the B cell pool. Am J Clin Nutr 53:1329-1335, 1991.
14. Chandra RK, Gupta S, Singh H. Inducer and suppressor T cell subsets in protein-energy malnutrition. Analysis by monoclonal antibodies. Nutr Res 2:21-26, 1982.
15. Abbott WC, Tayek JA, Bistrian BR, Maki T, Ainsley BM, Reid LA, Blackburn GAL. The effect of nutritional support on T-lymphocyte subpopulations in protein-caloric malnutrition. J Am Coll Nutr 5:577-584, 1986.
16. Roussel E. Immunoregulatory leucocyte subset typing and PHA response in relation to the nutritional state in cancer patients with gastrointestinali neoplasia. Diag Immunol 4: 10-16, 1986.
17. Garraud D, Daculsi R, Merlio JP, Lobera A, Legrand E. Detection of CD1 positive cells in the peripheral blood of patients suffering from cancer-associated malnutrition. Immunol Lett 15:73-76, 1987.
18. Joffe MI, Kew M, Robson AR. Lymphocyte subsets in patients with atopic eczema, protein-calorie malnutrition, SLE and liver disease. J Clin Lab Immunol 10:97-101, 1983.
19. Dagan R, Philip M, Sarov I, Skibin A, Epstein S, Kuperman O. Cellular immunity and T-lymphocyte subsets in young children with acute measles. J Med Virol 22:175-182, 1987.
20. Chandra RK. Malnutrition. In: Primary and Secondary Immunodeficiency Disorders (RK Chandra, ed). Churchill Livingston, New York, 1983, pp 187-203.
21. Chandra RK. McCallum Award Lecture. Nutrition and immunity: Lessons from the past and new insights into the future. Am J Clin Nutr 53:1087, 1990.
22. Chandra RK. Nutrition, immunity, and infection: Present knowledge and future directions. Lancet 2:688-691, 1983.
23. Heyworth B, Moore DL, Brown J. Depression of lymphocyte response to phytohaemagglutinin in the presence of plasma from children with acute protein energy malnutrition. Clin Exp Immunol 22:72-77, 1975.

24. Beatty DW, Dowdle EB. Deficiency in kwashiorkor serum of factors required for optimal lymphocyte transformation in vitro. Clin Exp Immunol 35:433-442, 1979.
25. Salimonne LS. Plasma inhibitory factors in protein calorie malnutrition. In: Nutrition and Immunology (RK Chandra, ed). Liss, New York, 1988, p 25.
26. Murphy PB. Enhanced inhibitory effect of UV on cell-cycle progression in cultures of lymphocytes from malnourished children. Experentia 39:144-145, 1983.
27. Bhaskaram P, Shivkumar B. Interleukin 1 in malnutrition. Arch Dis Child 61: 182-185, 1986.
28. Gupta S. Interleukins: Molecular and biological characteristics. In: Immunology of Rheumatic Diseases (S Gupta, N Talal, eds). Plenum Press, New York, 1985, pp 109-139.
29. Bruke M, Hesp R, Kark AE. The effect of undernutrition and disease site and stage on cell-mediated immunity in gastrointestinal cancer. Clin Oncol 9:203-211, 1983.
30. Toss G, Symreg T. Delayed hypersensitivity response and vitamin deficiency. Int J Vit Nutr Res 53:27-31, 1983.
31. Wyatt RJ, Farell M, Berry PL, Forristal J, Maloney MJ, West CD. Reduced alternative complement pathway control protein levels in anorexia nervosa: response to parenteral alimentation. Am J Clin Nutr 35:973-980, 1982.
32. Gross RL, Newberne PM. Role of nutrition in immunologic function. Physiol Rev 60: 188-302, 1980.
33. Chandra RK. Reduced secretory antibody response to live attenuated measles and poliovirus vaccine in malnourished children. Br Med J 2:583-585, 1975.
34. Watson RR, McMurray DN, Martin P, Reyes MA. Effect of age, malnutrition and renutrition on free secretory component and IgA in secretions. Am J Clin Nutr 42:281-288, 1985.
35. Chandra RK, Wadhaw M. Nutritional modulation of mucosal immunity. Immunol Invest 18:1190, 1989.
36. Garre MA, Boles JM, Youinou PY. Current concepts in immune derangement due to undernutrition. Gpn J Parenter Enteral Nutr 11:309-313, 1987.
37. Corman LC. Effect of specific nutrients on the immune response. Selected clinical application. Med Clin North Am 69:759-791, 1985.
38. Suskind RM. Malnutrition and the immune response. Beitr Infusiionther Klin Ernahr 19:1-25, 1988.
39. Chandra RK. Grace A. Goldsmith Award Lecture. Trace element regulation of immunity and infection. J Am Coll Nutr 4:5-16, 1985.
40. McMurray DN. Cell-mediated immunity in nutritional deficiency. Prog Food Nutr Sci 8: 193-228, 1984.
41. Zoppi G, Gaspirini R, Mantovanelli F, Gobio-Casali L, Astolfi R, Crovari P. Diet and antibody response to vaccination in healthy infants. Lancet 2:11-14, 1983.
42. Beisel WR. Single nutrient and immunity. Am J Clin Nutr 35 (Suppl):490-493, 1982.
43. Cowan MJ, Wara DW, Packman S, Ammann AJ, Yoshino M, Sweetman L, Nyhan W. Multiple biotin-dependent carboxylase deficiencies associated with defect in T-cell and B-cell immunity. Lancet 2:115-118, 1979.
44. Thoene J, Baker H, Yoshino M, Sweetman L. Biotin-responsive carboxylase deficiency associated with subnormal plasma and urinary biotin. N Engl J Med 304:817, 1981.
45. Meydani SN, Ribaya-Mercado JD, Russell RM, Sahyour N, Morrow FD, Gershaff SN. Vitamin B-6 deficiency impairs interleukin 2 production and lymphocyte proliferation in elderly adults. Am J Clin Nutr 53:1275, 1991.
46. Chavance M, Herbeth B, Fournier C, Jarot C, Vernhes G. Vitamin status immunity and infectious on an elderly population. Eur J Clin Nutr 43:827, 1989.
47. Stoerk HC. Effect of calcium deficiency and pyridoxin defiency on thymic atrophy (accidental involution). Proc Soc Exp Biol Med 62:90-96, 1946.
48. Axelrod AE. Immune processes in vitamin deficiency states. Am J Clin Nutr 24:265-271, 1971.

49. Hodges RE, Bean WB, Ohlson MA, Bleiler RE. Factors affecting human antibody response. IV. Pyridoxin deficiency. Am J Clin Nutr 11:180-186, 1982.
50. Hodges RE, Bean WB, Ohlson MA, Bleiler RE. Factors affecting human antibody response. V. Combined deficiencies of pantothenic acid and pyridoxin. Am J Clin Nutr 11:187-199, 1962.
51. Chandra RK, Au B, Heresi G. Serum thmic hormone activity in deficiencies of calories, zinc, vitamin A and pyridoxin. Clin Exp Immunol 42:332-336, 1980.
52. Robson LC, Schwartz MR. Vitamin B6 deficiency and the lymphoid system. I. Effects on cellular immunity and in vitro incorporation of 3H-uridine by small lymphocytes. Cell Immunol 16:135-144, 1975.
53. Willis-Carr JI, St. Pierre RL. Effect of vitamin B6 deficiency on thymic epithelial cells and T lymphocyte differentiation. J Immunol 120:1153-1159, 1978.
54. Gogos CA, Kapatais-Zoumbos KN, Zoumbos NC. Lymphocyte subpopulations in megaloblastic anemia due to vitamin B 12 deficiency. Scand J Haematol 37:316-318, 1986.
55. Kubota K, Arai T, Tamura J, Shirakura T, Morita T. Restoration of decreased suppressor cells by vitamin B 12 therapy in a patients with pernicious anemia. Am J Hematol 24:221-223, 1987.
56. Kätkä K, Eskola J, Granfors K, Koistinen J, Toivanen A. Serum IgA and anti-IgA antibodies in pernicious anemia. Clin Immunol Immunopathol 46:55-60, 1988.
57. Hitzig WH, Keung AB. The role of vitamin B 12 and its transport globulins in the production of antibodies. Clin Exp Immunol 20:105-111, 1975.
58. Yiagou M, Hadjipetrou-Kourounakis L. Effect of diet on adjuvant-induced disease and mitogen responses of fisher rats. Int Arch Allergy Appl Immunol 71:374-376, 1983.
59. Coovadia HM, Parent MA, Loening WE, Wesley A, Burgess B, Hallett F, Brian P, Grace J, Naidoo J, Smythe PM, Vos GH. An evaluation of factors associated with the depression of immunity in malnutrition and in measles. Am J Clin Nutr 27:665-669, 1974.
60. Bar-Shavit Z, Teitelbaum SL, Reitsma P, Hall A, Pegg LE, Trial J, Khan AJ. Induction of monocyte differentiation and bone reabsorption by 1,25-dihydroxyvitamin D3. Proc Natl Acad Sci (USA) 80:5907-5911, 1983.
61. Bermudex LEM, Young LS, Gupta S. 1,25-Dihydroxyvitamin D3 dependent inhibition of growth or killing of *Mycobacterium avium* complex is mediated by TNFα and GM-CSF. Cell Immunol 127:432-441, 1990.
62. Gupta S, Fass D, Shimizu M, and Vayuveglula B. Potentiation of immunosuppressive effect of cyclosporin A by 1,α-25 dihydroxyvitamin D3. Cell Immunol 121:290-297, 1990.
63. Chen W-C, Vayuvegula B, Gupta S. 1,25 dihydroxyvitamin D3-mediated inhibition of human B cell differentiation. Clin Exp Immunol 68:639-646, 1987.
64. Chandra S, Chandra RK. Nutrition, immune response and outcome. Prog Food Nutr Sci 10:1-65, 1986.
65. Bowman TA, Goonewardene M, Pasatiempo AMG, Ross AC, Taylor CE. J Nutr 120:1264-1276, 1990.
66. Watson RR, Prabhala RH, Plezia PM, Alberts DS. Effect of BeTa-carotene on lymphocyte subpopulation in elderly humans: Evidence for a dose-response relationship Am J Clin Nutr 53:90-94, 1991.
67. Prasad AS. Effect of vitamin E supplementation on leucocyte function. Am J Clin Nutr 33:606-608, 1980.
68. Kuvibidila S, Dardenne M, Saviro W, Lepault F. Influence of iron deficiency anemia on selected thymus functions in mice: Thymulin biological activity, T cell subsets, and Thymocyte proliferation. Am J Clin Nutr 51:228, 1990.
69. Bala S, Failla ML, Lunney JK. Alterations in lymphoid subsets and activation antigens in copper-deficient rats. J Nutr 121:745, 1991.
70. Fischbach M, Jenkinson S, Talal N, Lawrence R. Slenium deficient T cells are unresponsive to antigen stimulation. Clin Res 32:232A, 1984.

28
Influence of Nutrition on Immunocompetence in the Elderly

Ranjit K. Chandra
Memorial University of Newfoundland,
St. John's, Newfoundland, Canada

INTRODUCTION

Epidemiological and experimental observations indicate that nutritional status is a critical determinant of immunocompetence (1). This was first demonstrated in studies on young children with protein-energy malnutrition (PEM) in developing countries. There were consistent changes in cell-mediated immunity, complement system, phagocyte function, secretory immunoglobulin A (IgA) antibody response, and antibody affinity. These observations were then extended to young adults and now to the elderly. Furthermore, it was shown that deficiencies of single nutrients also impair immune responses; reduced intake of zinc, vitamin A, vitamin B_6, and other essential nutrients results in decreased immunocompetence.

In the elderly, many studies have documented the frequent presence of nutritional deficiencies. Besides general undernutrition due to reduced calorie intake, reduced intake and lower blood levels of iron, zinc, vitamin C, B vitamins, and vitamin E have been found (2-5). Socioeconomic deprivation, physical disability, isolation, dental problems, and increased nutrient needs due to underlying disease are common causal factors for nutritional problems in old age (6).

The immunological literature contains many reports demonstrating the common phenomenon of reduced immune responses with ageing (7-9). Cell-mediated immunity and phagocyte functions have been studied the most, and show significant alterations beyond 40-50 years of age in humans (10-11) and at corresponding periods in laboratory animals (9,12). However, this decline in the immune response is not an invariable occurrence. Almost one-third of the "healthy" elderly have immunological function at levels seen in younger age groups. This led us to postulate that nutritional deficiencies may contribute to the decline in immune responses seen in old age. Changes in neuroendocrine function (13) and in the "acute phase response" (14) have been observed in aging, and these responses as well may be affected by dietary influences. Intervention trials that attempted to correct nutritional deficiencies in the elderly demonstrated an improvement in immune responses, including antibody titer after prophylactic vaccination (1,15-18).

DEMOGRAPHIC CONSIDERATIONS

The increase in the proportion and absolute number of individuals above the age of 65 years has been documented in many industrialized countries. This age group constitutes at least 10-12% of the population, whereas the subset of the population above 75 years of age is expanding most rapidly. A number of factors have contributed to this demographic pattern; these include improved sanitation, better health care, decreased infant mortality, effective immunization, and reduced birth rate. It is noteworthy that ischemic heart disease, cerebrovascular accidents, and cancer are the leading causes of *death* in old age. However, infection is a common cause of *morbidity* (19). Respiratory infection, urinary tract infection, and, less frequently, gastrointestinal infection affect the elderly. There are recent studies that suggest that tuberculosis and tetanus are reemerging as important infectious causes of death in old age in the United States.

The World Health Organization Special Programme for Research in Ageing has emphasized that the number of elderly subjects is increasing in all countries. Since many developing countries have a very large population base, e.g., China, Mexico, and India, the absolute number of the elderly in the developing world easily exceeds that in the industrialized nations. Further, the rate of change in the number of elderly individuals will be far greater in the coming years in the economically less developed nations than in the economically affluent countries.

There is increasing fragmentation of the joint family system worldwide. In many economically developed countries, the majority of the elderly live independently. Those who cannot care for themselves live in nursing homes of varying sizes. This trend has reached a peak in North America, Europe, and Scandinavia. Interestingly, although Japan is among the top industrialized countries of the world, the elderly there continue to live with their children, at least at present. In most developing countries, the joint family system is still preserved, so that the elderly are cared for by their children and grandchildren. However, changing social and economic conditions, as well as progressive urbanization, is bound to influence this pattern. This will result in an enormous economic and health burden to the society that can ill afford to take on further stress. The cost of care for the elderly may further compromise economic advance in underprivileged populations.

IMMUNE RESPONSES IN OLD AGE

In the majority of the elderly, immune responsiveness declines soon after the age of 60 years. Some aspects, such as serum thymic hormone activity, begin to decrease after the age of 40 years. There is a correlation between age, immunocompetence, and survival. Those who show an absence of delayed cutaneous hypersensitivity have a much higher risk of impending death in the ensuing 3 years compared with those with a positive skin response. Much of the illnesses seen in old age, cancer and chronic infectious disease, may be direct consequences of reduced immunological vigor. Age-related changes in the immune response have been reviewed extensively (7-9,15) and are summarized here. It has been suggested that the prevention or correction of declining immunity in old age may delay or abort the onset of age-associated diseases (20). This suggestion gets some credence from experimental data in genetically at-risk mice in whom immunodeficiency, wasting, autoimmune renal and hematological disease, and amyloidosis can be prevented or at least postponed by reconstitution with young syngeneic thymus or spleen grafts.

The number of pluripotential stem cells is decreased in old animals. There is an impaired regenerative ability and clonal proliferation decreases. The generation of B cells and homing of precursor cells into the thymus is reduced. These changes may be relevant to the maintenance of homeostasis and the limitation of hematogenous spread of infection. It is known that the elderly have limited leukocytosis following sepsis. The expected shift to left of neutrophils does occur. Another interesting observation is the development of hemolytic anemia during infection in old animals but not in the young.

Delayed cutaneous hypersensitivity responses to common recall antigens are decreased in persons above 65 years of age (2,5,7,8). Even 2,4-dinitrochlorobenzene may fail to induce sensitization in some elderly subjects. The number of rosette-forming T cells in the peripheral blood is slightly reduced. The data on lymphocyte subsets are conflicting. The ratio of $CD4^+/CD8^+$ is generally reduced; this may be the combined result of decreased $CD4^+$ cells or increased $CD8^+$ suppressor cells or both (1,10). These changes in lymphocytes could explain the functional alterations—reduced lymphocyte proliferation response to mitogens and antigens, decreased production of lymphokines such as macrophage migration inhibition factor, impaired autologous mixed lymphocyte reaction, synthesis of interleukin-2, and natural killer cell activity—observed in several studies. Besides the immunological changes, a number of tissue changes and hormonal changes may explain the increased risk of infectious illness in the elderly (11,13,19).

Several studies have documented a reduction in thymic inductive factors in old age. Serum Facteur Thymique Serique as well as concentrations of thymopoietin and thymosin have been reported to be markedly decreased in samples obtained from individuals above the age of 60 years (21). Tissue culture experiments showed that thymic epithelium from young animals promoted the maturation and differentiation of bone marrow lymphocytes, whereas thymic epithelium from old donors fails to do this. There are qualitative changes in T cells with old age. (22). The density of receptors on T cells changes with age, and such receptors visualized by immunofluorescence as a continuous ring in young animals appear patchy and may be difficult to discern clearly. The rate of "capping" of three T-lymphocyte antigens is decreased. At the same time, new receptors appear. A terminal differentiation antigen appears on the surface of old cells, irrespective of the animals' age. This phenomenon may facilitate the removal of functionally ineffective cells from the body. Ultrastructural studies have shown swelling of mitochondria and the presence of myelinlike structures and a reduced number of cristae in cells from old individuals.

There are fewer changes in antibody response in old age (23,24). There is reduction in serum IgG concentration and an increase in serum IgA. The prevalence of autoantibodies increases, although the incidence of autoimmune *disease* is not increased. There is a slight reduction in B-cell proliferation response to mitogens. The recruitment of antibody-producing B cells is limited in old persons. In addition, antigens requiring T-cell help fare less well in antibody response. Further, the affinity of antibody is decreased. In some elderly, benign monoclonal gammopathy may be seen.

Neutrophils have reduced migration ability, but the ability to kill ingested bacteria is largely intact. Metabolic activity is decreased. Studies of macrophages obtained from old animals showed that most of the functions are intact, although antigen processing may be impaired to some extent. The production of interleukin 1 (IL-1), lysosomal enzyme activity, and cooperation with T and B cells to generate immune response are comparable in old and young animals. Interestingly, studies on elderly, malnourished patients in nursing homes have shown that neither IL-1 nor tumor necrosis factor (TNF) production were reduced in vitro compared to either age-matched or young controls (25). Thus, preservation of some aspects of immunity appears to occur even among elderly persons in nonoptimal conditions. However, cytokine production may be enhanced among elderly persons with experimentally increased vitamin E supplementation, as shown by Meydani et al. for IL-2 produced by T cells (26). Furthermore, it is important to consider that studying response in persons not challenged with environmental pathogen may not be predictive of the ability to mount a sufficiently vigorous reaction in face of an infectious challenge. Cannon et al. (14) noted a significant difference between older and younger persons in terms of neutrophil mobilization after exercise stress challenge, which may provide a useful parallel with infectious challenge. This difference was eliminated in elderly persons who received vitamin E supplementation.

IMMUNOLOGICAL FINDINGS IN PROTEIN-ENERGY MALNUTRITION

The subject of nutrition-immunity interactions has been the focus of an increasing number of publications in the last decade. Changes occurring in the immune system during the aging process have many similarities with the effects of some types of protein-calorie, or energy, malnutrition. Yet, in the absence of essential nutrient deprivation, energy intake restriction may actually retard aging (27). Implications for cancer development are discussed in Chapter 31.

Epidemiological studies have documented the adverse effect of protein-energy malnutrition (PEM) on morbidity and mortality (1). Pathological examination of tissues from children dying of PEM showed the frequent presence of several opportunistic microorganisms, including *Pneumocystis carinii*. Morbidity due to diarrheal disease is increased, particularly among those children whose weight-for-height is less than 70% of standard.

Lymphoid tissues show a significant atrophy (28). For instance, the size of the thymus is small. Histologically, there is a loss of corticomedullary differentiation, there are fewer lymphoid cells, and the Hassal bodies are enlarged, degenerated, and occasionally calcified. In the spleen, there is a loss of lymphoid cells around small blood vessels. In the lymph nodes, the thymus-dependent areas show depletion of lymphoid cells.

Delayed cutaneous hypersensitivity responses both to recall and new antigens are markedly depressed. There is a significant positive correlation between the size of skin response and visceral protein synthesis as judged by serum albumin concentration. It is not uncommon to have complete anergy to a battery of different antigens. These changes are observed in moderate deficiencies as well (29). Findings in patients with kwashiorkor were more striking compared with those in marasmus. One plausible reason for reduced cell-mediated immunity in PEM is the reduction in mature fully differentiated T lymphocytes that can be recognized by the classic technique of rosette formation or by the newer method of fluorescent labeling with monoclonal antibodies. The reduction in serum thymic factor activity observed in PEM may underlie the impaired maturation of T lymphocytes. There is an increase in the amount of deoxynucleotidyl transferase activity in leukocytes, a feature of immaturity. The recent availability of monoclonal antibodies has provided an excellent tool for the identification and enumeration of subsets of T cells. Cell flow methods showed that the number of helper $CD4^+$ cells was decreased markedly, often to values less than 50% of controls (1,10). The change in number of suppressor T cells is less marked (1). Thus, the helper/suppressor ratio is significantly decreased. Lymphocyte proliferation and synthesis of DNA are reduced, especially when autologous patient plasma is used in cell cultures. This may be the result of inhibitory factors as well as deficiency of essential nutrients lacking in patient's plasma.

Serum antibody responses are generally intact in PEM, particularly when antigens in adjuvant are administered or in the case of those materials that do not evoke T-cell response. Rarely, the antibody response to organisms such as *Salmonella typhi* may be decreased. This also bears similarities to findings in aging. Before impaired antibody response can be attributed to nutritional deficiency, one must carefully rule out infection as a confounding factor. Recently, we have found that antibody affinity is decreased in patients who are malnourished. This may provide an explanation for a higher frequency of antigen-antibody complexes found in such patients. As opposed to serum antibody responses, secretory IgA antibody levels after deliberate immunization with viral vaccines are decreased; there is a selective reduction in secretory IgA levels. This may have several clinical implications, including an increased frequency of septicemia in undernourished children (30,31). Related studies in aging persons should be done, as there is little information on secretory IgA in this setting.

The process of phagocytosis is also affected in PEM. Complement is an essential opsonin and the levels and activity of most complement components are decreased. The best documented is a reduction in complement C3, factor B, and total hemolytic activity. Although the ingestion of particles by phagocytes is intact, subsequent metabolic activation and destruction of bacteria is reduced. Finally, recent work in humans and animals has demonstrated that the production of interleukin-1 is decreased in PEM (31). This is apparently not the case in aging (32).

SELECTED NUTRIENT DEFICIENCIES: RELATION TO AGING

Clinical malnutrition in humans is usually a complex syndrome of multiple nutrient deficiencies. However, observations in laboratory animals deprived of one dietary element and findings in rare patients with a single nutrient deficiency have confirmed the crucial role of several vitamins and trace elements in immunocompetence, and thus finding certain deficiencies in elderly persons may imply decreased immune competence.

Deficiencies of pyridoxine, folic acid, vitamin A, vitamin C, and vitamin E result in impaired cell-mediated immunity and reduced antibody responses. Vitamin B_6 deficiency results in decreased lymphocyte stimulation response to mitogens such as phytohemagglutinin and is observed among elderly persons (5). A moderate increase in vitamin A intake enhances the immune response and affords partial protection against the development of certain tumors in animals.

Zinc deficiency, both acquired and inherited, is associated with lymphoid atrophy, decreased cutaneous delayed hypersensitivity responses and homograft rejection, and lower thymic hormone activity. In laboratory animal models, these findings can be confirmed, and in addition one can demonstrate a reduced number of antibody-forming cells in the spleen and impaired T-killer cell activity. Wound healing is impaired. Excess zinc also depresses neutrophil function and lymphocyte responses (33). Deficiency of iron is the commonest nutritional problem worldwide even in industrialized countries. On the one hand, free iron is necessary for bacterial growth: Removal of iron with the help of lactoferrin or other chelating agents reduced bacterial multiplication, particularly in the presence of specific antibody. On the other hand, iron is needed by neutrophils and lymphocytes for optimal function: Bacterial capacity is reduced in iron deficiency. Also, the lymphocyte proliferation response to mitogens and antigens is impaired: Response to tetanus toxoid and herpes simplex antigens was low in iron-deficiency subjects and iron therapy resulted in a significant improvement in their response. There are many molecular explanations for impaired lymphocyte and neutrophil function in iron deficiency, including the deficiency of myeloperoxidase and ribonucleotidyl reductase. However, iron overload may cause increased prostaglandin synthesis and thus downregulation of lymphocyte responsiveness, especially in older animals (34). Copper-deficient animals show a reduction in the number of antibody-producing cells compared to healthy and pair-fed controls.

Dietary deficiencies of selected amino acids decrease antibody responses; in other states of amino acid imbalance, the overall response may be enhanced, indicating that changes in suppressor cells may occur. The phagocytic clearance of macromolecules from the blood is reduced, as is antibody affinity in inbred animals.

The effect of a single nutrient deficiency on serum thymic hormone activity has been evaluated recently (see Chap. 33). Zinc is critical to the biological activity of thymic inductive factors; as much as 80% of such activity is lost when zinc is chelated. Vitamin B_6 also exerts a significant influence on thymic factor activity. On the other hand, the activity of thymulin is not affected significantly by deficiencies of copper, vitamin A, and selenium. It is generally considered that many of the deleterious effects of aging are related to alteration in thymic function and consequent effects on T lymphocyte-mediated immunity. To some degree, studies showing a positive effect of zinc supplementation support this point of view, although it is important to consider other possible actions of zinc as well. Furthermore, we know very little about the interactions of nutrients with each other, and this will probably be critical for beneficial supplementation programs in the elderly.

NUTRITION AND IMMUNITY IN OLD AGE: INTERVENTION

The critical role of nutrition in the modulation of immune responses has led to a few studies in which nutritional status has been correlated with immune responses in old age, although not all studies have found such a difference (35,36). Furthermore, intervention trials have attempted to improve immunocompetence by correction of nutritional abnormalities. In an early study, we looked at the nutritional and immunological status of a group of 'healthy' elderly subjects who had no evidence of an under-

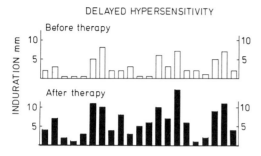

Figure 1

lying systemic disease. Among those with clinical, hematological, and biochemical evidence of nutritional deficiency, there was a significant reduction in delayed cutaneous hypersensitivity, T-cell number, and response to phytohemagglutinin (35a). Nutritional advice and supplement to increase the energy intake by approximately 500 kcal/day and to provide at least the recommended allowance of vitamins and trace elements for a period of 8 weeks resulted in improved skin test responses (Fig. 1) and an increase in the number of T cells and lymphocyte response to PHA (Table 1). The improvement in immunological function was associated with higher levels of albumin, prealbumin, retinol-binding protein, zinc, and iron. The individuals with abnormally low zinc and iron levels showed significantly impaired immunocompetence and improved after supplementation. Response to influenza virus vaccine was significantly enhanced in the group given appropriate nutritional supplements in a controlled study (Table 2) (17).

There are limited data on the influence of single-nutrient supplementation on immunocompetence in the elderly. The administration of 50-100 mg zinc daily for 4-6 weeks was associated with an increase in the number of circulating T cells and delayed cutaneous hypersensitivity responses (37). Serum IgG antibody to tetanus was higher in the supplemented group. In a double-blind placebo controlled trial, we observed the beneficial effects of zinc therapy on cell-mediated immunity in the elderly (38). About one-third of the treated group responded, which may reflect the prevalence of zinc deficiency in this age group. It is important to emphasize that moder-

Table 1 Effect of Nutritional Supplementation on Immunological Responses

	Number	Delayed cutaneous hypersensitivity (Number positive)	Stimulation index[a]	Rosetting T cells (%)
Before therapy	21	6	38 ± 14	41 ± 7
After therapy	21	12	79 ± 17	57 ± 5
p		<0.05	<0.05	<0.05

Values are given as mean ± SD.
[a]Maximum response was obtained with 10 ml PHA. Results obtained with this amount of PHA are shown.

Table 2 Response to Influenza Virus Vaccination in Nutritionally Supplemented Elderly and Nonsupplemented Controls

Group	Number studied	No. achieving seroconversion	Log reciprocal geometric mean antibody titer
Supplemented	15	14[a]	5.7 ± 1.2[b]
Nonsupplemented	15	9	2.5 ± 0.7

[a] $p < 0.05$.
[b] $p < 0.01$.

ately large supplements of zinc may impair immune responses, including T-cell proliferative capacity and neutrophil chemotaxis (Table 2) (33).

Vitamin supplementation has been tried in order to enhance immunity in old age. Vitamin C given in a dose of 500 mg/day for 1 month enhanced lymphocyte proliferation in vitro and skin reaction to tuberculin in vivo (39). There was no change in immunoglobulin levels or the proportion of rosetting T cells. Our recent work in this area suggests that selective specific correction of isolated vitamin deficiencies may be expected to improve immunocompetence in the elderly (15,23). On the other hand, in a recent study, the elderly receiving megadose vitamin C supplements tended to respond better on skin testing but the difference from the nonsupplemented controls were not significant (36). There were no changes in lymphocyte responses to mitogens in vitro. Subjects taking the supplements of vitamin B complex and vitamin E tended to lower lymphocyte counts than did controls. Multivitamin/mineral supplementation has also yielded promising results (40). Controlled experiments are clearly needed in this important area of considerable public health importance.

CONCLUSIONS

The frequent occurrence of nutritional problems is not in question nor is the significant decline in immune responses in the majority of the elderly individuals. Previous studies have confirmed the importance of nutrition in immunocompetence in children and young children. Thus, it is logical to try and attempt correction of nutritional deficiencies in the elderly with the aim of improving their immune responses and reducing the risk of infectious disease and other age-related disorders. At the same time, the wisdom and need of taking megadose supplements of vitamins and trace elements is questionable.

REFERENCES

1. Chandra RK. McCollum Award Lecture: Nutrition and immunity: Lessons from the past and new insights into the future. Am J Clin Nutr 1991;53:1087.
2. Bogden JD, Oleske JM, Munves EM, Lavenhar MA, Bruening KS, Kemp FW, Holding KJ, Denny TN, Louria DB. Zinc and immunocompetence in the elderly: Baseline data on zinc nutriture and immunity in unsupplemented subjects. Am J Clin Nutr 1987; 46:1037.
3. Payette H, Bola-Pleszcynski M, Ghadirian P. Nutrition factors in relation to cellular and regulatory immune variables in a free-living elderly population. Am J Clin Nutr 52:927.
4. Meydani SN, Meydani M, Blumberg JB. Antioxidants and the aging immune response. Adv Exp Biol Med 1990;262:57.

Table 3 Plasma, Zinc Levels, and Polymorphonuclear (PMN) Leukocyte Function

Time of sample	Plasma zinc, (g/dl)	Chemotactic migration,[a] PMNs per 10 HPF[b]	Ingestion of bacteria, No./100 PMNs	Bactericidal capacity, % Viable Bacteria
Baseline	83.0 ± 9.2[c]	493 ± 47[c]	3.1 ± 1.1[e]	
During zinc administration, wk				
2	101.1 ± 12.7[e]	585 ± 99[e]	386 ± 51[d]	3.9 ± 1.4[e]
4	181.5 ± 21.1[c]	355 ± 86[c]	272 ± 36[c]	4.6 ± 1.9[e]
6	199.7 ± 18.5[c]	292 ± 57[c]	251 ± 40[c]	3.8 ± 2.1[e]
Follow-up after cessation of zinc supplement, wk				
2	167.4 ± 20.3[c]	401 ± 71[c]	198 ± 43[c]	4.5 ± 2.3[e]
10	90.3 ± 10.0[c]	576 ± 114[c]	459 ± 56[c]	2.7 ± 1.2[e]

Value are given as mean ± SE.
[a]HPF indicates high-power field.
[b]Results are shown for migration at 120 min. Similar differences were observed at 60 and 180 min.
[c]$p < 0.01$ for differences between baseline or follow-up figures and values obtained during zinc administration.
[d]$0.5 < p < 0.1$.
[e]NS, $p > 0.1$.

5. Chavance M, Herbeth B, Fournier C, Jarot C, Vernhos G. Vitamin status, immunity, and infections in an elderly population. Eur J Clin Nutr 1989; 43:827.
6. Chandra RK. The relation between immunology, nutrition and disease in elderly people. Age and Aging 1990; 19:S25.
7. Kay MMB. Immunodeficiency in old age. In: Primary and Secondary Immunodeficiency Disorders (Chandra RK, ed). Edinburgh: Churchill Livingstone, 1983.
8. Chandra RK, ed. Nutrition, Immunity and Illness in the Elderly. New York, Pergamon Press, 1985.
9. Cinader B. Aging and the immune system. Clin Biochem 1983; 16:118-124.
10. Thompson JS, Robbins J, Cooper JK. Nutrition and Immune function in the geriatric population. Clin in Geriatr Med 1987; 3:309.
11. Lipschitz DA. Nutrition, aging, and the immunohematopoietic system. Clin Geriatr Med 1987; 3:319.
12. Hosokawa T, Hosono M, Higuchi K, Aoki A, Kawai K, Takeda T. Immune responses in newly developed short-lived SAM mice. I. Age-associated early decline in immune activities of cultured spleen cells. Immunology 1987; 62:419.
13. Meites J. Aging: Hypothalamic catecholamines, neuroendocrine—immune interactions, and dietary restriction Proc Soc Exp Biol Med 1990; 195:304.
14. Cannon JG, Orencole SF, Fielding RA, Meydani M, Meydani SN, Fiatarone MA, Blumberg JB, Evans WJ. Acute phase response in exercise: interaction of age and vitamin E on neutrophils and muscle enzyme release. Am J Physiol 259:R1214.
15. Chandra RK. Nutrition is an important determinant of immunity in old age. Prog Clin Biol Res 1990; 326:321.
16. Bogden JD, Oleske JM, Lavenhar MA, Munves EM, Kemp FW, Bruening KS, Holding KJ, Denny TN, Guarino MA, Holland BK. Effects of one year of supplementation with zinc and other micronutrients on cellular immunity in the elderly. J Am Coll Nutr 1990; 9:214.
17. Chandra RK, Puri S. Nutritional support improves antibody response to influenza virus vaccine in the elderly. Br Med J 1985; 291:705.
18. Peretz A, N'eve J, Desmedt J, Duchateau J, Dramarx M, Famaey JP. Lymphocyte response is enhanced by supplementation of elderly subjects with selenium-enriched yeast. Am J Clin Nutr 1991; 53:1323.
19. Harkness GA, Bently DW, Roghmann. Risk factors for nosocomial infections in the elderly Am J Med 1990; 89:457.
20. Siskind GW. Immunological aspects of aging: An overview In: Biological Mechanisms in Aging (Schmicke RT, ed.) USDA, TNIH, 1980, p 455.
21. Safieh B, Kendall MD, Norman JC, Metreau E, Dardenne M, Bach JF, Pleau JM. A new radioimmune assay for the thymic peptide thymulin and its application for measuring thymulin in blood samples. J Immunol Meth 1990; 127:255.
22. Schwab R, Weksler ME. Cell biology of the impaired proliferation of T cells from elderly humans. In: Aging and the Immune Response. (Goidl EA, ed). Marcel Dekker, New York, 1987, p 67.
23. Chandra RK. Nutritional regulation of immunocompetence and risk of disease in the elderly. In: Nutrition in the Elderly. Washington: World Health Organization, 1990, p. 243.
24. Cobleigh MA, Braun DP, Horris JE. Age dependent changes in human peripheral blood B cells and T cell subsets: correlation with mitogen responsiveness. Clin Immunol Immunopathol 1980; 15:162.
25. Bradley SF, Vibhsgoal A, Fabrick S, Terpenning MS, Kauffman CA. Monokine production by malnourished nursing home patients. Gerontol Psy 1990; 36:165.
26. Meydani SN, Barkland MP, Liu S, Meydani M, Miller CA, Cannon JG, Morrow FD, Rocklin R, Blumberg JB. Vitamin E supplementation enhances cell-mediated immunity in healthy elderly subjects. Am J Clin Nutr 1990; 52:557.

27. Walford RL, Harris SB, Weindruch R. Energy restriction and aging: Historical phases, mechanism and current directions. J Nutr 1987; 117:1650.
28. Keusch GT, Wilson CS, Waksal SD. Nutrition, host defenses, and the lymphoid system. Arch Host Def Mech 1983; 2:275-359.
29. McMurray DN. Cell-mediated immunity in nutritional deficiency. Prog Food Nutr Sci 1984; 8:193-228.
30. Islikar H, Schurch B. eds. The impact of malnutrition on immune defense in parasitic infestation. Bern, Hans Stuber, 1981.
31. Chandra RK. Nutrition, immunity, and infection: present knowledge and future directions. Lancet 1983; 1:688-691.
32. Inamiza T, Chang MP, Makinodan T. Influence of age on production and regulation of interleukin-1 in mice. Immunology 1985; 55:447.
33. Chandra RK. Excessive intake of zinc impairs immune responses. J Am Med Assoc 1984; 252:1443-1446.
34. Wu WH, Meydani M, Meydani SN, Barklund PM, Blumberg JB. Effect of dietary iron overload on lipid peroxidation, prostaglandin synthesis and lymphocyte proliferation in young and old rats. J Nutr 1990; 120:280.
35. Chandra RK, Joshi P, Au B, Woodford G, Chandra S. Nutrition and immunocompetence of the elderly. Effect of short-term nutritional supplementation on cell-mediated immunity and lymphocyte subsets. Nutr Res 1982; 2:223-232.
36. Goodwin JS, Garry JP. Relationship between megadose vitamin supplementation and immunological function in a healthy elderly population. Clin Exp Immunol 1983; 51: 647-653.
37. Duchateau J, Delepesse G, Vrijens R, Collet H. Beneficial effects of oral zinc supplementation on the immune response of old people. Am J Med 1981; 70:1001-1004.
38. Chandra RK. Nutritional regulation of immune function at the extremes of life: in infants and in the elderly. In: Malnutrition: Determinants and Consequences. New York: Liss, 1984; 245-251.
39. Kennes B, Dumont I, Brohee D, Hubert C, Neve P. Effect of vitamin C supplements on cell-mediated immunity in old people. Gerontology 1983; 29:305-311.
40. Subotičanec K, Stavlenič A, Bilič-Pešić L, Gorajščan M, Gorajščan D, Brubacher G, Buzina R. Nutritional status grip strength, and immune function in institutionalized elderly. Int J Vit Nutr Res 1989; 59:20.

Part IV
Issues and Implications in Nutrient Immune Interactions

29
Issues in Retinoid and Carotenoid Research

Adrianne Bendich
Hoffmann–La Roche, Inc., Nutley, New Jersey

FREE RADICALS AND IMMUNITY

Free radicals, molecules with one or more unpaired electrons, are used by the phagocytic cells of the immune system to aid in the killing of pathogens and tumor cells. Free radicals initiate the liberation of arachidonic acid from phospholipids from cellular membranes. Products of the arachidonic acid cascade are synthesized during free radical chain reactions. Recent evidence points to the requirement of free radical reactions in the initiation of cell-mediated immune responses (1,2). The research to determine the necessity of radical reactions for the formation of lymphokines, growth factors, and other regulatory molecules is in its infancy; 5 years ago, there were a handful of papers/year on this topic in the *Journal of Immunology*, currently, there can be several articles in each issue.

Free radical-mediated oxidative damage to immune activities is more fully documented than the data linking radical generation to normal immune functions. The majority of the findings of adverse effects of lipid peroxidation such as radical-induced cross-linking of DNA, enzyme and/or immunoglobulin inactivation, loss of mitochondrial integrity, receptor defects, and others have been documented in models of antioxidant deficit (3-5). The balance of required free radical reactions and antioxidant protection from the devastating effects of overabundance of radical reactions will continue to be the subject of research for many years to come.

DIETARY ANTIOXIDANTS

Antioxidants have the capacity of lowering the free radical burden either by interfering with the initiation of free radical formation or by inactivating the radicals once they are formed. Many of the antioxidants are not synthesized de novo in the body;

rather they must be consumed in the diet. Vitamin E is the major lipid-soluble antioxidant in serum and in cellular membranes. Vitamin C, which has been shown to be the most important water-soluble antioxidant in serum, is also found in high concentrations in neutrophils and macrophages. β-Carotene and a large number of the 500 or more carotenoids (with or without provitamin A activity) can lower the free radical levels and are very effective in deactivating singlet oxygen (6). Fewer than 10% of dietary carotenoids serve as precursors for vitamin A. Vitamin A, in contrast, is a poor antioxidant and cannot quench singlet oxygen. In addition, vitamin A has a smaller index of safety compared to the antioxidant vitamins and β-carotene (7). Yet, vitamin A deficiency can result in xerophthalmia and blindness. Furthermore, deficiency in children in developing countries has been associated with significant morbidity from infections, so that supplementation has been advised (8). Acute hypervitaminosis A may occur when more than 500,000 IU are ingested, significantly more than that used by Black and Zachrau in their pharmacological therapy in breast cancer (Chap. 26). Many factors which are poorly understood and include other dietary elements and vitamins (C, D, E, K) may affect the development of chronic hypervitaminosis A (8).

There are also three important antioxidant enzymes which require essential minerals for their activity; Cu/Zn and Mn-superoxide dismutases, Fe-catalase, and Se-glutathione peroxidase (9,10). Most research to date has been confined to examination of the immunological effects of single antioxidant micronutrients; future research should be focused on the interactions of the antioxidants, since many of these compounds are found in the same food sources and chemically the antioxidants interact with one another. Several lines of evidence suggest that toxic oxygen metabolites increase the aging process and that this underlies defective immune response. For example, defective detoxification by the glutathione peroxidase system in thymphocytes of aged rats has been found to cause reduced proliferative response (11).

CAROTENOIDS-SPECIAL CONSIDERATIONS

Carotenoids, such as β-carotene, in the crystalline form available commercially, are highly insoluble in aqueous media. Additionally, as antioxidants, they are prone to free radical attack and inactivation, with consequent bleaching of the yellow-red color. In vitro experiments with crystalline material are, therefore, fraught with problems of accurate assessment of concentration, formation of true solutions, and loss of bioactivity prior to addition of the cell cultures. Exposure to fluorescent light can also enhance inactivation. Without the measurement of carotenoid concentrations directly in the cells exposed to the carotenoid, it is very difficult to determine whether any effect seen is specific. This is equally true for any other micronutrient. The choice of the appropriate control is equally important. Is a saline control sufficient for a fat-soluble molecule? Should the carotenoid oxidatively inactivated be used as the control substance? Should homologous serum from carotenoid-fed animals be assayed for carotenoid concentration and the serum lipoproteins, the natural carriers of carotenoids, be used as the vehicle for adding carotenoids to cell cultures (especially if the culture system normally contains serum)?

There are water-soluble beadlet preparations of β-carotene and canthaxanthin and matched-control beadlets available for experimental use in vitro as well as in vivo; however, the concentration of the active component is only one-tenth the weight of the beadlet. There is a growing literature of animal experiments utilizing the beadlet forms. Consistency between carotenoid levels used in different experiments as well as type and concentration of dietary fat will be critical in determining the real effects of these compounds on immune responses. There are also problems with the use of rodents as experimental models because of their efficiency of conversion of β-carotene to vitamin A. The result of β-carotene supplementation at a level sufficient to result in measurable tissue carotenoid levels is a highly elevated liver vitamin A level and a decreased circulating level of vitamin E. All purified, defined protein source diets used in laboratory animal experiments contain virtually no β-carotene or other carotenoids and provide vitamin A in the vitamin premix added to the diet. Would β-carotene addition to these diets alter immune responses?

Protocols designed to differentiate between carotenoid and vitamin A effects are needed. However, it will be especially difficult to develop research projects in human populations, since non-vitamin A carotenoids, such as canthaxanthin, are not currently permitted in supplements in the United States, may be ill advised, and no other pure, single carotenoid is as yet available for human use. The effects of β-carotene on enhancement of certain immune functions in subjects with precancerous conditions as well as alterations in subset populations have been reported (12) (see Chapter 4), and further work in this area is strongly encouraged. These preliminary studies suggest a carotenoid effect on immune cells. The fact that some investigations have shown that β-carotene supplementation in vivo may increase immune function in vitro, whereas others have not (13), may reflect length of supplementation period (14) or other unidentified factors. The potential for a retinoid effect cannot be ruled out. Nevertheless, β-carotene represents a very safe, regulated delivery system for increasing vitamin A status with no possibility of acute hypervitaminosis A; and should there be a separate β-carotene immunoenhancing effect, the safety of supplemental β-carotene has already been well documented.

ANTIOXIDANT EFFECTS ON SPECIFIC ASPECTS OF IMMUNE FUNCTIONS

Currently, there is consensus that dietary deficiencies of vitamin C and/or vitamin E are associated with defects in phagocytic functions, especially chemotaxis (see Chapters 5 and 14) (15) and autooxidation. Supplementation of each vitamin separately has been shown to enhance phagocytic functions in individuals with genetically inherited defects, and in certain population groups prone to infections, such as children and the elderly. Cannon et al. (16) have recently shown that vitamin E affects neutrophil mobilization in a restorative fashion in the elderly after stress exercise.

The critical importance of vitamin A in lowering the morbidity of viral infections, such as measles (17), has been recently linked to the requirement of macrophages for cell-mediated responses to this and other potentially pathogenic microbes. Future research on the role of carotenoids in phagocytic functions and the examination of the requirement of antioxidant nutrients such as vitamins C and E in conditions which increase the free radical burden (such as seen with chronic infections, arthritis, and diabetes) should be given high priorities.

Promising results (such as described in Chap. 26) point to the potential for antioxidants to increase tumor immunity and thereby lower the tumor burden. The reports by several groups of enhancement of cytotoxicity and increased production of soluble molecules capable of killing tumor cells following the administration of vitamin E and/or carotenoids with or without vitamin A activity are quite interesting. Protocols need to be developed to examine these responses in the subjects involved in the placebo-double-blind trials currently sponsored by the National Cancer Institute to determine the chemopreventive effects of β-carotene as well as some of the other antioxidants. These studies are especially relevant in light of the growing consistent literature from epidemiological and intervention studies showing immunoenhancement of cell-mediated responses in individuals with high antioxidant status. Improving antioxidant status has been found to increase the immune response in the elderly and this may have an anticancer benefit (18).

There are many other examples of chronic diseases in which free radical levels are significantly increased because of the disease as well as treatment of the condition. Examples include emphysema, AIDS, chemotherapies, especially involving radiation, and degenerative diseases of the nervous system in which the drugs are metabolized by the liver's cytochrome P-450 system. In all cases, immunocompromise is an additional factor. Antioxidants may lower the free radical burden and enhance already compromised immune systems. Of particular importance is the examination of the effects of antioxidant micronutrient status (deficiency and supplementation) on the pathology of viral infections, especially HIV. Vitamin A deficiency in an experimental animal model has been found to produce decreased interferon production (19). The early findings of increased interferon production following vitamin C supplementation should be reexamined with the new, more sophisticated assays and reagents currently available. Research in this area is encouraged, since the antioxidant vitamins have been shown to be safe at levels well beyond 10 times the recommended daily allowance.

Acute, unpredictable conditions, such as severe burns, trauma, wounds, infections by pathogens, and even strenuous exercise and/or short-term exposure to UV light, have been shown to increase free radical generation and at the same time to depress many immune functions. Similarly, certain lifestyle habits (4), such as cigarette smoking and alcohol consumption, are also linked to increased oxidative stress and immunosuppression as well as lowered circulating levels of antioxidants such as vitamin C and β-carotene.

There is a growing list of assays which can document the effects of antioxidants on lowering free radical levels. Immunologically relevant indicators include prostaglandin E_2, serum lipid peroxides, and urinary DNA oxidation products. Studies which include indices of effects of antioxidants on immune functions which are also correlated with a lowering of free radical generated, immunosuppressive compounds are strongly recommended.

CONCLUSIONS

Future research on the immunological effects of antioxidant vitamin C and E and β-carotene are important to help to define the levels of the essential nutrients necessary for optimal immune activities. In vitro and laboratory animal investigations, although difficult with relatively unstable compounds such as antioxidants, are needed to define the mechanisms of action. The success of recent human trials involving supplemental levels of vitamin E are most exciting and should encourage other well-designed and controlled protocols in the near future.

REFERENCES

1. Bendich A, Chandra RK, Keusch GT, Cerami A, Takaku F. 1990. Micronutrients and immune functions/cytokines and metabolism. Ann NY Acad Sci 587.
2. Bendich A, Phillips M, Tengerdy RP, eds. 1990. Antioxidant Nutrients and Immune Function. New York: Plenum Press; (Advances in Experimental Medicine and Biology; v. 262).
3. Bendich A. 1990. Antioxidant vitamins and immune response. Am NY Acad Sci 587:168.
4. Machlin LJ, Bendich A. 1987. Free radical tissue damage: protective role of antioxidant nutrients. FASEB J 1:441-445, 1987.
5. Leibovitz B. 1990. Dietary supplements of vitamin E, β-carotene coenzyme Q10 and selenium protect tissues against lipid peroxidation in rat tissue slices. J Nutr 120:97.
6. Bendich A, Olson JA. 1989. Biological actions of carotenoids. FASEB J 3:1927-1932.
7. Bendich A, Langseth A. 1989. Safety of vitamin A. Am J Clin Nutr 49:358.
8. Vitamin A and malnutrition/infection complex in developing countries (editorial) Lancet 1:336-1349, 1990.
9. Spallholz JE. 1990. Selenium and glutathione peroxidase: Essential nutrient and antioxidant component of the immune system. Adv Exp Med and Biol 262:145.
10. Bendich A. 1990. Antioxidant nutrients and immune functions—introduction. Adv Exp Med Biol 262:1.
11. Franklin RA, Li YM, Arkins S, Kelley D. 1990. Glutathione augments in vitro proliferative responses of lymphocytes to concanavalin A to a greater degree in old than young rats. J Nutr 120:1710.
12. Prabhala RH, Garewal HS, Hicks MJ, Sampliner RE, Watson RR. 1991. The effects of 13-cis retinoic acid and β carotene on cellular immunity in humans. Cancer 67:1556.
13. Ringer TV, DeLoof MJ, Winterrowd GE, Francom SF, Gaylor SK, Ryan JA, Sanders ME, Hughes GS. 1991. Beta-carotene's effect on serum lipoproteins and immunologic indices in humans. Am J Clin Nutr 53:688.
14. Watson RR. 1991. Beta-carotene's effects on serum lipoproteins and immunologic indices in humans. Am J Clin Nutr 54:609.
15. Bendich A. 1988. Vitamin E and immune function. Basic Life Sci 49:615.
16. Cannon JG, Orencole SF, Fielding RA, Meydani M, Meydani SN, Fiatarone MA, Blumberg JB, Evans WJ. 1990. Acute phase response in exercise: Interaction of age and vitamin E on neutrophils and muscle enzyme release. Am J Physiol 259:R1214.
17. 1991. Vitamin A administration reduces mortality and morbidity from severe measles in populations nonendemic for hypovitaminosis A. Nutr Rev 49:89.
18. Meydani SN, Blumberg JB. 1991. Vitamin E supplementation and enhancement of immune responsiveness in the aged. In: Micronutrients in Health and in Disease Prevention; A Bendich and C E Butterworth, eds, Marcel Dekker, Inc. New York, NY, pp 289-306.
19. Bowman TA, Goonewardeene M, Pasatempo AMG, Ross AC, Taylor CE. 1990. Vitamin A deficiency decreases natural killer cell activity and interferon production in rats. J Nutr 115:1033.

30
Impact of Infectious Disease on the Interaction Between Nutrition and Immunity

William R. Beisel
The Johns Hopkins School of Hygiene and Public Health, Baltimore, Maryland

INTRODUCTION

As evidenced throughout this book, various forms of malnutrition can lead to anatomical and functional impairments of the immune system. See *in particular* chapters 18, 23, and 27. Metabolic and physiological components of the acute phase response to infectious diseases can cause large losses from the nutritional reserves of the body (1-4). It, therefore, follows logically, that infectious diseases can lead to immune system derangements as secondary consequences of malnutrition.

Despite the simplicity of this logic, the pathogenesis of the infection—malnutrition—immune system dysfunction sequence is complex, and much has yet to be learned about the mechanisms which produce such a dysfunction. Hopefully, methods to prevent or minimize this problem will emerge through future research.

We now possess detailed knowledge concerning immune system responses to various specific antigens introduced by infectious microorganisms. We know a great deal, even at the molecular level, about the cell-mediated and humoral mechanisms employed by the immune system to recognize and respond to such specific antigens. A good understanding has also been developed about the genesis of potentially harmful immunological responses to infection, such as those produced by immune complexes, autoimmunity, or allergy, or by the impairment of a key subset of lymphocytes, as seen in AIDS virus infections.

We have gained some insight into the molecular mechanisms during acute phase reactions that result in a broad, nonspecific stimulation of the immune system, and the activation of a wide array of antigenically nonspecific host defense mechanisms (5-10).

In contrast, relatively little is known about the details of the nutritional losses, or imbalances, that are induced by acute generalized infectious illnesses (2,3). Although a transient loss of delayed dermal hypersensitivity reactions has been noted in patients with infections such as measles or typhoid fever, no systematic studies have been conducted to evaluate the potential role of malnutrition in contributing to the derangements of immune system function that may accompany or follow a severe or prolonged infection. Recent studies have shown that HIV infection is accompanied by viral-associated malabsorption, leading to significant loss of body mass which can be partially corrected by total parenteral nutrition but apparently, only in patients without systemic infections (11).

THE ACUTE PHASE RESPONSE

The acute phase response during generalized infectious diseases includes many metabolic and physiological reactions. Activated monocytes, macrophages, and other body cells produce and release interleukin 1, which serves in a hormonelike role to trigger acute phase responses throughout the body (5-10). Three cytokines of leukocytic origin, IL-1, tumor necrosis factor (TNF), and interleukin 6 (IL-6) are the principal mediators of changes in intermediary metabolism causing decreased food intake, increased resting energy expenditure, gluconeogenesis, glucose oxidation, and hepatic synthesis of fatty acids and acute phase proteins, and altered fatty acid distribution and mineral metabolism. Fever is generated, accompanied by an increase in body oxygen consumption and metabolic rates. Anorexia, myalgia, somnolence, and lassitude are accompanying symptoms. Leukocytosis may occur, and numerous additional endocrine responses are seen (2,3,7).

Body metabolic processes are markedly affected by the acute phase response. Proteolysis of actin and myosin in skeletal muscle leads to the release of free amino acids, many of which are taken up by hepatocytes. The liver increases its synthesis of glucose, urea, and a large variety of proteins. Amino acids contribute as major substrates for this enhanced gluconeogenesis (2,3,7). And importantly, there is a broad, nonspecific, interleukin 1-induced stimulation of the immune system (5,6,8).

NUTRITIONAL COSTS OF THE ACUTE PHASE RESPONSE

Although the various components of the acute phase response appear to be purposeful, and of ultimate benefit to the host in helping to control the infectious process (8-10), the acute phase response is a costly one in terms of the body nutrients that are expended, destroyed, or lost. Current knowledge concerning the magnitude and composition of these nutritional losses remains grossly incomplete. Furthermore, the production of oxygen reactive species, vital to the bactericidal activity of phagocytic cells, must be balanced by production of endogenous scavengers so that the damaging effect of these species is mitigated. Dietary components such as lipids, ascorbic acid, and alpha-tocopherol (in membrane-bound form) strongly affect these interactions through prostaglandins and thromboxanes (12), and thus have long-term consequences for recovery from infections processes.

Some losses of nutrients from the body during infectious illness have been measured directly by metabolic balance studies (1,4). Losses of body nitrogen seem to vary in magnitude in relationship to the severity and duration of a generalized infection. Daily losses of "labile" nitrogen are greatest during the early febrile period (2, 7). But the body stores of labile nitrogen are finite and they can be exhausted rapidly, i.e., within several weeks. Any prolongation of the infectious process and its accompanying anorexia will then deplete additional protein components of body tissues, including the visceral organs (2,7).

Initial infection-induced losses of protein nitrogen appear to come from the body pool of labile nitrogen, which is largely contained within the somatic tissues. If an infection becomes subacute or chronic, nitrogen losses come from the visceral tissues as well (2,7). Eventually, daily nitrogen losses taper off exponentially, and a new phase of equilibrium in nitrogen balance is reestablished, albeit at a cachectic level. Since all body defensive measures, including the immune system, require nitrogen-containing amino acids to build new proteins, infection-induced cachexia will compromise these defenses (1-3,7).

Most of the studies on direct, infection-induced losses of body nutrients have focused on nitrogen (2,3,7). Far less is known about losses of other body minerals and electrolytes. Only a few studies have measured infection-induced losses of the principal intracellular elements—magnesium, potassium, and phosphorus (4). These elements seem to be lost in amounts proportional to losses of nitrogen, and the same may hold true for losses of zinc and sulfur from the body (2,4).

Hormonal responses during generalized infections usually lead to a renal retention of body salt and water (2,4,7). But, on the other hand, fecal losses of sodium, chloride, potassium, and bicarbonate will be seen if diarrhea is present. These losses may be extensive in severe secretory diarrheas, such as those caused by *Vibrio cholerae* or enterotoxigenic *Escherichia coli* (2).

Indirect losses of essential body nutrients, caused by their accelerated metabolism or consumption, are believed to occur during infectious diseases, but these losses are difficult to measure with certainty (1-3). Reductions in the tissue concentrations of vitamin A and vitamin C have been detected. Overt vitamin deficiency states such as scurvy, night blindness, pellagra, and beriberi have been triggered by acute infections (1). Despite these bits and pieces of data about the infection-induced depletion of body vitamins and essential trace (or ultratrace) elements, very little detailed information is at hand (1,2). Currently available technology does not allow for the widespread clinical assessment of marginal deficiency states of many of the vitamins, minerals, and trace elements.

Hopefully, new analytical methodologies will be developed to permit the clinical measurement of body nutrient stores and their derangements. Such knowledge should permit an accurate appraisal of body composition in health and disease, and should form the basis for prophylactic and corrective nutritional measures.

PREVENTIVE AND THERAPEUTIC STRATEGIES

Immunological and Infection-Related Strategies

Because the immune system can be affected by various forms of malnutrition, systematic studies of the entire spectrum of essential single nutrients, and of energy-producing substrates will be required (1,13,14). The threshold levels at which individual nutrients begin to affect immune system functions must also be identified (13).

It will be important to study various forms of acute infection to determine if changes in body composition and losses of body nutrients occur in a consistent pattern, or vary with the nature of the infection. It will also be important to determine the pathogenesis of such infection-induced nutritional losses when infections become subacute, or change into a chronic illness (1,7). It is likely that subacute infection may affect growth and development through a range of mechanisms, which need to be identified, and that age may play a role such that antibiotic prophylaxis can be beneficial at some periods and not at others (15).

Several corrective strategies should reduce the immune system dysfunctions caused by infection-induced loss of body nutrients. The overall magnitude of the problem can be reduced by measures which reduce the incidence of infectious illness. These include the continued development and use of vaccines and public health measures which reduce disease transmission. Prompt diagnosis and effective antimicrobial therapy can also minimize nutrient losses due to infection. These infection-related measures must continue to be improved and extended.

Nutritional Strategies

Another conventional approach requires the prompt correction of infection-induced nutritional deficits (1,2,13). Methods to speed up and improve nutritional rehabilitation must continue to be developed. As pointed out in earlier paragraphs, far too little is known about the magnitude and complexity of infection-induced malnutrition. A valid scientific basis must be created to establish truely effective programs of nutritional rehabilitation after severe or prolonged infectious illnesses (1,13).

Although nutritionally induced immunoincompetence is generally reversible, many questions still remain unanswered concerning the safest methods to prevent or correct nutritional deficits that may occur during an infectious process. If anorexia is a beneficial response, should forced feedings or intravenous alimentation be attempted during its presence? How great is the possibility that immune system imbalances may be created by the process of nutritional rehabilitation?

Are certain nutrients (such as zinc (16,17), other trace elements, or vitamins) of special importance during the early convalescent period when anorexia disappears and body nutrient stores are most depleted? What special or unusual dietary measures may be necessary if the degree of malnutrition is extremely severe (18)?

With respect to malnutrition and possible alterations in host susceptibility to infection, are any special precautions necessary during the correction of nutritional deficits? Severely malnourished patients may be afflicted by subclinical, inapparent infections, and these may flare up once nutritional rehabilitation reaches a level that will permit signs of illness (e.g., fever, leukocytosis, inflammation) to again become manifest. How great is the possibility that therapeutically administered iron will saturate nutritionally lowered plasma transferrin concentrations, and thus permit a massive growth of iron-requiring microorganisms (19)?

Other Future Strategies

A third, still theoretical, strategy is now becoming possible. If proven safe and effective, an entirely new approach will be opened for the restoration (or amplification) of immune system competence. This future approach is based on the therapeutic or prophylactic use of one or more biological response modifiers (i.e., naturally occurring endogenous mediators, hormones, immunostimulants, and antiviral agents) that are now becoming available through the use of recombinant DNA technology.

Although the potential role of various biological response modifiers is only now being explored, these substances hold great promise as therapeutic agents (20). Potential future uses include a wide role in the control of infectious diseases and in immunopotentiation. Gene cloning procedures, which now allow many of these natural human factors to be produced in quantity, are also providing finite knowledge of their identities, molecular structures, and specificities (20,21).

A family of closely related interferons is now undergoing clinical testing, but their ultimate role in the control of various infectious diseases has yet to be established. Because in high doses the interferons can induce fever, anorexia, and other components of the acute phase response, they do cause losses of body nutrients. However, ongoing research should eventually identify the true and useful range of the interferons, and their optimal doses, for helping to prevent or treat infectious illnesses.

Several of the interleukins have been cloned and made available for testing. Four species of interleukin 1 all seem to have similar functions. Although interleukin 1 triggers the acute phase response, this hormonelike mediator also activates lymphocytes and neutrophils. Functioning as an immunostimulant, interleukin 1 initiates an enhanced lymphocytic production and release of interleukin 2. Interleukin 2, in turn, stimulates the proliferation of lymphocyte populations. Clinical testing with interleukin 2 is currently underway, with the objective of enhancing immune system competence. Interleukin 3 also is becoming available (20,21). It acts to stimulate replication of the earliest stages of stem cells in the bone marrow.

Other new hormonelike biological response modifiers are also becoming available for testing. A number of different hematological growth factors, termed colony-stimulating-factors, act in concert with interleukin 2 and interleukin 3 to enhance a full spectrum of red and white blood cells. These factors include erythropoietin and colony growth stimulants for granulocytes and macrophages (20,21). These substances have a wide range of potential clinical uses, including the treatment of infectious diseases and immunosuppression (21).

Additionally, human growth hormone has now become available as a safe, cloned product. An increase in growth hormone concentrations in plasma has been demonstrated during acute infectious illnesses (3), but the physiological role of this response has yet to be clarified. It is possible that the administration of exogenous growth hormone could reduce the nutritional losses of infection, or speed up nutritional rehabilitation during convalescence.

CONCLUSIONS

Although infectious diseases generally stimulate an immune response, an adverse secondary effect on the immune system and other host defense mechanisms may be created by the large nutritional costs of infection. These costs include the actual loss of many nutrients from the body, and the loss of others which are destroyed by metabolic processes. These nutritional costs appear related to both the severity and duration of an infectious process. Because deficiencies in various individual nutrients can lead to different forms of reversible immune system dysfunction, much more detailed information must be gained about the nutritional costs of infection. Future strategies to prevent or correct the infection-malnutrition-immune dysfunction sequence have been discussed.

REFERENCES

1. Beisel WR, Blackburn GL, Feigin RD, Keusch GT, Long CL, Nichols BL (1977). Symposium on the impact of infection on nutritional status of the host. Am J Clin Nutr 30:1203-1371, 1439-1566.

2. Beisel WR. 1991. Nutrition and infection. In: Nutritional Biochemistry and Metabolism with Clinical Applications. 2nd Edition. M C Linder, ed. Elsevier, New York, pp 507-542.
3. Powanda MC, Canonico PG, ed. 1981. Infection: The Physiologic and Metabolic Responses of the Host. Elsevier/North Holland, New York.
4. Beisel WR, Sawyer WD, Ryll ED, Crozier D. 1967. Metabolic effects of intracellular infections in man. Ann Intern Med 67:744-779.
5. Editorial. 1985. Interleukin-1 in defense of the host. Lancet 1:536-537.
6. Dinarello CA. 1985. An update on human interleukin-1: From molecular biology to clinical relevance. J Clin Immunol 5:287-297.
7. Beisel WR. 1987. Humoral mediators of cellular response and altered metabolism. In: Trauma, Emergency Surgery and Critical Care. JH Siegel, ed. Churchill Livingstone, New York, pp. 57-78.
8. Dinarello CA. 1990. Interleukin-1 and its biologically related cytokines. In: Lymphokines and the Immune Response. ES Cohen, ed. CRC Press, Boca Raton, p 181.
9. Wan JM, Haw MP, Blackburn GL. 1989. Nutrition, immune function, and inflammation: an overview. Proc Nutr Soc 48:315.
10. Beisel WR. 1990. Intestinal aspects of the acute phase reaction. J Lab Clin Med 115:652.
11. Kotler DP, Tierney AR, Culpepper-Morgan JA, Wang J, Pierson RNJR. 1990. Effect of home total parenteral nutrition on body composition in patients with acquired immunodeficiency syndrome. J Parenter Enterol Nutr 14:454.
12. Foegh MC, Thomas G, Ramwell PW. 1990. Free radicals, arachidonic acid metabolites and nutrition. J Parenter Enterol Nutr 14:218S.
13. Chandra RK. 1990. Cellular and molecular basis of nutrition-immunity interactions. Adv Exp Med Biol 262:13.
14. Beisel WR. 1981. Single nutrients and immunity. Am J Clin Nutr 35(Feb Suppl):417-468.
15. Khin-Maung-U, Bolin TD, Duncombe VM, Pereira SP, Myo-Khin, Nyunt-Nyunt-Wai, Linklater JM. 1990. Effect of short term intermittent antibiotic treatment on growth of Burmese (Myanmar) village children. Lancet 336:1090-1094.
16. Castillo-Duran C, Heresi G, Fisberg M, Uauy R. 1987. Controlled trial of zinc supplementation during recovery from malnutrition: effect on growth and immune function. Am J Clin Nutr 45:602-608.
17. Beisel WR. 1990. Future role of micronutrient on immune function. Ann NY Acad Sci 587:267.
18. Beisel WR. 1989. Role of nutrition in immune system diseases. Comp Ther 13:13.
19. Sherman A. 1990. Influence of iron on immunity and disease resistance. Ann NY Acad Sci 587:140.
20. Kolata G. 1987. Clinical promise with new hormones. Science 236:517-519.
21. Oppenheim JJ, Shevach EM. 1990. Immunophysiology: The Role of Cells and Cytokines in Immunity and Inflammation. Oxford University Press, England.

31
Nutritional Indications for Cancer Prevention—Calorie Restriction

Ellen Lorenz
All Children's Hospital, St. Petersburg, Florida

Robert A. Good
All Children's Hospital and University of South Florida, St. Petersburg, Florida

INTRODUCTION

Several chapters in this book provide evidence that protein calorie malnutrition impairs immune function and produces susceptibility to infection. In the context of surgical procedures, the beneficial effect of arginine on the immune response and wound healing has been described (Chap. 3).

On the other hand, it has been found that giving certain types of lipid emulsions to cancer patients as an adjunct to surgery or chemotherapy—even in the context of genuine nutritional need—may actually promote tumor development. Thus, nutritional supplementation is a two-edged sword. These issues are critical when we consider nutritional therapy in aging, where, as described by Chandra, immune dysfunction even in healthy persons, has parallels with protein calorie malnutrition.

There is a growing body of evidence that caloric restriction in the absence of essential nutrient deficiencies may slow the aging process. Further, as we discuss here, caloric restriction appears to have a direct benefit in host defense against cancer.

In the more than 50 years since Clive McCay undertook investigations of the effects of underfeeding on the incidence of cancer in laboratory mice, diet has come to be appreciated as one of the chief contributors to cancer incidence and mortality. Indeed, Doll and Peto (1) have estimated that from 75 to 80% of cancers may be attributed to lifestyle and that, in fully one-third or more, diet is the chief contributor in the etiology of malignancy. Thus, after cigarette smoking, dietary factors appear to represent the single most important—and potentially controllable—cause of cancer.

Epidemiological studies have been of limited use in helping to determine which strategies would be most effective in preventing cancer by dietary manipulation, whereas results of more than 5 decades of experiments with laboratory animals, in particular, the venerable mice and rats, have permitted us to begin to sort out the respective roles of dietary components in the development of cancer. A growing number of animal studies indicate that calorie intake is the single most critical variable in the influence of nutrition on the development of cancer.

DIETARY RESTRICTION AND DISEASE: EARLY FINDINGS

In the 1930s, McCay and his colleagues showed that dietary restriction could delay the onset of diseases associated with aging, prolong life span, and lower the incidence of spontaneous tumors in mice (2-4), which was attributed to the action of underfeeding in retarding growth and development.

Recent evidence indicates that dietary restriction may block cancers at the cellular and molecular levels.

The first systematic investigations of the effects of dietary restriction on experimental carcinogenesis were begun by Tannenbaum in the late 1930s, who reported that underfeeding reduced the incidence of spontaneous breast tumors from 40 to 4% in virgin DBA mice and from 30 to 7% in a population heterogeneous for both virgin and parous mice (5-7). Moreover, Tannenbaum demonstrated that dietary restriction could effectively prevent tumorigenesis even when initiated rather late in life.

Based on these and later investigations, Tannenbaum concluded that calorie restriction during the phase of tumor promotion appeared to be the most efficacious means to the inhibit growth of spontaneous mammary tumors.

In separate investigations during the same period, Visscher (8) studied spontaneously occurring mammary tumors in C3H mice and observed no tumors in the calorie-restricted mice compared to a 67% incidence of tumor formation in the ad libitum fed mice, and concluded that underfeeding worked through reduced calorie intake rather than changes in dietary composition.

Ross and Bras (9), in extensive studies employing approximately 1000 Charles River rats, reported that food restriction inhibited the development of spontaneously occurring cancers (most notably lymphomas, fibrosarcomas, fibromas, and pancreatic islet cell tumors) in exponential proportion to the level of caloric intake. Varying levels of dietary protein and carbohydrate was also tried. Although life span was increased and incidence of degenerative disease such as glomerulonephritis was reduced by restriction of protein and carbohydrate as well as calories, tumor occurrence was affected only by total calorie intake (9).

In investigations of spontaneously occurring mammary tumors in Fischer 344 rats, Tucker (10) showed that restricting calorie intake (25-40%) inhibited the formation of tumors at a number of susceptible sites. Moreover, the number of tumors developed per rat was significantly reduced in both male and female rats.

Many of the earliest efforts at dietary restriction used a rather rudimentary methodology of simply feeding experimental animals smaller portions of the same diet fed to ad libitum mice. As nutritional investigations progressed and became more refined, protein and carbohydrate intakes were adjusted so that experimental animals received proportionately equivalent amounts of these macronutrients. However, micronutrients were not usually adjusted, so that unrecognized nutrient deficits may have affected those early studies. Over the past 2 decades, we and others (11-18) have refined the preparation of experimental rations so that animals placed on restricted diets consume all micronutrients and trace elements at the same level as do the ad libitum animals. Such techniques have permitted close analysis of the independent influences of macronutrients; namely, calories versus fat, in relation to life span and prevention of cancer.

ENERGY DERIVED FROM CALORIES VERSUS ENERGY DERIVED FROM FAT

Numerous investigations have attempted to analyze the respective roles of fat and calories in the onset and progression of tumors in experimental systems. Kritchevsky, Klurfeld, and their colleagues have stated rather strongly the case for the critical influence of calorie intake rather than dietary fat in tumor formation in rats (19-21). In 7,12-dimethylbenz[a]anthracene-induced colon tumors and mammary adenocarcinoma, a most significant reduction of tumorigenesis occurred when calorie intake was restricted by 40% (whether dietary fat composition was 3.9% of total calories or more than three times this level).

This group also fed DMBA-treated rats diets that contained 5% fat (in the form of corn oil) and were calorie restricted (20, 30, or 40%). Mammary tumor incidence was only marginally reduced by a 20% restriction in calories. In contrast, tumor occurrence was significantly inhibited with 30-40% restriction.

Bouissoneault et al. (22) studied chemically induced (DMBA-induced) breast cancer in Fischer F344 rats and demonstrated that mammary tumor induction was influenced by a multifactorial combination of energy intake, energy utilization, and body size, with calorie intake playing a key role.

In our own investigations over the past 15 years (13,15,16,23,24), we have employed calorie restriction, or as we have termed it, chronic energy intake restriction (CEIR), in a number of genetically short-lived strains of mice, and have established that restriction of energy intake is the most important factor in the extension of life span and the prevention of diseases of aging. To achieve optimal results, CEIR, was imposed at time of weaning in a diet reduced 40% in calories but enriched to provide essential vitamins, minerals, and nutrients. Such calorie restriction could regularly double, triple, or even quadruple life span in mice of these genetically autoimmune-prone strains; e.g., B/W, NZB, MRL/lpr lpr, kdkd, and BXSB mice. CEIR delays or prevents development of immunologically based hyalinizing renal disease, vascular lesions, and certain malignancies. We have shown that CEIR can be initiated as late as midlife, or even after successful reproduction and lactation, and still provide this dramatic effect.

To determine whether calorie source or total calorie intake was more critical, we tested diets which varied in composition from very high-fat/no carbohydrate, high-carbohydrate, very low fat, moderate-fat, or moderate-carbohydrate diets (15, 16,25). No significant differences in life span were found. However, when each diet was fed at a restricted calorie level, both the median longevity and maximal life span of mice of each strain studied were significantly increased. The most significant shift in life span was observed when the diet was relatively low in fat and relatively high in carbohydrate. However, we did note a secondary effect of a high-fat diet whereby mice which consumed a high-fat, calorie-restricted diet lived approximately twice as long as the ad libitum fed animals. In contrast, calorie-restricted mice on high-carbohydrate, low-fat diet lived up to four times longer than ad libitum fed mice (25,26). This deleterious effect of fat, secondary to the influence of the level of calorie intake, has important implications for prevention of disease by dietary means.

We also employed isocaloric CEIR diets in which fat or carbohydrate represented the principal energy source to study the prevention of mammary tumors in C3H/Ou mice (27). Mice on purified iso caloric diets which varied in energy source (fat or carbohydrate) were compared to mice fed both diets at an ad libitum or restricted level. We found that calorie intake exerted the most dramatic influence on tumor formation. Full-fed mice developed breast cancer within 6 weeks of feeding whether they consumed the high-fat diet or a diet containing only enough fat to meet minimum essential fatty acid requirements. On the other hand, only 5 of 86 mice fed the calorie-restricted diet developed tumors. Although we found that full feeding of fat-based diets appeared to promote a slightly earlier onset of tumors among either full-fed or CEIR diets, this difference lacked statistical significance compared to full feeding or calorie restriction. Thus, fat may have some promoting effect, independent of the level of calorie consumption. These results are consistent with recent biostatical analyses by Freedman et al. (28) of more than 100 animal studies who found that calorie intake was the most significant variable in the development of mammary cancer, but that there was a specific enhancing effect of dietary fat as well. Another recent report has confirmed that feeding high levels of dietary fat can significantly increase mammary carcinogenesis, but only in those animals fed ad libitum (29). With respect to breast cancer, this secondary effect of fat appears particularly to influence tumor latency (27).

FOCUS: DIET AND BREAST CANCER

The effect of diet on mammary cancer has been a special focus of research in our laboratories (11,30,31). We have used spontaneously occurring breast cancer attributable to murine mammary tumor virus infection as a model system. Our work began with studies with Fernandes and Yunis in which we imposed a 40% energy (calorie) restriction in C3H/Umc mice and observed a dramatic decrease in the occurrence of mammary tumors (11). Within 500 days, tumors had developed in 71% of ad libitum fed mice but in none of the CEIR mice.

We found (30) that calorie restriction not only dramatically reduced the incidence of mammary tumors, but also greatly inhibited the associated development of precancerous minimal alveolar lesions, the so-called hyperplastic alveolar nodules within the mammary tissue. Here, we also observed a significant reduction in the formation of type A and type B retroviral particles within the mammary gland. This could not be attributed to obvious hormonal changes such as alteration of estrus cycle, inhibition of thyroid-stimulating hormone production, or disturbances in somatotropin production. The only hormonal influence of CEIR that could be demonstrated readily was a highly significant decrease in the circulating levels of prolactin. In subsequent studies, we discovered the fundamental influence of calorie restriction on circulating prolactin in C3H mice (27). Mice fed a diet high in calories had elevated serum prolactin levels, elevated levels of circulating immune complexes, and elevated levels of antibodies to the mouse mammary tumor virus. We then analyzed the effect of calorie restriction (40%) on proviral messages of endogenous mouse mammary tumor virus (32), and found that calorie restriction inhibits proviral DNA transcription and suppresses MMTV messages not only in the mammary gland, but also in a number of other tissues, including liver, kidney, lung, and small intestine. Moreover, CEIR appeared to reduce the expression of the putative proto-oncogenes *int*-1, *int*-2, and *ras*, suggesting a key potential mechanism for the influence of CEIR on the development of cancer.

The effect of CEIR on prolactin was underscored in subsequent in vivo investigations (33) in which mice fed calorie-restricted diets received adenohypophyseal grafts to elevate circulating prolactin levels, and mice fed ad libitum were treated with the dopamine analog actahydrogbengo[g]quinolone to reduce serum prolactin levels. This manipulation of circulating prolactin overrode the control of MMTV mRNA expression by calorie restriction. In the mice fed a CEIR diet but subjected to adenohypophyseal grafting, we observed a linear correlation between prolactin levels and MMTV mRNA; in the ad libitum fed mice given the dopamine analog, MMTV proviral expression was significantly reduced compared to that observed in unmanipulated full-fed mice. Koizumi et al. (34) recently reported that CEIR decreased the level of mRNA for the mouse mammary tumor virus present in both mammary glands and uteri of C3H mice; mean MMTV mRNA levels in mammary glands from ad libitum fed mice was five times higher than in mammary glands taken from the calorie-restricted mice.

These recent findings on the influences of diet on prolactin levels, mammary tumor virus activity, and mammary tumor formation point to an important role for prolactin in the nutritional regulation of cellular proliferation and indicate the need for further detailed investigations. Like other nonapeptide hormones whose multifaceted immunological and physiological roles are still being elucidated, i.e., thymulin and oxytocin, it appears that prolactin may be an important multifunctional physiological mediator. For example, there have been a number of reports which link prolactin to a possibly essential role in cellular proliferation (35,36). Prolactin has been shown to be comitogenic with certain phytomitogens, and to exert a crucial influence in the regenerative proliferation of hepatic cells that occurs after partial hepatectomy in experimental systems (36a,37). Prolactin also influences protein kinase C translocation in the preproliferative state for epithelial cells, suggesting that prolactin's effects on mammary tumors and hyperplastic alveolar nodules may be related to regulation of protein kinase C, which in turn has been assigned a possible role in the etiology of cancer (37a).

Russell et al. also reported that prolactin can induce activation of ornithine decarboxylase (35), the principal rate-limiting enzyme in polyamine biosynthesis and an enzyme which is thought to play an important role in the promotion of tumors (38). In studying the effects of calorie restriction on chemically induced colon cancer in F344 rats, Kumar et al. (39) recently reported that calorie restriction lowered ornithine decarboxylase activity in the colonic mucosa in rats and inhibited the rise of colonic mucosal ornithine decarboxylase activity that normally occurs subsequent to chemical (azoxymethane) stimulation.

Epidemiological studies of human breast cancer data have found an association between prolactin levels, perhaps interrelated with dietary factors, and the incidence of mammary cancer. In a recent study of Australian women, Ingram et al. (40) found that elevated prolactin values were associated with a more than twofold increase in the risk of breast cancer. An influence of diet on prolactin levels also was noted in premenopausal women who reported high consumption of saturated fats (fat intake rather than calorie intake still being a more common parameter of analysis in epidemiological studies of breast cancer). If it can be assumed, as is most likely, that such high fat intake reflected a diet relatively high in calories, then these recent observations strengthen the association between calorie intake, prolactin levels, and their influence on mammary tumorigenisis.

CALORIES MAY CONTROL CELLULAR PROLIFERATION

The concept that dietary restriction exerts its inhibitory influence on cellular proliferation is strengthened by a number of other recent studies. We studied the effects of 40% calorie restriction on the rate of cellular replication within the epithelial layer along the entire length of the gastrointestinal tract and also within thymus, liver, and spleen (41). CEIR dramatically decreased the rate of cellular proliferation within these tissues, as measured by the incorporation of [^{3}H]thymidine. In related investigations, we demonstrated that CEIR could limit proliferation of a subset of B lymphocytes, the Ly-1B lymphocytes or CD5 B lymphocytes, that has been shown to exhibit an increased capacity for oligoclonal or neoplastic expansion (42). Albanes and Winnick (43) have demonstrated a similar inhibitory effect of CEIR on the proliferative rate of cells of the colonic mucosa, and their findings have been confirmed by other investigators (44,45). Furthermore, these investigators reported that calorie restriction is even able to reduce the ultimate mass or numbers of epithelial cells in the colon. Given that hyperplastic cell growth has been observed in human subjects at familial risk for colon cancer (46), the findings discussed above underscore the fact that calorie restriction may be a most effective approach to the dietary prophylaxis of cancer, particularly in high-risk populations.

Recent reports indicate that a genetic predisposition toward such hyperplastic cell growth may be an important factor in women who have a significantly increased risk of breast cancer through family history (47) in whom proliferative breast disease appears to function as a precursor lesion for the development of breast cancer. Our own investigations (30-33) showing that dietary restriction could significantly reduce the formation of hyperplastic alveolar nodules appear to be an important corollary in the mouse of benign proliferative breast disease in the human female. These studies point to the potential of nutritional approaches to prevention of cancer.

MORE MECHANISMS, AND A UNIFYING THEORY?

In addition to the control of the rate of cellular proliferation, a number of other actions at the cellular and molecular level have been proposed as a basis for the life-extending influences of calorie restriction. In studies with genetically short-lived mice, we have found that CEIR slows down the immunological involution that accompanies aging (48), reduces the formation of circulating immune complexes and deposition of gp70-anti-gp70 immune complexes in a capillary distribution within the glomeruli (49), inhibits the age-related decrease of interleukin 2 (IL-2) responsiveness and IL-2 production (50), and selectively enhances the activity of radical scavenging enzymes, thereby limiting the deleterious effects of oxidative stress that occurs in aging (51).

In their work with animals of more long-lived strains, Walford, Weindruch, and their colleagues found that calorie restriction can increase intestinal absorption of vitamin A (52) and presumably augment its antioxidative abilities, increases catalase activity (53), enhances NK cell function (54), and slows the age-related decline in DNA repair by lymphoid cells (55). Klurfeld, Kritchevsky, and their group (56) have found that calorie restriction lowers serum insulin levels and also lowers levels of insulinlike growth factors, suggesting that calorie restriction may delay or prevent mammary cancer at least in part through this mechanism. Cerami has theorized that glucose serves as an important biological mediator of aging through its role in the glycation of nonenzymatic protein and the formation of the end products of glycosylation (57,58). Masoro et al. have found that plasma glucose can regularly be lowered as a function of calorie restriction (59), suggesting yet another important means by which dietary restriction can inhibit cancer and many of the physiological effects of aging.

Walford and Crew have put forth a theory of the action of calorie restriction that may encompass yet extend far beyond the numerous cellular and molecular mechanisms noted above (60). According to their integrative hypothesis, calorie restriction causes an organism to redirect energy from a number of biological processes and to channel that energy into essential maintenance and repair processes at the cellular and molecular level. Most notably, energy may be redirected from reproduction, as observed when calories are reduced more than 50% and the estrus cycle is interrupted, and from basal or unstimulated levels of cellular proliferation (42), as well as from other physiological processes (e.g., reduced formation of circulating immune complexes). The redirection of energy into biological repair and preventive maintenance may be reflected in the capacity of CEIR to enhance DNA-repair processes, upregulate the action of certain radical-scavenging enzymes (53), and to regulate gene expression (32). Specifically, Walford and Crew suggest that this intensification of maintenance and repair occurs through the regulation of *trans*-acting factors which bind to shared sequences on specific genes the expression of which is involved in maintenance/repair processes. Thus, calorie restriction may actually embody a form of gene therapy for the control of cancer and the extension of the spans of life and health.

CEIR: A PRESCRIPTION FOR LONGEVITY?

Based on the many beneficial influences of CEIR discussed above, a cautionary note should be sounded about much of the current received wisdom regarding prudent nutritional practice. In the United States and other Western countries, concern about the role of diet in coronary vascular disease has led to a modest reduction of dietary fat, but perhaps all too often the emphasis has been directed toward substitution of polyunsaturated or monounsaturated fats for saturated fats without a significant accompanying reduction in total fat intake. Yet, as Willett has pointed out (61), a modest reduction in dietary fat and the avoidance of obesity appears unlikely to have any significant impact on the incidence of breast cancer. It seems likely, too, that more stringent dietary changes will be needed to be of true merit in the nutritional prophylaxis of any cancer.

In light of the discussion presented here, it seems appropriate to question current guidelines encouraging the limiting of fat intake to approximately 30% of total calories (sometimes a 20% limit is exhorted). Far more spectacular progress might be made if we were to advocate a 30-40% reduction in total calories, with fat intake representing well under 20% of this amount. Such seemingly draconian changes in diet could be achieved by means of a high-nutrient, low-calorie diet as described by Walford (62). Moreover, such a diet would almost by necessity increase consumption of fruits and vegetables, which have been found to contain cancer-preventing factors (e.g., β-carotene, indoles, isoflavones, lignans, terpenes).

The obstacles to large-scale trials of such an approach to preventive nutrition may seem formidable, but the benefits could be so very great. Already genetic susceptibilities to some of our most common deadly forms of cancer, i.e., breast and colon cancer, have been described. The rapid development of molecular biological analyses promises to help us soon to be able to identify those individuals at greatest risk for malignant disease. In such populations, nutritional trials will be especially meaningful and offer much hope in the prevention of disease.

REFERENCES

1. Doll R, Peto R. The Causes of Cancer. Oxford, England, Oxford University Press, 1981.
2. McCay CM, Crowell MF, Maynard LA. The effect of retarded growth upon the length of life span and upon the ultimate body size. J Nutr 10:63-79, 1935.
3. McCay Cm, Maynard LA, Sperling G, Barnes LL. Retarded growth, life span, ultimate body size and age changes in the albino rat after feeding diets restricted in calories. J Nutr 18:1-13, 1939.
4. McCay CM, Ellis GH, Barnes LL, Smith CAH, Sperling G. Chemical and pathological changes in aging and after retarded growth. J Nutr 18:15-25, 1939.
5. Tannenbaum A. The initiation and growth of tumors. Introduction. I. Effects of underfeedings. Am J Cancer 38:335, 1940.
6. Tannenbaum A. The genesis and growth of tumors. II. Effects of calorie restriction per se. Cancer Res 2:460, 467, 1942.
7. Silverstone H, Tannenbaum A. The dependence of tumor formation on the composition of the calorie-restricted diet as well as on the degree of restriction. Cancer Res 5:616-625, 1945.
8. Visscher MB, Ball ZB, Barnes RH, Siversten I. The influence of caloric restriction upon the incidence of spontaneous mammary carcinoma in mice. Surgery 11:48, 1942.
9. Ross MH, Bras G. Lasting influence on early caloric restriction on prevalence of neoplasms in the rat. J Natl Cancer Inst 47:1095-1113, 1971.
10. Tucker MJ. The effect of long-term food restriction on tumours in rodents. Int J Cancer 23:803, 1979.
11. Fernandes G, Yunis EJ, Good RA. Influence of diet on survival of mice. Proc Natl Acad Sci USA 83:1279-1283, 1976.
12. Fernandes G, Yunis EJ, Good RA. Suppression of adenocarcinoma by the immunological consequences of calorie restriction. Nature 263:504, 1976.
13. Fernandes G, Friend P, Yunis EJ, Good RA. Influence of dietary restriction on immunologic function and renal disease in (NZBxNZW) F1 mice. Proc Natl Acad Sci USA 75:1500-1504, 1978.
14. Fernandes G, Good RA. Inhibition by restricted diet of lymphoproliferative disease and renal damage in MRL/lpr mice. Proc Natl Acad Sci USA 83:6144-6148, 1984.
15. Kubo C, Johnson BC, Day NK, Good RA. Calorie source, calorie restriction, immunity and aging of (NZB/NZW)F1 mice. J Nutr 114:1884-1899, 1984.
16. Kubo C, Johnson BC, Gajjar A, Good RA. Crucial dietary factors in maximizing life span and longevity in autoimmune-prone mice. J Nutr 117:1129-1135, 1987.
17. Weindruch R, Walford RL, Fligiel S, Guthrie D. The retardation of aging in mice by dietary restriction: Longevity, cancer, immunity and lifetime energy intake. J Nutr 116:641-654, 1986.
18. Weindruch R, Walford RL. The Retardation of Aging and Disease by Dietary Restriction. Springfield, Illinois, Charles C Thomas, 1988, pp 1-454.
19. Kritchevsky D, Weber MM, Klurfeld DM. Dietary fat versus caloric content in initiation and promotion of 7,12-dimethylbenz[a]anthracene-induced mammary tumorigenesis in rats. Cancer Res. 44:3174-3177, 1984.
20. Klurfeld DM, Weber MM, Kritchevsky D. Calories and chemical carcinogenesis. In: Dietary Fiber (GV Vahouny, D Kritchevsky, eds). New York, Plenum Press, 1985, pp 441-447.
21. Klurfeld DM, Welch CB, Davis MJ, Kritchevsky D. Determination of degree of energy restriction necessary to reduce DMBA-induced mammary tumorigenesis in rats during the promotion phase. J Nutr 119:286-291, 1989.
22. Boissoneault GA, Elson CE, Pariza MW. Net energy effects of dietary fat on chemically induced carcinogenesis in F344 rats. J Natl Cancer Inst 76:335, 1986.
23. Fernandes G, Yunis EJ, Miranda M, Smith J, Good RA. Nutritional inhibition of genetically determined renal disease and autoimmunity with prolongation of life in kd/kd mice. Proc Natl Acad Sci USA 75:2888-2892, 1978.

24. Mark DA, Alonso DR, Quimby F, Thaler T, Kim YT, Gernandes G, Good RA, Weksler ME. Effects of nutrition on disease and life span. I. Immune responses, cardiovascular pathology and life span in MRL mice. Am J Pathol 117(1):110-124, 1984.
25. Gajjar A, Kubo C, Johnson BC, Good RA. Influence of extremes of protein and energy intake on survival of B/W mice. J Nutr 117:1136-1140, 1987.
26. Kubo C, Johnson BC, Misra HP et al. Nutrition, longevity, and hepatic enzyme activities in mice. Nutr Reps Int 35:1184-1194, 1987.
27. Engelman RW, Day NK, Chen RF, Tomita Y, Bauer-Sardiña I, Dao ML, Good RA. Calorie consumption level influences development of C3H/Ou breast adenocarcinoma with indifference to calorie source. Proc Soc Exp Biol Med 193:23-30, 1990.
28. Freedman LS, Clifford C, Messina M. Analysis of dietary fat, calories, body weight, and the development of mammary tumors in rats and mice: A review. Cancer Res 50:5710-5719, 1990.
29. Welsh CW, House JL, Herr BL, Eliasberg SJ, Welsch MA. Enhancement of mammary carcinogenesis by high levels of dietary fat: a phenomenon dependent on ad libitum feeding. J Natl Cancer Inst 82:1615-1620, 1990.
30. Dong ZW, Witkin SS, Fernandes GF, Sarkar NH, Good RA, Day NK. Circulating immune complexes, antigens, and antibodies related to the murine mammary tumor virus in C3H mice. J Immunol 129:872-877, 1982.
31. Sarkar NH, Fernandes G, Teland NT, Kourides IA, Good RA. Low-calorie diet prevents the development of mammary tumors in C3H mice and reduces circulating prolactin level, murine mammary tumor virus expression, and proliferation of mammary alveolar cells. Proc Natl Acad Sci USA 79:7758-7762, 1982.
32. Chen RF, Good RA, Engelman RW, Hamada N, Tanaka A, Nonoyama M, Day NK. Suppression of mouse mammary tumor proviral DNA and proto-oncogene expression: Association with nutritional regulation of mammary tumor development. Proc Natl Acad Sci USA 87:2385-2389, 1990.
33. Hamada N, Engelman RW, Tomita Y, Chen RF, Iwai H, Good RA, Day, NK. Prolactin effects on the dietary regulation of mouse mammary tumor virus proviral DNA expression. Proc Natl Acad Sci USA 87:6733-6737, 1990.
34. Koizumi A, Wada Y, Tsukada M, Kamiyama S, Weindruch R. Effects of energy restriction on mouse mammary tumor virus mRNA levels in mammary glands and uterus and on uterine endometrial hyperplasia and pituitary histology in C3H/SHN F1 mice. J Nutr 120:1401-1411, 1990.
35. Russell D, Snyder SH. Amine synthesis in rapidly growing tissues: Ornithine decarboxylase activity in regenerating rat liver, chick embryo and various tumors. Proc Natl Acad Sci USA 60:1420, 1968.
36. Russell DH, Mills KT, Talamantes FJ, Bern HA. Neonatal administration of prolactin antiserum alters the developmental pattern of T- and B-lymphocytes in the thymus and spleen of BALB/c female mice. Proc Natl Acad Sci USA 85:7406-7407, 1988.
36a. Buckley AR, Putnam CW, Russell DH. Prolactin as a mammalian mitogen and tumor promoter. Adv Enzyme Reg 27:371-391, 1988.
37. Buckley AR, Putnam CW, Evans R et al. Hepatic protein kinase C: Translocation stimulated by prolactin and partial hepatectomy. Life Sci 41:2827-2834, 1987.
37a. Weinstein IB. The Origins of human cancer: molecular mechanisms of carcinogenesis and their implications for cancer prevention and treatment. Cancer Res 48:4135-4143, 1988.
38. Boutwell RK. Evidence that an elevated level of ornithine decarboxylase activity is an essential component of tumor promotion. Adv Polyam Res 4:127-134, 1983.
39. Kumar SP, Roy SJ, Tokumo K, Reddy BS. Effect of different levels of calorie restriction on azoxymethane-induced colon carcinogenesis in male F344 rats. Cancer Res 50:5761-5766, 1990.
40. Ingram DM, Nottage EM, Roberts AN. Prolactin and breast cancer risk. Medical Journal of Australia 153(8):469-73, 1990.

41. Ogura M, Ogura H, Ikehara S, Dao ML, Good RA. Decrease by chronic energy intake restriction of cellular proliferation in the intestinal epithelium and lymphoid organs in autoimmunity-prone mice. Proc Natl Acad Sci USA 86:5918-5922, 1989.
42. Ogura M, Ogura H, Ikehara S, Good RA. Influence of dietary energy restriction on the numbers and proportions of Ly-1$^+$ B lymphocytes in autoimmune-prone mice. Proc Natl Acad Sci USA 86:4225-4229, 1989.
43. Albanes D, Winick M. Are cell number and cell proliferation risk factors for cancer? J Natl Cancer Inst 80:772-775, 1988.
44. Lok E, Scott FW, Mongeau R, Nera EA, Malcolm S, Clayson DB. Calorie restriction and cellular proliferation in various tissues of the female Swiss Webster mouse. Cancer Lett 51:67-73, 1990.
45. Bruce WR. Short-term tests and long-term prospects for colon cancer prevention. Med Oncol Tumor Pharmacother 7:131-136, 1990.
46. Lipkin M, Blattner WA, Gardner EJ, Burt RW, Lynch H, Deschner E, Winawar S, Fraumeni JF Jr. Classification and risk assessment of individuals with familial polyposis, Gardner syndrome and familial non-polyposis colon cancer from [3H−)dThd-labeling patterns in colonic epithelial cells. Cancer Res 44:4201-4207, 1984.
47. Skolnick MH, Cannon-Albright LA, Goldgar DE, Ward JH et al. Inheritance of proliferative breast disease in breast cancer in kindreds. Science 250:1715-1719, 1990.
48. Ogura M, Ogura H, Lorenz E, Ikehara S, Good RA. Undernutrition without malnutrition restricts the numbers and proportions of Ly-1$^+$ B lymphocytes in autoimmune (MRL/1 and BXSB) mice. Proc Soc Exp Biol Med 193:6-12, 1990.
49. Izui S, Fernandes G, Hara I, McConahey PJ, Jensen FC, Dixon FJ, Good RA. Low-calorie diet selectively reduces expression of retroviral envelope glycoprotein gp70 in sera of (NZB xNZW) F1 hybrid mice. J Exp Med 154:1116-1124, 1981.
50. Jung LKL, Palladino MA, Calvano S, Mark DA, Good RA, Fernandes G. Effect of calorie restriction on the production and responsiveness to interleukin 2 in (NZB X NZW) F1 mice. Clin Immunol Immunopathol 25:295-301, 1982.
51. Franklin RA, Yong ML, Arkins S, Kelley KW. Glutathione augments in vitro proliferative responses of lymphocytes to concanavalin A to a greater degree in old than young rats. J Nutr 120:1710, 1990.
52. Hollander D, Dadufalza V, Weindruch R, Walford RL. Influence of life-prolonging dietary restriction on intestinal vitamin A absorption in mice. Exp Gerontol 9:57-60, 1986.
53. Koizumi A, Weindruch R, Walford RL. Influences of dietary restriction and age on liver enzyme activities and lipid peroxidation in mice. J Nutr 117:361-367, 1987.
54. Weindruch R, Devens BH, Raff HV, Walford RL. Influence of dietary restriction and aging on natural killer cell activity in mice. J Immunol 130:993-996, 1983.
55. Licastro F, Walford RL. Aging, proliferative potential and DNA repair capacity in short-lived and long-lived mice. Mech Ageing Dev 31:171-186, 1985.
56. Ruggieri BA, Klurfeld DM, Kritchevsky D, Furlanetto RW. Caloric restriction and 7,12-dimethylbenz[a]anthracene-induced mammary tumor growth in rats: Alterations in circulating insulin, insulin-like growth factors I and II, and epidermal growth factor. Cancer Res 49:4130-4134, 1989.
57. Cerami A, Vlassara H, Brownlee M. Glucose and aging. Sci Am 256:90-96, 1987.
58. Brownlee M, Vlassara H, Kooney A, Urich P, Cerami A. Aminoguanidine prevents diabetes-induced arterial wall protein cross-linking. Science 232(4758) 1629:32, 1986.
59. Masoro EJ. Physiological consequences of dietary restriction: An overview. In: Biological effects of dietary restriction (L. Fishbein, ed). Springer-Verlag, New York, 1991, pp 115-122.
59a. Masoro EJ. Assessment of nutritional components in prolongation of life and health by diet. Proc Soc Exp Biol Med 193(1):31-4, 1990.
60. Walford RL, Crew M. How dietary restriction retards aging: An integrative hypothesis (editorial). Growth Dev Aging 53:139-140, 1989.
61. Willett W. The search for the causes of breast and colon cancer. Nature 338:389-394, 1989.
62. Walford RL. Maximum Life Span. New York, WW Norton, 1983, pp 1-256.

32
Circulation and Distribution of Iron: A Key to Immune Interaction

Maria de Sousa
Abel Salazar Institute for the Biomedical Sciences, Oporto, Portugal

It is thus demonstrated that a perpetual motion of the blood in a circle is brought about by the beat of the heart. What shall we say? Is this for the purpose of nutrition?

William Harvey

IRON AND ITS CIRCULATING PROTEINS

According to Robb-Smith, it was Menghini in 1747 who first showed that iron was present in the blood, "separating it from the ash with the aid of a magnet" (1).

Because an iron atom can exist in two states of valency, ferrous and ferric, iron became the primordial partner of oxygen in evolution. Like many other long-standing partnerships, this one, to survive, had to surround itself with protective devices that would not allow the toxicity of either partner in the presence of the other to be expressed. These devices have a most refined development in hemoglobin and the red cell and in useful and practical forms in ferritin and transferrin.

It is the acknowledged job of the iron-storing and -binding proteins, ferritin and transferrin, and of hemoglobin within the red cell, to protect the body from the toxicity of iron in the presence of oxygen, to ensure that oxygen is transported and delivered, and to make iron continuously available, not only for the biosynthesis of hemoglobin and erythropoiesis, but for all the other enzymatic pathways requiring it (2).

The amount of iron excreted per day is negligible: 0.5-1.0 mg. Even in a normal woman with a hemoglobin of 14 g/100 ml of blood, with an estimated periodic menstrual loss of 20-23 mg of iron, the daily additional loss is another 0.5-1.4 mg, not exceeding 1.5 mg/day (3). During pregnancy, the requirements of the growing fetus impose an estimated loss of 2.4 mg of iron per day over the three trimesters. These small amounts contrast with the total amount of iron recycled every day: 30–35 mg, of which only 1 mg comes from absorption (3).

Normally the amount of iron in the body is kept constant at the absorption level which takes place largely through the upper sections of the small intestine (Table 1). The total body iron in a 70-kg man has been estimated to be 4.2 g, distributed as follows: hemoglobin (74.3%), ferritin (16.4%), myoglobin (3.3%), haptoglobin-hemoglobin (0.2%), catalase (0.11%), cytochrome c (0.08%), transferrin (0.07%).

After absorption, iron travels on the serum protein transferrin, which carries it to the bone marrow; in the bone marrow, iron is incorporated in the biosynthetic pathway of hemoglobin. Transferrin, however, has been identified also as a major nutritional requirement for lymphocyte proliferation in vitro, in response to stimulation by antigens and mitogens (4-6), and for the proliferation in vitro of malignant T cells (7-9). Hemoglobin is the almost exclusive constituent of the red cell (95% of its dry weight). Mammalian hemoglobin free in the plasma would have been expected to have a half-life of about 40 min and would easily be lost through the kidneys and the reticuloendothelial system (10). Through having evolved to travel in a cell that acts simultaneously as a protective environment and a carriage, the life expectancy of hemoglobin increased to the greater life expectancy of the red blood cell itself; in humans this is about 120 days. Human senescent red cells, representing about 0.7% of all erythrocytes, are selectively removed by macrophages; macrophages ensure iron's recycling and reentry into the circulating pool of transferrin. In the adult, 2-3 million red blood cells are produced and broken down per second.

IRON AND THE MODELING OF THE IMMUNE SYSTEM

The possibility that iron can contribute to the modulation of the immune response is amply illustrated in Chapter 7 and elsewhere (11). In light of the complexity of its interaction with the immune system, however, iron may also be considered as having a direct modeling effect on the immune system itself, analogous to the effect of an external antigen (12). Iron, as a product of red cell breakdown and recycling can thus be regarded as a target of immune surveillance (12-15). In human states of iron overload, immune cell functions are altered (16), reflecting this process.

Table 1 Zonal Grading of Iron Absorption and Number of IgA/Positive Cells in the Small Intestine

Zone	Fe absorption[a]	IgA-positive cells
Duodenum	69.8 + 6.05	1,953 (1,588-2,429)
Mid jejunum	28.6 + 4.08	1,235 (1,005-1,652)
Jejunum-ileum	9.2 + 3.08	—
Ileum	2.1 + 0.64	963 (712-1,404)

[a]Expressed as % of dose of 59 Fe injected directly into the bowel.
Source: Slightly modified from de Sousa (20), based on data from Duthie (21) and Husband and Gowans (22) in rats.

IRON AND LYMPHOCYTE MIGRATION

One red blood cell contains 400 million molecules of hemoglobin; that signifies that 2-3 million times that number of molecules of hemoglobin are recycled through the immune system per second. The macrophages of the red pulp of the spleen are central to the removal of effete red cells (17,18). This continuous process is thus the most significant and the most substantial illustration of an interaction between iron and the immune system. The two systems, however, "coexist" at two other major anatomical sites: Iron absorption takes place at an area of the small intestine richest in lymphoid tissue, the duodenum (see Table 1). Iron delivery for erythropoiesis occurs at the major site for cell differentiation within the lymphomyeloid system; i.e. the bone marrow (13).

Iron Absorption and the Distribution of Immunoglobulin A-Positive Cells

Comparing data on the amount of iron absorbed in the duodenum, the mid jejunum, and the jejunum-ileum (19) and data from separate experiments on numbers of IgA-positive cells seen in the same areas of the small intestine (20), it becomes apparent that there is a similar zonal grading of the two (see Table 1); the highest amount of iron is absorbed in the duodenum, the highest average numbers of IgA-positive cells are seen in the same region, followed by the mid jejunum and the ileum. This anatomical coexistence may provide a basis for the results of a study of the effect of iron-fortified formula on secretory IgA of the gastrointestinal tract in early infancy (21). In a study comparing the amount of fecal IgA measured at birth, 2, 4, and 8 weeks in two groups of infants, one receiving a standard formula (Enfamil) and another receiving Enfamil with iron, the authors found significantly higher amounts of IgA at 2, 4, and 8 weeks in the group that had received the iron-fortified formula (Table 2); a higher percentage of the infants receiving the iron-fortified formula had demonstrably higher amounts (>1 mg/dl) of fecal IgA from 2 weeks of age onwards (Fig. 1). This result could indicate that the oral administration of iron has stimulated the development of the intestinal microbial flora.*

Table 2 Effect of the Administration of an Iron-Fortified Formula on Amount of Fecal Secretory IgA in Early Human Life

GROUP	n	1	2	3	4
+ Fe	15	0	3.8[a] (0-20)	7.37 (0-30)	23 (6-68)
− Fe	15	0	0	1.62 (0-8.3)	4.4 (0.5-14)

Stages
1: At birth. 2: 2 wks. 3: 4 wks. 4: 8 wks.
[a]mg/dl.
Source: Data Ref. 25.

---

*Clearly, this does not imply that iron requirements for the infant are in question. Indeed recent data show that iron fortification is needed for development (47).

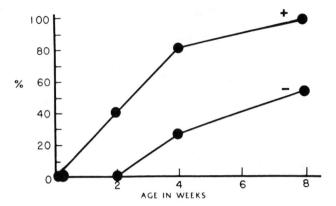

Figure 1 Percentage of infants (%) with fecal sIgA levels higher than 1 mg/dl. +: group (n = 15) that received iron-fortified formula (Enfamil). —: group (n = 15) that received Enfamil only. Age groups correspond to stages 1, 2, 3, and 4 in Table 2. (Modified from Ref. 21.)

Lymphocyte Migration and Iron Distribution in Fetal Organs

Studies of lymphocyte migration in the fetus are comprehensibly, few. Cahill and his coworkers have undertaken studies of the fetal lymphocyte circulation in sheep (22,23). Lymphocytes obtained from the intestinal or prescapular lymph in the fetus or in the adult animal were radioisotopically labeled and traced in their respective age-matched recipients.

A comparison of the percentage of radioactivity recovered in the spleen and the liver in the two groups (Table 3) shows that in the fetus, lymphocytes migrate predominantly to the liver (32.6%) in contrast with the adult where recovery in the liver is 4.4%. The reverse situation is observed in the spleen: In the adult, a higher number of lymphocytes is recovered in the spleen (20%) than in the liver (4.4%). Studies of the human fetus have demonstrated that the amount of iron in the fetal liver is always significantly higher than that found in the spleen (24). Differences were also noted in the proportions of lymphocytes recovered in the small intestine in the fetus and in the adult. These differences occurred exclusively with the lymphocytes obtained

Table 3 Lymphocyte Migration to Liver, Spleen, and Small Intestine in Adult Sheep and the Fetal Lamb

Source of lymphocytes infused	Liver	Spleen	Small intestine
Foetus			
intestinal lymph	32.6[a]	12.2	3.0
prescapular lymph	23.7	11.7	2.5
Adult			
intestinal lymph	4.4	20	12.9
prescapular lymph	2.8	25.7	1.4

[a]Expressed as mean % radioactivity: three animals used in each group.
Source: Data from Ref. 26.

Circulation and Distribution of Iron

from the intestinal lymph. A higher percentage of labeled intestinal lymphocytes were found in the adult small intestine (see Table 3) than in the fetus. No differences were seen with the lymphocytes obtained from the prescapular lymph. The differences observed between the fate of the lymphocytes derived from the two different sources are a reflection of the possible separate effect exerted by microbial antigens on lymphocyte migration.

The definitive clarification of the possible part played by iron absorption on the modulation of the migration of intestinal lymph lymphocytes to the intestine can only be established in experiments done in pathogen-free conditions.

Lactation

Lactation is another physiological process where T lymphocytes, IgA-producing cells, and iron interact.

The most striking changes take place within the first days of lactation and consist of marked declines in numbers of T lymphocytes, lactoferrin concentration, and IgA concentration (25-27).

Available data on the changes of iron content of human and rat breast milk during the first week of lactation (26,28) indicate that the changes in iron concentration parallel the changes in numbers of lymphocytes (Fig. 2). Data pooled from studies of Zn concentration during lactation indicate that Zn too declines (29). No changes seem to occur in the copper levels during lactation.

Iron and the Synovium

There is a considerable body of evidence dating from 1939 indicating that exposure to the systemic administration of iron, either in drinking water (30) or intravenously, causes alterations in the synovium, and exacerbation of arthritis in RA patients (31). We have approached this question more directly by examining the changes in the numbers of T lymphoid cells appearing in the synovium after injecting ferric citrate in-

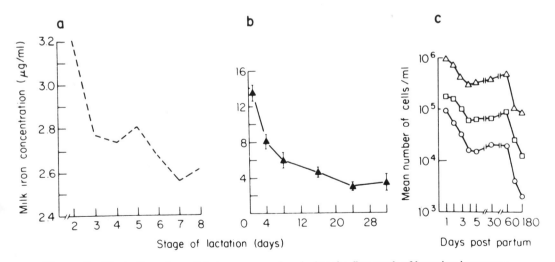

Figure 2 Illustration of parallel changes occuring during the first week of lactation in women (a,c) and female rats (b) in iron concentration of milk (a,b), mononuclear cells (△), total (□), and T lymphocytes (○). (From Ref. 18. Data from Refs 24, 25, 26; used with permission.)

Table 4 Changes in Numbers of Rat T Lymphocytes Identified in the Synovium After IV Injection of Ferric Citrate

Time after injection (hr)	No. of W3/13$^+$ cells[a]
0	10.4
8	13.6
24	34.2

[a]Number of peroxidase positive cells per 10 microscopic fields detected with a pan-T monoclonal antibody.
Source: Data from Ref. 32.

travenously in rats in a quantity sufficient to cause a transient oversaturation of transferrin (32). After a single intravenous injection of ferric citrate, a series of transient changes occurred in the synovial capillaries and synovial cells, including the appearance of increasing numbers of T lymphocytes at 8 and 24 hr after the injection, which were detected by immunocytochemistry (Table 4). These experiments represent the closest direct indication of iron acting as a "motivating" signal for lymphocyte migration (32). Subsequent studies in which iron was given to animals undergoing an inflammatory joint process (collagen arthritis) confirmed and extended the original findings, indicating that the lymphocyte subsets represented at the inflammatory site varied with the timing of the injection of iron (33) and could be correlated with exacerbation or suppression of the inflammatory process (34).

CONCLUSIONS

The data briefly reviewed above indirectly or directly point in a direction suggesting that physiological changes in iron concentration in tissues and breast milk go hand-in-hand with similar changes in numbers of lymphocytes found at those sites. This coincidence could signify that lymphocytes go to those sites for the purpose of their own nutrition. This is a plausible interpretation, particularly for activated normal lymphocytes and transformed lymphocytes, which are known to express receptors for transferrin-iron (6,17,35). Moreover, transferrin and iron have been identified as indispensable nutritional requirements for lymphocyte growth in vitro (4-9). For those envisaging the circulation of lymphocytes with a surveillance function developing in response to the potential toxicity of iron, lymphocyte numbers could parallel the concentration of iron to balance iron concentration at the local site. Further, iron may directly affect lymphocyte surface antigen expression (36). In association with this possibility, it may be noted that cells of the lymphomyeloid system contribute to the production of the proteins capable of binding iron. A subset of activated T lymphocytes, the CD4$^+$ cells, have been shown to synthesize transferrin (37). Earlier work, using immunofluorescence to detect the association of iron binding proteins with cells of the immune system, demonstrated that a higher percentage of T than B cells contained intracytoplasmic transferrin and that after overnight culture, transferrin was seen outside the cells (38).

Much earlier, in 1966, Phillips and Thorbecke (39), studying the origin of the serum proteins in rat to mouse radiation chimeras, had demonstrated that the serum transferrin in the chimeras derived from the repopulating donor rat bone marrow cells. In the same study, it was shown that the recipient tissues that produced the highest amounts of transferrin in culture were the spleen, the peritoneal macrophages, and the thymus (39). Our own work on the synthesis of ferritin by lymphocytes demonstrated that normal T lymphocytes synthesized a ferritin richer in H than L subunits (40), and that in response to increasing concentrations of iron in culture, macrophages increased the synthesis of H and L subunits, whereas T lymphocytes did not (13,41). Pattanapanyasat et al. (42) have confirmed in a lymphocyte activation model that mitogen-activated T lymphocytes increase the synthesis of H-rich ferritin by five- to sevenfold in contrast with a threefold increase in L-rich ferritin. Regarding secretion of these proteins, by applying an indirect hemolytic plaque assay to the study of ferritin secretion, we have shown that macrophages secrete ferritin, and that after mitogen activation in the presence of ferric citrate, plaque formation appeared to be regulated by HLA phenotype (43). From "short-term" in vitro studies, it has been suggested that the T cell-derived transferrin could be an important nutritional element for supporting the growth of other activated T cells expressing Tf receptors (37). Activated B cells, however, are also known to express Tf receptors (44). A nutritional role for T cell-derived transferrin is attractive and could be envisaged as a bridge of importance in Tv-B cell interactions.

In conclusion, iron can be considered unique among "antigens" being presented to the immune system, as part of heme within hemoglobin, at the rate of 2-3 million times 400 million molecules per second. It is hard to imagine this number of molecules of hemoglobin containing 4 times that number of atoms of iron, with no place to go. The reality nearest to such a picture is perhaps seen in the β-thalassemias, where the requirement of lifetime blood transfusions leads to the development of an iron load, well beyond the capacity of the macrophage system. Such iron overload is incompatible with life; only after the development of effective iron chelation in recent years has the life expectancy of these patients been increased to the third decade (45).

The best illustration of the incompatibility of iron overload with life is, however, apparent in neonatal hemochromatosis (46), a rare disease of unknown pathogenesis. In 25 cases reviewed by Kinsley et al., survival ranged from minutes after birth to 9 days, with a mean of 2.7 days (46).

Thus, we see in iron a prototype nutritional element of major importance for the structural configuration of the immune system, formative in its development and differentiation, and unique in its modulation of immune function (48).

ACKNOWLEDGMENTS

Throughout the years work by the author on iron and the immune system was done with the support of the following institutions: Cardinal Fund (Sloan-Kettering Cancer Research Institute), the Cancer Research Institute (New York), and the American-Portuguese Biomedical Research in the United States. Work on iron and the rat synovitis is funded by grant #709.85.25 from the Portuguese Funding Agency for Science & Technology (JNICT).

I wish to thank my colleague, Coralia Vicente, for her generous help in the final "word processing" of the manuscript and Barbara Brown for its final typing.

REFERENCES

1. Robb-Smith AHT. The growth of knowledge of the functions of the blood. In: The Functions of the Blood. Macfarlane, AHT Robb-Smith, eds. Blackwell, 1961.

2. Beinert H. Development of the field and nomenclature. In: Iron Sulfur Proteins. W Lovenberg, ed. Academic Press, New York, 1973, pp 1-36.
3. Harris JW, Kellermeyer RW. The Red Cell. Harvard University Press, Cambridge, Massachusetts, 1974.
4. Tormey DC, Imrie RC, Mueller GC. Identification of transferrin as a lymphocyte growth promoter in human serum. Exp Cell Res 74:163, 1972.
5. Dillner-Centerlind ML, Hammarstrom S, Perlman P. Transferrin can replace serum for in vitro growth of mitogen stimulated T lymphocytes. Eur J Immunol 9:942, 1979.
6. Trowbridge IS, Newman RA. Monoclonal antibodies to transferrin receptors. In: Monoclonal Antibodies to Receptors: Probes for Receptor Structure and Function. MF Greaves, ed. Chapman and Hall, London, 1984, pp 237-261.
7. Taetle R, Rhyner K, Castagnola J, To D, Mendelsohn J. Role of transferrin, Fe and transferrin receptors in myeloid leukemia cell growth studies with an anti-transferrin receptor monoclonal antibody. J Clin Invest 75:1061, 1985.
8. Kitada S, Hays EF. Transferrin-like activity produced by murine malignant T-lymphoma cell lines. Cancer Res 45:3537, 1985.
9. Basset P, Zwiller J, Revel MD, Vincendon G. Growth promotion by transformed cells by iron in serum-free culture. Carcinogenesis 6:355, 1985.
10. Crosby WH. The metabolism of hemoglobin and bile pigment in hemolytic disease. Am J Med 18:112, 1955.
11. Bryan CF, Stone MJ. The immunoregulatory properties of iron. In: Nutritional Modulation of the Immune Response. S. Cunningham-Rundles, ed. Marcel Dekker, New York, 1992.
12. de Sousa M. Lymphoid cell positioning: A new proposal for the mechanism of control of lymphoid cell positioning. Symp Soc Exp Biol 32:393, 1978.
13. de Sousa M, Martins Da Silva B, Dorner M, Munn CG, Nishiya K, Grady RW, Silverstone A. Iron and the lymphomyeloid system: Rationale for considering iron as a target of immune surveillance. In: The Biochemistry and Physiology of Iron. P Saltman, J Hegenauer, eds. Elsevier North Holland, Amsterdam, 1982, p 687.
14. de Sousa M. Iron and the lymphomyeloid system: Old frontier new perspective. Microbiology, pp 322-326, 1983.
15. de Sousa M. Lymphocyte Circulation: Experimental and Clinical Aspects. Wiley & Chichester, England, 1981.
16. de Sousa M. Immune cell functions in iron overload. Clin Exp Immunol 75:1, 1989.
17. Rifkind R. Destruction of injured red cells in vivo. Am J Med 41:711, 1976.
18. de Sousa M. Cell Traffic. In "Receptors and Recognition". Series A vol. 2. ed. P. Cuatrecases and M. F. Greaves, Chapman and Hall, London. p 105, 1976.
19. Duthie HL. The relative importance of the duodenum in the intestinal absorption of iron. Brit J Haematol 10:59, 1964.
20. Husband AJ and Gowans JL. The origin and antigen-dependent distribution of IgA containing cells in the intestine. J Exp Med 148:1146, 1978.
21. Koutras AK, Vigorita VJ and Quiroz E. Effect of iron fortified formula on SIgA of gastrointestinal tract in early infancy. J Pediatr Gastroenterol & Nutr 5:926, 1986.
22. Cahill RNP, Poskitt DC, Hay JB, Heron I and Trnka Z. The migration of lymphocytes in the fetal lamb. Eur J Immunol 9:251, 1979.
23. Cahill RNP and Trnka Z. Growth and development of recirculating lymphocytes in the sheep fetus. Monographs in Allergy. 16:38, 1980.
24. Singla PN, Gupta VP and Agarwal KN. Storage iron in human foetal organs. Acta Pediatr Scan 74:701, 1985.
25. Fabiano A. Valori siderimetrici del latte materno e tratamento marziale. Ann Obstr Ginecologia 78:1043, 1956.
26. Ezekiel E and Morgan EH. Milk iron and its metabolism in the lactating rat. J Physiol 165:336, 1963.

27. Ogra SS, Ogra PL. Immunologic aspects of human colostrum and milk. J Pediatr 92:550, 1978.
28. McClelland DB, McGrath J and Samson RR. Antimicrobial factors in human milk. Acta Scand Suppl 271, 1978.
29. Picciano MF, Guthrie HA. Copper, iron and zinc content of mature human milk. Am J Clin Nutr 29:242, 1976.
30. Hiyeda K. The cause of Kaschin-Beck's disease. Jpn J Med Sci 4:91, 1939.
31. Blake D, Lunec J, Ahern M, Ring EFJ, Bradfield J, Gutteridge JMC. Effect of intravenous iron dextran on rheumatoid synovitis. Ann Rheum Dis 44:183, 1985.
32. de Sousa M, Breedveld F, Dynesius-Trentham R, Mota-Garcia F, Teixeira Da Silva M, Trentham ED. Activation of the rat synovium by iron. Arthritis Rheum 31:653, 1988.
33. de Sousa M, Breedveld F, Dynesius-Trentham R, Trentham DE, Lum J. Iron, the iron binding proteins and immune system. Cells Ann New York Acad Sci 526:310, 1988.
34. Breedveld FC, Dynesus-Trentham R, DeSousa M. Collagen arthritis in the rat is initiated by CD_4 + T cells and can be amplified by iron. Cell Immunol 121:1, 1989.
35. Neckers LM, Crossman J. Tf Receptor induction in mitogen stimulated human T lymphocytes is required for DNA synthesis and cell division is regulated by IL-2. Proc Natl Acad Sci USA 80:3493, 1983.
36. Bravo I, Carvalho GS, Barbosa MA, de Sousa M. Differential effects of eight metal ions on lymphocyte differentiation antigens in vitro. J Bio Med Mater Res 24:1059, 1990.
37. Lum J, Infante AJ, Makker DM, Yang F, Bowman BH. Transferrin synthesis by inducer T lymphocytes. J Clin Invest 77:841, 1986.
38. Nishiya K, Chiao JW, de Sousa M. Iron binding proteins in selected human peripheral blood cell sets: Immunofluorescence. Br J Haematol 46:235, 1980.
39. Phillips ME, Thorbecke GJ. Studies on serum proteins of chimeras. Int Arch Allergy 29: 553, 1966.
40. Dorner M, Silverstone A, Nishiya K, de Sostoa A, Munn CG, de Sousa M. Ferritin synthesis by human T lymphocytes. Science 209:1019, 1980.
41. Dorner MH, Silverstone AE, Sostoa A, Munn CG, de Sousa M. Relative subunit composition of the ferritin synthesized by selected human lymphomyeloid cell populations. Exp Hematol 11:866-872, 1983.
42. Pattanapanyasat K, Hoy TG, Jacobs A. The response of intra cellular and surface ferritin after T-cell stimulation in vitro. Clin Sci 73:605-611, 1987.
43. Pollack MS, Martins Da Silva B, Moschief RD, Groshen S, Bognacki J, Dupont B, de Sousa M. Ferritin secretion by human mononuclear cells: association with HLA phenotype. Clin Immunol Immunopathol 27:124-134, 1983.
44. Brieva JA, Stevens RH. Involvement of the transferrin receptor in the production of NK induced suppression of human antibody synthesis. J Immunol 133:1288, 1984.
45. Orkin SH. Disorders of hemoglobin Synthesis: The thalassemias. In: The Molecular Basis of Blood Diseases. Stammatoyannopoulos G, Nienhuis AM, Leder P, Majerus PW. Saunders, Philadelphia, p 122, 1987.
46. Knisley AS, Magid MS, Dische NR, Cutz E. Neonatal Hemochromatosis Birth Defects: original article series 23:75-102, 1988.
47. Lozoff B, Jimerez E, Wolf AW. Long-term developmental outcome of infants with iron deficiency. N Engl J Med 325:687, 1991.
48. de Sousa M, Reimao R, Ponto G, Grady RW, Hilgartner MW, Giardina P. Iron and lymphocytes: reciprocal regulatory interactions. Coll. Stud. Hematol. Blood Transf. 58:171-177, 1991.

33
Rationale for the Mechanism of Zinc Interaction in the Immune System

Mireille Dardenne and Jean-François Bach
Hôpital Necker, Paris, France

INTRODUCTION

Zinc is a ubiquitous trace metal essential to the development and maintenance of the immune system and influencing both lymphocyte and phagocyte cell functions.

Aspects of the interaction of zinc with the immune system have been described in Chapter 33. Indeed, zinc appears to have a particularly selective association in immune cell interactions. Although other divalent cations have been shown to cause at least a low level of lymphocyte mitogenesis, the effects have been more limited in scope. In this book, Cook-Mills and Fraker (Chap. 8) have shown that zinc deficiency was associated with reduced mononuclear phagocyte response to *Trypanosoma cruzi*, which led to 85% mortality in the infected group, and Vruwink et al. (Chap. 17) have demonstrated that the effect of perinatal zinc deficiency is transmitted into successive generations as reduced immunoglobulins and plaque-forming cell response. The work of Castro and Sevall (Chap. 9) indicates a possible principal impact of zinc deficiency at the gene level. Prasad was the first to show that zinc deficiency occurs in humans with major consequences for the immune system, and in this book (Chap. 24), he has contributed interesting studies on the effect of zinc deficiency on immune function in sickle cell anemia. Cunningham-Rundles et al. have shown that therapeutically induced zinc deficiency as a side effect of iron chelation may cause marked changes in immune response (Chap. 25). In this chapter, we will explore the possible basis of the critical nature of the interaction of zinc with the immune system.

The influence of nutritional factors on the immune system is now generally accepted. Many authors have reported an abnormal prevalence of infection and consistence atrophy of lymphoid organs in zinc-deprived children. Converging evidence suggests a role of zinc deficiency in this type of immune deficit (1,2). Zinc appears to influence both lymphocyte and phagocyte cell function (3). Its abnormal absorption or excretion has been incriminated in diseases such as acrodermatitis enteropathica and drepanocytosis as well as in many situations in which decreased zinc plasma levels are associated with T-cell deficit.

CONSEQUENCES OF EXPERIMENTAL ZINC DEFICIENCY

Zinc deficiency severely depresses immune responses. Experimental zinc deprivation (with all other nutritional elements at normal levels) leads to thymic involution, particularly of the cortex, whereas other lymphoid elements, the spleen, and the lymph nodes are less involved. It has been shown that this atrophy is not due to stress, since similar effects have been observed in adrenalectomized animals (4).

T-Mitogen responses (phytohemagglutinin and concanavalin A) are very significantly decreased (5), as is the production of lymphokines (6) and that of antibodies directed against T-dependent antigens (sheep red blood cells and hemocyanin). We have recently reported that infection-related thymic involution is not glucocorticoid dependent (7).

With regard to antibody production, both primary responses (immunoglobulin M, IgM) and secondary responses (immunoglobulin G, IgG) are involved. Zinc deficiency also inhibits autoantibody production in autoimmune mice such as the NZB strain (8); this production can be restored by injection of thymocytes from nondeficient animals.

Cytotoxic T-cell production is also decreased after in vivo administration of allogenic cells (4); however, it paradoxically remains normal in vitro when the allogenic stimulus is present during mixed lymphocyte reaction, no doubt because of the presence of zinc traces in the culture medium.

Other parameters of the immune response are less modified. This is the case for the serum immunoglobulin level, which is only slightly decreased. On the contrary, the rosette formation inhibition test shows that the serum level of thymulin, a thymic hormone, is considerably altered (9-11), and that the number of autologous rosettes is increased, as is observed after thymectomy.

These abnormalities increase in severity as zinc deprivation occurs earlier in life, indicating that postnatal lymphocyte development is zinc dependent. In the case of early deficit, abnormal immunoglobulin levels are observed; i.e., low IgM, IgG2a and IgA, and high IgG_1 and IgG2b.

Although the main consequences of zinc deficiency are focused on functional development of T lymphocytes, it also affects other cell lines (12). Responses to lipopolysaccharide (LPS), a polyclonal B-cell activator, are little affected, as are responses to T-independent antigens. K Cell activity is increased, whereas that of natural killer (NK) cells has been reported by various authors to be either increased or decreased (4). In addition, phagocyte cell function is altered and monocytosis is often observed (12).

It thus appears clear that zinc deficiency has multiple consequences on the immune system, and that they are similar to those observed after thymectomy, either neonatal thymectomy in extreme cases of deficiency where zinc deprivation is total and occurs very early, or thymectomy in the young adult when deficiency is induced during adulthood. It is known that thymectomy in the very young adult (2-3 weeks in the mouse) induces numerous anomalies in T-cell function, as does zinc deficiency, whereas when it is performed later (around 2 months of age), its consequences are much more limited.

It should also be mentioned that chelating agents such as EDTA or diethylthiodicarbamate inhibit various lymphocyte functions in vivo. These anomalies are totally and immediately corrected in vitro by the addition of zinc. This observation indicates that zinc can have immediate effects on lymphocytes (probably by modifying their metabolism), which differ from the alterations observed after prolonged zinc deficiency in that the latter are more severe and require repeated zinc administration.

RELATIONSHIP BETWEEN ZINC AND THYMIC HORMONES

Various mechanisms can explain the early thymic atrophy observed in zinc-deprived mice. Rapidly replicating lymphocytes in the thymus could be particularly sensitive to the functional anomaly of zinc-rich metalloenzymes required for lymphocyte proliferation. Another hypothesis could be that the epithelial function of the thymus could be specifically altered. A third involves direct action of thymulin, a thymic hormone molecule. Several authors have reported (6,9,11) that the serum level of the thymic hormone thymulin was abnormally decreased in zinc deficiency, both in the mouse (9,11) and in humans.

Interactions Between Zinc and Thymulin: Biochemical Aspects

It has now been directly demonstrated that the thymulin molecule contains zinc and that this metal is indispensable for the biological activity of the hormone (13). Synthetic or natural thymulin loses its biological activity when it is treated by a chelating agent (Chelex-100), and this activity is restored by the addition of zinc, or to a lesser degree, by the addition of other metals (Cu^{2+}, Al^{2+}). Experiments using labeled molecules showed that thymulin activation is secondary to zinc fixation to the peptide. This fixation is stoichiometric. The peptides thus exists in two conformations, one without zinc, which is biologically inactive, and the other bound to zinc (1:1), which is biologically active in vitro and in vivo. The effect of zinc on the conformation of thymulin was recently confirmed by nuclear magnetic resonance, which also showed that zinc binds to the peptide by C-terminal asparagine group and the two hydroxyl and serine 4 and 8 groups (14). In addition, it was shown that zinc has an affinity of approximately 10^{-7} M for the peptide, and that the two structures can be distinguished by monoclonal antibodies recognizing epitopes particular to each of them (15). These unexpected results are essential for the pharmaceutical development of the peptide. They could have a more farreaching impact and be applied to other peptides.

Zinc Deficiency, Zinc Supplementation, and Thymulin

Experimental Zinc Deprivation

The zinc/thymulin relationship was further investigated using two models of in vivo zinc deprivation. First, active thymulin levels were studied in sera from mice subjected to a long-term marginally zinc-deficient diet. In spite of the absence of thymic atrophy, a significant decrease in the serum levels of thymulin was observed as early as 2 months after beginning the diet. However, these levels could be consistently restored after in vitro addition of ZnC12 (13). These findings strongly suggest that the nonactive zinc-deprived peptide is secreted in these experimental conditions. Interestingly, analysis of thymuses from Zn-deprived mice showed that, in spite of the absence of major changes in thymic epithelial cells, there was a progressive increase in the number of thymulin-containing cells, suggesting an increase in the production of the hormone. These observations indicate a compensatory phenomenon, similar to a classic feedback response. It has been recently shown in normal mice that an experimental decrease of circulating thymulin, obtained by injections of antithymulin monoclonal antibodies, induces an increase in the number of thymulin-containing cells (16). In the case of marginal Zn deficiency, this feedback effect could be stimulated by the decline of the hormone in its active form, suggesting that the biological regulatory system only recognizes the peptide containing zinc. This hypothesis is in agreement with the fact that all the thymulin functions investigated to date require the presence of zinc in the molecule (17).

More recently, similar observations were made in human volunteers submitted to zinc-deficient diets. Their thymulin levels, which were in a normal range at the beginning of the diet, dropped very rapidly during zinc deprivation, in close parallel with zinc plasma levels and were restored to normal after in vivo zinc repletion. In addition, the low thymulin levels observed during zinc deprivation could also be restored to normal values by in vitro addition of zinc chloride (18). These results represent a further argument in favor of natural coexistence of the active (zinc-containing) and inactive (zinc-deprived) forms of thymulin in the serum, the latter being predominant in zinc-deficient conditions.

Our recent studies have shown that thymulin secretion is affected by at least one monokine, prostaglandin E (19), and by thyroid and steroid hormones (20,21), suggesting neuroendocrine involvement in the modulation of thymic epithelium. Thus, zinc requirement at the tissue level may reflect the interaction of different regulators through effects on the endocrine function of the thymus.

Zinc Deficiency in Pathological Situations

NEPHROTIC SYNDROME AND CHRONIC RENAL FAILURE: Thymulin levels were recently studied in various pathological situations with zinc deficiency. The first study was performed in young children with the nephrotic syndrome, in which we observed low thymulin levels compared to age-matched subjects. These low levels of thymulin activity were restored to normal after remission of the disease or after in vitro addition of zinc salts to the serum under study (22).

Similar observations were made in patients with chronic renal failure (CRF) treated by hemodialysis by Travaglini et al. (23). First, they found, as had others, that men with CRF undergoing hemodialysis had serum zinc levels significantly lower than those found in normal individuals. Second, the hemodialyzed men with CRF had plasma thymulin levels that were much lower than those in age-matched men. Third, they demonstrated that thymulin levels increased significantly after oral zinc supplementation.

The effects of zinc supplementation on thymic endocrine activity were particularly evident in aged patients with CRF, in whom the plasma thymulin levels during zinc treatment reached values usually found in normal young men. These data confirm previous observations suggesting that the age-dependent involution of the thymus is not an irreversible phenomenon. Thus, low serum zinc levels seem to play a major role in causing thymic failure in patients with CRF. For example, the impaired cellular immunity in uremic patients (24) is restored to normal by zinc administration (25). Whether such an effect is mediated through its action remains to be established (26).

SICKLE CELL ANEMIA PATIENTS: Similar studies were performed in subjects with sickle cell anemia (see Chap. 24). Studies have shown that several parameters of cellular immune function may be altered in such patients and related to a zinc deficiency. In these patients, thymulin levels were found to be significantly lower than in age-matched healthy subjects. However, as previously observed in human volunteers in whom restricted zinc intake induced a mild specific deficiency of zinc, paralleled with low thymulin levels, it was observed that zinc supplementation or in vitro zinc activation restored normal thymulin values (18).

TYPE 1 DIABETES: In a recent report, Mocchegiani et al. (27) investigated the serum levels of zinc and the plasma levels of thymulin in a series of young patients suffering from type 1 (insulin-dependent) diabetes, since low serum and tissue zinc values have been reported to occur in diabetic conditions.

Serum zinc levels were significantly decreased and the active form of thymulin strongly reduced in diabetic patients as compared to normal age-matched individuals. In vitro zinc addition to plasma samples from patients induced a return of thymulin to values comparable with those observed in healthy controls, suggesting that low thymulin levels recorded in diabetic conditions were not due to thymic failure in synthesizing and secreting thymic hormone, but as previously mentioned in other situations, to a peripheral defect in zinc binding to the hormone molecules. This failure might account for the immunological abnormalities associated with type 1 diabetes.

DOWN'S SYNDROME: Recent findings regarding the endocrine function of the thymus in individuals with Down's syndrome were published by Franceschi et al. (28).

First, the authors found markedly reduced concentrations of circulating thymulin in plasma from these persons. This observation was attributed to a defect in bioavailability of zinc ions consequent to a marginal zinc deficiency, since the in vitro addition of nanomolar quantities of zinc salt to plasma samples restored thymulin levels to normal values.

Second, on the basis of their results obtained in vitro, these authors demonstrated the beneficial effect of zinc supplementation on thymic endocrine function, immune parameters, and clinical status. Interestingly, these results have been achieved using low doses of zinc, thus excluding a pharmacological action of this element.

The mechanism of action of zinc in vivo in these situations is still unclear. In particular, it is still open to question whether zinc simply activates preexisting thymulin molecules, or whether it might also increase the production of thymulin by thymic epithelial cells. Nevertheless, these observations that zinc is required to render thymulin biologically active (29) suggest that functional thymulin deficiency could contribute significantly to the immune deficiency induced by lack of zinc intake.

ZINC, A MITOGENIC AGENT OF LYMPHOCYTES

Lymphocytes cultured in the presence of zinc have increased synthesis of DNA and RNA and are transformed into lymphoblasts (30). Optimal stimulation occurs at a 0.1-mmol concentration of Zn^{2+}. Synthesis of nucleic acids increases after 2 or 3 days of culture and reaches its maximum at 6 days. It is inhibited by the addition of actinomycin D or by the blocking of protein synthesis. The mitogenic effect is not due to a change in the concentration of cations produced by the addition of the metal to the lymphocyte cultures, since neither Ca^{2+} nor Mg^{2+} affects DNA synthesis. Aside from direct mitogenic effects, zinc is essential to the action of other mitogens such as PHA. Thus, the EDTA inhibition of transformation induced by PHA is totally reversible after the addition of zinc.

ZINC AND SELECTIVE T-CELL DEFICIENCIES

Zinc deficit can be severe, as in acrodermatitis enteropathic (31), a familial disease caused by zinc malabsorption (1,2). Immunologically, this disease is characterized by thymic atrophy, deficiency of cellular immunity with reduced levels of T lymphocytes, decreased mitogen response, and a decrease in delayed hypersensitivity reactions.

The plasma zinc level is very low and all clinical symptoms as well as immunological anomalies are rapidly corrected by zinc administration. A highly similar picture is observed in patients receiving only parenteral feeding without addition of zinc (2). Such patients also have reduced T-cell levels as well as T-cell functional anomalies which disappear after administration of zinc.

Undernourished children have thymic atrophy which seems to be due to zinc deficiency, since it can be selectively corrected by zinc absorption.

Perhaps more interesting because of its frequent observation is the minor zinc deficiency observed in a large number of diseases such as immune deficits (Di George syndrome, severe combined immune deficiency), certain types of cancer (head and neck cancer, breast cancer, bronchial cancer), hemopathies (Hodgkin's disease, leukemia), and infectious diseases (2). There are disorders in which a modest but significant deficit in cellular immunity is frequently observed; in many cases, it can be related to zinc deficiency. In addition, a correlation is observed between the serum zinc level and the degree of immune deficit. Pediatric patients with Di George may show improved immune response with repletion of low serum zinc (S. Cunningham-Rundles, personal communication).

HYPOTHESES CONCERNING THE MODE OF ACTION OF ZINC ON THE IMMUNE SYSTEM

All of the mechanisms involved in the relationship between zinc and the immune system are not yet elucidated. Although not exclusive, five hypotheses appear most likely:

1. Zinc is essential to the activity of many enzymes; over 100 metalloenzymes are inactive in its absence because zinc is fixed at the active site and participates in the catalytic process. For this reason, zinc is necessary for the action of enzymes such as TDT, DNA polymerase, thymidine kinase, and 5' nucleotidase, which play a role in nucleotide metabolism. The implication of these enzymes in nucleic acid synthesis could explain the effects of zinc on lymphocyte proliferation (2).

2. The activity of certain humoral immune mediators requires the presence of zinc. This has been clearly demonstrated for the thymic hormone thymulin, but could also apply to other factors such as lymphokines or some lymphocyte growth factors. It should be noted that zinc is an essential consituant of the nerve growth factor (NGF).

3. Zinc could contribute to membrane stabilization by acting at the cytoskeletal level. For example, it reacts with cytochalasin B, which has well-known membrane

effects. The effect of zinc on membranes could also be explained by its inhibitory effect on membrane enzyme activity such as calcium-dependent ATPase and phospholipase A_2, thus being responsible for the increased integrity of the membrane structure.

Some observations suggest that zinc affects membrane structures in a manner analogous to that of vitamin E. It could act as a antagonist of calmodulin, which is a protein binding calcium, thus triggering a series of intracellular events. The antagonism between zinc and calcium would in fact be the result of the inhibitory effect of zinc on functions mediated by calmodulin. In addition, putative binding sites for zinc in the regulatory domain of protein kinase C have been proposed, suggesting an important role in cell activation (32).

The effect of zinc on membranes would explain its interaction with phagocytic cells and with certain T-cell membrane receptors. The hypothesis should be underlined whereby one of the intracellular roles of interleukin 2 (IL-2) would be to induce phenotypic expression of receptors having a high affinity for transferrin, the major carrier of zinc toward T lymphocytes.

4. Zinc could be the regulator of messenger RNA, responsible for the de novo synthesis of metallothionein in intestinal cells. It has been suggested that metallothionein would regulate the movement of zinc within intestinal cells and would play an important role in the regulation of the absorption and/or excretion of zinc, cadmium, and copper (2).

5. Finally, zinc could act directly by its mitogenic effect as a polyclonal activator of T (and possibly B) cells.

REFERENCES

1. Good RA. Nutrition an immunity. J Clin Immunol 1981; p 3-10.
2. Prasad AS. Clinical, endocrinological and biochemical effects of zinc deficiency. Clin Endocrinol Metab 1985; 14:567-589.
3. Vruwink KG, Fletcher MP, Keen CL, Golub MS, Hendrickx AG, Gershwin MG. Moderate zinc deficiency in rhesus monkeys. An intrinsic defect of neutrophil chemotaxis corrected by zinc repletion. J Immunol 1991; 146:244-249.
4. Chandra RK, Au B. Single nutrient deficiency and cell-mediated immune responses. Am J Clin Nutr USA 1980; 33:736-738.
5. Good RA, Fernandez G, Cunningham-Rundles C, Cunningham-Rundles S, Garofalo JA, Murali Kirshna Rao K, Incefy GS, Iwata T. The relation of zinc deficiency to immunologic function in animals and man. In: Primary Immunodeficiencies INSERM Sumposium N°6. M Seligmann, WH Hitzig, eds. Amsterdam, Elsevier North Holland, 1980, pp 223-233.
6. Bendzen K, Mayland L. Role of Zn^{2+} and other divalent metal ions in human lymphokine production in vitro. Scand J Immunol 1982; 15:81-86.
7. Leite de Moraes MC, Hontebeyrie-Joskowicz M, Lebounlenger F, Savino W, Dardenne M, Lepault F. Studies on the thymus in Chagas disease. II. Thymocyte subset fluctuations in trypanosoma cruzi-infected mice: Relationship to stress. Scand J Immunol 1991; 33:267-275.
8. Beach RS, Gershwin ME, Hurley LS. Nutritional factors and autoimmunity I. Immunopathology of zinc deprivation in New Zealand mice. J Immunol. 1981; 126:1999-2006.
9. Dardenne M, Savino W, Wade S, Kaiserlian D, Lemonnier D, Bach JF. In vivo and in vitro studies of thymulin in marginally zinc-deficient mice. Eur J Immunol 1984; 14:454-458.
10. Fernandez G, Madvhavan N, Kazunori O, Tanaka T, Floyd R, Good RA. Impairment of cell-mediated immunity functions by dietary zinc deficiency in mice. Proc NY Acad Sci 1979; 76:457-461.

11. Iwata T, Incefy GS, Tanaka T, Fernandez G, Menendez-Botet JC, Pih K, Good RA. Circulating thymic hormone levels in zinc deficiency. Cell Immunol 1979; 47:100-105.
12. Chvapil M, Zukoski CF, Hattler B, Stankova G, Montgomery L, Carlson EC, Ludwig JC. Zinc and cells. In: Trace Elements in Health and Diseases: Zinc and Copper. AS Prasad, D Oberleas, eds. Academic Press, New York, pp 269-281.
13. Dardenne M, Pléau JM, Nabarra B, Lefrancier P, Derrien M, Choay J, Bach JF. Contribution of zinc and other metals to the biological activity of the serum thymic factor. Proc Natl Acad Sci USA 1982; 79:5370-5373.
14. Cung MT, Marraud M, Lefrancier P, Dardenne M, Bach JF, Laussac JP. NMR study of a lymphocyte differentiating thymic factor. An investigation of the Zn (II)-nonapeptide complexes (thymulin). J Biol Chem 1988; 263:5574-5580.
15. Dardenne M, Savino W, Berrih S, Bach JF. A zinc-dependent epitope on the molecule of thymulin, a thymic hormone. Proc Natl Acad Sci USA 1985; 82:7035-7038.
16. Savino W, Huang PC, Corrigan A, Berrih S, Dardenne M. Thymic hormone containing cells. V. Immunohistological detection of metallothionein within the cells bearing thymulin (a zinc containing hormone) in human and mouse thymuses. J Histochem Cytochem 1984; 32:942-946.
17. Bach JF, Dardenne M. Thymulin, a zinc dependent hormone. Med Oncol Tumor Pharmacol 1989; 6:25-29.
18. Prasad AS, Meftah S, Adballah J, Kaplan J, Brewer GJ, Bach JF, Dardenne M. Serum thymulin in human zinc deficiency. J Clin Invest 1988; 82:1202-1210.
19. Homo-Delarche F, Gagnerault MC, Bach JF, Dardenne M. Thymic hormones and prostaglandins. II. Synergistic effect on mouse spontaneous rosette forming cells. Prostaglandins 1990; 39:299.
20. Dardenne M, Savino W, Gagnerault MC, Itoh T, Bach JF. Neuroendocrine control of thymic hormonal production. I. Prolactin stimulates in vivo and in vitro the production of thymulin by human and murine thymic epithelial cells. Endocrinol 1989; 125:3-12.
21. Dardenne M, Savino W, Bach JF. Modulation of thymic hormone function by thyroid and steroid hormones. Int J Neuroscience 1988; 39:325-334.
22. Bensman A, Dardenne M, Morgant C, Vasmant D, Bach JF. Decreased biological activity of serum thymic hormone (thymulin) in children with nephrotic syndrome. Int J Pediatric Nephrol 1983; 201-204.
23. Travaglini P, Moriondo P, Togni E, Bochicchio D, Conti A, Ambroso G, Ponticelli C, Mocchegiani E, Fabris N, Faglia G. Effect of oral zinc administration on prolactin and thymulin circulating levels in patients with chronic renal failure. J Clin Endocrinol Metab 1989; 68:186-192.
24. Raskova J, Ghobrial I, Shea SM, Ekert EC, Eisinger RP, Raska JR, KT. Cells in patients undergoing chronic hemodialysis: mitogenic responses, suppressor activity and interleukin 2 production. Diagn Immunol 1986; 4:209-213.
25. Antoniou LD, Shaloub RJ, Schechter GP. The effect of zinc on cellular immunity in chronic uremia. Am J Clin Nutr 1981; 34:1912-1919.
26. Fraker PJ, De Pasqueale-Jardieu P, Zwikel CM, Luecke RW. Regeneration of T helper cell function in zinc-deficient adult mice. Proc Natl Acad Sci USA 1978; 75:5660-5684.
27. Mocchegiani E, Boemi M, Fumelli P, Fabris N. Zinc-dependent low thymic hormone level in type 1 diabetes. Diabetes. 1989; 12:932-937.
28. Franceschi C, Chiricolo M, Licastro F, Masi M, Mocchegiani E, Fabris N. Oral zinc supplementation in Down's Syndrome: restoration of thymic endocrine activity and of some immune defects. J Ment Defic Res 1988; 32:169-181.
29. Bach JF. The multi-faceted zinc dependency of the immune system. Immunol Today 1981; 225-227.
30. Berger NA, Skinner AM. Characterization of lymphocyte transformation induced by zinc ions. J Cell Biol 1974; 61:45-55.

31. Brummerstedt E, Flagstad T, Basse A, Andresen E. The effect of zinc on calves with hereditary thymus hypoplasia (lethal trait A46). Acta Pathol Microbiol Scand 1971; A79: 686-687.
32. Forbes IJ, Zalewski PD, Giannakis C, Betts WH. Zinc induces specific association of PKC with membrane cytoskeleton. Biochem Int 1990; 22:741-748.

34
Interactions Between Cytokine Production and Inflammation: Implications for Therapies Aimed at Modulating the Host Defense to Infection

Lyle L. Moldawer and Stephen F. Lowry
The New York Hospital, Cornell University Medical Center, New York, New York

INTRODUCTION

As a result of bacterial, viral, or parasitic infection, surgical injury, trauma, or some forms of cancer, the host undergoes a series of responses that result ultimately in the loss of lean tissue and body fat. This wasting response is now known to be initiated and integrated in part by an interdependent network of cytokines released by activated inflammatory cells. Interleukin 1 (alpha and beta), tumor necrosis factor alpha (or cachectin), and interleukin 6 (beta$_2$ interferon) all interact to effect many of the changes in somatic tissue metabolism that characterize the dynamic response to inflammation or injury.

When considered in toto, this acute phase response serves an important function in promoting survival. By altering the metabolism of somatic tissues and activating immune system cells, cytokines play central roles in enhancing inflammatory responses to provide additional metabolic substrates for immune tissues, reduce tissue damage, promote wound healing, and stimulate new growth. This process requires intense mobilization of nutrient substrates. However, prolonged cytokine release can also lead to tissue wasting, cachexia, and immune system dysfunction. When the finely tuned cytokine network is not closely controlled, as may occur during endotoxemia or overwhelming gram-negative infection, excessive release of tumor necrosis factor alpha and interleukin 1 can lead to shock, tissue damage and, death. Exhaustion of body nitrogen stores and nutrients may contribute to overall morbidity.

In general, cytokines play pivotal roles in how the host responds to invasive stimuli. The future lies in modulating the impact of cytokine production to potentiate beneficial tissue responses and minimize adverse tissue damage as well as to spare energy expended in substrate mobilization (1). Only through a better understanding of cytokine production and actions can a rational approach toward manipulation of the host response be achieved.

ROLE OF CYTOKINES IN ACUTE PHASE REACTION

During the past 5 years, a greater appreciation has developed for the role that cytokines play in effecting the host response to infection, injury, and trauma. First characterized almost 30 years ago as *leukocyte endogenous mediator(s)*, or *endogenous or leukocytic pyrogen*, proteinaceous products of activated leukocytes were shown to induce many components of the acute phase response of inflammation, including changes in leukocyte populations, hepatic protein synthesis, and trace mineral redistribution (reviewed in Refs. 2 and 3). Certain minerals such as iron may affect immune cell distribution (see Chap. 32). These early studies emphasized that the response to infection was not directly due to the invading pathogens or their products, but rather resulted from the action of such endogenous leukocytic factors. In the past 5 years, the isolation, purification, and cloning of several factors, now termed cytokines, has permitted a more detailed characterization of the roles of individual mediators comprising the inflammatory cytokine network. Relationship of cytokine network interaction with nutrients is discussed in Chapter 2.

As recently as 1985, it was generally assumed that a single family of endogenous mediators (presumably interleukin 1) was responsible for the many changes in body temperature, food intake, and the redistribution of hepatic proteins, trace minerals, structural somatic proteins, and circulating leukocytes characteristic of inflammation (4,5). Thought to act primarily in a classic hormonal manner, interleukin 1 was proposed to be secreted by blood monocytes or tissue macrophages into the systemic circulation where it acted on distant tissue sites to induce these changes.

Evidence accumulated in the past several years has not refuted this earlier view entirely, but has revealed that the pattern of cytokine action is much more complex than originally proposed. It is now clear that the functional term *leukocyte endogenous mediator* must now include several families of cytokines with overlapping and complimentary biological actions. For example, the actions of tumor necrosis factor alpha (cachetin) and interleukin 6 (beta$_2$ interferon) overlap considerably with interleukin 1 in their mutual capabilities to induce fever, hepatic acute phase protein regulation, anorexia, and prostaglandin release (6-9). In some cases, functions previously attributed to interleukin 1, such as neutrophil activation (10), skeletal muscle protein degradation (11,12), and many components of hepatic acute phase protein response (13), rightly belong to tumor necrosis factor, interleukin 6, or some still-undescribed cytokines. For example, we have recently reported that interleukin 8 is produced in response to endotoxemia or proinflammatory cytokine stimulation and appears to be associated with restoration of neutrophils in the peripheral blood compartment following septic shock (14).

It is also recognized that monocytes and macrophages are not the only cell types which synthesize inflammatory cytokines; rather a variety of cell types can and do release these mediators under physiological conditions. For example, skin keratinocytes, endothelial cells, renal mesangial cells, some glial cell populations, large granular lymphocytes, B cells, and even neutrophils are all capable of synthesizing interleukin 1 (8,9,15). A similar variety of tissue types, although somewhat less extensive, synthesize and release tumor necrosis factor and interleukin 6 (15,16). In fact, interleukin 6 (beta$_2$ interferon) was first described as a product of activated fibroblasts and was only later shown to also be produced by tissue macrophages.

Only a few years ago, cytokines were thought to act principally like classic macrohormones, communicating via the systemic circulation as endocrine hormones.

Although systemic appearance of cytokines frequently occurs, as during endotoxemia or gram-negative infection (17), such a phenomenon is by no means the only mechanism by which these proteins exert their effects. The revelation that interleukin 1 is synthesized locally in many tissues where it may act suggested an important function at the paracrine level. This seems especially true in both the central nervous system and the skin where interleukin 1 acts as a local growth factor (18,19). The importance of paracrine action is supported by the observation that almost 80% of interleukin 1β is retained intracellularly as an inactive precursor molecule (20). Almost half of newly synthesized interleukin 1α is found in a membrane-bound form where it may serve in the monocyte's antigen presentation role for T lymphocytes (21,22). The precursor molecules of both interleukin 1α and β are rapidly cleaved from their precursor molecules to active mature hormones by serine proteases (22). Thus, the local wound or abscess environment, containing numerous enzymes released by activated or destroyed neutrophils and macrophages, serves as a prime environment for the release and activation of interleukin 1. The availability of key substrates such as L-arginine (see Chap. 3) may affect this process (23).

Although tumor necrosis factor is more readily secreted than interleukin 1, its hydrophobic signal sequence is unusually long (6). More importantly, Kriegler and associates have reported the isolation of a larger molecular weight (26 kDa) membrane-bound form of tumor necrosis factor from human blood monocytes that possesses biological activity only in the context of cell-cell contact (24). Such evidence also suggests important paracrine or autocrine function for tumor necrosis factor. When we exposed healthy human volunteers to an endotoxin bolus, net cachectin efflux from splarchnic organs showed that these tissues were producing large amounts of this cytokine (25). This regional influence suggests paracrine control of splanchnic tissue. To date, our knowledge concerning interleukin 6 remains too sparse to draw many conclusions regarding the relative significance of its paracrine versus endocrine functions. However, preliminary data suggest that, unlike interleukin 1, interleukin 6 is readily released into the circulation of infected or endotoxemic patients where its concentration may reach 100 ng/ml versus 500 pg/ml for interleukin 1 or tumor necrosis factor (25-27). Since interleukin 6 production can be induced by interleukin 1 or tumor necrosis factor alpha in vitro (28), some investigators have suggested that interleukin 6 serves as the predominant endocrine mediator in response to the locally released interleukin 1, and perhaps tumor necrosis factor. Using a monoclonal antibody against the interleukin 1 receptor, we have recently shown that IL-1 orchestrates weight loss and body composition changes during inflammation and contributes to induction of interleukin 6 (29). On the other hand, antibodies to cachectin/tumor necrosis factor strongly attenuate both interleukin 1 and interleukin 6 response in vivo (30).

BENEFICIAL ROLE OF CYTOKINES IN THE RESPONSE TO INFECTION

Despite evidence that cytokines in some cases contribute to morbidity and even to mortality, there is indisputable evidence that these mediators play a net beneficial role in ensuring host survival in the face of invasive stimuli. Some of the controversy may be related to the fact that cytokine levels parallel degree of injury or severity of the septic state (31) where the likelihood of mortality is also increased. Early studies demonstrated that pretreatment with crude medium conditioned by activated peritoneal macrophages protected rats from subsequent gram-negative infections (32). The timing of such cytokine administration is critical. Pretreatment from 4 to 24 hr prior to infection conferred survival advantage, whereas simultaneous treatment or treatment 1-6 hr after infection had no effect. More recent studies by Czuprynski and colleagues demonstrated that 12- to 24-hr intraperitoneal pretreatment of rats with purified or recombinant interleukin 1 significantly improved survival against intracellular *Listeria* infections (33). Intravenous administration of interleukin 1 simultaneously with the *Listeria* also conferred survival advantage and significantly reduced the number of viable bacteria in the circulation.

Moldawer and colleagues took an alternative approach to demonstrating the role of interleukin 1 as an immunomodulator (34). Noting that protein depletion in both hospitalized patients and experimental animals is associated with reduced endogenous pyrogen production, we proposed that protein-depleted animals subject to bacterial infections be given similar quantities of partially purified interleukin 1 to those which would normally be produced endogenously. We subsequently demonstrated that treatment with interleukin 1 significantly increased in vivo bactericidal capacities both in guinea pigs subject to protein depletion, and also in rats immunosuppressed by splenectomy and portocaval anastomosis (35,36).

Van der Meer and Dinarello also found that interleukin 1 treatment of cyclophosphamide-induced neutropenic mice improved survival to gram-negative infections (37). Although one of interleukin 1's biological actions is to induce the synthesis of multiple lineage colony-stimulating factors (38,39), the mechanism of action was not due to interleukin 1 enhancing granulopoiesis. Rather the authors postulate a nonimmunological mechanism, suggesting that interleukin 1 pretreatment reduces the deleterious effects on endothelial tissue of a subsequent infection-related cytokine burst.

Nenciani and colleagues have investigated synthetic peptide fragments of the interleukin 1 molecule for their immunological activities (40). They have synthesized a dodecapeptide from the carboxy region of interleukin 1 which possesses immunostimulatory properties, but does not induce a fever in vivo. Such a construct raises the possibility that it will soon be possible to separate other beneficial and deleterious responses of the molecule. Since there now appears to be at least two distinct interleukin 1 receptors with differing affinities (41), studies must determine whether the separation of host responses by this interleukin 1 construct is attributed to a differential receptor binding. As noted previously, inhibition of the IL-1 receptor with an antibody competing for a binding site common to both α and β caused marked decrease in IL-6 production (29).

Although preliminary studies with partially purified, and more recently recombinant-derived, interleukin 1 have demonstrated an immune modulatory role that promotes survival to subsequent infection, similar studies have not been performed with interleukin 6. However, there is some indirect evidence to suggest that an endogenous tumor necrosis factor or other cytokine response may contribute to immune potentiation. Polk and colleagues, for example, have demonstrated that muramyl dipeptide, a synthetic product structurally similar to lipopolysaccharide, stimulates antimicrobial responses in normal and immune-suppressed animals (42). Although the authors have not fully delineated the underlying endogenous mechanism of muramyl dipeptide's immune stimulatory capacity, they postulate a cytokine response as one possible mechanism. Since muramyl dipeptide is a potent inducer in vitro of both interleukin 1 and tumor necrosis factor, its in vivo effects may be simply due to a secondary synthesis and release of these cytokines. Because of their overlapping biological functions, as well as their synergy, both tumor necrosis factor or interleukin 6 are also good candidates to stimulate host responses against microbial invasion, or to accentuate the immune stimulatory effects of interleukin 1. Further, tumor necrosis factor given experimentally has been found to increase liver weight and protein synthesis and to elicit IL-1 production (43).

The vast majority of experience with in vivo administration of tumor necrosis factor has been in patients or experimental animals with cancer. Under these conditions, the primary action of tumor necrosis factor is to induce a direct hemorrhagic necrosis of solid tumors via thrombosis of supporting neovasculature (44).

However, many of the putative beneficial responses (45) of tumor necrosis factor are aimed at improving the antimicrobial and antitumor actions of leukocyte populations. In this regard, some biological actions previously attributed to interleukin 1 have now been more accurately ascribed to tumor necrosis factor. For example, tumor necrosis factor, and not interleukin 1, appears to be responsible for neutrophil degranulation, superoxide production, and lysozyme release (10).

Other investigators report that tumor necrosis factor, like interleukin 1, promotes release of neutrophils from bone marrow, resulting in neutrophilia (46). However, tumor necrosis factor also promotes the activation and margination of neutrophils into pulmonary epithelium, which might explain the neutropenia secondary to sepsis and bacteremia (47). Although interleukin 1 can produce similar effects, interleukin 1 appears to induce margination through a prostanoid-dependent pathway, whereas the effects of tumor necrosis factor are both prostaglandin dependent and independent (46). As noted previously, the relatively later appearance of IL-8 is associated with recovery of neutrophil numbers (14).

Tumor necrosis factor also appears to induce the differentiation of myelogenous cell lines along a monocyte/macrophage pathway (47,48). Bone marrow cytology from animals treated chronically with tumor necrosis factor shows an almost complete replacement of erythroid precursors with myeloid cells (49). In contrast, although IL-1 reduces red cell life span, no anemia is produced (50). Acutely, macrophages responding to invasive stimuli in a local wound environment could recruit additional cells to respond by enhancing their differentiation from precursor populations at the expense of the synthesis of other cell types. Furthermore, tumor necrosis factor transforms resting mature macrophages into an activated state (51) capable of inhibiting viral and parasitic replications intracellularly (52). Virus-infected cells also appear to be more sensitive to tumor necrosis factor-induced cytolysis and tumor necrosis factor-activated macrophages exhibit increased cytotoxicity against transformed and infected cells (51). Tumor necrosis factor is essential for initiation and amplification of interleukin 1 and interleukin 6 release (30).

Studies by Sehgal and Van Damme suggest that antimicrobial actions of interleukin 1 or tumor necrosis factor may be mediated by the synthesis and release of interleukin 6 (53). Interleukin 6 is induced in fibroblasts and monocytes/macrophages by either interleukin 1 or tumor necrosis factor, and interleukin 6 can in itself block viral replication of infected cells and reduce the overall viral burden. Since under in vivo conditions it is difficult if not impossible to have a systemic interleukin 1 or tumor necrosis factor alpha response in the absence of interleukin 6, it is presently unresolved what contribution interleukin 6 makes to the immune responses associated with bacterial or viral invasion. These questions can only be resolved when sufficient quantities of recombinant protein and monoclonal antibodies become available.

PATHOLOGY ASSOCIATED WITH EXCESSIVE OR CHRONIC CYTOKINE PRODUCTION

Although cytokines have central and pivotal roles in the beneficial host responses to invasive stimuli, an excessive or chronic production of these monokines causes considerable pathology (54). Recent studies suggest that overproduction of either interleukin 1 and/or tumor necrosis factor may be an underlying cause in the development of several chronic and acute inflammatory diseases, including rheumatoid arthritis, cancer cachexia, atherosclerosis, sarcoidosis, Reye's syndrome, Kawasaki's syndrome, and endotoxin-induced or gram-negative infection-induced shock. The nutritional costs of this overproduction or indeed, even "normal" production during an acute phase response have been discussed in Chap. 30.

The evidence that interleukin 1 and tumor necrosis factor are central to the pathogenesis of rheumatoid arthritis is particularly strong. Elevated levels of both cytokines have been recovered from plasma and synovial fluid, and both interleukin 1 and tumor necrosis factor stimulate synovial protease, prostaglandin, and collagenase activity (55-58).

Similarly, our knowledge regarding the proximal role that tumor necrosis factor plays in the pathogenesis of septic shock has increased considerably (31). Such studies were originally predicated on the observation of Tracey et al. that tissue responses to high doses of recombinant human tumor necrosis factor were remarkably similar to those seen in clinical injury and infection (59). These experiments revealed first in rats (59) and subsequently in dogs (60) that infusion of tumor necrosis factor is sufficient to reproduce many, if not all, of the pathological sequelae typical of lethal endotoxemia. In rats, high-dose tumor necrosis factor produces lethargy, piloerection without chills, bloody diarrhea, and tachypnea within minutes. Treated animals expire with severe metabolic acidosis and respiratory arrest, and postmortem examination reveals significant inflammatory damage to vital organs. The lungs are diffusely hyperemic with histopathological evidence of focal hemorrhagic areas. Arterial occlusion by polymorphonuclear leukocytic thrombi is also evident with margination of polymorphonuclear leukocytes through the walls of the pulmonary vessels, accompanied by severe interstitial and peribronchiolar pneumonitis. Segmental ischemia and regional hemorrhage and necrosis of the large bowel are also present. In addition, congestion of the kidneys attributable to acute tubular necrosis is seen.

Investigations have demonstrated that these potent effects are not fully shared by the other principal, early inflammatory monokine, interleukin 1. Administration of recombinant human interleukin 1β to rabbits produces a transient decline in hemodynamic performance, but the changes are reversible and do not lead to tissue damage or shock (61). However, like tumor necrosis factor, interleukin 1 can produce transient lung damage through a prostaglandin-mediated margination of neutrophils in the pulmonary epithelium. Not surprisingly, a combination of the two cytokines results in severe lung damage at doses far lower than observed when each cytokine is given separately (61). Neutralization of tumor necrosis factor by antibodies did not prevent weight loss or acute phase response in an inflammatory model; however, antibody blockade of the IL-1 receptor preserved lean body mass in subsequent challenge (29).

Kettelhut, Goldberg, Dinarello, and their coworkers report that cytokine-induced shock is completely reversible by prostaglandin synthesis inhibitors (61,62). Since tumor necrosis factor is a potent inducer of prostanoid synthesis (55), a putative mechanism of tumor necrosis factor-mediated shock is excessive production of prostaglandin E_2 and thromboxane B_2, which together lead to vasoconstriction and neutrophil margination. Support for this observation comes from the studies of Pomposelli and Bistrian, who report that guinea pigs fed a chronic fish oil diet high in omega-3 fatty acids produce less thromboxane B_2 and have less lung damage to intravenously administered endotoxin (63). In addition, omega-3 fatty acids have been found to reduce cytokine production (interleukin 2) independently of the cyclooxygenase pathway (64). See also Chap. 13, this volume. Another contributing factor to shock may be a tumor necrosis factor-mediated alteration in procoagulant activity by vascular endothelium (65). Such alterations are thought to promote a hypercoagulopathy which can be further aggravated by interleukin 1 (65).

The role of these cytokines in other chronic inflammatory diseases, such as cancer cachexia, is controversial, but is an area of active research. Cytokine changes in tumor-bearing animals ressemble the septic state (54,66). Patients with malignancies often present with weight loss, body fat depletion, hypertriglyceridemia, and alterations in serum trace metals and hepatic acute phase protein levels consistent with an active inflammatory response (67). Such changes do not appear to be attributed to anorexia alone. For example, albumin degradation increases but is not attributable to malnutrition (68). Furthermore, many of the changes in host physiology can be reproduced in experimental animals by cytokine administration alone (69,70). Furthermore, inhibition of cachectic/tumor necrosis factor response in a tumor model reduced tissue wasting (71).

As discussed in Chapter 23, nutritional support of cancer patients with lipid emulsions did increase interleukin 2 production but decreased overall survival, which raises important questions about the impact of cytokines on malignant cell growth. Recent studies have also been able to demonstrate increased cytokine production in several experimental and human malignancies (54,66). For example, in an earlier study, Norton et al. demonstrated in parabiotic rats that a humoral factor produced by the Meth A sarcoma-bearing rat and present in their serum induced anorexia and weight loss in the non-tumor-bearing parabiote (72). Later, the same authors detected tumor necrosis factor-like bioactivity in the serum of Meth A tumor-bearing rats with large tumor burden (73). We have also been able to demonstrate spontaneous interleukin 1 and tumor necrosis factor alpha production from mice bearing a cachexia-inducing sarcoma (66,74). Both tumors and spleens from such animals had increased quantities of interleukin 1α and tumor necrosis factor mRNA as well as immune reactive protein. Furthermore, under some circumstances, we have observed that IL-1 and tumor necrosis factor may act as growth factors promoting tumor development (75).

Elevated serum levels of tumor necrosis factor have also been observed in one study of patients with malignancy (76). In addition, Aderka et al. reported that blood mononuclear cells from patients with cancer have spontaneous tumor necrosis factor production in vitro and produce elevated quantities when stimulated with endotoxin (77).

Although tumor necrosis factor has been detected in the serum of patients and animals with cancer-associated cachexia, other cytokines, including interferon-γ are also present (78). Several approaches have been recently employed to test whether tumor necrosis factor is a causative factor in the development of weight loss and cachexia. In an ingenious study, Oliff and associates implanted a human xenograft that constitutively produces tumor necrosis factor into nude mice and observed marked weight loss and cachexia (79). We have demonstrated that treating mice bearing a Lewis lung adenocarcinoma with antibodies against murine tumor necrosis factor (antimurine cachectin immunoglobulin) can significantly attenuate the development of carcass lipid depletion, as well as the serum hypertriglyceridemia seen during progressive tumor growth (80). Rather surprisingly, anticachectin antibodies did not impact on the development of tumor-induced anemia or an hepatic acute phase response in this tumor model. In other studies with a transplanted, low differentiated, rapidly growing tumor, we also found that anti-tumor necrosis factor treatment and anti-IL-1 receptor treatment had no effect on the acute phase response, whereas reducing tumor growth and increasing food intake (75). However, in contrast to the results that we obtained when mice were treated with anti-murine cachectin immunoglobulin without effect on tumor-induced anemia, subsequent treatment of rats with recombinant human cachectin/tumor necrosis factor (in comparison with recombinant IL-1 or endotoxin) showed a significant effect on anemia. Tumor necrosis factor decreased red cell synthesis and survival, whereas IL-1 had no effect on synthesis and only a modest effect on survival (50). Thus, an experimental approach including such factors as species specificity, purity, and concentration of cytokine may affect the way these substances interact in the host. There is a general need for complementary experimental design in the study of cytokine regulation if the goal of positive intervention is to be attained.

FUTURE CONSIDERATIONS FOR THERAPEUTIC MODULATION

More than forty years after the initial description of *leukocytic pyrogen* by Beeson and Bennett (81), our understanding of the role that cytokines play in the inflammatory and systemic host responses to infection, injury, and some forms of cancer is still incomplete. However, it is now apparent that an interdependent network of cytokines with both distinctive and overlapping biological activities mediate most, if not all, of the host responses to invasive stimuli. Future studies will further delineate the contribution specific cytokines make to individual components of the host response.

The actions of these cytokines are often two sided. At a very low concentrations (10^{-12} M), interleukin 1 or tumor necrosis factor play an important role in the communication between different cell types in a single tissue. One such example is the local production of interleukin 1 by keratinocytes, which is an essential growth factor for the developing dermal cells. Yet interleukin 1 at higher concentrations in the skin or at similar concentrations but in another location, a joint, for example, can induce considerable pathology. Interleukin 1 production in the synovium leads to excessive tissue remodeling and arthritis.

The availability of recombinant human-derived cytokines and monoclonal antibodies directed against cytokines and/or their receptors has raised considerable excitement as potential tools for therapeutic interventions in specific disease processes.

Although the prospect of modulating the immune response is great, caution must be exercised until a thorough understanding of the multiple biological actions of individual cytokines is achieved. For example, proposals to administer either recombinant interleukin 1 or tumor necrosis factor as an immune adjuvant or inducer of erythropoiesis will need to consider the obvious pathology associated with excessive production or administration. Indeed patients receiving either interleukin 1 or tumor necrosis factor will have to be closely monitored for hemodynamic and respiratory changes, coagulopathy, gastrointestinal pathology, and anemia, among others. Clinical efficacy will be counterbalanced against toxicity, and doses will be closely titrated for maximal response with minimal side effects. Patients on total parenteral nutrition may have different responses (82).

Conversely, efforts to block the pathological effects of interleukin 1 and tumor necrosis factor during chronic inflammation will also require close scrutiny. In cases of acute sepsis and endotoxic shock, administration of antibodies against tumor necrosis factor confer survival and hemodynamic stability (83). In those cases, an excessive production of tumor necrosis factor, which leads subsequently to hemodynamic instability and hypercoagulopathy, is directly pathological to the host. In addition, antibodies blocking an endogenous tumor necrosis factor response in cerebral malaria appears to reduce the pathology associated with this intracellular infection (84). However, blocking an endogenous tumor necrosis factor, or for that matter an interleukin 1 or interleukin 6 response, in sublethal bacterial or viral infections may not be beneficial, and may even prolong the infectious period. If indeed these cytokines are closely regulated and function to promote antimicrobial responses in the host, altering this interdependent network of cytokine feedback with antibodies or antagonists could theoretically lead to immune suppression, bacterial overgrowth, and ultimately death. Further experimental work is required to ascertain whether blocking an endogenously controlled-cytokine response is detrimental to the host.

REFERENCES

1. Fong Y, Moldawer LL, Shires GT, Lowry SF. The biological characteristics of cytokines and their implications in surgical injury. Surg Gynecol Obstet 170:363, 1990.
2. Kampschmidt RW. Leukocyte endogenous mediator/endogenous pyrogen. In: Infection: The Physiologic and Metabolic Responses of the Host (edited by Powanda, MC, Canonico PG), New York, Elsevier-North Holland, 1981.
3. Bodel P. Studies on the mechanism of endogenous pyrogen production. I. Investigation of new protein synthesis in stimulated human blood leukocytes. Yale J Biol Med 43:145-163, 1970.
4. Dinarello CA. Interleukin 1. Rev Infect Dis 6:51-94, 1984.
5. Dinarello CA. Interleukin 1 and the pathogenesis of the acute phase response. N Engl J Med 311:1413-1418, 1984.
6. Moldawer LL, Lowry SF, Cerami A. Cachectin, its impact on metabolism and nutritional status. Ann Rev Nutr 8:585-609, 1988.
7. Kohase M, May LT, Tamm I, Vilcek J, Sehgal PB. A cytokine network in human diploid fibroblasts. Interactions of beta-interferons, tumor necrosis factor, platelet-derived growth factor and interleukin 1. Mol Cell Biol 7:273-280, 1987.
8. Beutler B, Cerami A. Cachectin: More than a tumour necrosis factor. N Engl J Med 316: 379-385, 1987.

9. Le J, Vilcek J. Tumour necrosis factor and interleukin 1: Cytokines with multiple overlapping biological activities. Lab Invest 56:234-248, 1987.
10. Georgielis K, Schaefer C, Dinarello CA, Klempner MS. Human recombinant interleukin 1 beta has no effect on intracellular calcium or on functional responses of human neutrophils. J Immunol 138:3403-3407, 1987.
11. Moldawer LL, Svaninger G, Gelin J, Lundholm K. Interleukin 1 (alpha or beta) and tumour necrosis factor-alpha do not regulate protein balance in skeletal muscle. Am J Physiol 253:C766-C773, 1987.
12. Goldberg AL, Kettlehut IC, Furuno K, Fagan JM, Baracos VM. Activation of protein breakdown and prostaglandin E_2 production in rat skeletal muscle in fever is signalled by a macrophage product distinct from interleukin 1 and other known cytokines. J Clin Invest 81:1378-1381, 1988.
13. Baumann H, Onorato V, Gauldie J, Jahreis GP. Distinct sets of acute phase plasma proteins are stimulated by separate human hepatocyte stimulating factors and monokines in rat hepatoma cells. J Biol Chem 262:9756-9768, 1987.
14. Van Zee KJ, DeForge LE, Fischer E, Marano MA, Kenney JS, Remick DG, Lowry SF, Moldawer LL. IL-8 in septic shock, endotoxemia, and after IL-1 administration. J Immunol 146:3478, 1991.
15. Nathan CF. Secretory products of macrophages. J Clin Invest 79:319-326, 1987.
16. Sehgal PB, May LT, Tamm I, Vilcek I. Human B_2 interferon and B-cell differentiation factor BSF-2 are identical. Science 235:731-732, 1987.
17. Hesse DG, Tracey KJ, Fong Y, Manogue KR, Dinarello CA, Cerami A, Lowry SF. Cytokine appearance in human endotoxemia and nonhuman primate bactermia. Surg Gyn Obstet 1987.
18. Giulian D, Lachman LB. Interleukin 1 stimulation of astroglial cell proliferation after brain injury. Science 228:497-499, 1985.
19. Sauder DN. Biologic properties of epidermal cell thymocyte activating factor (ETAF). J Invest Dermatol 85:1765-1772, 1985.
20. Dinarello CA. Biology of interleukin 1. FASEB J 2:108-115, 1988.
21. Dinarello CA. Interleukin-1 and its biologically related cytokines. In: Lymphokines and the Immune Response. (Edited S Cohen). CRC Press, Boca Raton, Florida, p. 181, 1990.
22. Intracellular localization of human monocyte associated interleukin 1 (IL-1) activity and release of biologically active IL-1 from monocytes by trypsin and plasmin. J Immunol 136:2883-2891, 1986.
23. Barbul A, Lazarou SA, Efron DT, Wasserkreig HL, Efron G. Arginine enhances wound healing and lymphocyte immune responses in humans. Surgery 108:331, 1990.
24. Kriegler M, Perez C, DeFay K, Albert I, Lu SD. A novel form of TNF/cachectin is a cell surface cytotoxic transmembrane protein: Ramifications for the complex physiology of TNF. Cell 53:45-53, 1988.
25. Fong YM, Marano MA, Moldawer LL, Wei H, Calvano SE, Kenney JS, Allison AC, Cerami A, Shires GT, Lowry SF. The acute splanchnic and peripheral tissue metabolic response to endotoxin in humans. J Clin Invest 85:1896, 1990.
26. Fong Y, Moldawer LL, Marano MA, Wei H, Tatter SB, Clarick RH, Santhanam U, May LT, Sehgal PB, Lowry SF. Endotoxemia elicits increased circulating B_2-interferon/interleukin 6 in man. J Immunol 142:2321, 1989.
27. Fong Y, Moldawer LL, Marano M, Wei H, Tatter SB, Clarick RH, Santhanam Y, Sherris D, May LT, Sehgel PB. Endotoxemia elicits increased circulating beta 2-INF/IL-6 in man J Immunol 142:2321, 1989.
28. Kohase M, Henriksen-DeStefano D, May LT, Vilcek J, Sehgal PB. Induction of interferon-beta 2 by tumour necrosis factor: Homeostatic mechanism in the control of cell proliferation. Cell 45:659-667, 1986.

29. Gershenwald JE, Fong YM, Fahey TJ III, Calvano SE, Chizzonite R, Kilian PL, Lowry SF, Moldawer LL. Interleukin-1 receptor blockade attenuates the host inflammatory response. Proc Natl Acad Sci USA 87:4966, 1990.
30. Fong Y, Tracey KJ, Moldawer LL, Hesse DG, Manogue KB, Kenney JS, Lee AT, Luo GC, Allison AC, Lowry SF. Antibodies to cachectin/tumor necrosis factor reduce interleukin 1 beta and interleukin 6 appearance during lethal bacteremia. J Exp Med 170:1627, 1989.
31. Marano MA, Fong Y, Moldawer LL, Wei H, Calvaro SE, Tracey KJ, Barie PS, Manogue K, Cerami A, Shires GT. Serum cachectin/tumor necrosis factor in critically ill patients with burns correlates with infection and mortality. Surg Gynecol Obstet 170:32, 1990.
32. Kampschmidt RF, Pulliam LA. Stimulation of antimicrobial activity in the rat with leukocyte endogenous mediator. J Reticuloendoth Soc 17:162-169, 1975.
33. Czuprynski CJ, Brown JF. Recombinant murine interleukin 1 alpha enhancement of nonspecific antibacterial resistance. J Immunol 55:2061-2065, 1987.
34. Moldawer LL, Sobrado J, Blackburn GL, Bistrian BR. A rationale for administering leukocyte endogenous mediator (interleukin 1) to protein-malnourished, hospitalized patients. J Theoret Biol 106:119-133, 1984.
35. Moldawer LL, Hamawy KJ, Bistrian BR, Georgieff M, Drabik M, Dinarello C, Blackburn GL. A therapeutic use for interleukin 1 in the protein depleted animal. Br J Rheumatol 24(suppl) 220-224, 1985.
36. Hamawy KJ, Yamazaki K, Georgieff M, Dinarello CA, Moldawer LL, Blackburn GL, Bistrian BR. Improvements in host immunity by partially purified interleukin 1 in rats with portocaval anastomosis and splenectomy. J Parenter Enter Nutr 10:146-150, 1986.
37. Van der Meer JWM, Barza M, Wolff SM, Dinarello CA. A low dose of recombinant interleukin 1 protects granulocytopenic mice from lethal gram negative infection. Proc Natl Acad Sci USA 85:1620-1623, 1988.
38. Vogel SN, Douches SD, Kaufman EN, Neta R. Induction of colony stimulating factor in vivo by recombinant interleukin 1 alpha and recombinant tumor necrosis factor-alpha. J Immunol 138:2143-2148, 1987.
39. Anderson L, Weiner RS. Interleukin 1 stimulates fibroblasts to produce granulocyte-macrophage colony stimulating activity and prostaglandin E2. J Clin Invest 77:1857-1863, 1986.
40. Nenciani L, Villa L, Tagliabue A, Antoni G, Presentini R, Perin R, Silvestri S, Boraschi D. In vivo stimulatory activity of the 161-173 peptide of human IL-1 beta. J Immunol 139:800-804, 1987.
41. Lowenthal JW, MacDonald HR. Binding and internalization of interleukin 1 by T cells: Evidence for high- and low-affinity classes of interleukin 1 receptor. J Exp Med 164:1060-1074, 1987.
42. Polk HC Jr. The enhancement of host defenses against infection-search for the Holy Grail. Surgery 99:1-6, 1987.
43. Moldawer LL, Andersson C, Gelin J, Lundholm KG. Regulation of food intake and hepatic protein synthesis by recombinant-derived cytokines. Am J Physiol 254:G450, 1988.
44. Old LJ. Tumor necrosis factor. Sci Am 258:59-75, 1988.
45. Moldawer LL. Nutrition and immunology: Challenge for the 1990s (editorial). Nutr Clin Pract 5:187, 1990.
46. Ulich TR, Castillo JD, Keys M, Granger GA, Ni RX. Kinetics and mechanism of recombinant human interleukin 1 alpha and tumour necrosis factor alpha induced changes in circulating numbers of neutrophils and lymphocytes. J Immunol 139:3406-3415, 1987.
47. Munker R, Gassoon J, Ogawa M, Koeffler HP. Recombinant human TNF induces production of granulocyte-macrophage colony stimulating factor. Nature 323:729-732, 1986.
48. Sato K, Kasono K, Fujii Y, Kawakami M, Tsushima T, Shizuma K. Tumour necrosis factor type alpha (cachectin) stimulates mouse osteoblast-like cells (MC3T3-E1) to produce macrophage colony stimulating activity and prostaglandin E2. Biochem Biophys Res Commun 145:323-329, 1987.

49. Tracey KJ, Wei H, Manogue KR, Fong Y, Hesse DG, Nguyen HT, Cotran RS, Cerami A, Lowry SF. Cachectin/TNF induces cachexia, anorexia and inflammation. J Exp Med 1988.
50. Moldawer LL, Marano MA, Wei H, Fong Y, Silen ML, Kuo G, Marogue KR, Vlassara H, Cohen H, Cerami A, et al. Cachectin/tumor necrosis factor-alpha alters red blood cell kinetics and induces anemia in vivo FASEB J 3:1637, 1989.
51. Philip R, Epstein LB. Tumour necrosis factor as immunomodulator and mediator of monocyte cytotoxicity induced by itself, gamma interferon and interleukin 1. Nature 323:86-89, 1986.
52. Wong GHW, Goeddal DV. Tumour necrosis factors alpha and beta inhibit virus replication and synergize with interferons. Nature 323:819-821, 1986.
53. Van Damme J, De Ley M, Van Snick J, Dinarello Billiau A. The role of interferon B1 and the 26 kD protein (interferon B2) as mediators of the antiviral effect of interleukin 1 and tumor necrosis factor. J Immunol 139:1867-1872, 1987.
54. Moldawer LL, Sherry B, Lowry SF, Cerami A. Endogenous cachectin/tumour necrosis factor-alpha production contributes to experimental cancer-associated cachexia. Cancer Surveys 8:859, 1989.
55. Dayer JM, Beutler BM, Cerami AC. Cachectin/tumor necrosis factor stimulates collagenase and prostaglandin E2 production by human synovial cells and dermal fibroblasts. J Exp Med 162:2163-2168, 1985.
56. Dayer JM, deRochemonteix B, Burrus B, Demczuk S, Dinarello C. Human recombinant interleukin 1 stimulates collagenase and prostaglandin E2 production by human synovial cells. J Clin Invest 77:645-649, 1986.
57. Saklatvala J. Tumor necrosis factor stimulates resorption and inhibits synthesis of proteoglycan in cartilage. Nature 322:547-549, 1986.
58. Saklatvala J. Interleukin 1: purification and biochemical aspects of its action on cartilage. J Rheumatol 14:52-54, 1987.
59. Tracey KJ, Beutler B, Lowry SF, Merryweather J, Wolpe S, Milsark IW, Hariri RJ, Fahey TJ III, Zentella A, Albert JD, Shires GT, Cerami A. Shock and tissue injury induced by recombinant human cachectin. Science 234:470-474, 1986.
60. Tracey KJ, Lowry SF, Fahey TJ, Fong Y, Hesse D, Beutler B, Manogue K, Calvano SE, Wei H, Albert JD, Cerami A, Shires GT. Cachectin/tumour necrosis factor induces lethal septic shock and stress hormone responses in the dog. Surg Gynec Obstet 164:415-422, 1987.
61. Okusawaol S, Gelfand JA, Ikejima T, Connolly RJ, Dinarello CA. Interleukin 1 induces a shock-like state in rabbits. J Clin Invest 81:1162-1172, 1988.
62. Kettlehut IC, Fiers W, Goldberg AL. Toxic effects of tumour necrosis factor in vivo and their prevention by cyclooxygenase inhibitors. Proc Natl Acad Sci USA 84:4273-4277, 1987.
63. Pomposelli JJ, Flores EA, Bistrian BR, Blackburn GL, Zeisel S. Fish oil enriched diets ameliorate the metabolic acidosis induced by endotoxin in guinea pigs. FASEB J 2:1692A, 1988.
64. Santoli D, Zarier RB. Prostaglandin E precursor FAs inhibit human IL-2 production by a prostaglandin E-independent mechanism. J Immunol 143:1303, 1989.
65. Bevilacqua MP, Pober JS, Majeau GR, Fiers W, Cotran RS, Gimbrone MA Jr. Recombinant tumour necrosis factor induces procoagulant activity in cultured human vascular endothelium: characterization and comparison with interleukin 1. Proc Natl Acad Sci USA 83:4533-4537, 1986.
66. Lonnroth C, Moldawer LL, Gelin J, Kindblom L, Sherry B, Landholm K. Tumor necrosis factor-alpha and interleukin-1 alpha production in cachetic tumor bearing mice. Int J Can 46:889, 1990.
67. Moldawer LL, Georgieff M, Lundholm KG. Interleukin 1, tumour necrosis factor-alpha and the pathogenesis of cancer cachexia. Clin Physiol 7:263-274, 1987.

68. Andersson CE, Lonnroth IC, Gelin CJ, Moldawer LL, Lundholm KG. Pretranslational regulation of albumin synthesis in tumor bearing mice. The role of anorexia and undernutrition. Gastroenterology 100:939, 1991.
69. Ternell M, Moldawer LL, Lonnroth C, Gelin J, Lundholm K. Plasma protein synthesis in experimental cancer compared with paraneoplastic conditions including monokine administration. Cancer Res 47:5825-5830, 1987.
70. Fong Y, Moldawer LL, Wei H, Barber A, Manogue K, Tracey KJ, Kuo G, Fischman DA, Cerami A et al. Cachectin/TNF on IL-1 alpha induces cachexia with redistribution of body proteins. Am J Physiol 256:R659, 1989.
71. Sherry BA, Gelin J, Fong Y, Marano M, Wei H, Cerami A, Lowry SF, Landholm KG, Moldawer LL. Anticachectin/tumor necrosis factor- alpha antibodies attenuate development of cachexia in tumor models. FASEB J 3:1956, 1989.
72. Norton JA, Moley JF, Green MV. Parabiotic transfer of anorexia/cachexia in male rats. Cancer Res 45:5547-5552, 1985.
73. Stavroff MC, Fraker DL, Norton JA. Cachectin levels in the serum of cachectic tumor bearing rats. Soc Surg Onc 96A, 1988.
74. Lonnroth C, Moldawer LL, Sherry B, Mizel SB, Lundholm K. Spontaneous interleukin 1 and cachectin production by tumours of cachectic, sarcoma-bearing mice. Cancer Res 1988.
75. Gelin J, Moldawer LL, Lonnroth C, Sherry B, Chizzonite R, Lundholm K. Role of endogenous tumor necrosis factor alpha and interleukin 1 for experimental tumor growth and the development of cancer cachexia. Cancer Res 51:415, 1991.
76. Balkwill F, Osborne R, Burke F, Naylor S, Talbot D, Durbin H, Tavernier J, Fiers W. Evidence for tumour necrosis factor/cachectin production in cancer. Lancet 2:1229-1231, 1987.
77. Aderka D, Fisher S, Levo Y, Holtmann H, Hahn H, Wallach D. Cachectin/tumor necrosis factor production by cancer patients. Lancet 2:1190-1191, 1985.
78. Krause R, Humphrey C, VonMeyerfeldt M. A central mechanism for anorexia in cancer. Cancer Treat Rep 65:15-23, 1981.
79. Oliff A, Defeo-Jones D, Boyer M, Marinez D, Kiefer D, Vuocolo G, Wolfe A, Socher, SH. Tumors secreting human TNF/cachectin induce cachexia in mice. Cell 50:555-563, 1987.
80. Moldawer LL, Sherry BE, Fong Y, Marano M, Wei H, Tracey K, Cerami A, Lowry SF. Anticachectin antibodies attenuate carcass lipid depletion in Lewis lung adenocarcinoma bearing mice. Surg Forum 39:429, 1988.
81. Bennett IL Jr, Beeson PB. Studies on the pathogenesis of fever. J Exp Med 98:477-491, 1953.
82. Fong YM, Marano MA, Barber A, He W, Moldawer LL, Bushman BD, Coyle SM, Shires GT, Lowry SF. Total parenteral nutrition and bowel rest modify the metabolic response to endotoxin in humans. Ann of Surg 210:449, 1989.
83. Tracey KJ, Fong Y, Hesse DG, Manogue KR, Lee AT, Kuo GC, Lowry SF, Cerami A. Anti-cachectin/TNF monoclonal antibodies prevent septic shock during lethal bacteremia. Nature 1987.
84. Grau GE, Fajordo LF, Piguet PF, Allet B, Lambert PH, Vassali P. Tumour necrosis factor (cachectin) is an essential mediator in murine cerebral malaria. Science 237:1210-1212, 1987.

35
Human Milk Antibodies and Their Importance for the Infant

Lars Å. Hanson, Ingegerd Adlerberth, Barbro U. M. Carlsson, and Mirjana Hahn-Zoric
University of Göteborg, Göteborg, Sweden

Lotta Mellander
East Hospital, Göteborg, Sweden

F. Jalil and S. Zaman
King Edward Medical College, Lahore, Pakistan

D. M. Roberton
Children's Hospital, Adelaide, Australia

INTRODUCTION

Milk, as the first nutrient source in postnatal life, provides key elements for the developing infant and supplies essential immune protection through antibodies and receptor analogs (1-4). In addition, milk contains factors (proteins, enzymes, trace elements, substrates, growth factors, and cytokines that may directly activate and regulate the immune system during this critical formative period (5,6). The role of some of these factors, such as antioxidants, including certain vitamins such as β-carotene, α-tocopherol, and ascorbate, as well as other anti-inflammatory agents such as antiproteases, lysozyme, and lactoferrin, are not well understood, but are notably absent or reduced in cow's milk and most formula (6).

As discussed in another chapter, human milk has contrasting effects on the immune system of the infant through the stimulation of general responsiveness by cytokines present in milk and by reducing certain aspects of specific response by antigen exclusion. In studies by Cunningham-Rundles in this book, an indication of the significance of bovine casein and gamma globulin in eliciting immune network interactions in instances such as selective immunoglobulin A (IgA) deficiency where macromolecular absorption from the gastrointestinal tract can occur is given. This type of study also provides further support for the relative beneficial effect of human milk.

Thus, the study of milk provides a model system for conceptualizing key aspects of the development of human immunity and identifying vital keys for positive intervention.

HUMAN MILK ANTIBODIES

Human milk is very rich in antibodies. Several years ago, it was demonstrated that these antibodies were primarily composed of secretory IgA (sIgA) antibodies and especially adapted for the defense of mucosal membranes (1). A fully breast-fed infant receives as much as 0.5-1.0 g sIgA daily, which should be compared with the about 2.5 g synthesized daily by an adult. The milk sIgA is produced as part of the common mucosal immune defense system. This means that the sIgA is synthesized in the mammary glands by lymphocytes which have homed mainly from the gut-associated lymphoid tissues, GALT or Peyer's patches, but also possibly from the BALT (bronchus-associated lymphoid tissue). As a result, human milk contains sIgA antibodies against the many microorganisms present within the mother's gut, and probably also her lungs. Therefore, the breast-fed baby receives large amounts of sIgA antibodies against the microbial agents most likely to be present on mucous membranes after birth. We have recently shown in an experimental system that the nature of the antigen and the stage of maturation of the responding lymphocytes affects homing and appearance of various antibodies in different secretions (7).

Human milk also contains IgG and IgM antibodies, but at much lower concentrations than sIgA (8). Some of the milk IgG and IgM may also be locally produced, although this has not been settled (1,9,10). The IgM transferred to the infant via the milk is only a few milligrams per day, whereas about 20 mg/day of IgG is obtained during early lactation and thereafter declining, often becoming undetectable (8).

MODE OF FUNCTION OF HUMAN MILK ANTIBODIES

The sIgA antibodies function mainly by binding microbes, preventing their contact with mucosal membranes primarily in the respiratory and gastrointestinal tracts. Without that contact viruses and bacteria cannot initiate infection. This type of defense protects without involving host tissues, as happens when IgG-IgM-complement-neutrophils as well as T lymphocytes-lymphokines-macrophages mediate their protective, but tissue-damaging, inflammation. Not only sIgA, but also many other defense factors in milk, provide their effects in a noninflammatogenic manner, which presumably is advantageous to the infant (6,11).

THE EFFECT OF BREAST-FEEDING ON INFECTIONS AND COLONIZATION OF THE INFANT

There is overwhelming evidence that breast-feeding protects against gastroenteritis. Actually, the risk of morbidity and mortality in diarrhea is increased manyfold in the non–breast-fed infant (12-14). There are also suggestions that breast-feeding can protect against otitis media and various respiratory tract infections (12,15-18). Recent studies show that even partial breast-feeding protects against neonatal sepsis in a developing country (19).

Among the host defense factors in human milk, only sIgA has been completely proven to be protective (20). Thus, Glass et al. (21) showed that the protection of breast-fed infants against cholera related to the level of sIgA antibodies in the mothers' milk to *Vibrio cholerae* O antigen and enterotoxin. It has been demonstrated similarly that milk sIgA protects the baby against diarrhea caused by *Campylobacter* (22) and enterotoxin-producing *Escherichia coli* (23).

One factor that may influence the efficiency in the protective capacity of milk sIgA is binding efficiency, measured as avidity. We have noticed that avidity of milk sIgA antibodies to poliovirus and diphtheria toxin was significantly higher in Swedish than Pakistani mothers (24). Furthermore, the Swedish mothers kept their higher levels of avidity rather constant during the first several weeks of lactation, whereas the Pakistani mothers first showed increasing avidity, but then decreased again. It is not clear whether this difference is due to inadequate nutrition and/or heavy microbial exposure in the Pakistani compared to the Swedish mothers. It is of importance to try to determine whether or not the antibodies of lower avidity may confer immunity less well. We also found that the naturally exposed Pakistani women responded well to parenteral but not to oral *V. cholerae* and *S. typhimurium* vaccines (25).

It was a surprise to note that fully breast-fed infants were colonized with *E. coli* against which there were sIgA antibodies in the mothers' milk, both against the O and the K antigens (26,27). The explanation may be that the gut is a large reservoir containing such enormous numbers of microorganisms that it becomes impossible for any amount of antibodies to affect the presence of the bacteria. Their most important function is presumably not to keep the bacteria away, but to try to keep their numbers down and to prevent or limit attachment to the gut mucosa. Artificial colonization with a particular strain of *E. coli* possessing type 1 fimbriae has been found to block subsequent growth of other strains with the same type of fimbriae (28), and this observation supports the hypothesis of limitation.

Recent preliminary studies of colonization of the oral cavity by pneumococci and *Haemophilus influenzae* in breast-fed and non–breast-fed infants suggest that in this much smaller fluid volume (about 2 ml in an adult) the milk immune factors may even affect the colonization (29). The inhibitory activity was associated with human milk kappa casein for *Sreptococcus pneumoniae* and with whole casein for inhibition of *H. influenzae*.

Most recently, it was actually suggested that sIgA antibodies induced by oral vaccination against *Streptococcus mutans* can in fact depress the appearance of these cariogenic bacteria in the oral cavity (30). This would suggest that at local sites milk sIgA may also influence colonization.

A requirement for sIgA antibodies to function especially in the gut is their stability. Two studies have indicated that in spite of this stability part of the milk sIgA consumed by the breast-fed infant is destroyed during its passage through the gut. Prentice et al. (31) showed that about 20% of the milk sIgA remained unaffected in the stool, whereas Davidsson and Lönnerdahl (32) found between 10 and 80% to be still detectable. However, it is not quite excluded that intact SIgA antibodies could still remain attached to the innumerous bacteria in the stool.

Human milk contains several oligosaccharides, glucoproteins and glycolipids. Among these has been identified a disaccharide which is an analogue of the receptor for pneumococci on pharyngeal epithelial cells (33). Human milk as well as this oligosaccharide can prevent pneumococci from adhering to such epithelial cells (34). Furthermore, milk contains a not yet fully identified macromolecule which can prevent the attachment of *H. influenzae* to such cells (29,34). Human milk also contains components which can block adherence of *V. cholerae* and *E. coli* enterotoxins to gut epithelium (35–37). It is possible that such receptor analogs in the milk can be important for the prevention of otitis media, respiratory infections, and gastroenteritis. It may well be that they are also important for regulation of the early colonization of the gut in the newborn. In Pakistani infants, we have seen a rapid appearance in the stool of several species of enterobacteria, clearly earlier than in Swedish infants (4). It is likely that the receptor analogs in the milk are of considerable significance for infants who are heavily exposed to microbes directly after birth. Our knowledge about these components in the milk is, however, very limited. A role for oligosaccharide receptor analogs in inhibiting attachment of bacteria causing urinary tract infections has been postulated (3,38). Further, neutral oligosaccharides have been found to block adhesion of *E. coli* to uroepithelial cells (38), which may underly our experience that breast-feeding showed a negative correlation with pyelonephritis in young children (3).

In addition to the passive protective effect of milk sIgA on the breast-fed infant, the possibility also exists that anti-idiotypic antibodies in the milk may prime the infant for production of the corresponding idiotype. In preliminary studies, we have in fact found evidence for anti-antipoliovirus antibodies in human milk as well as in commercial immunoglobulin (39). Furthermore, Stein and Söderström (40) showed in mice that monoclonal anti-idiotypic antibodies against the *E. coli* K13 polysaccharide capsule, transferred to the offsprings via the milk, could prime them for this antigen.

It has been demonstrated (41-43) that breast-fed infants have more sIgA in their urine than non–breast-fed. We noticed that the response in salivary sIgA antibodies to vaccination with diphtheria and tetanus toxoid as well as poliovirus type 1 was significantly higher in breast-fed than formula-fed infants (44). Several studies have suggested that breast-fed infants may have lower serum IgA levels than non–breast-fed (45,46). The reason for this is not clear, but may be due to an increased exposure to food and microbial antigens in the non–breast-fed.

Koutras and Vigorita (47) observed enhanced fecal sIgA in breast-fed compared to non–breast-fed infants by 2 weeks of age, which, however, was not strictly related to the level of sIgA in breast milk and appeared attributable to the stimulatory effect of breast milk on immunological development of the gastrointestinal tract. The non–breast-fed infants received an iron-free formula. As noted in Chapter 32, the addition of iron to their formulas may also increase fecal sIgA in infants. Whether this relates to increased gut colonization by bacteria or direct stimulation of the immune system is debatable. However, as noted previously, the protective qualities of breast milk are apparently not mediated through prevention of particular bacterial species from entry to the infant gastrointestinal milieu, but more probably by reducing the degree of colonization and influencing the balance of species.

BREAST-FEEDING AND ALLERGY

It has been considered that breast-feeding could result in antigen avoidance and protect the infant against food allergy, but this has not really been substantiated in spite of several studies. However, ongoing projects suggest that a diet for the breast-feeding mother under certain circumstances may have effect (48,49).

The level of sIgA antibodies in milk to a food antigen relates to the mother's intake of that food (50,51). Machtinger and Moss (52) showed interestingly that the risk of development of cow's milk allergy in breast-fed infants was inversely related to the level of IgA antibodies to cow's milk protein in the mothers' milk.

VACCINATION AND HUMAN MILK ANTIBODIES

Parenteral cholera vaccination of mothers who had been naturally exposed and already had a sIgA response gave a booster in milk as well as saliva (53). A similar booster effect was induced by parenteral poliovirus vaccination, but not by peroral poliovaccination, which often decreased the milk sIgA anti-polio antibodies (54). Peroral exposure to an *E. coli* 083 and a live *Shigella* vaccine gave sIgA antibodies in the milk (55,56), as did a *S. mutans* vaccine (30). A cowpea protein induced milk sIgA antibodies whether or not the mothers were undernourished (57).

An earlier study suggested that infants on a low-protein formula responded less well than breast-fed infants or infants on a high-protein formula to tetanus and diphtheria toxoid as well as to poliovirus vaccination (57). We have recently demonstrated, however, that the serum IgG, IgA, and IgM antibody responses to these three vaccines were not significantly different in infants fed a formula with only 1.1 g/100 ml of protein compared to a group fed a formula with 1.5 g protein/100 ml (44), although the low-protein formula group had a much higher serum neutralizing titer to polio virus after the second vaccine dose. In contrast, the breast-fed group showed better serum responses to peroral and parenteral vaccines at 21-40 months of age than either of the formula-fed groups. Secretory responses were better shortly after the vaccinations. One explanation for this difference could be the presence of anti-idiotypic antibodies in transplacental Ig and milk sIgA, in combination, so that the immune system of the breast-fed infant would be more responsive to subsequent immunization (39).

CONCLUSIONS

It is quite clear that human milk contains several components of importance for the passive protection of the infant, especially against gastroenteritis, but also against respiratory tract infections. Among these components so far only sIgA has been proven to provide protection, although a role for oligosaccharide receptor analogs is strongly indicated (29,34,78). The receptor analogs blocking microbial attachment to mucosae and present in milk can block or impede bacterial colonization on mucosal membranes and potentially act against, e.g., urinary tract infections (58) and may well prevent other infections, as yet unrecognized, as well.

Vaccination can be used to increase the specific sIgA antibodies in the mother's milk. Such antibody responses may include anti-idiotypic antibodies (39) which may prime the breast-fed infant to active immunity.

ACKNOWLEDGMENTS

Our studies were supported by grants from the Swedish Medical Research Council (No. 215), the Ellen, Walter and Lennart Hesselman Foundation for Scientific Research, first of May Flower Campaign and the Medical Faculty of Göteborg University. This paper was written while L Å H was the first Sir Clavering Fison Visiting Professor at the Institute of Child Health in London.

REFERENCES

1. Hanson L Å, Adlerberth I, Carlsson B, Coffman K, Dahlgren U, Nilsson K, Jalil F, Roberton D (1988). Mucosal immunity—from past to present. Monogr. Allergy 24:1.

2. Hanson LÅ, Adlerberth I, Carlsson B, Zaman S, Hahn-Zoric M, Jalil F 1990. Antibody-mediated immunity in the neonate. Padiatr und Padolog 25:371.
3. Mårild S, Jodal U, Hanson LÅ. 1990. Breast feeding and urinary tract infection. Lancet 336:942.
4. Adlerberth K, Carlsson B, deMan P, Jalil F, Khan SR, Larsson P, Mellander L, Svanborg Edén C, Wold AE, Hanson LÅ. Intestinal colonization with *Enterobacteriaceae* in Pakistani and Swedish hospital-delivered infants. Acta Paediatr Scand 80:61.
5. Mincheva-Nilsson L, Hammarström P, Juto P, Hammarström S 1990. Human milk contains proteins that stimulate and suppress T lymphocyte proliferation. Clin Exp Immunol 79:463.
6. Goldman AS, Goldblum RM, Hanson LÅ. 1990. Anti-inflammatory systems in human milk. Adv Exp Med Biol 262:69.
7. Dahlgren UI, Wold AE, Hanson LÅ, Midtvedt T. 1990. The secretory antibody response in milk and bile against fimbriae and LPS in rats monocolonized or immunized in the Peyer's patches with *Escherichia coli*. Immunology 71:295.
8. McClelland DBL, McGrath J, Samson RR. 1978. Antimicrobial factors in human milk. Studies of concentration and transfer to the infant during the early stages of lactation. Acta Paediatr Scand 67(suppl 271):1.
9. Brandtzaeg P. 1983. The secretory immune system of lactating human mammary glands compared with other exocrine organs. Am NY Acad Sci 409:353.
10. Keller MA, Heiner DC, Kidd RM, Myers AS. 1983. Local production of IgG4 in human colostrum. J Immunol 130:1654.
11. Goldman AS, Thorpe LW, Goldblum RM, Hanson LÅ. 1986. An hypothesis: anti-inflammatory properties of human milk. Acta Paediatr Scand 75:689.
12. Feachem RG, Koblinsky MA. 1984. Interventions for the control of diarrhoeal diseases among young children: Promotion of breastfeeding. Bull WHO 62:271.
13. Hanson LÅ, Bergström S. 1990. The link between infant mortality and birth rates—The importance of breast feeding as a common cause. Acta Paediatr Scand 79:481.
14. Hanson LÅ, Adlerberth I, Carlsson B, Castrignano SB, Dahlgren LH, Jalil F, Khan SR, Mellander L, Edén CS, Svennerholm AM, Wold A. 1989. Host defense for the neonate and the intestinal flora. Acta Paediatr Scand 351:122.
15. Saarinen UM. 1982. Prolonged breastfeeding as prophylaxis for recurrent otitis media. Acta Paediatr Scand 71:567.
16. Kovar MG, Serdula MK, Marks JS, Fraser DW. 1984. Review of the epidemiologic evidence for an association between infant feeding and infant health. Pediatrics 74(suppl):615.
17. Cochi SL, Fleming DW, Heightower AW, Broome CV. Reply to: Rulin DH, Palmer LS, Menasse L, Erenberg FG. 1987. Does breast-feeding protect infants from *Haemophilus influenzae* infection? J Pediatr 110:162.
18. Victora CG, Vaughn JP, Lombardi C, Fuchs SM, Gigante LP, Smith PG, Noble LC, Teixeira AMB, Moreira LB, Banos FC. 1987. Evidence for protection by breast-feeding against infant deaths from infectious diseases in Brasil. Lancet 2:319.
19. Ashraf RV, Jalil F, Zaman S, Karlberg J, Khan SR, Lindblad BS, Hanson LÅ. 1991. Breast feeding and protection against neonatal spesis in a high risk population. Arch Dis Child 66:488.
20. Hanson LÅ, Ashraf R, Cruz JB, Hahn-Zoric M, Jalil F, Nave F, Reimer M, Zaman S, Carlsson B. 1990. Immunity related to exposure and bacterial colonization of the infant. Acta Paediatr Scand 365:38.
21. Glass RE, Svennerholm A-M, Stoll BJ, Khan MR, Hossain KMB, Huq MI, Holmgren, J. 1983. Protection against cholera in breast-fed children by antibodies in breast milk. N Engl J Med 308:1389.
22. Ruiz-Palacios GM, Calva JJ, Pickering L, Lopez-Vidal Y, Volkow P, Pezzarozi H, West MS. 1990. Protection of breast-fed infants against *Campylobacter* diarrhea by antibodies in human milk. J Pediatr 116:707.

23. Cruz JR, Gil L, Cano P, Caceres P, Pareja G. 1988. Breast milk anti-*Escherichia coli* heat-labile toxin IgA antibodies protect against toxin-induced infantile diarrhea. Acta Paediatr Scand 77:658.
24. Roberton DM, Carlsson B, Coffman K. Hahn-Zoric M, Jalil F, Jones C, Hanson L Å. 1988. Avidity of IgA antibody to *Escherichia coli* polysaccharide and diphtheria toxin in breast milk from Swedish and Pakistani mothers. Scand J Immunol 28:783.
25. Hahn-Zoric M, Carlsson B, Jalil F, Mellander L, Germanier R, Hanson L Å. 1989. The influence on the secretory IgA antibody levels in lactating women of oral typhoid and parenteral cholera vaccines given alone or in combination. Scand J Infect Dis 21:421.
26. Carlsson B, Gothefors L, Ahlstedt S, Hanson L Å, Winberg J. 1976. Studies of *Escherichia coli* O-antigen specific antibodies in human milk, maternal serum and cord blood. Acta Paediatr Scand 65:216.
27. Carlsson B, Kaijser B, Ahlstedt S, Gothefors L, Hanson, L Å. 1982. Antibodies against *Escherichia coli* capsular K-antigens in human milk and serum. Their relation to the *E. coli* gut flora of the mother and neonate. Acta Paediatr Scand 71:313.
28. Slaulkova M, Lodinová Zádniková R, Hanson L Å, Adlerberth I, Carlsson B, Wold AE, Svanborg Edén C. 1990. The influence of artificial colonization with *E. coli* strain 083 on the intestinal flora in infants. Folio Microbiol 35:266.
29. Aniansson G, Andersson B, Lindstedt R, Svanborg C. 1990. Antiadhesive activity of human casein against *Streptococcus pneumoniae* and *Haemophilus influenzae*. Microb Pathol 8:315.
30. Gregory RL, Filler SJ. 1987. Protective secretory immunoglobulin A antibodies in humans following oral immunization with *Streptococcus mutans*. Infect Immun 55:2409.
31. Prentice A, Ewing G, Roberts SB, Lucas A, MacCarthy A, Jargon LMA, Whitehead RG. 1987. The nutritional role of breast-milk IgA and lactoferrin. Acta Paediatr Scand 76:592.
32. Davidson LA, Lönnerdal B. 1987. Persistence of human milk proteins in the breast-fed infant. Acta Paediatr Scand 76:733.
33. Andersson B, Dahmén J, Frejd T, Leffler H, Magnusson G, Noori G, Svanborg Edén C. 1983. Identification of an active disaccharide unit of glycoconjugate receptor for pneumococci attaching to human pharyngeal epithelial cells. J Exp Med 158:559.
34. Andersson B, Porras O, Hanson L Å, Lagergård T, Svanborg Edén C. 1986. Inhibition of attachment of *Streptococcus pneumoniae* and *Haemophilus influenzae* by human milk and receptor oligosaccharides. J Infect Dis 153:232.
35. Holmgren J, Svennerholm A-M, Åhrén C. 1981. Non-immunoglobulin fraction of human milk inhibits bacterial adhesion (hemagglutination) and enterotoxin binding of *Escherichia coli* and *Vibrio cholerae*. Infect Immun 33:136.
36. Holmgren J, Svennerholm A-M, Lindblad M. 1983. Receptor-like glycocompounds in human milk that inhibit classical and El Tor *Vibrio cholerae* cell adherence (hemagglutination). Infect Immun 39:147.
37. Otnaess AB, Laegreid A, Ertesvåg K. 1983. Inhibition of enterotoxin from *E. coli* and *V. cholerae* by gangliosides from human milk. Infect Immun 40:563.
38. Coppa GV, Gabrielli O, Giorgi P, Catassi C, Montanari MP, Varaldo PE, Nicholas BC. 1990. Preliminary study of breast feeding and bacterial adhesion to uroepithelial cells. Lancet 335:569.
39. Hanson L Å, Carlsson B, Ekre HP, Hahn-Zoric M, Osterhaus AD, Roberton D. 1989. Immunoregulation mother-fetus/newborn, a role for anti-idiotypic antibodies. Acta Paediatr Scand 351(suppl):38.
40. Stein KE, Söderström T. 1984. Neonatal administration of idiotype and anti-idiotype primes for protection against *E. coli* K13 infection in mice. J Exp Med 160:1001.
41. Goldblum RM, Schanler R, Garza C, Goldman AS. 1987. The effect of feeding human milk on the development of immunity in low birth weight infants. In: Human Lactation 3. The Effects of Human Milk on the Recipient Infant. Eds. A Goldman, S Atkinson, L Å Hanson. Plenum Press, New York, p. 246.

42. Prentice A. 1987. Breastfeeding increases concentrations of IgA in infants urine. Arch Dis Child 62:792.
43. Schanler RJ, Goldblum RM, Garza C, Goldman AS. 1986. Enhanced fecal excretion of selected immune factors in very low birth weight infants fed fortified human milk. Pediatr Res 20:711.
44. Hahn-Zoric M, Fulconis F, Minoli I, Moro G, Carlsson B, Böttiger M, Räihä N, Hanson L Å. 1990. Antibody responses to parenteral and oral vaccines are impaired by conventional and low protein formulas as compared to breast feeding Acta Paediatr Scand 79:1137.
45. Savilahti E, Järvenpää AL, Räihä N. 1983. Serum immunoglobulins in preterm infants: Comparison of human milk and formula feeding. Pediatrics 72:312.
46. Saarinen UM, Pelkonen P, Siimes MA. 1979. Serum immunoglobulin A in healthy infants: an accelerated postnatal increase in formula-fed, compared to breast-fed infants. J Pediatr 95:410.
47. Koutras AK, Vigorita VJ. 1989. Fecal secretory immunoglobulin A in breast milk versus formula feeding in early infancy. J Pediatr Gastroenterol Nutr 9:58.
48. Chandra RK, Puri S, Suraiya C, Cheema PS. 1986. Influence of maternal food antigen avoidance during pregnancy and lactation on incidence of atopic eczema in infants. Clin Allergy 16:563.
49. Hattevig G, Kjellman B, Sigurs N, Björksten B, Kjellman NM. 1989. The effect of maternal avoidance of eggs, cow's milk and fish during lactation upon allergic manifestations of infants. Clin Exp Allergy 19:27.
50. Hanson L Å, Ashraf R, Carlsson R, Jalil F, Strannegård IL, Porras O, de Soto M, Zaman S, Ahlstedt S. 1990. The immunologist and the developing world. Scand J Immunol 31: 127.
51. Cruz JR, Garcia B, Urrutia JJ, Carlsson B, Hanson L Å. 1981. Food antibodies in human milk from Guatemalan women. J Paediatr 99:600.
52. Machtinger S, Moss R. 1986. Cow's milk allergy in breastfed infants: the role of allergen and maternal secretory IgA antibody. J Allergy Clin Immun 77:341.
53. Svennerholm A-M, Hanson L Å, Holmgren J, Lindblad BS, Nilsson B, Quereshi F. 1980. Different secretory IgA antibody response to cholera vaccination in Swedish and Pakistani women. Infect Immun 30:427.
54. Svennerholm A-M, Hanson L Å, Holmgren J, Lindblad BS, Khan SR, Nilson A, Svennerholm B. 1981. Milk antibodies to live and killed polio vaccines in Pakistani and Swedish mothers. J Infect Dis 143:707.
55. Goldblum RM, Ahlstedt S, Carlsson B, Hanson L Å, Jodal C, Lidin-Janson G, Sohl-Åkerlund A. 1975. Antibody forming cells in human colostrum after oral immunization. Nature 257:797.
56. Hanson L Å, Carlsson B, Cruz JR, Garcia G, Holmgren J, Raza Kahn S, Lindblad BS, Svennerholm A-M, Svennerholm B, Urrutia JJ. 1979. The immune response of the mammary gland. In: Immunology of Breast Milk. Eds. PL Ogra, DH Dayton. Raven Press, New York, p 145.
57. Cruz JR, Hanson L Å. 1986. Specific milk immune response of rural and urban Guatemalan women to oral immunization with a food protein. J Pediatr Gastroent Nutr 5:450.
58. Zoppi G, Mantovanelli F, Astolfi R, Gasparini R, Gobio-Casak L, Crovari P. 1983. Diet and antibody response to vaccinations in healthy infants. Lancet 2:11.
59. Mårild S, Jodal U, Mangelus L. 1989. Medical histories of children with acute pyelonephritis compared with controls. Pediatr Infect Dis J 8:511.

36
Dietary Antigens and Regulation of the Mucosal Immune Response

Warren Strober
*National Institute of Allergy and Infectious Diseases,
National Institutes of Health, Bethesda, Maryland*

INTRODUCTION

Certain chapters in this volume focus attention on the spectrum of interactions occurring between the mucosal immune system and the antigens in the mucosal environment. On the one hand, Troncone and his colleagues in Ferguson's laboratory consider the mucosal immune processes that led to either unresponsiveness to nonpathogenic mucosal antigens or a responsiveness that might be a cause of disease, such as gluten-sensitive enteropathy. On the other hand, Cunningham-Rundles discusses in detail the mucosal immune processes that leads to exclusion of antigens from the internal milieu, which if defective because of IgA deficiency, leads to autoantibody formation and possible autoimmune disease. These processes quite obviously involve very different aspects of mucosal immune function; nevertheless, they may be related to one another by the cellular mechanisms that underlie mucosal antibody responses. In this chapter, this possibility is examined and, in doing so, some of the more unique aspects of the mucosal immune system are explored.

ANTIGEN-SPECIFIC REGULATION OF MUCOSAL IMMUNE RESPONSES

As alluded to by Troncone and his colleagues, an important aspect of stimulation of the mucosal immune system is that such stimulation frequently causes overall immune unresponsiveness (oral tolerance) (1,2). To date, the most clearly documented explanation of this phenomenon is that oral antigen administration leads to an immune response (in the Peyer's patches) dominated by antigen-specific suppressor T cells, which, following systemic dissemination, prevent responses to the antigen administered by any route (1,2). Suppressor T cells in Peyer's patches (and in other lymphoid sites) have in the past been thought to arise from an elaborate suppressor T-cell network composed of interacting T cells triggered in an ordered fashion by particular kinds of antigen-presenting cells either directly or via antigen-specific or idiotype-specific suppressor factors; in addition, it was thought that some of the antigen-specific suppressor factors were the actual mediators of suppression (2-4). However, this concept can no longer be regarded as tenable in view of the inability of investigators in the field to define the aforementioned suppressor factors in molecular terms and/or to relate such factors to well-defined T-cell recognition molecules, i.e., T-cell receptors. Another possibility, one that has yet to be proven, is that certain forms of antigen presentation to T cells induce the latter to synthesize and secrete antigen-nonspecific suppressor cytokines or lymphokines. In this view, the apparent antigen specificity of the suppressor T cells results from the fact that specific antigen is necessary to obtain the cell-cell interactions necessary for suppressor effects. This second mechanism has the advantage that it preserves the validity of antigen-specific suppressor phenomena, whereas dispensing with the nettlesome idea that such phenomena are necessarily mediated by a unique class of suppressor factors.

In that our knowledge of antigen-specific immune suppression mediated by T cells is still uncertain, we are hard put to identify the reason why suppressor T-cell development is favored over helper T-cell development in the Peyer's patches. Are the antigen-presenting cells that interact with T cells in the patches somehow better able to induce suppressor T cells than helper T cells? If so, how do these antigen-presenting cells differ from those present elsewhere in the immune system? Alternatively, are the T cells developing in the patches more likely to become T cells capable of mediating suppression regardless of how they are presented with antigen, and if this is the case, what factors do these suppressor T cells produce that bring about suppression? Clearly, these questions must be answered if we are to gain a full understanding of a key aspect of mucosal immune function.

IMMUNOGLOBULIN CLASS-SPECIFIC REGULATION OF MUCOSAL IMMUNE RESPONSES

An important and somewhat surprising feature of the immune unresponsiveness that follows oral antigen administration is that it is to some extent Ig class specific. Thus, while IgG and IgE responses may become profoundly suppressed following oral antigen administration, IgA responses may be less suppressed, unaffected, or even enhanced (5). One striking example of this is seen when antigen is fed to mice for long periods of time (6). In this situation there is an initial IgG antibody response which is followed (after several weeks) by suppression of the response unless agents are administrated which abrogate the development of suppressor T cells such as cyclophosphamide. In contrast, the initial IgA antibody response is not suppressed during the same time period either in the presence or absence of cyclophosphamide.

The basis of this Ig class-specific suppression is also not well understood, but probably is the result of induction of regulatory T cells which effect IgG and IgA responses in different ways. This view is favored by the findings of Richman et al. (and later by Mattingly), who showed some years ago that oral immunization with ovalbumin induced a predominantly helper T-cell response for IgA anti-ovalbumin responses and, a little later, a predominantly suppressor T-cell response for IgG anti-ovalbumin responses (7,8). A possible mechanism of this differential regulatory T-cell function is suggested by the studies of Kiyono et al., in which it was shown that T-cell hybridomas bearing IgA-Fc receptors provide preferential help for IgA synthesis as opposed to IgG synthesis (9). Such T cells may influence IgA responses via release of a factor that binds to secretory IgA (sIgA) on sIgA-bearing B cells (10). Alternatively, it is possible that T cells bearing IgA-Fc receptors are better able to undergo isotype-specific cell-cell interactions with IgA B cells than T cells not bearing IgA-Fc receptors, and that these interactions allow focusing of isotype-nonspecific regulatory lymphokines such as interleukin 5 (IL-5) and IL-4 on sIgA-bearing B cells rather than on cells bearing other surface isotypes.

These data relating to IgA-specific helper cells are complemented by data presented by Lynch and his colleagues on Ig class-specific suppressor cells in general (11). In the relevant studies these investigators have shown that T-cell populations obtained from mice with plasmacytomas contain increased numbers of T cells bearing Fc receptors of the isotype of the plasmacytoma, and that such T cells have isotype-specific suppressor activity (11). Taken in conjunction with those of Kiyono et al., these findings suggest that the enhancement of IgA responses following oral antigen challenge is due to the induction of IgA-specific (?IgA-Fc receptor-bearing) helper T cells which regulate sIgA-bearing B cells in a positive fashion and, conversely, the concomitant suppression of IgG responses is due to the presence of IgG-specific suppressor T cells regulating sIgG-bearing B cells in a negative fashion.

A final mechanism of preferential help for IgA, one unrelated to IgA-Fc receptor-bearing T cells, is suggested by recent findings that a particular lymphokine, tumor growth factor beta (TGF-β), has the ability to induce IgM to IgA isotype switching, whereas at the same time suppressing expression of other isotypes (12). This finding allows one to entertain the possibility that IgA-specific help at mucosal sites is due to release of particular cytokines.

SIGNIFICANCE OF IMMUNOGLOBULIN CLASS-SPECIFIC REGULATION

An important outcome of the fact that the mucosal immune system is oriented toward suppression of IgG responses but not IgA responses is that the overall mucosal antibody output consists largely of IgA, an antibody class exquisitely tailored to an antigenic environment in which the task of the immune system is not necessarily to kill pathogens, but rather to prevent their colonization of the mucosal surface. In this regard, it is well established that secretory IgA is specifically delivered to and focused on the mucosal surface (via secretory component-mediated transport), that secretory IgA is multivalent (and thus can agglutinate potential pathogens), and that secretory IgA is resistant to digestive enzymes (13). In addition, it is known that IgA antibodies induce complement activation poorly, and thus greatly reduce the potential of the multitude of substances in the mucosal area to induce inflammation (14).

A second way in which the simultaneous suppression of IgG responses and preservation of the IgA responses in the mucosal immune system may be advantageous to the organism relates to the possibility that such a response profile guards against the development of autoimmunity. To understand how this is so we must digress to a brief discussion of the abnormal immune processes that are currently thought to be responsible for the development of certain forms of (systemic) autoimmune disease.

It is now well established that the normal B-cell repertoire contains cells that produce polyspecific antibodies that react with both biochemically simple environmental antigens and self-antigens (15,16). For the most part, these B cells utilize germline V-region genes and produce IgM-class antibodies that react with self-antigens with relatively low affinity. Recently, it has been shown that these B cells may undergo antigen-driven somatic mutation and selection to develop into B cells producing IgG-class antibodies that react with high affinity with conventional (exogenous) antigens and that do not react at all with self-antigens (17). On this basis, it is useful to think of the B cells producing polyspecific antibodies as a reservoir of cells from which the normal immune system can rapidly derive its usual complement of memory cells.

These polyspecific B cells pose no threat to normal individuals, since, as suggested above, they do not produce antibodies with capacity for immune injury. There is growing evidence, however, that in autoimmune states such B cells (a) undergo isotype switching to develop into IgG-producing cells that retain V-region germline configuration and polyspecificity; and (b) undergo somatic mutation and isotype switching to develop into IgG-producing cells that have an altered V-region configuration and a high affinity for self-antigens. The precise mechanism of this abnormal development is unknown, but it is clear that it can only occur in the presence of an abnormal T-cell regulatory environment, and that in addition some clonally distributed B-cell abnormality must also be present (16). Overall, then, certain forms of autoimmunity can be the result of the abnormal differentiation of normally occurring B cells with autoimmune potential, and therefore the key defect in these forms of autoimmunity is a problem in T-cell regulation of particular B cells rather than the de novo occurrence of autoimmune B cells.

These considerations relate to mucosal immune responses because the mucosal environment is replete with simple antigens such as those mentioned above that react with polyspecific B cells capable of producing autoantibodies (18). Thus, it seems reasonable to suggest that the T cell-mediated suppression of IgG responses so prominent in normal mucosal tissues plays a dual role: It prevents potentially inflammatory (IgG-mediated) responses in the mucosa and, more germane to this discussion, it prevents the emergence of autoimmune B cells that produce high-affinity IgG antibodies. In the same vein, the ability of mucosal T cells to direct differentiation into an IgA pathway may be a way of allowing the development of B cells that react with high affinity to biochemically simple antigens (and concomitant high-affinity reactivity to self-antigens) without at the same time allowing development of "inflammatory" IgG antibodies that could mediate autoimmune disease.

Evidence that supports the above viewpoint has been gathered in numerous studies of mouse models of autoimmune disease (16). One example that is particular relevant to the mucosal immune response relates to an animal model of IgA nephropathy in which glomerulopathy is caused by deposition of immune complexes in the kidney (6). In these studies, it has been shown that IgA nephropathy can be induced in certain mouse strains by chronic feeding of protein antigens provided that normal suppressor T-cell responses are intact. Thus, if mice are fed antigen, IgA but not IgG antibody-antigen complexes are subsequently deposited in the kidney, presumably because of differential isotype regulation; in this case, no disease develops. In contrast, if mice are fed antigen and at the same time are treated with the anti-T-cell agent cyclophosphamide (which abrogates the suppressor T-cell response), both IgA and

IgG complexes are deposited in the kidney; in this case, disease develops. Thus, it appears that channeling of responses into an IgA pathway leads to the avoidance of autoimmune disease.

Yet another aspect of mucosal immune function that relates to autoimmunity concerns the well-known fact that circulating IgA can be taken up in the liver (19,20). In rodents, it can be shown that hepatic uptake is mediated by secretory component receptors on biliary epithelial and hepatic parenchymal cell surfaces (19). In contrast, in humans, hepatic uptake is mediated by asialoglycoprotein receptors present on hepatic parenchymal cells (20). Whatever uptake mechanism is involved, these findings suggest that IgA is a key component of a clearance pathway that prevents antigens that manage to breach the mucosal barrier from reaching systemic lymphoid tissues. Since, as alluded to above, systemic lymphoid tissue may have a greater tendency to mount helper T-cell responses than mucosal lymphoid tissues, IgA-mediated antigen clearance becomes another way of shunting responses to mucosal antigens (that may mimic self-antigens) into the controlled regulatory environment of the Peyer's patch.

RELATION OF MUCOSAL REGULATORY MECHANISMS TO SPECIFIC DISEASE

The above discussion sets the stage for a reconsideration of gluten-sensitive enteropathy and IgA deficiency as well as the relationship between these diseases. We can now see that gluten-sensitive enteropathy is best considered an antigen-specific "break" in the general tendency of the mucosal immune system to react to common environmental antigens with suppressor T cell-dominated responses, with the result that there is the production of T-cell and/or B-cell effector cells with the capacity to induce mucosal injury. The basis of this type of disorder relates to the cellular mechanisms governing the regulation of mucosal responses and, as such, cannot be precisely defined as yet. A clue to the nature of this abnormality derives from the fact, discussed in more detail below, that gluten-sensitive enteropathy is associated with certain major histocompatibility complex (MHC) class II genes. This finding allows the suggestion that gluten-sensitive enteropathy is due to the presence of an "immune response gene" that favors cell-cell interactions leading to T-cell help rather than suppression with respect to a particular ingested antigen, gliadin. Such a defect is formally equivalent to an autoimmune response because gliadin, by virtue of its capacity to be taken up and reexpressed by mucosal epithelial cells (as is any food antigen) can in effect be considered a self-antigen.

Whatever cellular mechanism is ultimately shown to be the cause of the abnormal mucosal immune response in gluten-sensitive enteropathy, the ultimate result of the response must be the elaboration of either B-cell or T-cell effectors which actually bring about damage to the absorptive epithelial surface. One might postulate that these consist, at least in part, of B cells producing IgG or IgA antigliadin antibodies, with the former bringing about tissue damage, as in the case of IgA nephropathy. Evidence in favor of this idea is that B cells producing antigliadin can be identified in the lamina propria, and complement is found in the basement membrane zone of lesional tissue (21,22). More likely, however, is the possibility that the effector mechanism consists of gliadin-specific T cells that mediate either direct or indirect lysis of epithelial cells. This latter possibility is consistent with the fact that the villous atrophy of gluten-sensitive enteropathy can be reproduced in animals by activation of mucosal T cells by a mitogen, and that the number of intraepithelial lymphocytes are increased in the disease (23,24).

Like gluten-sensitive enteropathy, IgA deficiency can also be characterized as a defect in the regulation of the mucosal immune response; in this case, involving an entire Ig class rather than a single antigen-specific response. This view represents a departure from the conventional view that the disease is due to an intrinsic defect of IgA B cells. However, it is justified on the basis of emerging evidence that IgA deficiency is part of a spectrum of immunodeficiencies (which include common variable immunodeficiency) that have as their fundamental cellular defect, a failure to secrete the lymphokines necessary for terminal B-cell differentiation (25). This mechanism of IgA deficiency is consistent with the observation that in IgA deficiency, IgM B cells do in fact undergo isotype switching to IgA B cells, so that the defect is one involving terminal expansion of an existing isotype class.

In asserting that IgA deficiency is a T-cell regulatory defect we can draw certain parallels between this disease and gluten-sensitive enteropathy. First, from the discussion above in which the coordinate regulation of IgG and IgA responses in the mucosal system was noted, the possibility arises that both IgA deficiency and gluten-sensitive enteropathy are diseases involving different but related aspects of T-cell function as manifested in the secretion of regulatory lymphokines. It may seem paradoxical that inappropriate upregulation of an antigen-specific response (in this case to gliadin) can be related to abnormal downregulation of an entire Ig class. However, if we assume that suppression of IgG responses and enhancement of IgA responses may depend on secretion of particular (antigen-nonspecific) cytokines, it becomes possible to resolve this paradox. It is possible, for instance, that in both gluten-sensitive enteropathy and in IgA deficiency an abnormality in the production of a cytokine with differential regulatory properties (such as TGF-β) can be instrumental in both diseases. Second, IgA deficiency, like gluten-sensitive enteropathy can also be considered a "break" in mucosal unresponsiveness, although in this case the break is not a primary feature of the disease, but rather a secondary feature occurring as a consequence of a deficient intestinal barrier that leads to a bypass of the suppressor T-cell mechanisms in the Peyer's patches. In this case, because of the more generalized nature of the defect, we see the formation of antibodies against many food antigens, not just gliadin.

A third relationship between IgA deficiency and gluten-sensitive enteropathy, one that in fact solidifies those already discussed, is based on mounting evidence that the two diseases have a common genetic basis. This first became evident in epidemiological studies and family studies in which it was found that the two diseases tend to occur together far more frequently than would be predicted by chance, and there exists certain families in which members develop IgA deficiency, gliadin sensitivity, and certain forms of autoimmunity in different combinations (26). Later, it was established that both diseases (as well as certain forms of autoimmunity) are frequently associated with the same "extended" MHC haplotypes (combinations of MHC alleles which are in linkage disequilibrium) (27-30). The role of these extended haplotypes in the pathogenesis of either gluten-sensitive enteropathy or IgA deficiency is an intriguing and unanswered question. Such haplotypes also occur in large numbers of normal individuals, suggesting that they ordinarily provide some sort of selective advantage, such as a more effective response to certain environmental pathogens. On this basis, one can postulate that they somehow lead to a T-cell regulatory function which is tilted toward certain kinds of increased immune responses. If this is indeed the case, then it is possible that these extended MHC haplotypes, when they occur in association with other genetic (or environmental factors), lead to disease. In gluten-sensitive enteropathy, for instance, the hyperresponsiveness provided by the extended MHC haplotypes may be accompanied by genes that direct the hyperresponsiveness into an abnormal pathway leading to reactivity to gliadin. In IgA deficiency, on the other hand, one might postulate that the extended MHC haplotype, in association with other genetic factors, leads to unbalanced IgG/IgA regulation and IgA deficiency. Obviously, these explanations are still too vague to provide a truly satisfying synthesis of disease pathogenesis. The latter will have to await further insights into the cellular and molecular mechanisms responsible for gluten-sensitive enteropathy and IgA deficiency as well as into the "disease genes" that are responsible for such mechanism.

CONCLUSIONS

In conclusion, gluten-sensitive enteropathy and IgA deficiency represent related abnormalities because they are caused by defects in different but associated aspects of mucosal function, one concerning regulation of antigen-specific responses and another concerning regulation of Ig class-specific responses. In addition, the two diseases have genetic features in common which may ultimately lead to a molecular definition of their interrelatedness. The challenge to further research in this important area of abnormal immune function will be to more specifically define the molecular mechanisms responsible for these diseases, so as to derive more rational and effective treatment.

REFERENCES

1. Strober W, Richman LK, Elson CO (1981). The regulation of gastrointestinal immune responses. Immunol Today 2:156.
2. Mowat AMcl (1987). The regulation of immune responses to dietary protein antigens. Immunol Today 8:93.
3. Asherson GL, Colizzi V, Zembala M (1986). An overview of T-suppressor cell circuits. Ann Rev Immunol 4:37.
4. Gautan SC, Battisto JR (1985). J Immunol 135:2975.
5. Saklayer MG, Pesce AJ, Pollak VE, Michael JG (1984). Kinetics of oral tolerance: Study of variables affecting tolerance induced by oral administration of antigen. Int Arch Allergy Appl Immunol 73:5.
6. Gesualdo L, Emancepator SN, Lamm ME (1990). Defective oral tolerance promotes nepretogenesis in experimental IgA nephropathy induced by oral immunization. J Immunol.
7. Richman LK, Graeff AS, Yarchoan R, Strober W (1981). Simultaneous antigen-specific IgA helper T cell and IgG suppressor T cell induction in the murein Peyer's patch following protein feeding. J Immunol 126:2079-2083.
8. Mattingly JA (1983). Cellular circuiting involved in orally induced systemic tolerance and local antibody induction. Ann NY Acad Sci 409:204.
9. Kiyono H, Cooper MD, Kearney JF et al (1984). Isotype specificity of helper T cell clones. Peyer's patch Th cells preferentially collaborate with mature IgA B cells for IgA responses. J Exp Med 149:798-811.
10. Kiyono H, Mosteller-Barnum LM, Pitts AM, et al (1985). Isotype-specific immunoregulation IgA-binding factors produced by Fcα receptor-positive T cell hybridomas regulate IgA responses. J Exp Med 161:731-747.

11. Williams KR, Lynch RG (1988). Tumor models of isotype-specific regulation. In: Mucosal Immunity and Infections at Mucosal Surfaces. Strober W, Lamm ME, McGhee JR, James SP, eds. New York, Oxford University Press, pp 74-79.
12. Coffman RL, Lebman DA, Shrader B (1989). Transforming growth factor β specifically enhances IgA production by lipopolysaccharide-stimulated murine B lymphoytes. J Exp Med 170:1039.
13. Strober W, Brown WR (1988). The mucosal immune system. In: Immunological Diseases. 4th ed. Samter M, Talmage DW, Frank MM, Austen KF, Claman HN, eds. Little, Brown, Boston/Toronto, p79.
14. Kilian J, Mestecky J, Russel MW (1988). Defence mechanisms involving Fc-dependent functions of immunoglobulin A and their subversion by bacterial immunoglobulin A proteases. Microbiol Rev 52:296.
15. Cairns E, St Germain J, Bell DA (1985). The in vitro production of anti-DNA antibody by cultured peripheral blood or tonsillar lymphoid cells from normal donors and SLE patients. J Immunol 135:3839.
16. Schwartz RS, Datta SK (1989). Autoimmunity and autoimmune diseases. In: Fundamental Immunology. 2nd ed. Paul WE, ed. Raven Press Ltd. New York, p 819.
17. Naparstek Y. Andres-Schwartz J, Manser T, Schwartz RS (1986). A single germline VH gene segment of normal A/J mice encodes autoantibodies characteristic of systemic lupus erythematosus. J Exp Med 164:614.
18. Carroll P, Stafford D, Schwartz RS, Stollar BD (1985). Murine monoclonal anti-DNA autoantibodies bind to endogenous bacteria. J Immunol 135:1086.
19. Underdown BJ, Schiff JM (1986). Immunoglobulin A: Strategic defence initiative at the mucosal surface. Ann Rev Immunol 4:389.
20. Tomana M, Kulhavy R, Mestecky J (1988). Receptor-mediated binding and uptake of immunoglobulin A by human liver. Gastroenterology 94:672.
21. Lycke N, Kilander A, Nilsson L-Å, Tarkowski A, Werner N (1989). Production of antibodies to gliadin in intestinal mucosa of patients with coeliac disease: A study at the single cell level. Gut 30:72.
22. Halstensten TS, Brandtzaeg P (1990). Personal Communication.
23. MacDonald TT, Spencer J (1988). Evidence that activated mucosal T cells play a role in the pathogenesis of enteropathy in human small intestine. J Exp Med 167:1341.
24. Kuitenen P, Kosnai I, Savilahti E (1982). Morphometric study of the jejunal mucosa in various childhood enteropathies with special reference to intraepithelial lymphocyte. J Pediatr Gastroenterol Nutr 1:525.
25. Sneller MC, Strober W (1990). IgA deficiency. Ann Allergy.
26. Van Thiel DH, Smith WI, Rabin BS, Fisher SE, Lester R (1977). A syndrome of immunoglobulin A deficiency diabetes mellitus, malabsorption and a common HLA haplotype. Immunologic and genetic study of forty-three family members. Ann Int Med 86:10.
27. Strober W (1990). Gluten-sensitive enteropathy. In: The Genetic Basis of Common Disease. King R, Motolsky A, Rotter J, eds. New York, Oxford University Press (in press).
28. Wilton AN, Cobain TJ, Dawkins RL (1985). Family studies in IgA deficiency. Immunogenetics 21:333.
29. Bugawan TL, Angelini G, Larrick J, Auricchio S, Ferrara GB, Erlich HA (1989). A combination of a particular HLA-DPβ alleles and a HLA-DQ heterodimer confers susceptibility to coeliac disease. Nature 339:470.
30. Schaffer FM, Palermos J, Zhu ZB, Barger BO, Cooper MD, Volenakis JE (1989). Individuals with IgA deficiency and common variable immunodeficiency share polymorphisms of major histocompatibility complex class II genes. Proc Natl Acad Sci USA 86:8015.

Index

Absorption, gastrointestinal
  after bone marrow transplantation, 354
  bovine casein in hypogamma-
    globulinemia, 347
  dietary antigens in IgA deficiency, 340
  dietary peptides, 346
  high iron (*see* hemochromatosis)
  hyperabsorption, 340, 351, 352
  infancy, 354
  measurement of, 349–350
  milk in IgA deficiency, 340
  polyethylene glycol absorbtion test, 351
Acetominophen and Vitamin A, 69
Acquired immunodeficiency syndrome,
  AIDS, 55, 67, 68, 256, 259, 444
Acrodermatitis enteropathica, 273, 400, 506
Acute phase response, 476
  excessive, 516–518
  nutritional costs of, 476–477
  role in inflammation, 512–513
Adenosine deaminase (ADA), 406
Adenovirus, response in vitro and vitamin
  C, 98, 99
Adjuvant immunotherapy
  of breast cancer with vitamins, 423–437
  in cancer, 369

Adoptive cellular immunotherapy, 95, 375,
  376, 377
Adrenal, 266
Aging
  and caloric restriction, 481, 486
  and carotenoids, 67
  and vitamin E, 226
AIDS (*see* acquired immunodeficiency syndrome)
Albumin, 370
Alcohol
  alcoholic hepatitis, 255
  chronic, 258
  combined with retroviral infection,
    259
  delayed type hypersensitivity, 255
  effect on immune function, 255–262
  lymphocyte subsets, 256, 257, 258
  murine model, 257
  and zinc deficiency, 127
Alkaline phosphatase and zinc deficiency,
  394–95
Allergies
  effect of infant diet on, 312–314, 528
  IgA deficiency and, 340
Allogeneic response, 107

Alpha linoleic acid (flax seed oil), 382
Alphatocopherol, 476
Amino acids
  arginine, 47–61
  citrulline, 49
  dietary deficiency and tumor rejection, 360
  glutamine, 47
  ornithine, 49, 50, 51, 53
  phenylalanine, 47, 154, 360
  synthetic, 155
  tyrosine, 47, 154, 360
Aminoplex, 381
Amyloidosis
  and lipids, 212
  and vitamin E, 226, 231
Anaphylatoxins, 161
Anemia, 413, 505 (*see also* iron)
Anergy, 370
Anorexia in cancer, 376
Anorexia nervosa, 360
Antibody
  absence in hypogammaglobulinemia, 347
  affinity decreased in elderly, 458
  antimilk antibody, 341
  in autoimmune model, 156
  to beta-casomorphin, 347
  to dietary antigens, significance of in IgA deficiency, 345
  and lipid emulsions, 374
  and low protein diet, 360
  and methionine deficiency, 93
  in milk, 302, 525–532
  in primary iron overload, 114
  production, 156, 264, 265, 266, 268
  production and oxysterols, 192
  response and iron, 106, 108
  and vitamin A deficiency, 63
Antibody dependent cellular cytotoxicity, 106, 108, 128
Anti DNA Antibodies, 156
Anti-idiotype
  anticasein antibodies, 345–346
Antioxidants
  butylated hydroxytoluene, 224
  carotenoids and, 67
  free radical-scavenging and vitamin C and E, 82
  N,N-diphenyl-p-phenylenediamine (DPPD), 224
  tocopherol quinone, 224
  torolox C, 224
  vitamin C, 76, 94
  vitamin E, 94, 223–238

Antitumor, 68, 128, 375 (*see also* cytotoxicity)
Antirachitic substance, 3
Apolipoprotein E, 169, 175
  inhibitory activity, 175
  immunoregulatory properties, 169–180
  network, 172
  plasma levels in disease, 175
Apoprotein B, 163, 174
Apoprotein E, 163
Apotransferrin, 117
Arachidonic acid, 132, 133, 158, 163, 211–216, 372
  synthesis from cis-linoleic acid, 134
Arginine
  AIDS, 55
  biosynthesis, 48
  effect on insulin, 49
  effect on prolactin, 49
  effect on thymic involution, 51
  and lymphocyte subsets, 52
  nutrient need in injury, 49
  nutrient requirement, 49
  operative support, 53, 371
  protective role in infection, 51
  relationship to polyamines, 50
  requirement for lymphocyte proliferation, 50
  role in protein synthesis, 48
  and tumor induction, 51, 52
Arteriosclerosis, 157, 194
  polyunsaturated fats and, 386
  and vitamin E, 226
Arthritis
  adjuvant induced, 207–208
  animal studies, 212–213
  and fatty acids, 201–221
  human studies, 214–216
  immune complexes in IgA deficiency and, 342
  and iron intake, 495
  and prostaglandins, 201–221
  rheumatoid, 162, 516
Arthus reaction, 204, 212
Ascorbic acid, ascorbate (*see also* vitamin C)
  detoxification of histamine, 94–95
  detoxifying effects and vitamin E, 92
  depolymerization effects, 92
  and free radical damage, 83
  in infectious disease, 476
  relative tissue levels, 92
  uptake by phagocytes, 76–77
Asialoglycoprotein receptors, 537

Index

Aspirin, 204
Atopic dermatitis, 162
Atopy, 340
Atransferremia, 116
Autoimmune hemolytic anemia, 156, 157
Autoimmune-prone NZB/NZW mice, 227
    (*see also* New Zealand Black mice)
Autoimmunity, 153-167
    anti DNA antibodies and diet, 160
    development of, 536
    fish oil and, 160
    IgA deficiency and, 340
    immune complexes in IgA deficiency, 345
    immune nephritis and, 160
    iron deficiency and, 111
    pathological mechanisms, 160
    protection against, 535
    mouse model, 536
    retroviral gp70 immune complexes and, 160
    role of prostaglandins, 158
    steroids and, 160
Autooxidation, 183 (*see* cholesterol)

Bacterial infections
    clearance and lipid emulsions, 373
    in PCM, 361
Bacterial killing, 81, 130-132 (*see also* phagocytosis)
Balb/3T3 tumor cells
    and vitamin E, 229
B cell (bone marrow derived) (*see also* antibody)
    in elderly, 457
    in mucosal immune response, 536-537
    and zinc deficiency, 128
B cell differentiation factor, 383, 386
B cell growth factor, 374, 383
B cell response (*see also* antibody)
    Bromelian treated RBC response, 157
    and LDL-In, 172
    lipid emulsions and, 374
    in malnutrition, 443, 447
Beef tallow, 160, 212
Beta carotene, 64
    and NK cells, 66
Biological response modifiers, 369, 376
Biotin, 448
Bone and vitamin D_3, 10
Bone marrow
    effect of vitamin D_3 on differentiation, 9
    in PCM, 363

Bone marrow transplantation
    allograft rejection, 25
    in malnutrition, 360
    mucosal immunity in reconstitution, 353
Borage seed oil, 160, 215
Border cells, 339
Bovine antigen absorption in hypogammaglobulinemia, 347, 348
Bovine beta casomorphin, 346
Bovine casein, 340
Bovine casomorphin, 346
Bovine gamma globulin, 340
Bovine milk proteins, 340
Bovine rhinotracheitis virus, 226
Bovine serum albumin in milk, 302
Bradykinin, 203-204
Breast cancer
    adjuvant use of vitamins, 423-439
    aggressive potential, 423
    autologous reactivity to tumor, 424
    and high fat, 485
    prognostic significance of reactivity to tumor, 429-430
    and prolactin, 485
    vitamin therapy and second primary, 433-434
Breast milk, human
    antibodies in, 302, 525-532
    effect on immunological development, 302-312
    effect on vaccinations, 307-311
    iron content, 495
    lymphocytes in, 302
    macrophages in, 302
    modulation of cell function by, 303, 313
    relationship to allergies, 312-314
    relationship to infant mortality, 302
    transfer of tuberculin sensitivity via, 303
    versus infant formulas, 301-318, 525-532
Bronchopulmonary displasia, 231
Burn, 68

Cachectin, 511-519
Calcium, 21, 143, 163
Caloric restriction, 272
    in autoimmunity, 154
    cancer prevention, 481-490
Calorie source, 483 (*see* intravenous feeding fat versus calorie)
Cancer, 164
    adjuvant vitamin therapy of breast cancer, 424
    beta carotene and cancer, 64, 67

Cancer (*continued*)
cachexia, 517
and caloric restriction, 481–490
chronic granulocytic leukemia and vitamin C, 84
colorectal and TPN, 379
effect of arginine on tumor growth, 52
effect of low protein on antitumor response, 360
factors influencing host defense, 64
gastrointestinal, 370, 376
hepatoma and iron, 114–115
Hodgkins disease, 274
human promyeloycytic HL-60, 6–9
immunotherapy and, 375
leukemic myeloid cell differentiation and 1,25-dihydroxyvitamin D_3, 11, 12
lung cancer, 95
malnutrition, 369, 370
mammary tumors and caloric restriction, 482
melanoma, 376
preleukemia and vitamin D_3 therapy, 13–15, 24
sarcoma and TPN, 380
skin test anergy, 370
TPN and immune response, 374, 375
vitamin A, 68
and vitamin C, 95
and vitamin E, 226, 231
Candida albicans, 81, 111
Capping, effect of fatty acids, 384, 385
Carbohydrate TPN, 374, 380
Carbonic anhydrase and zinc deficiency, 394
Carotene (*see* beta carotene, carotenoid, vitamin A)
Carotenoids, 66, 67 (*see also* beta carotene)
Carrageenin, 203–204
Casein, 301, 302, 347, 349
kappa-caesin, 347
Casomorphin, beta-, 347
Catalase, 83
Celiac disease, 319, 322–326, 340
Cell mediated immune CMI, response
antitumor, 423
low protein and, 360
Cell mediated lympholysis, and iron, 106
Cellular cytotoxicity (*see* cytotoxic T lymphocyte)
Chaga's disease, 129, 130, 137
Chediak-Higashi, 79

Chelation, 109, 411–421 (*see also* deferioxamine)
Chemotaxis, 76, 79, 84, 95, 159, 160, 373
Children, iron deficiency and, 110
Cholesterol, 163, 385
effect on macrophage cholesterol, 169
in food, 185
hypercholesterolemia, 170, 194
and LDL-In, 173
loading and Apo E production, 176
synthesis, 185
Chromatin, 270
and zinc, 141–150
Chronic energy intake restriction (CEIR), 483
Chronic granulomatous disease (CGD), 79, 80
Chronic renal failure, 504
Cirrhosis, 255, 340
Cis retinoic acid, 65, 66
Cis-unsaturated fatty acids, 163
Cobalt, 136
Coconut oil (myristic acid), 159
Collagen, type II, 160, 212
Colon cancer, hyperplastic cell growth and caloric restriction, 486
Colonization, microbial, 527, 535
Colorectal carcinoma and TPN, 379
Columnar epithelial cells, 339
Common variable immunodeficiency (*see* hypogammaglobulinemia)
Complement
C_3, 348
C_3 A, 370
Clq and vitamin C deficiency, 93–94
Common varied immunodeficiency, 340
Concanavalin A, Con A
as a mitogen, 224
Congenital immune disorders, 340
Copper, 239–254
and chelation therapy, 416
in chromatin conformation, 143
copper deficient rat model, 239, 240, 242
copper/zinc superoxide dismutase, 135, 241
cytochrome c oxidase activity, 241
effect of gender, 242
effect of low copper on food intake, 242
and IL-1, 39
interaction with iron, 240, 245
lymphocyte subsets, 254
macrophages and copper deficiency, 248

Copper (*continued*)
  Menkes syndrome, 239
  plasma ceruloplasmin, 240
  requirement in development, 272
Corn oil, 158, 159
Cow milk
  antigenicity of, in infants, 302
  versus breast milk, 301–318
  in IgA deficiency, 340–345
Crohn's disease, 340, 351
Cyclic AMP, 79, 92
Cyclic GMP
Cyclooxygenase, 132, 133, 158, 212
  pathway, 159, 385
Cyclophosphamide, 68, 521, 534, 536
Cytokine
  in breast milk, 525
  colony stimulating factors (CSF), 5
  excessive nutrients and, 39
  granulocyte-monocyte colony stimulating factor (GM-CFS), 5
  in inflammation, 511–523
  inhibitory cytokines, factors, 38
  interferon alpha, 33, 362
  interferon beta, 33
  interferon gamma (INF gamma), 22, 23, 33, 36, 361, 376, 383
  interleukin-1 (IL-1), 32, 257, 265
  interleukin-2 (IL-2), 15, 16, 33, 154, 156, 265, 379, 383, 403
  interleukin-2 receptor (IL-2r), 18, 257, 259
  interleukin-4 (IL-4), 386
  interleukin-6 (IL-6), 32
  iron binding proteins, 118
  lymphocyte inhibition factor (LIF), 32, 35
  lymphokines, 32
  macrophage inhibitor factor (MIF), 32, 35
  monokines, 33
  nutrient deficiencies and, 31–45, 265
  production enhanced with vitamin supplements, 458
  severe and moderate protein deficiency and, 40
Cytoskeletal defects and vitamin E, 233
Cytotoxic T lymphocyte (CTL), 51, 161
  antitumor lymphocytotoxicity, 369
  low protein diet and, 360
  and sterols, 188–190
  and vitamin A, 68
Cytotoxicity, 360

Deferioxamine (DF), 109, 412–416
Degranulation, 77
Dehydroascrobate, 77, 80
Delayed cutaneous hypersensitivity (DCH)
  in cancer, 370
  decreases with zinc deficiency, 128, 460
  effect of flax seed oil, 382
  effect of lipids,
  effect of vitamin A, 68
  effect of vitamin C, 97
  in elderly, 456, 457, 460–461
  in infants, 227, 230–231
  from infectious disease, 476
  in lupus model, 208
Delayed type hypersensitivity, 68, 94, 156, 296
  mucosal, 320–321
DNA and histones, effect of zinc, 142
Deoxythymidine kinase and zinc deficiency, 394
Dermatitis herpetiformis, 326–330, 340
Diabetes, 155
  and vitamin E, 232
  and zinc, 505
Dicylglycerol lipase, 133, 134
Diet
  cholesterol, 192–193
  high-fat, 158
  low-fat, 158
  restriction and mouse mammary tumor virus, prolactin, 485
  vitamin A, 68
  vitamin E in corn oil versus fish oil diet, 227–228
  and zinc deficiency, 127
  zinc deficient and chromatin structure, 142
Dietary antigens, 339, 347
Dietary fat, 153–167
  versus calorie in tumor formation, 483
  role of lipoproteins in immune cell function, 171
Dietary lipids, clinical implications, 386
Dietary protein (*see also* bovine)
  absorption in primary humoral immunodeficiency, 340–353
  immune complexes containing, 340
  and tumor-specific cytotoxicity, 360
  dietary restriction and experimental tumorigenesis, 482
Dihomo-gamma-linoleic acid, 134, 135, 160

1-25-Dihydroxyvitamin D_3, 3–29
  administration in myelodysplastic syndromes, 13–15
  and bone modulation, 10
  calcium and phosphorus homeostasis, 4
  effect on normal human myeloid cells, 9
  effects on Th cells, 17
  gene circuitry hypothesis, 5
  HL-60 cell growth and differentiation, 6–9
  and Ig response, 19–21
  and IL-2 response, 18
  increased production, extra renal synthesis, 23
  inhibitory effects on immune response, 15, 16
  mechanism of immune cell interaction, 24
  metabolism, 3–5
  and myeloid cell differentiation, 5
  plasma concentrations, 10, 23
  production of in lymphomas, 13
  receptors, 5, 15
  and sarcoid, 21
  and sunlight, 3
  synthesis by monocytes/macrophages, 21, 22
  vitamin D binding protein, 3
  vitamin D resistant rickets, 10
  vitamin D_3 analogs, 8, 10
docosahexaenoic acid, 212
Dolichol, 185
Down's syndrome, 274, 505
Duodenum iron absorption, 493

Eczema, 351
Edema formation, 203–204
Egg albumen, 212
Eicosanoids, 162
  and arthritis, 201–221
  regulator of acute inflammation, 201–206
  regulator of chronic inflammation, 206–211
Eicosapentaenoic acid (EPA) (menhaden oil), 159, 160, 162, 212–216
Elderly
  causes of morbidity, 456
  relationship of diet and immune response, 455–465
Endogenous pyrogen (see cytokine)
Endotoxin, 206, 512, 513
Energy redirection hypothesis, 487
Energy supplementation, 461

Enteral feeding, 370
enteropathy, protein-sensitive, 319–336
  in animals, 320
  gluten, 537–539
EPA (see eicosapentaenoic acid)
Epidermal growth factor
  enhances gut maturation, 304
  in milk, 303
Epinepherine, 92
E-rosette
  in malnutrition, 445
  receptor, 287
Escherichia coli
  antibodies to, in infants, 304
Essential fatty acids, 158, 372
Eye, 63
Exercise, 64
Excess nutrients (see also iron, iron overload)
  arginine, 50
  and cytokine production, 39
  fat, 155–158
  lipid emulsion use, 373
  saturated versus unsaturated, 154–158
  vitamin A excess, 63, 70–72
Experimental allergic encephalanyelitis, 94

Fat intake, preventive benefit of reduction, 487
  and plasma lipoprotein regulation of immunity, 171
Fatty acid
  and arthritis, 201–221
  in parenteral nutrition, 369
  profile and immune effects, 382–384
  saturated versus unsaturated, 384
  unsaturated, 163
Fc receptors, 373, 418
Ferric citrate, 106
Ferrioxamine, 412
Ferritin, 106, 497
Fetal cord blood plasma lipoproteins, 174
Fever and iron, 109
Fish oil, 159, 212, 379
Flax seed oil, alpha linolenic acid, 382
Folic acid, 449
Free fatty acids and LDL-In, 174
Free radicals (see antioxidant)
Fungi, 81

Gamma-linoleic acid (GLA), 160
Gastroenteritis and breast milk, 526

Index

Gastrointestinal barrier, 339
Gastrointestinal cancer, TPN and, 376–378
Gene expression and zinc, 141–150
GLA (see gamma-linoleic acid)
Gliadin, 319–336, 537
Glomerulopathy, 536
Glomeruonephritis, 153, 156
Glucocorticoid, 411
Glucose metabolism
  and aging, 486–487
  and arginine, 49
  energy source in TPN, 371
Glutathione, 131
Glutathione peroxidase, 80
Glutathione reductase, 80, 83
Glutathione synthetase deficiency, 232
Gluten-free diet mouse colony, 331–336
Gluten-sensitive enteropathy, 527–539
  in dermatitis herpetiformis, 326–330
  dose-dependent, 326–330
  gluten challenge, 322–326
Goblet cells, 339
Gp55, gp 55-like determinant in breast cancer, 428
  effect of vitamins on response to, 434–435
Graft versus Host (GvH), 68, 321, 352, 353
Gram-negative bacteria
  cytokines, 512, 513
  and iron, 109
Granulocyte (see neutrophil, phagocyte)
Granulomas, hypersensitivity and foreign body type, 210–211
Growth retardation, 413
Gut, 339
Gut colonization, effect of infant diet, 527
Gut permeability of infants, 302, 304
Glycerol, 371

Haber-Weiss reaction, 81, 82, 131, 136
Hassall's corpuscles, 445
Heart disease, 164
Helper T cell activity
  and low protein diet, 360
  and repletion in PCM, 364
  and vitamin E, 225
Hemagglutination (HA), 224
Hemin, 106
Hemochromatosis, neonatal, 497 (see also hereditary hemochromatosis)

Hemodialysis, chronic, 112
Hemoglobin
  and iron deficiency, 109–110
  and mixed lymphocyte culture, 107–108
Hemolytic anemia, 231
Henoch-Shonlein purpura, 340
Hepatitis, 116
Hepatotoxins and vitamin A, 69
Heptoma, 115, 116
Hereditary hemochromotosis (HH), 111–115, 116
Hexose monophosphate shunt, 80, 373
Histamine, 94, 203
Histamine decarboxylase, 95
Histones, 142
  and dietary zinc deficiency, 144, 145
Histoplasma capsulatum, 363
HLA, 107, 111–112, 116
Hodgkin's disease, 274
Hormone
  1,25-dihydroxyvitamin D_3
  thymic hormones, 292–293, 364
  thymulin, 155, 404
Human immunodeficiency virus (HIV)
  beta carotene supplementation and, 68
  nutrient malabsorption, 476
  risk of transmission via breast milk, 302
Human supplementation
  arginine, 52, 53
  orninthine, 53
  vitamin C, 79
  zinc deficiency, 274, 395–396
Humoral immune response (see antibody, B cells)
Humoral immunodeficiency, 340
Hydrogen peroxide, 80, 83, 130
3-Hydroxy-3-methylglutaryl-Co A reductase, 183, 185
Hydroxycholesterol, 191
Hydroxyl radical formation and vitamin C, 82
Hypercalcemia, 21
Hyperzincuria, 394
Hypogammaglobulinemia, 347
  bovine antigens in sera of, 348
Hypohalous acid, 132

Ibuprofen, 160
Ileojeunal bypass, 340
Immune complex, 156, 340, 341
  absence in hypogammaglobulinemia, 347
  chronic circulating in IgA deficiency, 345

Immune complex (*continued*)
  bovine proteins in IgA deficiency, 345
  in chronic GvH disease, 354
  nephritis, 153, 156
Immune response, general components, 105
  and lipoproteins, network, 172
Immunization, 447
Immunoglobulin
  cellular mechanism of, 538
  class involvement in mucosal immune response, 534–536
  effect of TPN, 370
  and fat level in autoimmune model, 156
  IgA, 339
    deficiency, 340, 344
    dietary antigens, 340–345
    and iron absorption, 493
    and lactation, 495
    levels in elderly, 457
    in milk, 302, 526–529
    in mucosal immune response, 533–540
    nephropathy, 340
    post transplantation, 353
    salivary, 340, 342
    secretory, 340, 526–529
    secretory, and infant formulas, 493–494
    secretory in PEM, 361, 447
    urinary secretion of in infants, 303
  IgG
    to cow milk proteins, 302
    levels in breast-fed versus bottle-fed infants, 304, 526
    in mucosal immune response, 534
  IgM, 535–536
    levels in elderly, 457, 461
    levels in infants, 304–307, 309–311
    in malnutrition, 447
    in milk, 526
    secretory, 340
  infusion
    dietary antigen in blood in hypogammaglobulinemia, 348
    intravenous versus intramuscular, 348
  immune complex formation, 342
  salivary immunoglobulins, 344
  serum immunoglobulins, 344
  subclasses, 268, 269
  synthesis and lipoproteins, 172
  in zinc deficiency, 268
Immunotherapy
  nutritional support and, 375

Inanition, 32
  effect of low copper on food intake, 242
  zinc deficiency and, 393
  vitamin C deficiency and, 94
Indomethacin, 204
Infants, 110
Infections
  and iron, 108–109, 111
  and PCM, 361
  and vitamin C deficiency, 94
  sinopulmonary and IgA deficiency, 340
  and zinc deficiency, 128, 129
Infectious diseases, effect of, 475–480
Inflammation, 160
  and cytokines, 511–523
  and eicosanoids, 201–207
  mediators, 159
Influenza, in vitro response and vitamin C, 98–100
Infusion of intralipid, 373
Insulin, 49
  effect of protein deficiency, 37
  and prostaglandin, 39
  and trace mineral levels, 34, 36, 37, 39
Interferon, 156
  addition to in vitro culture in PCM, 362
  in infants, 311
  INF-gamma, 161, 207, 376
  malnutrition and therapeutic use, 376
  production by milk lymphocytes, 303
  production and vitamin C, 95, 100
  in protein calorie malnutrition, 361
  and vitamin A, 63
Interleukin-1 (IL-1), 32, 160, 206, 446
  in infectious disease, 476, 479
  in inflammatory response, 511–519
  retinyl palmitate and, 69
Interleukin-2 (IL-2), 32, 33, 161
  caloric restriction in autoimmune mouse model, 153
  and deferioxamine, 414
  effect of alcohol, 257
  effect of TPN, 374
  effect of vitamin and mineral deficiency, 36
  fat and, 156
  high dose, therapeutic use, 375
  and iron, 120
  and linoleic acid, 213
  lipid emulsions and, 377, 380
  in malnutrition, 446
  production affected by vitamin E, 227, 231

Index

Interleukin-2 (IL-2) (*continued*)
and prostaglandin, 206
  receptor and beta carotene, 67
  receptor, lipid effects on expression, 384
  retroviral infection, 258
  therapy and hypovitaminosis C, 95
  and tranferrin, 118
  and vitamin C, 98-99
  vitamin D_3 and IL-2 response, 18
  zinc deficiency and, 128, 265, 266, 403
Interleukin-5 (IL-5), 535
Interleukin-6 (IL-6), 476, 511-515
Intestine
  hypersensitivity of, 319-336
  permeability, assessment of, 349-350
Intralipid, 371, 373, 381, 385
Intravenous feeding (*see also* parenteral nutrition, and total parenteral nutrition)
  glucose solutions, 370
  lipid emulsions, 369-391
Ionizing radiation, 84
Iron, 491-499
  absorption, 492, 493
  circulating proteins, 491-492
  delivery, 493
  distribution, 492
  excretion, 491-492
  in fetal organs, 494-495
  fortified infant formulas, 493
  in Haber-Weiss reaction, 82, 136
  and host defense against microorganisms, 108-109
  immunoregulation, 105-126
  importance in lymphocyte proliferation, 460
  iron deficiency, 109-110
  iron excess, 112
  and lactation, 495
  and lymphocyte migration, 493
  and lymphocyte proliferative response, 107
  modeling of the immune system, 492
  partition inactivated lymphocytes, 119
  overload, 112, 412-414
  and synovium, 495
  and T cell surface marker expression, 107
  transferrin, 492, 163
Iron dextran and sepsis, 110
Isopentenyl adenosine (IPA), 185

Jejunum
  in gluten intolerance, 319
  and iron absorption, 493

Ketone bodies, 371
Kupfer cells, 69, 70, 71
Kwashiorkor, 283-300, 359, 361, 362, 446

Lactation, 267, 273 (*see* milk)
  interaction with iron, 495
Lactoferrin, 106, 108
LAK (*see* lymphokine activated killer cells)
Lauric acid, 159
Lead, 411-412
Lectin, 330
Leukemic cells and sterol synthesis, 186
Leukocytes (*see also* neutrophil)
  phagocytosis and vitamin C, 79, 81
  chemotaxis, 95
Leukotrienes, 132, 133, 158, 212 (*see also* eicosanoids)
  LTB_4, 159, 202-203, 214-216
  LTC_4, 159
  LTD_3, 159, 160
  LTD_4, 159
  LTD_5, 159, 160
  LTE_4, 159
LFA-3, 114
Lieber-Carli diet, 256
Linoleic acid, 158, 159, 212-215, 371, 372
Lipid emulsions, 369-391
  incorporation into cell membranes, 385
  infant feeding, 385
  immune response to, 372
  immunosuppression and, 372
  lipid based TPN in cancer, 376-377
  rationale for use, 371
  and sepsis in immunocompromised patients, 373
Lipidosis, 372
Lipids, 155, 158, 162
  effect on inflammatory diseases, 212-216
  infectious disease, 476
  and phagocytes, 170
Lipofundin, 382
Lipopolysaccharide (LPS),
  as a mitogen, 224
Lipoprotein lipase system, 373
Lipoproteins, 161, 162, 163, 169-181, 370, 386 (*see also* plasma lipoproteins)
  circulating levels, 170
  high density lipoprotein (HDL), 163, 174, 177
  influence on autoimmune processes, 161
  low density lipoprotein (LDL), 163, 169-174, 194

Lipoproteins (*continued*)
  very low density lipoprotein (VLDL), 163, 194
Lipotropes, 272
Lipoxygenase, 133, 134, 158
  pathway, 159, 385
Listeria infections and iron, 115
Low density lipoprotein (LDL), 169
Low density lipoprotein inhibitor (LDL-In), 171–173
Lung microembolization, 205
Lupus, 158
Lymphocyte migration
  in fetal organs, 494
  and iron, 491–499
  T lymphocytes and lactation, 495
Lymphocyte proliferative response
  and apo E, 175
  and chelation therapy, 414
  and cyclic AMP, 206
  effect of alcohol, 256
  effect of breast versus bottle milk, 303, 307
  effect of fat in autoimmune model, 156
  effect of zinc, 505–506
  in elderly, 457
  enhanced by vitamin C, 463
  flax seed oil (alpha linoleic acid) and, 382
  higher overall rate in infants, 307–309
  and iron, 107–108, 119
  and LDL inhibitor, 170
  and LDL-In, 172
  and lipid emulsions, 377, 381
  in malnutrition, 296, 444–454
  synthesis of cholesterol, 186, 187
  and transferrin, 492
  and vitamin C, 97–100
  in vitro, 307
  and zinc deficiency, 128
Lymphocyte subsets
  and chelation therapy, 416–417
  in diseases of iron overload, 112, 115
  effect of low protein diet, 360
  effect of TPN regimen, 374
  in elderly, 457
  in granulomas, 210–211
  and iron, iron binding proteins, 106, 112
  lipid emulsions and, 372
  lipoproteins and, 163
  in protein-energy malnutrition, 290–291, 441–444, 446, 459
  and vitamin A (retinoic acid), 65, 66
  and vitamin C deficiency, 94

Lymphocyte transformation, 119, 206
Lymphoid aggregates, 68, 128, 288–289
Lymphokine
  in elderly, 457
  iron and, 118
  in mucosal hypersensitivity, 321
  and prostaglandin, 206
  zinc and, 502
Lymphokine activated killer (LAK) cells, 96, 100, 375, 377
Lymphopenia, 445
Lysozyme, 79

Macromolecular antigen absorption, 339
Macrophage activation, 68, 94, 114, 118, 207 (*see also* monocyte, and phagocyte)
  and apo E, 169
  retinoids, carotenoids, 63–74
  and zinc, 127–130
Magnesium, 143, 144
Major histocompatibility complex (MHC) Class I, Class II (Dr/Ia), 161, 187, 189, 445, 537, 538
Malabsorption
  and zinc deficiency, 400
Malaria, 109–110, 185
Malnutrition (*see also* protein calorie malnutrition, marasmus, and kwashiorkor)
  alcoholism and immunity, 255
  and cytokine production, 35, 36
  effect on interferon gamma production, 36
  effect on lymphocyte subsets, 38, 359, 441–446
  effect on NK cell activity
  during fetal development, 268, 272, 273
  due to human immunodeficiency virus, 476
  incidence in gastrointestinal cancer, 370
  due to infectious disease, 475–480
  marginal, 273
  neonatal, 267
  plasma inhibitory factors and, 364
  protein deficiency, 35, 36, 38, 274
  repletion, 363, 111
  repletion in cancer associated malnutrition, 375, 376
  and thymus gland, 283–300
Mammary cancer (experimental) and diet, 484
Manganese, 136

Index

Marasmus, 284–300, 359, 361, 362, 446
Marine lipid diets, 212–216
Mast cells, 203–204
MCT, 382, 384, 386
Measles, severe, and vitamin A, 63
Megadose vitamins
  in elderly, 96
  vitamin C, 95
Melanoma, 376
Membrane fluidity, 163
Membranous epithelial cells, 339
Membrane signal transduction and fatty acids, 384
Membrane structure, fluid mosaic, 183
Menhaden oil (eicosapentaenoic acid, EPA), 159
Menkes syndrome, 239
Metallothionein, 271
Metals, 411–421
Methionine deficiency, vitamin C and antibody deficiency, 93
Mevalonate, 185
Microbial killing, 81
Micrococcal nuclease, 144
Micronutrient deficiency and experimental cancer, 482
Migration inhibitory factor (MIF), 209
Migration, polymorphonuclear, 373
Milk
  antibodies in, 525–532
  breast versus bottle, 525–532
  casomorphin in, 346
  effect of ingestion in IgA deficiency, 340–343
  effect of maternal diet on, 266
  immune complex formation in IgA deficiency, 340
  intolerance, 302
Minerals, 450
Mitogen response
  in malnutrition, 446
  zinc, 502, 505–506
Monocyte, 114, 373
  activation and ascorbate, 77
  cholesterol loading and immune cell function, 171
  iron binding protein secretion, 118
  and oxidation of cholesterol linolate, 186
  stimulation with carotenoids and retinoids, 65
  synthesis of apo E, 175
Mononuclear phagocytes (MNP), zinc and parasitic infections, 128–130

Morphine (*see* beta casomorphin)
Mouse mammary tumors and caloric restriction, 483
Mouse mammary tumor virus and prolactin, 485
Mucosal immune system, 319–336, 339–345, 533–540
  IgA deficiency, 340
  regulation of, 321–322
Mucosal permeability, 340–347
Mucous membranes, 339
Muramyl dipeptide, 514–515
Murine leukemia virus (MuLV), 257
Myelodysplastic syndromes
  treatment with vitamin D_3, 13–15
Myeloid cells, 515
Myeloperoxidase, 80, 81, 132
Myelopoesis and lactoferrin, 108
Myocardial infarction, 96
Myopathy and vitamin E, 225
Myristic acid (coconut oil), 159

n-3 fatty acids, 212
N,N-diphenyl-p-phenylenediamine (DPPD), 224
NADPH oxidase, 80, 132, 133, 134, 135
Natural killer cell, 359
  activity and reduced tyrosine and phenylalanine, 47
  and arginine supplementation, 50
  and autoimmunity, 156
  and beta carotene, 66
  and chelation therapy, 414–417
  effect of lipid emulsions, 374, 377, 380
  and infection in PCM, 361, 362, 363
  and interferon production in PCM, 361
  and iron, 106, 108
  plasma inhibitory factor and, 364
  reduced activity in malnutrition, 36, 292, 359, 361
  reduced activity in zinc deficiency, 266, 402, 502
  repletion and recovery in PCM, 363–364
  vitamin A deficiency, 33, 63
Neonatal
  zinc deprivation, 268
Nephritis, 157, 212
Nephrotic syndrome, 110, 504
Neuraminidase, iron, and CD2 epitope, 114
Neutralizing factor, 162
Neutropenia
  and prostaglandin, 205
  and vitamin E, 225

Neutrophils
  lactoferrin and, 108
  and lipid infusion, 373
  in prostaglandin treated subjects, 205
  reduced migration ability in elderly, 458
  and vitamin C, 77–79
  and vitamin E, 228
Newborns
  absorption of immunoglobulins from milk, 303–304
  development of immune system, 302–312
  lymphocyte proliferation in, 307–309
  response to gut antigens, 304
Newcastle disease virus, 361
New Zealand Black mice, autoimmune model, 153 (*see also* autoimmune prone NZB/NZW)
  effect of caloric restriction, 154, 483
  effect of low protein diet, 360
Nitrogen loss in infectious disease, 476–477
Nitrogen sparin, 370
Nonhistone proteins, 270
Nonsteroidal antiinflammatory, 160
Norepinephrine, 92
Nuclear grade (NG), 423
Nucleoside phosphorylase activity, 271, 402, 403
Nucleoside phosphorylase (PNP), 402, 403, 406
Nucleosomal fiber, 142
5′-ecto-Nucleotidase (5′NT), 406
Null cell, 290
Nutrient requirements, 52, 272
Nutritional support
  in cancer, 369

Oleic acid, 371, 377
Omega-3 fatty acids (fish oil), 47, 160, 162, 517
Omega-6 fatty acids, 47
Oncogenes, 147, 484
Opioid, *see* beta casomorphin, 346
Opsonin, 77, 110
Oral antigens, 533–540
Oral refeeding, iron, 110
Ornithine decarboxylase, 485
Osteoclast activation factor, 207
Otitis media and breast milk, 526
Ovalbumin, 321
Oxidative metabolism, 373
Oxidative stress, 83
Oxygen, in respiratory burst, 79, 80, 131–132

Oxygen reactive species, 77, 129–131, 132–133, 134, 136, 372
Oxygenated derivatives of cholesterol, 183–199
Oxysterols, 185–189
  auto-oxidation, 191
  in diet, 193
  effect on lymphocyte activation, 190
  inhibitory components in serum, 191

Palmitic acid, 371, 373
Pannus, synovial, 213
Parasitic infection and zinc deficiency, 128–130
Parenteral nutrition, 37 (*see* protein calorie malnutrition (PCM), and protein energy or protein calorie malnutrition (PBM))
  arginine, 47, 55
  and delayed type hypersensitivity, 48
  FreAmine II, 53
  FreAmine III, 54
  importance of formulation, 384–385
  iron and, 110
  lipid emulsions, postoperative, 373
  lipid emulsions, preoperative, 378–379
  need for zinc, 274
  Nephramine, 53
  peroxidase and vitamin C, 84 (*see also* intravenous feeding)
  in shock, 47
  and tumor growth, 47, 377–378, 379
Peyer's patch, 526, 533
Phagocytes, 75
Phagocytosis, 69, 71, 77, 110, 114, 128, 129, 130, 131, 156, 170, 363
Phagoliposomes, 373
Phagolysosome, 131
Phagosome, 131–132
Phorbol myristate acetate, 7, 132
Phospholipase A,C, 132, 134
Phospholipid, 132, 133, 163, 371, 385
Phytate, 273
Phytohemagglutinin (PHA), 224
Plaque-forming cells (PFC), 157, 224
Plasma inhibitory factor, 364
Plasmalemmal lipids, 385
Plasma lipoproteins, 169, 192
  constituents, 173
  and immune response, 169–170
  low density lipoprotein inhibitor, 170
Plasma membranes, 184–185
Plasmocytoma, 535

Index

Platelet
  activating factor (PAF), 205, 214
  aggregation, 213
Polyamines, 50, 51, 485
Polyarthritis, diet and, 160
Polyethylene glycol (PEG), 349–351
Polyhydroxamic acid, 412
Polymorphonuclear (PMN) leukocytes
  in elderly, 462
  mediators of inflammation, 202–203
Polyunsaturated fatty acids (PUFA), 158, 162, 372, 386
Primrose seed oil, 215
Proinflammatory (*see* leukotrienes)
Prolactin, 49, 485
Prostacyclin, 160, 202, 205–206
Prostaglandin (PG), 34, 38, 158, 160, 363
  and arthritis, 201–221
  association with respiratory burst, 133
  dietary lipids and, 378–379
  dietary manipulation of, 211–212
  in infectious disease, 476
  local versus systemic effects of administration, 203–204
  PDG_2, 159
  PGE_1, 158, 204, 208–211
  PGE_2, 158
  PGF_2, 159, 210–211
  PGI_2, 159
  production by mammary cells, 303
  suppresses inflammatory cells, 202
  synthesis affected by vitamin E, 224, 227, 232
  and zinc, 504
Protein
  allergens, 155
  low protein diet and immune response in NZB mice, 360
  malnutrition, 448 (*see* milk, bovine, and dietary)
  restriction and autoimmunity, 154
Protein calorie malnutrition (*see* protein energy malnutrition)
Protein-energy malnutrition (PEM), 284–300, 445–447, 458–459
  discussion of caloric energy versus fat energy, 483
  graft rejection in, 360
  iron and, 111
  NK cell activity in, 359–368
  null cells in, 359
  and secretory IgA, 361
  susceptibility to infection, 363

Protein kinase, 79, 485
Provitamin A, beta carotene, 64
Psoriasis, 162
Pyridoxine, 272, 448

RIII-gp 55, 424
Reactive oxygen metabolites, 77
Recall skin test antigens, 370
Reid-Briggs Teklad diet, 94
Replacement (*see* repletion)
Repletion
  iron and, 111
  in PCM, 363–364
Respiratory burst, 79, 130–131, 373
  membrane events, 133
Retinoids, 63–74 (*see also* vitamin A)
Retinol, 64
Retinol esters, toxicity and excess vitamin A, 63
Retinyl palmitate, 68
Retrovirus, 13, 23, 55, 256, 259, 154
  type A and type B, 484
  type C, 162
Rheumatoid arthritis, 84, 155, 162, 351, 516
Rickets 3, 10
Rosette formation and iron, 106, 107
Rotrolental fibroplasia syndrome, 231

Safflower oil, 158, 159, 160
Salivary immunoglobulins, 344
Sarcoid, 21
Sarcoma, 379–380
Saturated fat, 162, 377
Schistosoma mansoni, 363
Scorbutic guinea pigs, 94
Scurvy, 91
Secretory immune system, 339, 353, 361
Secretory IgA (*see* Immunoglobulins)
Secretory IgM, 340
Selective IgA deficiency, 340
Selenium, 35, 39, 64, 272, 450
Sepsis, 82, 110, 370, 372, 516
Serum immunoglobulins, 344
Serum thymic hormone
  in elderly, 457, 459, 460
Sickle cell anemia, sickle cell disease, 112, 273, 393–410, 413, 505
Siderophore, 109
Sjögren's syndrome, 155, 157, 158
Skin graft rejection, 68
Skin test (*see* delayed cutaneous type hypersensitivity)

Skin window (SK), 424
  effect of vitamins, 426, 429–430, 433
  prognostic significance in breast cancer, 429–432
  types of reactions, 425
Soya hypersensitivity, 320
Soybean oil, 371
Spleen
  in malnutrition, 288–289
  removal of red blood cells, 493
Splenic lipidosis, 372
Staphylococcus aureus, vitamin C in Chediak Hiashi, 82
Starvation, 360
Steric acid, 371
Steroids, 160
Sterol, 184 (*see* cholesterol)
Sterol biosynthesis, 185
Superoxide, 136, 137
Superoxide anion production, 79
Superoxide dismutase (SOD), 83, 131, 134–136
Supplementation, 67, 79, 96, 97, 381, 382
Suppressor cells, 157
  and carotenoids in vitro, 67
  in low protein diet, 360
  plasma inhibitory factor and, 364
Surgery, nutrient support in (*see* parenteral nutrition)
Synovium
  and iron, 495
  pannus, 213
Systemic lupus erythematosus (SLE), 153, 202, 204
  animal model of, 208–209, 212
  human studies, 214–216
  SLE, PFUA and, 162

T cells
  chelation therapy, 414
  circulating, in malnutrition, 285, 287, 289–292
  effect of low protein diet, 360
  function, 433, 533–540
  function in vitamin C deficiency, 94
  PCM and, 361
  plasma inhibitory factor and, 364
  receptor expression and iron, 106
  suppressor, 533–534
T cell receptor, 105–106, 107
Terminal deoxynucleotidyl transferase (TdT), 290

Thalassemia
  chelation therapy, 411–421
  intermedia, 112, 115
  major, 112, 115
Theophylline, 207, 208
Thermostable erythrocyte rosette (TER), 112
Thrombocytopenia, 205
Thromboxane, 159, 160, 476
  thromboxane A_2, 159, 212
  thromboxane B_2, 159, 207
Thymectomy, effects of, 502–503
Thymic factors, 93, 361, 364
Thymidine kinase and zinc deficiency,
Thymocytotoxic antibody, 156
Thymopoetin, 294, 407, 457
Thymosin in elderly, 457
Thymosin fraction 5, 294–295
Thymulin, 292, 404, 445, 502–505
Thymus
  and arginine, 51
  in autoimmune model, 153
  histopathology, 284–287
  in malnutrition, 283–300, 361, 444
  and ornithine, 51
  thymocytotoxic antibody, 156
  and vitamin A, 64
  and zinc, 266, 502–505
Tonsils, 288–289
Total parenteral nutrition (TPN), 369 (*see also* parenteral nutrition)
  effect of constituents on immune response, 381
  immunotherapeutic use in cancer, 376, 377
  lipid versus carbohydrate, 374
  and metastasis, 379
  preoperative, 370
Transcription factor, 147
Transferrin
  and beta carotene, 66
  and lipoproteins, 163
  and lymphocyte proliferation, 492
  plasma, 110, 116
  and primary iron overload, 114
  receptor for, 106, 117, 413
Transfusion related immunosuppression, 380
Triglycerides, 371, 373, 382
Trypanosomiasis, 129, 363
Tuberculin, 303
Tumor
  cell lines, 372
  growth and calorie restriction, 482

Index

Tumor (*continued*)
  growth and lipoprotein, 173
  growth in malnutrition, 360
  growth and oxysterols, 186
  rejection, 68
  tumor blocking antibody in protein deficiency, 360
  tumor directed lymphocytoxicity and TPN, 376-377
Tumor cytolytic factor (TCF), 65
Tumor growth factor beta (TGF), 535
Tumor necrosis factor (TNF), 32, 34, 50, 161, 380, 476
  in inflammatory response, 511-519 (*see also* cachectin)
  in malnourished elderly, 458

Ubiquinone, 185
Underfeeding (*see* dietary restriction, calorie restriction)
Unsaturated fatty acids, 163, 377, 385

Vaccination
  affected by diet in infants, 307-311, 528-529
  in elderly, 461, 463
Vascular permeability, 203-205
Vasculitis, 204
Viral infections and iron, 111
Vitamin A, 33, 39, 47
  adjuvant use in breast cancer, 423-439
  deficiency and infections, 63, 361
  effects on macrophages, 68
  and immunosuppression, 68
  and infectious disease, 477
  liver toxicity, 69-72
  and malnutrition, 450
  and NK cell activity, 361
  retinoic acid and lymphocyte subsets, 65
  and TCF production, 65
Vitamin B
  biotin and malnutrition, 448
  B12 and malnutrition, 448
  effect of supplements in elderly, 463
  folic acid and malnutrition, 448
  pyridoxine and malnutrition, 448
Vitamin C, 47
  ascorbate redox system, 83
  and *C. albicans*, 82
  deficiency and differentiation of lymphoid organs, 93
  effect on chemotaxis in Chediak Higashi syndrome, 79

Vitamin C (*continued*)
  effect on chemotaxis in chronic granulomatous disease, 79
  effect of supplements in elderly, 96, 463
  guinea pigs, 92, 93
  human vitamin C deficiency, 95
  and interleukin-2, 98, 99
  and iron uptake, 96
  levels in phagocytes, 75
  and malnutrition, 449
  and rheumatoid arthritis, 84
  and sepsis, 82, 477
  and stress, 92, 96
  supplementation in institutionalized persons, 97
  supplementation and neutrophil motility, 79, 96
  vitamin C and phagocytes, 75-90
Vitamin D, 1-29
  1,25-Dihydroxyvitamin D_3, 3-29
  and malnutrition, 449-450
Vitamin E, 47
  adjuvant use in breast cancer, 423-439
  administration, oral versus intramuscular, 225, 226
  animal studies, 224-228
  and buccal cancer, 436
  cell culture studies, 228-229
  effect on aging, 226, 463
  effect on cell surface glycosphingolipids, 228
  effect on delayed cutaneous hypersensitivity, 227, 230-231
  effect on lipid peroxidation, 227
  effect on lymphocyte proliferation, 225
  in elderly, 230-231
  enhancing anticancer host defense, 64
  human studies, 229-231
  increases risk of tumors, 227
  inhibition of prostaglandin synthesis, 224, 227, 232
  limits of efficacy, 229
  in malnutritioin, 450
  megadoses of, 231
  as a mitogen, 224, 226, 227
  in newborns, 230
  with oxone exposure, 225
  protection against effect of neutrophils, 228
  role in disease states, 231-233
  role in immune function, 223-228
  with selenium deficiency, 225
  supplements, 224, 225, 226, 227, 231, 463

Wheat intolerance, 319

Yersinia infection, 115, 351

Xerophalamia, 63

Zinc, 127, 501–509
  acrodermatitis enteropathica, 400
  and chromatin, 141, 144, 270
  and dark adaptation, 398
  deficiency, 502–504
  deficiency and AIDS, 402
  deficiency and anergy, 402
  deficiency and autoimmunity, 155
  deficiency and cellular immunity, 265, 402, 450–451
  deficiency and delayed type hypersensitivity, 400, 460
  deficiency and infections, 128, 129, 266, 401
  deficiency and interleukin-2 production, 265, 403
  deficiency and lymphocyte subpopulations, 264, 265, 404, 406
  deficiency and NK cell function, 265, 266, 402, 414, 502
  deficiency and lymphoid atrophy, 460
  deficiency and nucleoside phosphorylase activity, 402, 403
  deficiency and sickle cell disease, 393–410

Zinc (continued)
  deficiency and T cell proliferation, 265, 400–401
  and delayed puberty, 393
  effect on endocrine function, 266, 271, 395
  elderly, 400
  growth, 393, 394, 399, 264
  homeostasis, 127, 272
  hyperammonemia, 397
  and IL-1, 265, 39
  and lymphocyte development, 502
  metallothionein, 271
  mitogenic properties, 270, 502, 505–506
  mode of action in immune response, 506–507
  and ornithine carbamoyaltransferase, 398
  and oxygen burst, 132–136
  perinatal, 263–279
  poor wound healing, 394
  relationship to IgA levels, 461
  relationship to polymorphonuclear leukocytes, 462
  retinal reductase, 398
  serum thymulin, 155, 404–405, 502–505
  supplementation in deficiency, 287, 395–396
  uremic patients, 400
  zinc dependent enzymes, 127, 270, 394, 395
Zinc-binding domains, 147
Zymosan, 77, 132, 133

About the Editor

SUSANNA CUNNINGHAM-RUNDLES is Director of the Immunology Research Laboratory at The New York Hospital-Cornell University Medical Center, New York, New York, and Associate Professor of Immunology in the Pediatrics Department of Cornell University Medical College, New York, New York. The author or coauthor of over 100 professional papers and a member of the American Association of Immunologists, the American Society for Histocompatibility and Immunogenetics, the Clinical Immunology Society, the Transplantation Society, the American Society for Clinical Nutrition, and the American Institute for Clinical Nutrition, she is an editor of the journal *Biotechnology Therapeutics* (Marcel Dekker, Inc.) and serves on the editorial board of *Nutrition and Immunology*. Her research is focused on regulation of immune response in acquired immunodeficiency, cancer, and AIDS. She is Vice Chair of the Program Committee of the New York Academy of Sciences and Chair Elect of the Division of Clinical and Diagnostic Immunology of the American Society for Microbiology. Dr. Cunningham-Rundles received the Ph.D. degree (1974) in biochemical genetics from New York University, New York, New York. She received her postdoctoral training in clinical immunology and immunogenetics at Memorial Sloan-Kettering Cancer Center, New York, New York.